130.00

Reduction Mammaplasty

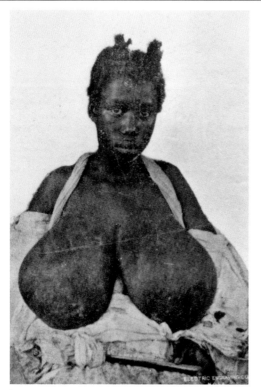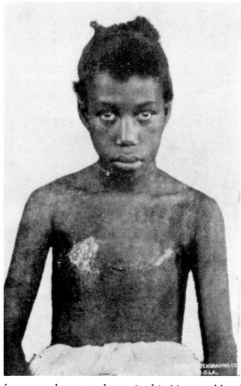

A century ago mastectomy was a common treatment for severe hypertrophy, as in this 14-year-old girl. (From E.D. Martin. Simple hypertrophy of mammary glands. New Orleans M. & S. J. 22:8, 1894–5.)

Reduction Mammaplasty

Edited by **Robert M. Goldwyn, M.D.**
Clinical Professor of Surgery, Harvard Medical
School; Head, Division of Plastic Surgery, Beth
Israel Hospital; Surgeon, Brigham and Women's
Hospital, Boston; Editor, *Plastic and Reconstructive Surgery*

Little, Brown and Company
Boston/Toronto/London

Library of Congress Catalog Card No. 89-62816

ISBN 0-316-31977-5

Printed in the United States of America

HAL

To Jacob Goldwyn, M.D. (1901–1985)
With gratitude for his love and example

Contents

Preface

Despite the many changes in the content and practice of plastic and reconstructive surgery during the past several decades, reduction mammaplasty* continues to be an operation frequently requested and performed. In 1988, an estimated 40,000 were done in the United States. The emphasis on physical and emotional well-being, exercise, and thinness have contributed to the increasing popularity of the procedure. Recent fashion trends have emphasized more exposure of the body; going braless is a desideratum for many. The openness — to the point of obsession — with which our society discusses corporeal and sexual matters has freed the breast from taboo. A major consequence of the feminist movement has been to encourage women to discuss matters that bother them and not to accept passively and needlessly a mental or physical condition that is correctable. The worldwide availability of plastic surgeons trained to perform reduction mammaplasty both answers and stimulates the need for this procedure.

Yet our results are not always what we and our patients would like them to be. Compared to the results of what even a singular surgeon like Jacques Josephs could achieve, our outcomes are considerably better. However, if reduction mammaplasty could be done routinely with satisfaction and without complications or controversy, this book would not have been written. Reduction mammaplasty has not yet become an ordinary procedure like the drainage of an abscess.

This is a multi-authored book, the kind our British colleagues often criticize as being the unfortunate prototype of American medical writing and publishing. In its defense — and mine — the principal reason for this type of book is my belief that no one surgeon, if honest, can in the course of a usual professional lifetime have gained sufficient experience with more than just a few methods of breast reduction. In fact, most surgeons adhere to one or perhaps two types of procedures for macromastia. These chapters will show how good surgeons can obtain good results for their patients with various methods. The common denominator may indeed be the surgeon's skill, yet executing well a poorly conceived technique seldom leads to triumph. Even a wise man will look silly at the end of a fool's errand.

The comments following many of the chapters are to give the reader additional knowledge and perhaps a different perspective. An originator or proponent of a procedure frequently fails to discern its limitations, whereas another person, not wedded by reputation to a particular operation, may be more objective.

Because this book brings together most of the major methods of reduction mammaplasty, it should spare the busy plastic surgeon from having to spend time searching through journals and books for needed information.

Finally, that an entire volume should be devoted to the large breast and not specifically to the breast with ptosis only is an interesting commentary on how our specialty and our books develop in response to our patients' needs.

R.M.G.

---

* The publisher and I prefer *mammaplasty* to *mammoplasty*, although either spelling is acceptable according to William R. Hensyl of Williams & Wilkins, who has shepherded many editions of *Stedman's Medical Dictionary*.

Acknowledgments

I wish first to express my gratitude to those who contributed chapters and commentaries to this book. Without these gracious individuals, there obviously would have been no book.

My profound appreciation to Elizabeth Willingham for her many skills and helpful suggestions. She made this project almost a pleasure.

My thanks also to Julia B. Figures, indexer, for improving the quality and usefulness of this volume.

To Susan F. Pioli, Senior Editor, I am most appreciative of her continuing support and enthusiasm.

Anita LoConte, my secretary, prepared the manuscript in addition to everything else she has to do in our office. I wish to thank her publicly as I have done so often privately for her competence. I am also extremely grateful to my other secretaries, Mary Mangiaracine and Ann Ricci, who also helped with the book while discharging their numerous other duties with their usual expertise and equanimity as well as good humor.

Contributing Authors

Antonio Roberto Bozola, M.D.
Professor of Plastic Surgery, Fund. Fac. Reg. de Medicina; Surgeon, Department of Plastic Surgery, Hospital de Base, São Jose do Rio Preto, Brazil

Nathalie Bricout, M.D.
Surgeon, Plastic Surgery Department, Hôpital Saint-Louis, Paris, France

Forst E. Brown, M.D.
Professor of Clinical Surgery (Plastic Surgery), Dartmouth Medical School; Chairman, Section of Plastic Surgery, Dartmouth-Hitchcock Medical Center, Hanover, New Hampshire

Melchiades Cardoso de Oliveira, M.D.
Professor, São Jose do Rio Preto School of Medicine; Chief, Plastic Surgery, Image Institute for Plastic and Reconstructive Surgery, São Jose do Rio Preto, Brazil

Carolyn J. Cline, M.D., Ph.D.
San Francisco, California

A. MacLeod Cloutier, M.D.C.M.
Assistant Professor of Surgery, McGill University Faculty of Medicine; Attending Surgeon, Plastic Surgery Department, Montreal Children's Hospital, Montreal, Canada

Eugene H. Courtiss, M.D.
Assistant Clinical Professor of Surgery, Harvard Medical School; Consultant in Surgery, Massachusetts General Hospital, Boston

Rollin K. Daniel, M.D.
Clinical Professor of Surgery, Division of Plastic Surgery, University of California, Irvine, California College of Medicine; Division of Plastic Surgery, Hoag Memorial Hospital, Newport Beach, California

Milton T. Edgerton, M.D.
Professor of Plastic Surgery, University of Virginia School of Medicine; Attending Plastic Surgeon, University of Virginia Health Sciences Center, Charlottesville

Arnoldo Fournier, M.D.
Attending Plastic Surgeon, Biblic Hospital, San José, Costa Rica

Gregory S. Georgiade, M.D., F.A.C.S.
Associate Professor of General Surgery and Plastic, Maxillofacial, and Reconstructive Surgery, Duke University Medical Center, Durham, North Carolina

Nicholas G. Georgiade, D.D.S., M.D., F.A.C.S.
Professor Emeritus and Former Chief, Division of Plastic, Maxillofacial Reconstructive, and Oral Surgery, Duke University Medical Center, Durham, North Carolina

Robert M. Goldwyn, M.D.
Clinical Professor of Surgery, Harvard Medical School; Head, Division of Plastic Surgery, Beth Israel Hospital; Surgeon, Brigham and Women's Hospital, Boston; Editor, Plastic and Reconstructive Surgery

Gilbert P. Gradinger, M.D.
Associate Professor of Plastic Surgery, Stanford University School of Medicine, Stanford, California; Chief, Division of Plastic Surgery, Peninsula Hospital, Burlingame, California

Frederick M. Grazer, M.D., F.A.C.S.
Associate Clinical Professor, University of California, Irvine, California College of Medicine; Clinical Associate Professor of Surgery, Pennsylvania State College of Medicine, Hershey; Chairman, Baromedical Committee, Hoag Memorial Hospital, Newport Beach, California

Yaron Har-Shai, M.D.
Resident, Department of Plastic Surgery, Rambam Medical Center, Haifa, Israel

Daniel J. Hauben, M.D.
Head and Director, Department of Plastic Reconstructive Surgery and Burns Unit, Beilinson Medical Center, Petah Tikva, Israel

Bernard Hirshowitz, F.R.C.S.
Professor of Plastic Surgery, Faculty of Medicine, Technion, Israel Institute of Technology; Head, Department of Plastic Surgery, Rambam Medical Center, Haifa, Israel

Saul Hoffman, M.D.
Clinical Professor of Surgery, Mount Sinai School of Medicine of the City University of New York; Attending Surgeon, Plastic Surgery Department, Mount Sinai Hospital and Beth Israel Medical Center, New York

John G. Kenney, M.D.
Associate Professor of Plastic Surgery, University of Virginia School of Medicine; Attending Plastic Surgeon, University of Virginia Health Sciences Center, Charlottesville

Ulrich Kesselring, M.D., F.M.H.
Centre de Chirurgie Plastique, Lausanne, Switzerland

Jean-Pierre Lalardrie, M.D.
Associate Professor of Surgery, Medical College of Paris; Head, Department of Plastic Surgery, Hôpital Péan, Paris, France

Claude Lassus, M.D.
Attending Plastic Surgeon, University Hospital, Nice, and Hospital of Cannes, France

Gordon Letterman, M.D., F.A.C.S.
Professor of Surgery (Plastic), George Washington University School of Medicine and Health Sciences, Washington, D.C.

Gaston-François Maillard, M.D.
Assistant Professor, Department of Surgery, University of Lausanne, Lausanne, Switzerland; Attending Surgeon, Hôpital de Morges, Vaud, and Hôpital Daler, Fribourg, Switzerland

Daniel Marchac, M.D.
Consultant Plastic Surgeon, Hôpital Necker Enfants Malades, Paris, France

Rodolphe Meyer, M.D.
Postgraduate Professor International Society of Aesthetic Plastic Surgery; Centre de Chirurgie Plastique; Former Associate Professor, Ear, Nose, and Throat Department, University Hospital, Lausanne, Switzerland

Robert D. Midgley, M.D.C.M., F.R.C.S.(C)
Active Staff Plastic Surgeon, Queen Elizabeth Hospital, Prince Edward Island, Canada

Rony Moscona, M.D.
Deputy Head, Department of Plastic Surgery, Rambam Medical Center, Haifa, Israel

Roger Mouly, M.D.
Associate Professor, College de Médecine des Hôpitaux de Paris, Paris, France

Lennart Ohlsén, M.D.
Associate Professor of Plastic Surgery, Uppsala University Faculty of Medicine; Consultant, Department of Plastic Surgery, University Hospital, Uppsala, Sweden

Jean-M. Parenteau, M.D., F.R.C.S., F.A.C.S.
Private Practice, Montreal, Canada

Gerardo Peixoto, M.D.
Professor of Plastic Surgery, Catholic University of Salvador, Salvador, Brazil

Ivo Pitanguy, M.D.
Head Professor of Plastic Surgery, Pontifícia Universidade Católica; Head Surgeon and Director, Plastic Surgery Department, Santa Casa de Misericórdia, Rio de Janeiro, Brazil

Ronaldo Pontes, M.D.
Professor, Faculdade de Medicina Universidade Federal Fluminense; Attending Surgeon and Director, Clínica Fluminense de Cirurgia Plástica, Rio de Janeiro, Brazil

Jorge M. Psillakis, M.D.
Professor of Plastic Surgery, University of São Paulo; Attending Plastic Surgeon, Oswaldo Cruz Hospital, São Paulo, Brazil; Distinguished Professor, University of Alabama School of Medicine, Birmingham

Paule C. Regnault, M.D., F.R.C.S.(C)
Former Professor Agrégé de Clinique, University of Montreal Faculty of Medicine; Former Chief of Plastic Surgery, Hôpital Saint-Luc, Montreal, Canada

Liacyr Ribeiro, M.D.
Former Head, Plastic Surgery Department, Hospital Universitário Antonio Pedro and Faculdade de Medicina Universidade Federal Fluminense; Attending Surgeon and Director, Clínica Fluminense de Cirurgia Plástica, Rio de Janeiro, Brazil

Ronald E. Riefkohl, M.D., F.A.C.S.
Associate Professor of Plastic, Maxillofacial, and Reconstructive Surgery, Duke University Medical Center, Durham, North Carolina

Thomas H. Robbins, F.R.C.S., F.R.C.S.E., F.R.A.C.S.
Consultant Plastic Surgeon, Division of Surgery, Sandringham Hospital, Melbourne, Australia

Sharon Romm, M.D.
Assistant Professor of Plastic Surgery, Georgetown University School of Medicine and Georgetown University Hospital, Washington, D.C.

Steven K. Sargent, M.D.
Assistant Professor of Radiology, Dartmouth Medical School; Attending Radiologist, Dartmouth-Hitchcock Medical Center, Hanover, New Hampshire

William E. Schatten, M.D., F.A.C.S.
Associate Clinical Professor, Division of Plastic Surgery, Emory University School of Medicine; Chief, Department of Plastic Surgery, West Paces Ferry Hospital, Atlanta

Maxine Schurter, M.D., F.A.C.S.
Clinical Professor of Surgery, George Washington University School of Medicine and Health Sciences, Washington, D.C.

Valdemar Skoog, M.D.
Associate Professor of Immunology, Uppsala University Faculty of Medicine; Senior Registrar, Department of Plastic Surgery, University Hospital, Uppsala, Sweden

Scott L. Spear, M.D.
Associate Professor and Deputy Director, Division of Plastic Surgery, Georgetown University Medical Center, Washington, D.C.

Melvin Spira, M.D.
Professor and Head, Division of Plastic Surgery, Cora and Webb Mading Department of Surgery, Baylor College of Medicine, Houston

Jan Olof Strömbeck, M.D.
Assistant Professor of Plastic Surgery, Karolinska Institutet; Chief, Department of Plastic Surgery, Sabbatsbergs sjukhus, Stockholm, Sweden

Rondi K. Walker, M.D.
Resident Physician, Department of Plastic and Reconstructive Surgery, Georgetown University School of Medicine and Georgetown University Hospital, Washington, D.C.

Daniel L. Weiner, M.D.
Attending Plastic Surgeon, New York Eye and Ear Hospital, New York

Reduction Mammaplasty

1

Jorge M. Psillakis and
Melchiades Cardoso de Oliveira

History of Reduction Mammaplasty

"Human vanity is the impulse of human evolution."

The mechanism of creativity in surgery is based on the experience of the surgeon associated with the need to improve the result without reducing safety. In general, various minor modifications of previous procedures is the rule of surgical evolution. Sometimes a major modification is described; then again, multiple minor changes bring the improvement.

In writing this chapter, our goal is to give credit to those authors who first create a new procedure and, more important, to follow the evolution of medical concepts to avoid repeating errors of the past. Experience shows that many times this goal is difficult to achieve for several reasons well known in our profession: (1) techniques are published by different authors, almost at the same time, in different journals or countries with minor variations; (2) ideas are learned by famous "traveler surgeons" in a country and published in a well-known journal; (3) information or ideas received in meetings or in its corridors are credited to the one who was first published; (4) the same idea evolves at the same time in different places by coincidence; (5) techniques from the past are revived with new improvements and names; (6) techniques created but never published by a surgeon are published later by one of his or her former assistants; (7) techniques are created by an unknown surgeon and published together with a well-known surgeon who receives the credit; and so on.

In the evolution of reduction mammaplasty, it seems that from the beginning uncertainty over priority has been the rule, since Thorek [129] discussed in detail the controversy of the paternity or maternity of many techniques in the past, of which we also have many examples today. The evolution of medical concepts, which is the real history of any chapter of medical science, is the revision of papers published in books and in traditional or well-known international journals filed in libraries. Oral communications and papers published in minor local journals sometimes had not been filed, and they are difficult to obtain to track the evolution of thoughts.

Our history is based on the publications we could find and on our experience since 1962. We read the original papers and some of the translations of the originals. As this book focuses on reduction mammaplasty, our references concentrate on only those techniques that describe some reduction in volume of the breast, even though many are also correcting the ptosis. Techniques that correct only breast ptosis were not included.

Previous chapters in other texts on the history of mammaplasty [59, 62, 73, 118, 129] made our work easier, even though sometimes the information was inconsistent. To reduce the possibility of mistakes, we tried to follow exactly the words of authors and the descriptions of those who lived during that period. However, inadvertently, we may have made some mistakes.

The surgery of reduction mammaplasty developed during this century. We didactically divide the history of reduction mammaplasty into five periods: (1) the past, before 1900; (2) the pioneers, 1901 to 1930; (3) the "trend" period, 1931 to 1960; (4) the period of safety, 1961 to 1979; and (5) the period of refinement, 1980 until today.

Before 1900

Even though mammary deformities were of great interest in ancient cultures, which can be seen in sculptures and paintings, there is no record of early attempts to correct breast hypertrophies compared to what we find with regard to old methods of reconstructing noses. In the first comprehensive textbook published in plastic surgery by Edward Zeis [138, 139], *Handbuch der Plastischen Chirurgie* (Berlin, 1838) and *Die Literatur und Geschichte der Plastischen Chirurgie*, there is no record on the subject of breast reduction.

There are descriptions of reducing the breast for different reasons such as that of Paulus of Aegineta (1538) [3], who described the correction of male gynecomastia. The first description of an attempt to reduce a female breast was by Will Durston (1670) [34–36, 63] to correct sudden and excessive swelling of a woman's breast. He treated this patient with emollients and warm packs and a 2.5-in. incision for drainage, but he failed to achieve his goal.

Velpeau (1854) [133] in France published the first systematic book on breast pathology and surgery and described breast hypertrophy. He stated:

There are several types of hypertrophy: the organ may be of the fat element, glandular, or fibrocellular in structure . . . the treatment of diffuse hypertrophy of the breast still leaves much to be desired. . . . tartar emetic all kinds of astringent local applications, have been employed. Like others I have tried these plans several times without success . . . I have ended by renouncing them altogether . . . methodical compression either as a principal or accessory remedy nevertheless failed. I do not know a single example of breast hypertrophy cured by compression.

It is supposed that this book exerted a great influence on the future evolution of breast surgery in France, since the first attempts at breast reduction surgery were made in that country.

T. Gaillard Thomas (1882) [46, 124] from New York was a gynecologist who first described the incision on the mammary sulcus to remove benign tumors. He said:

I have practiced thus far in a dozen cases . . . a semicircular line is drawn with pen and ink exactly in the fold which is created by the fall of the organ upon the thorax . . . with a bistoury the skin and areolar tissue are cut through . . . the line of incision is closed by interrupted suture . . . the line of incision is covered with gutta-percha, collodium and the ordinary antiseptic dressing . . . the only sign of the operation . . . is a delicate cicatricial semicircular line, which is in great degree concealed by the folding of the skin.

Later, this incision was used by French surgeons (Guinard and Morestin) to reduce breast hypertrophies.

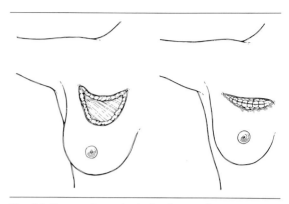

Fig. 1-1. Pousson's method of reduction by transverse semilunar resection.

Pousson (1897) [102, 103] from France first described a surgical procedure with the intention to reduce the breast by a transversal semilunar resection of skin and breast tissue in the anterior superior area of the breast (Fig. 1-1). He was the first surgeon to build a bridge between the ablative breast surgery and plastic surgery.

Verchère (1898) [134], also from France, based on Pousson's technique, followed the principle of resecting the breast in the anterior superior part but with a less visible scar. He described:

I examined her . . . and she really had a very large breast . . . She was 29 years old . . . and she was an artist, one of our best singers who exposed professionally the superior part of the breast for the eyes of the spectators . . . I refused to do the surgery on her . . . but after insistency I promised to give her a solution . . . I began to do studies in cadavers . . .

He performed a resection of skin and breast tissue in the lateral border of the breast near the axilla.

1901 to 1930: The Pioneers

The evolution of anesthesia aided the evolution of surgery in general as well as that in breast reduction. Morally the surgeons had first to face the fact that breast hypertrophies and pendulous abdomens were not only aesthetic problems but also deformities with impairment to the health of patients. This concept gave them moral and medical support to perform this type of surgery. In the beginning only very large breasts were reduced in size; these are still the most difficult. Partial amputation was initially done, and, progressively, famous surgeons accepted the morality of the procedure that allowed and consolidated surgical research.

From 1901 to 1930, almost all the technical possibilities were attempted; some were based on anatomic knowledge and others completely ignored the vascular blood supply of the breast.

Small and medium-sized breasts could be reduced with a great margin of safety with transposition of the areola, but surgeons had difficulties in transposing the areola safely in large breasts; this difficulty also occurred with surgeons in the second period, 1931 to 1960, when large-breast reductions were made by partial amputations and areola graft or by two surgical procedures for safe transposition of the nipple. Only after 1960 could large hypertrophies be more safely performed in a single surgical stage.

Important contributions from the pioneer period remain today with the improvement of modern surgical methods: (1) partial amputation of large breasts and nipple-areola graft, (2) transposition of the areola to a higher position, (3) deepithelialization of the skin around the areola, (4) wedge resection of breast tissue under the areola, and (5) oblique wedge resection on the lateral pole and final scar indifferent shapes—inverted "T", "L", horizontal on the sulcus, vertical from the areola to the sulcus, and only a periareolar scar.

The contributions for this period that have been abandoned today include undermining of the skin of the breast tissue, resections of breast tissue in the superior pole, resections of breast tissue in the surface of the gland, and resections of breast tissue in different poles during the same procedure. Unfortunately, we sometimes encounter in regional meetings or publications "re-creation" of these concepts that were abandoned because of the higher risk of areola-nipple and tissue necrosis.

European surgeons, who dominated medicine in this period, made the majority of contributions, followed by surgeons in the United States. The evolution of ideas had the following course:

Guinard (1903) [47] from France did reduction mammaplasty by an elliptical skin resection on the mammary sulcus and a truncated cone resection of breast tissue. He described:

1200 grams were resected on the right and 1400 grams on the left side . . . as there was excess skin, one semilunar

incision was made in each side of the mammary sulcus . . . after the breast was undermined from the pectoral muscle, breast tissue was resected in a truncated cone shape at the base of the breast; after I finished only the apex of the cone like a cap remained which naturally rested in the major pectoral muscle.

Morestin (1905) [88, 89], also in France, did a similar procedure, but he resected the breast in a discord shape. He wrote:

After the undermining of the deep layer . . . I cut in a vertical-transversal plan in the overall width and height in such a way to remove a disc with two transversal fingers in thickness.. . . . several months after the surgery the right breast began to grow again but with pain symptoms. I did not hesitate to perform a second operation similar to the first one . . . after a certain period of time . . . there was no more pain . . . the volume of the breasts was stable two years after the left breast surgery and one year after the second right breast surgery.

The advantage of this method was safety, but it produced a flat breast.

Villandre (1911) [135] from France according to Thorek [129] from Chicago, Illinois, made the first transposition of nipple through a buttonhole opening in the skin higher up.

The transposition of the nipple-areola complex into a higher position was the principle that allowed different surgeons to create a great variety of procedures. It was a major contribution to breast reduction surgery, and it is difficult to establish whether its paternity was Morestin, Villandre, Aubert, or Passot.

Lexer (1912) [64], from Freiburg, Germany, described the reduction of the breast of a 20-year-old woman in the following manner: "Two diverging incisions extending from the middle mammary gland to the mammary sulcus. Excess of skin and breast were removed. The remaining breast was raised by sutures so the operated breast had a completely normal form, if the absence of the nipple could be ignored."

Kausch (1916) [54], from Germany, described a circular resection of skin and breast tissue around the areola, from the skin to the pectoral muscle. As expected, he had a total necrosis of the nipple-areola complex. After his lack of success, he suggested performance of his procedure in two stages.

Nitter (1922) [91], also from Germany, believed that it was justified to amputate both breasts in a girl 21 years of age; when removed, they weighed 6.0 kg and 4.7 kg.

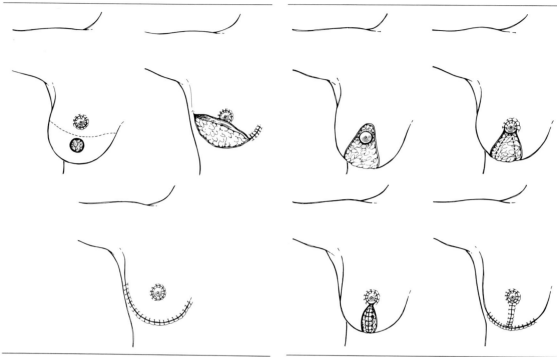

Fig. 1-2. Thorek's method of nipple-areola transplantation.

Fig. 1-3. Lexer-Kraske method.

Thorek (1922) [131] described the ablation on breast hypertrophy in a 27-year-old singer with nipple transplant. He wrote, "The nipples were then transplanted from the ablated breasts to the newly constructed ones. The patient returned to the stage, mentally and physically much improved and fully able to follow her vocation" (Fig. 1-2).

This principle of nipple-areola transplantation was also a major contribution for large-breast hypertrophy reduction. Its paternity is also discussed in the literature. It seems that Lexer performed only the first areola graft, and later Thorek and Dartigues performed the nipple and areola graft, probably in an independent way. Thorek described the method first, and, in the majority of publications, paternity is attributed to him. Many articles followed [1, 2, 27, 29, 41, 66, 67, 72, 74, 75, 99, 104, 114, 125–129, 132].

Von Kraske (1923) [57], from Freiburg, working with Lexer, published in detail his method of breast reduction. The areola was incised, and a strip of skin and subcutaneous tissue was resected from the superior pole of the areola to the future position of the nipple. From the mammary sulcus, two incisions were made up to the areola. After skin resection in this area, excess breast tissue was resected in a wedge. Sutures approximated the wound edges of the breast tissue and skin, and subcutaneous tissue was closed (Fig. 1-3). Lexer (1925) [65], also from Germany, later discussed briefly this technique, which is today well known as the Lexer-Kraske operation. This method was also a great contribution, and there is no controversy about paternity. The great contribution was the wedge resection in the inferior pole, absence of separation of the skin from the breast tissue, conification of the breast, and transposition of the nipple to a higher position.

Lotsch (1923, 1928) [69, 70], from Magdeburg, Germany, described a similar procedure of skin resection. The difference is that he undermined completely the skin from the breast and removed the fat layer in a radial direction. In this "shave" type of reduction, he could reduce 250 to 500 gm of breast tissue. In 1923, he published the method for the correction of breast ptosis without reduction and, in 1928, for breast reduction.

Aubert (1923) [8], from Marseille, described resecting the totality of skin from the inferior part of the breast from the inframammary sulcus up to above the areola. The areola was maintained on the breast. The remaining skin was undermined to the level of the clavicle. The resection of the mammary gland was made in a wedge in the lateral pole. The superior edge of the gland was sutured to the pectoral fascia as high as possible. The skin was brought down over the gland, and a 2-cm piece of skin was excised in the new position of the nipple and areola.

Passot (1925) [93], in France, described a similar method of skin resection but removed the breast tissue in a different way. He said, " . . . It is necessary to resect the inferior pole . . . by an oblique wedge resection in the posterior surface of the breast in the retromammary space." The resection is similar to "the discord shape of Morestin." The nipple was transposed in a higher position in the same way as described by Villandre and Aubert.

Dufourmentel (1925) [33], also in France, described a similar method.

Axhausen (1926) [10], from Berlin, likewise evolved the same principles with resection of the breast tissue on the anterior surface of the breast.

Hollander (1924) [48], also from Berlin, used a lateral resection of the breast tissue with a final L-shaped scar. The first incision began at the axilla and continued to the areola. A second incision was made from the first in the axilla of the mammary sulcus to the lower extent of the breasts and upward to the areola. The resection included skin and breast tissue to the fascia. Sutures brought together the tissue edges. Another incision was made around the upper edge of the areola, resecting skin and subcutaneous tissue; the nipple was transposed upward (Fig. 1-4). He stated, "I based my procedure on the Lexer-Kraske technique." This is also a contribution that remained in history, even though the author changed only the position of the wedge resection of the breast previously described.

Dartigues (1925) [30, 31], from France, published his second method for correction of a second-degree severely ptotic breast. Through a vertical subareola incision, he excised the necessary amount of skin and breast tissue and fixed it in a

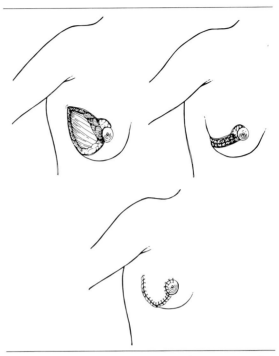

Fig. 1-4. Hollander's method of lateral resection with L-shaped scar, based on the technique of von Kraske-Lexer.

higher position in the pectoralis muscle. He obtained at the end of the operation only a vertical scar. He pointed out the value of this technique in selective cases with skin of proper quality and consistency (Fig. 1-5). It seems that he was the first to describe the vertical scar from the areola to the sulcus, which has recently been rediscovered by modern surgeons.

Many procedures failed to take into consideration the variability of the blood supply to the breast with frequent necrosis of the nipple. To diminish this risk, Joseph [51, 52], from Berlin, described a two-stage procedure in which the nipple areola complex was transposed by a cutaneous bridge. He was the first surgeon to maintain the supply of the nipple-areola complex in the inferior pedicle and to utilize two stages for larger hypertrophies. Using two surgical stages to transpose the areola was the method chosen by the majority of surgeons until 1960.

Kuster (1926) [58] described two methods of resection of skin and breast tissue down to the fascia in a U-shape. In the first, the nipple remained in

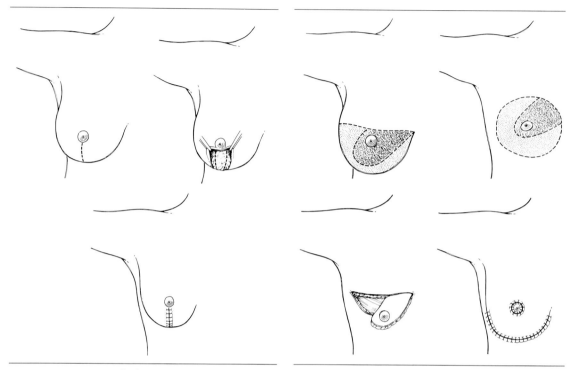

Fig. 1-5. *Dartigue's method of correcting second-degree ptosis, using vertical incision from areola to sulcus.*

Fig. 1-6. *Schwarzmann's method based on dermal vascularization of nipple and areola.*

the lateral pole. Because he encountered necrosis, he described a second one where the pedicle remained in the superior pole.

Monard (1926) [86], in France, by a submammary incision, undermined a cutaneous flap from the breast tissue up to the superior pole and maintained the nipple and areola in the breast tissue. To reduce in volume and to give conicality, he removed a wedge-shaped area of breast tissue in the inferior pole without reaching the areola. He described this method for breast reduction and for resection of benign tumors.

Biesenberger (1928, 1930) [16, 17], from Vienna, after complete dissection of the skin, resected the outer half of the parenchyma of the breast and adipose tissue, by an S-shaped incision. The incision began in the axilla and extended to the lower pole under the areola. To rebuild the conical shape of the breast, the lower portion of the breast segment carrying the nipple was displaced upward and outward. After having obtained the desired form of the breast, the skin was replaced and the excess removed with a final inverted T scar. He believed that with his method he could repair all types of ptosis and hypertrophic breasts safely.

It is interesting that this method remained so popular for many years with all the misconceptions regarding the blood supply of the nipple. Even with the modification of Schwarzmann [116], many surgeons described total necrosis of the nipple. Although other safer methods had already been described, this method continued to be used until 1960.

Schreiber (1929) [112], from Vienna, described a two-stage method based on Lexer-Kraske-Lotsch principles. In the first stage, he resected breast tissue in the superior pole and moved the nipple to a higher position. In the second stage, a wedge resection inferior to the nipple was made and excess skin was removed. At the end of the operation he obtained an inverted T scar.

Schwarzmann (1930) [116], also from Vienna, introduced a new concept on the blood supply of the nipple that is still used today. He believed that the vascularization of the areola and nipple was carried by the dermis. Like Biesenberger, he based his procedure on a medial pedicle alone, with resection of the inferior and part of the lateral pole of the breast. The flap carrying the nipple was rotated in an upward direction, and an oval hole in the superior skin was made to be the new site of the areola. By this means, he obtained a horizontal scar in the inframammary sulcus (Fig. 1-6).

Bames (1930) [12], from Los Angeles, used different methods according to the degree of ptosis of the breast. In major cases, he removed the entire skin from the inferior pole of the breast, up to the projection of the mammary sulcus, to the anterior surface of the breast. The resection of the breast was on the lateral side of the nipple. His drawings are not very clear and have been interpreted in different ways. He said:

Any superfluous fat is picked up away until we have a clean, well defined gland, attached to its base by an elongated pedicle of 4 to 5 inches in diameter. If the gland is still too large after removal of all superfluous fat, a radial section or several such sections, taking the entire thickness of the gland from periphery to areola, may be safely excised. These sections are taken from the lower half of the gland to minimize size and weight below the nipple.

The principle to perform different procedures for different breasts was to be routine in the following period.

1931 to 1960: The "Trend" Period

The experiences of the first period increased the number of patients "in the market" for breast reduction. Large series of patients were common in publications. Even though this period does not show creativity in the development of new techniques, like the first one, it was innovative in the practical sense. Surgeons looked carefully at their failures and had a better understanding of the variations of the blood supply; also they looked at breast hypertrophies as a deformity variable in degree with different approaches for each one. Different sizes of breast hypertrophy were treated in different ways by different surgeons, and several classifications were described. A better knowledge of the blood supply supported the surgical technique, and in small or medium-sized breasts, nipple transposition was made safely in one stage with deepithelialization of the skin around the areola. The nipple-areola graft was more commonly used for large hypertrophies because it was

safer. When, in these cases, transposition of the nipple was used, two surgical stages instead of one were used due to the high incidence of necrosis in a single one, since total undermining of the skin from breast tissue was routine.

At the end of this period, two important contributions occurred: a reduction in the area of skin separated from the breast tissue to reduce risks of necrosis, and utilization of dermofat flaps pedicled in the areola or in the mammary sulcus, which are used today in many modern techniques.

From the editorial point of view, many books were published due to the increasing popularity of this surgery. We were able to collect 12 books specifically on this subject, but many more chapters were also published in general surgery texts. Six books were published in France [21, 26, 77, 87, 92, 136], three in Germany [15, 50, 55], two in the United States [73, 129], one in Brazil [105], and one in Argentina [81]. Many publications were also found in journals from different countries. Among these we can find contributions that improved this procedure, step by step, for the safety and quality of results that will mark the following period.

Von Fraenkel (1932) [43], from Germany, reduced large-breast hypertrophies in two stages, first with the Lotsch operation and second with Biesemberger's.

Dartigues (1933) [28] said:

Until some years ago the breast was looked upon by the surgeon only from the pathological point of view and then for extirpation of benign and malign tumors. With the influence of modern evolution that demanded from a person a better physical aspect . . . plastic surgeries to correct the breast were made with great frequency . . . I divided breast ptosis in several degrees: first degree, light deformity but visible, when the breast loses its firmness . . . it is the beginning of the decline of the body.

He classified breast deformities in four degrees and used different procedures for each one: first degree, Passot method or an elliptical vertical resection under the areola as he described; the second and third degree, vertical resection of breast tissue and skin under the areola; and fourth degree, partial amputation of the breast and nipple-areola graft.

Burian (1934, 1938) [19, 20], from Prague, said:

This report is based on personal experience of 161 operations of various degrees of ptosis and hypertrophies of mammals . . . in order to prevent necrosis it is neces-

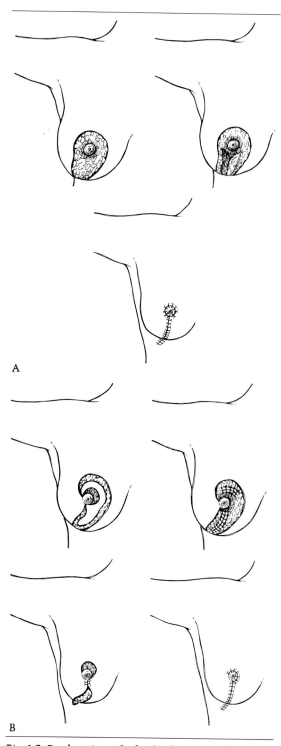

A

B

Fig. 1-7. Prudente's methods of reduction with incision going completely around the areola (A) and incision partially around areola (B).

sary to preserve the periareolar vessels especially the venous flow of the blood. The "circulus venosus" must remain intact, for a necrosis is always an infarct from the venostasis . . . this way a protective zone of 2–3 cm in width is formed around the areola . . . but large scars meant a serious drawback; the inner parts of submammary scars are especially very trying to women. These scars also are frequently inclined to hypertrophy. None of the published methods was quite free from any of the disadvantages mentioned above.

He maintained a wide dermal flap around the areola and resected the breast tissue on the inferior lateral and, in larger hypertrophies, also in the superior segments. The gland was rotated laterally, and the excess of skin resected with a final inverted T-shaped scar.

Prudente (1936) [105], from São Paulo, divided breast deformities into five groups: simple ptosis, atrophic ptosis, fat ptosis, hypertrophic ptosis, and asymmetric ptosis. He divided the surgical techniques into five types: classical method (Morestin, Villandre, Passot, Dufourmentel, and Axhausen); vertical resection of breast tissue with incision around the areola; vertical resection of breast tissue with partial incision around the areola; T method; and method in two stages (Fig. 1-7).

Eitner (1935) [37, 38], from Vienna, did two different cuts to correct the position and shape of the breast, depending on the size of the breast. He said, " . . . [I]n small breasts an oral circumcision of the areola . . . only the layer of the epidermis is removed . . . completely around the areola, and the skin separated as usual . . . separate the breast from the cutaneous envelope and remove a retromammary wedge-shaped portion of breast tissue." At the end of the operation, he had only a scar around the areola. He believed that the skin envelope would adapt to the breast (Fig. 1-8). For large breasts, he operated in two stages: in the first stage, he transposed the areola to a higher position in a similar way for small breasts, and in the second stage, he removed breast tissue in the inferior pole with a final inverted T scar. It seems that this was the first description to end a breast reduction surgery with a final scar only around the areola and to allow the skin to adapt to breast tissue. This principle was to be published again later.

Fomon (1936) [42], from New York, described in detail the anatomy of the breast and the procedure of Biesenberger.

Schwarzmann (1937) [115] presented a series of 180 operations and stated, "In large hypertrophies

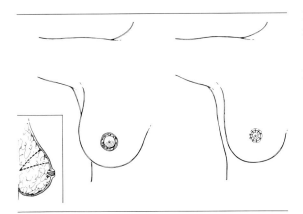

Fig. 1-8. Eitner's method of circumareolar incision and resection. Final result depended on future shrinkage of the skin envelope.

and ptosis of the breast, in spite of all prophylactic measures taken, a partial or total necrosis of the nipple can occur. Based on a large series of cases, in 1930 I recommended not to remove the dermis around the areola where we found the veins and nerves necessary for the vitality of the areola."

McIndoe (1938) [82], from London, wrote, "This review is based on an analysis of 80 cases of mammary hypertrophy operated on by Sir Harold Gillies and myself . . . today there is little need to justify plastic surgical procedures on the pendulous breast . . . measured in terms of human happiness to the patient few surgical operations are as satisfactory . . . " He divided mammary hypertrophy into five types: (1) long heavy pendulous breasts, (2) broad heavy breasts associated with obesity, (3) sac-like dependent breasts, (4) true gynecomastia with marked hypertrophy of the glandular elements, and (5) asymmetry.

The procedure should be fully explained to the patient and the nature of the scars shown to her, if possible by means of photographs . . . the one stage or Biesenberger operation is reserved for a moderate degree of ptosis where there is good opportunity of obtaining an attractive cosmetic result with complete safety . . . in marked hypertrophy the two stage procedure with an interval of 3–4 months has been the rule and is justified by the greater degree of safety and the higher aesthetic standard."

He condemned the Biesenberger method for large

hypertrophies since he had breast tissue necrosis in all his five cases.

Nedkoff (1930) [90], from Bulgaria, said, "Every surgeon who is dealing with cosmetic surgery has had the experience, that especially in this branch of surgery you have to fulfill the wishes of your quite ambitious patients." He resected the skin from the mammary sulcus up to the new nipple site in an inverted T-shaped area. Breast tissue was resected only in the inferior pole.

Gillies and McIndoe (1939) [45] described their experience with two methods: the Biesenberger technique for medium hypertrophies and, for the fatty breast, a double pedicle technique, with resection of breast tissue over the areola. They wanted to preserve the lateral thoracic vessels as well as those of the second and third intercostal space. They stated, "Partial necrosis of skin flaps is an annoying complication . . . necrosis of a portion of the pedicle will be evidenced by an abscess pointing underneath the skin . . . nipple sensation becomes fully established in 70% of the cases."

Ragnell (1946) [106], from Sweden, used resections of breast tissue only superiorly to the nipple in moderate hypertrophies; in large ones, he also did a resection on the inferior pole.

Bames (1948) [11], from Los Angeles, removed the epithelium around the areola; the skin was undermined from the breast tissue, which was resected in a wedge shape in the inferior lateral part; in larger hypertrophies, he resected a triangle in the medial part, and the areola remained based on a superior and inferior pedicle (Fig. 1-9).

Aufricht (1949) [9], from New York, wrote:

In planning mammaplastic operations there are two approaches: the improvised and preoperatively geometrically planned. In the first without specific presurgical mensuration except reliance on experience . . . many surgeons use only their eyes and digital estimations . . . the second approach consists of presurgical planning . . . various single abstract geometric figures, measurements and calculations were devised . . . The methods should complement each other rather than be relied on singly. With the most careful presurgical planning it may be discovered that the selected measurements prove impracticable.

He described in great detail the manner in which he planned a breast reduction.

Koechlin (1950) [56], from Geneva, concluded:

10

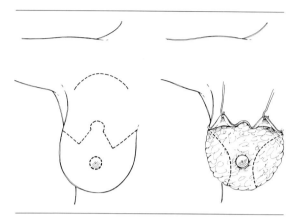

Fig. 1-9. Bames' method.

We have shown in more than 400 cases that it did not lead to any ill consequences . . . a very superficial circular incision is made . . . it must not be forgotten that the nutrient vessels to the nipple are quite near the surface . . . if the scalpel cuts a little too deeply it may produce necrosis of the nipple . . . I have practiced about 800 times without seeing any necrosis of the nipple . . . I have removed glandular masses weighing as much as 2-½ kilograms, but in ordinary cases the resections have a weight of 700 to 1500 grams.

He used lateral resection of the breast as in the Biesenberger method.

Tamerin (1951) [122], from New York, described a modification of the Lexer-Kraske procedure. He stated, "Unlike the accepted transposition techniques, however, the skin of the upper part of the breast is not separated from the gland so that the vascularity of the flaps from which the breast is to be formed is undisturbed." Resection of the skin extended up to the level of the nipple with a block wedge resection of breast tissue, skin, and part of the areola. The circular shape of the areola was rebuilt by suture of the margins. If the final position of the areola was too low, a second operation was performed. Under local anesthesia, resection of the epithelium in a semilunar shape was performed to allow suturing of the areola in a higher position.

Marc (1952) [78], from France, revived the oblique method with skin and breast tissue resection on the external pole.

In 1952 and 1953, four similar papers were published on dermofat flaps to remodel the breast and nipple-areola graft. The paternity of each is difficult to establish, but we can determine from their order of publication how this principle evolved. These flaps have been used and described in more modern procedures in different shapes and sizes.

Marino (1952) [80], from Buenos Aires, published for the first time the "total" breast resection for benign disease and used a dermofat flap based superiorly to rebuild the breast along with a nipple-areola graft.

Conway (1952) [22], from New York, described his method to correct large breast hypertrophies with partial breast amputation and remodeling the breast with superiorly based flaps and areola and nipple graft.

Longacre (1953) [68], also from New York, used the superiorly and inferiorly based dermofat flaps to rebuild the volume of breasts resected for the treatment of benign diseases. The nipple and areola were grafted. The illustrations on his paper are superb.

Maliniac (1953) [76], from New York, proposed the use of the inferiorly based pedicle flap to reshape the breast volume after resection of all breast tissue in diffuse cystic disease. The nipple and areola were grafted.

Penn (1955) [96], from Johannesburg, in an important contribution, recommended a reduction in the area of skin undermining to avoid skin necrosis.

Wise (1956) [137], from Texas, finding difficulty in how safely a breast could be reduced in size and the difficulty in symmetric planning in breasts of different sizes, conducted an interesting study to find a pattern to plan his surgery. He based his thinking on the idea "that the brassiere was made to fit and contribute to the desirable shaping of the breast, it followed that the breast might be made to fit in a particular brassiere." The makers of a specific type of brassiere popular in his time gave him the forms and patterns to fashion a brassiere; this enabled him to develop a pattern to mark the incision to reduce a breast.

Arié (1957) [6], from São Paulo, revived in a modern way the Lexer-Kraske technique based on the experience he had when he worked with Prudente. We had the opportunity to see this excellent surgeon performing his technique many times. After he marked the new nipple position, the epidermis was resected around the areola; skin and breast tissue were resected in one block inferiorly to the nipple up to the mammary sulcus in a

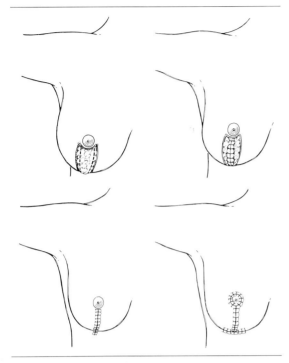

Fig. 1-10. Arié's method.

"shield" shape with two slight convex incisions (Fig. 1-10). The mammary gland was resected in a wedge shape up to the pectoralis muscle posteriorly and to the level of the nipple superiorly. The breast was undermined from the pectoralis fascia; the margins of the wound were sutured to obtain the conical shape; the breast tissue was fixed by sutures to the periosteum of the ribs. In his publication, he ended the surgery with a vertical scar that extended under the mammary sulcus, but, later, when the fashion of bathing suits changed from one piece to two pieces, he finished with an inverted T scar, removing more skin at the level of the mammary sulcus. Large hypertrophies were reduced in two surgical stages at 6-month intervals with the same procedure. His method was very popular in South America at this time because of its safety based on his correct conclusions that "the mammary gland is a cutaneous gland . . . it is very important not to undermine the skin of the breast tissue to avoid necrosis in the nipple-areola and skin . . . the main blood supply of the nipple was variable and a double pedicle supply was necessary to avoid necrosis . . . the resection of

breast tissue had to respect the directions of the mammary ducts to maintain the function of the organ." In a period of time when Biesenberger's procedure was the choice of the majority of the surgeons, he was a voice of dissent that made possible the creation of the new techniques from Brazil.

1961 to 1979: The Period of Safety

Whereas in the preceding time periods, large breast reductions had to be performed in two surgical stages, the period from 1961 to 1979 was characterized by the descriptions of large-breast reduction techniques in a single surgical procedure; different concepts are revived with improvements. Refinements in the techniques to obtain more pleasant aesthetic results are also described, and a high degree of safety was the goal.

The key to safety was based on the principles of Lexer-Kraske and Schwarzmann with a larger area of skin and breast tissue resection. Blood supply and innervation of the areola-nipple complex were maintained by medial and lateral pedicles, with deepithelialization of the skin around the areola and without separation of the skin from the breast tissue.

At the same time, Strombeck (1960) [121], from Stockholm, and Pitanguy (1960, 1961, 1963) [98–100], from Rio de Janeiro, presented two techniques similar in principle with different ways to perform and with a high degree of safety even in large hypertrophies.

Tamerin (1963) [123], from New York, added to the Lexer-Kraske technique the resection of breast tissue on the posterior aspect of the breast; Skoog (1963) [119], from Uppsala, Sweden, presented his technique based on Schwarzmann's procedure; McKissock (1972) [83], from Torrance, California, described the vertical dermal flap, based on Strombeck's procedure. His pattern of breast tissue resection is similar to the one described by Bames.

Pontes (1973) [101], from Rio de Janeiro, improved the late aesthetical results, based on Pitanguy's technique, changing the pattern of skin and breast resection on the lateral and medial pole.

The lateral resection described by Hollander is revived by several authors: Dufourmentel and Mouly (1968) [32]; Perel (1962) [97] and Elbaz (1975) [39] from France; Mir y Mir (1968) [85] from Barcelona; Schatten et al (1971) [111] from Atlanta; Regnault (1974) [108] from Montreal; Meyer and Kesserling (1975) [84] from Lausanne,

Switzerland; and Ely (1976) [40] and Horibe et al (1976) [49] from Brazil.

A third technique was improved with the areola and nipple based on an inferior dermofat pedicle described and used by several authors: Ribeiro (1975) [109]; Jurado (1976) [53] from Brazil; Courtiss and Goldwyn (1977) [23], Robbins (1977) [110], Smith and Schmidt (1979) [120], Georgiade et al (1979) [44], Ariyan (1980) [7], Schultz and Markus (1981) [113], and Crepeau and Klein (1982) [24].

A fourth technique for medium breasts in young patients was presented by Andrews et al (1975) [5] from São Paulo, based on Arie's technique. He described a procedure with a final periareolar scar only with resection of breast tissue on the inferior pole. This publication drove surgeons to search for techniques with small scars, which became the goal for the following period.

After 1980: The Period of Refinement

The period after 1980 has been characterized by surgical techniques with a reduced final scar but with the same standard of aesthetic quality and safety.

Publications from Peixoto (1980, 1985) [94, 95], Sepulveda (1981) [117], Bozola et al (1982) [18], Andrews (1984) [4], and Basile (1986) [13] from Brazil; Regnault (1980) [107] from Canada; Marchac and Olarte (1982) [79] and Lassus (1986, 1987) [60, 61] from France; Crow (1983) [25] from the United States; Maillard (1986) [71] from Switzerland; and Berrino et al (1988) [14] from Italy are examples of techniques with short scars.

Many of the techniques cited during these last two periods will be described by their authors in this book and are a part of our actual history; therefore, we refrain from reporting these in detail here.

The history of reduction mammaplasty is a small quantity of sand in the building of human creations. Each tiny grain of sand describes a new surgical procedure by a new creator, and each one is of great importance for many patients to lead a more content life.

References

1. Adams, W.M. Free composite grafts of the nipples in mammaryplasty. *South. Surgeon* 13:715, 1947.
2. Adams, W.M. Free transplantation of the nipples and areolae. *Surgery* 15:186, 1944.
3. Aegineta, P. On male breasts resembling the female. In *The Seven Books of Paulus Aegineta*, Vol. 2, Book 6, Sect. 46. F. Adam (trans.). London: Sydenham Society, 1846. P. 334.
4. Andrews, J.M. A technique for reduction mammaplasty. *Aesthetic Plast. Surg.* 8:55, 1984.
5. Andrews, J.M., et al. An areolar approach to reduction mammaplasty. *Br. J. Plast. Surg.* 28:166, 1975.
6. Arié, G. Una nueva tecnica de mastoplastia. *Rev. Lat. Am. Cir. Plast.* 3:23, 1957.
7. Ariyan, S. Reduction mammaplasty with the nipple-areola carried on a single, narrow inferior pedicle. *Ann. Plast. Surg.* 5:167, 1980.
8. Aubert, V. Hypertrophie mammaire de la puberte. Resection partielle restauratrice. *Arch. Franco-Belg. Chir.* 26:284, 1923.
9. Aufricht, G. Mammaplasty for pendulous breasts. *Plast. Reconstr. Surg.* 4:13, 1949.
10. Axhausen, G. Uber Mammaplastik. *Med. Klin.* 22:1437, 1926.
11. Bames, H.O. Reduction of massive breast hypertrophy. *Plast. Reconstr. Surg.* 3:560, 1948.
12. Bames, H.O. The correction of pendulous breasts. *Am. J. Surg.* 10:83, 1930.
13. Basile, R.A. Mammaplasty: Large reduction with short inframammary scars. *Plast. Reconstr. Surg.* 76:130, 1986.
14. Berrino, P., Galli, A., Rainero, M.L., and Santi, P. Unilateral reduction mammaplasty sculpturing the breast from the undersurface. *Plast. Reconstr. Surg.* 82:88, 1988.
15. Biesenberger, H. *Deformitaten und kosmetiche Operationen der weiblichen Brust.* Vienna: Wilhem Mandrich, 1931.
16. Biesenberger, H. Eine neue methode der Mammaplastik. *Zentralbl. Chir.* 55:2382, 1928.
17. Biesenberger, H. Eine neue methode der Mammaplastik. *Zentralbl. Chir.* 57:2971, 1930.
18. Bozola, A.R., Oliveira, M.D., and Sanches, V.M. Mamoplastia em "L." Contribuicao pessoal. *AMRIGS* 26:207, 1982.
19. Burian, F. Our experience with mammaplasties. *Rev. Chir. Structive* 8:35, 1938.
20. Burian, F. Plastic surgery of the breast. *Cas. Lek. Cesk.* 73:397, 1934.
21. Claoue, C., and Bernard, I. *Plastique Mammaire.* Paris: Maloine, 1933.
22. Conway, H. Mammaplasty: Analysis of 110 consecutive cases with end results. *Plast. Reconstr. Surg.* 10:303, 1952.
23. Courtiss, E.H., and Goldwyn, R.M. Reduction mammaplasty by the inferior pedicle technique. *Plast. Reconstr. Surg.* 29:500, 1977.
24. Crepeau, R., and Klein, H. Reduction mammaplasty with inferiorly based glandular pedicle flap. *Ann. Plast. Surg.* 9:463, 1982.
25. Crow, R.W. Refinements of reduction mammaplasty. *Plast. Reconstr. Surg.* 71:205, 1983.
26. Dartigues, L. *Chirurgie Reparatrice: Plastique et Esthetique de la Poitrine, des Seins et de L'abdomen.* Paris: Lepine, 1936.
27. Dartigues, L. De la greffe autoplastique libre areolo-mamelonnaire combinee á la mammectomie bilateral totale: Les raisons de sa prise. *Paris Chir.* 21:11, 1929.

28. Dartigues, L. Estado actual de la cirurgia plastica mamaria. *Clin. y Lab.* 23:737, 1933.

29. Dartigues, L. Mammectomie totale et autogreffe libre areolo-mamelonnaire: Mammectomie bilaterale esthetique. *Bull. Mem. Soc. Chir. (Paris)* 20:739, 1928.

30. Dartigues, L. Procede de mastopexie par incision et resection cutanees verticales subareolaires. *Bull. Mem. Soc. Chir. (Paris)*, Seance, 1924.

31. Dartigues, L. Traitement chirurgical du prolapsus mammaire. *Arch. Franco-Belg. Chir.* 28:313,1925.

32. Dufourmentel, C., and Mouly R. Plastie mammaire par la methode oblique. *Ann. Chir. Plast.* 6:45, 1961.

33. Dufourmentel, L. La mastopexie par deplacement souscutanee avec transposition du mamelon. *Bull. Mem. Soc. Chir. (Paris)*, March 20, 1925 (cited by Maliniac).

34. Durston, W. Concerning a very sudden and excessive swelling of a woman's breasts. *Philos. Trans. R. Soc. London* IV:1047, 1670.

35. Durston, W. Concerning the death of the big-breasted woman. *Philos. Trans. R. Soc. Lond.* IV:1068, 1670.

36. Durston, W. Observations about the unusual swelling of the breasts. *Philos. Trans. R. Soc. Lond.* IV:1049, 1670.

37. von Eitner, E. Uber Hangebrustplastik aus kosmetischer Indikation. *Wien. Med. Wochenschr.* 46:1572, 1927.

38. von Eitner, E. Uber verwendung von Kutislappen bei kosmetischen Mammaplastiken. *Zentralbl. Chir.* 11:625, 1935.

39. Elbaz, J.S. A technique of mammaplasty with "J" scar. *Ann. Chir. Plast.* 20:101, 1975.

40. Ely, J.F. Mamaplastia obliqua. *Ann. XIII Congr. Bras. Cir. Plast.* Emma (ed.), 1976. P. 15.

41. Farina, R., and Villano, J.B. Reduction mammaplasty with free grafting of the nipple and areola. *Br. J. Plast. Surg.* 25:393, 1972.

42. Fomon, S. Surgical treatment of idiopathic hypertrophy of the breast. *Arch. Surg.* 33:253, 1936.

43. von Fraenkel, L. Uber Mammaplastik. *Feutr. Gynak.* 25:1506, 1932.

44. Georgiade, N.G., Serafin, D., Morris, T., and Georgiade, G. Reduction mammaplasty utilizing an inferior pedicle nipple-areolar flap. *Ann. Plast. Surg.* 3:211, 1979.

45. Gillies, H., and McIndoe, A.H. The technique of mammaplasty in conditions of hypertrophy of the breast. *Surg. Gynecol. Obstet.* 68:658, 1939.

46. Goldwyn, R. Theodore Gaillard Thomas and the inframmary incision. *Plast. Reconstr. Surg.* 76:495, 1985.

47. Guinard, R. In discussion of Morestin, M.H. Hypertrophie mammaire traitée par la resection discoide. *Bull. Soc. Chir. (Paris)* 33:651, 1907.

48. Hollander, E. Die Operation der Mammahypertrophie und der Hangebrust. *Dtsch. Med. Wochenschr.* 41:1400, 1924.

49. Horibe, K., Spina, V., and Lodovici, O. Mamaplastia reductora: Nuevo abordaje del metodo lateral oblicuo. *Cir. Plast. Ibero-Lat. Am.* 2:7, 1976.

50. Joseph, J. *Nasenplastik und Sonstige Gesichtsplastik nebst Mammaplastik.* Leipizig: C. Kabitzsch, 1928.

51. Joseph, J. Zur Beseitigung der einfachen und der hypertrophischen Hangebrust. *Dtsch. Med. Wochenschr.* 53:1853, 1927.

52. Joseph, J. Zur operation der hypertrophischen Hangebrust (Mastomiopexie). *Dtsch. Med. Wochenschr.* 51:1103, 1925.

53. Jurado, J. Plasticas mamarias de reducao baseadas em retalho dermico vertical monopediculado. *Ann. XIII Cong. Bras. Cir. Plast.* Emma (ed.), 1976. P. 29.

54. Kausch, W. Die Operation der Mammahypertrophie. *Zentralbl. Chir.* 43:713, 1916.

55. Kleinschmidt, O. Allgemeine und spezielle Operationslehre. In Martin Kirscher (ed.), *Band III, Die Eingriffe au der Brust und Brusthohle.* Berlin: Springer-Verlag, 1940.

56. Koechlin, H. The bleeding nipple and operation for pendulous breast. *Plast. Reconstr. Surg.* 6:387, 1950.

57. von Kraske, H. Die Operation der atropischen und hypertrophischen Hangebrust. *Munchen Med. Wochenschr.* 60:672, 1923.

58. Kuster, H. Operation bei Hangebrust und Hangeleib. *Monatsschr. Geburtshilfe Gynakol.* 73:316, 1926.

59. Lalardrie, J.P., and Jouglard, J.P. *Plasties Mammaires Pour Hypertrophie Et Ptose.* Masson et Cie., 1973. Pp. 46–86.

60. Lassus, C. Breast reductions: Evolution of a technique — a single vertical scar. *Aesthetic Plast. Surg.* 11:107, 1987.

61. Lassus, C. Reduction mammaplasty with very short inframammary scar. *Plast. Reconstr. Surg.* 77:680, 1986.

62. Letterman, G., and Schurter, M.A. A History of Mammaplasty with Emphasis on Correction of Ptosis and Macromastia. In R.M. Goldwyn (ed.), *Plastic and Reconstructive Surgery of the Breast.* Boston: Little, Brown, 1976. Pp. 3–36.

63. Letterman, G., and Schuster, M. Will Durston's mammaplasty. *Plast. Reconstr. Surg.* 53:48, 1974.

64. Lexer, E. Hypertrophie beider Mammae. *Munchen Med. Wochenschr.* 59:1702, 1912.

65. Lexer, H. Zur operation der Mammahypertrophie und der Hangebrust. *Dtsch. Med. Wochenschr.* 51:26, 1925.

66. Lodovici, O. Bases racionais do tratamento da hipertrofia mamaria. *Rev. Lat. Am. Cir. Plast.* 13:17, 1969.

67. Lodovici, O. Indicacoes das tecnicas de mastoplastias da hipertrofia mamaria. *Rev. Hosp. Clin. Fac. Med. (São Paulo)* 29:300, 1974.

68. Longacre, J.J. The use of local pedicle flaps for reconstruction of the breast after subtotal or total extirpation of the mammary gland and for the correction of distortion and atrophy of the breast due to excessive scar. *Plast. Reconstr. Surg.* 11:380, 1953.

69. Lotsch, F. Uber Hangebrustplastik. *Klin. Wochenschr* 7:603, 1928.

70. Lotsch, F. Uber Hangebrustplastik. *Zentralbl. Chir.* 50:1241, 1923.

71. Maillard, G. Mammaplasty with minimal scarring. *Plast. Reconstr. Surg.* 77:66, 1986.

72. Maliniac, J.W. A mammaplastic substitute for amputation in hypertrophy. *Surgery* 26:573, 1949.

73. Maliniac, J.W. *Breast Deformities and Their Repair.* New York: Grune & Stratton, 1950. Pp. 85–135.

74. Maliniac, J.W. Critical analysis of mammectomy and free transplantation of the nipple in mammaplasty. *Am. J. Surg.* 65:364, 1944.

75. Maliniac, J.W. Harmful fallacies in mammaplasty: With special reference to partial mammectomy with free grafting of nipples. *Conn. Med.* 25:1, 1961.

76. Maliniac, J.W. Use of pedicle dermofat flap in mammaplasty. *Plast. Reconstr. Surg.* 12:110, 1953.

77. Marc, H. *La Plastic Mammaire Par La Méthode Oblique.* Paris: G. Doin, 1952.

78. Marc, H. La plastique mammaire par la methode oblique. *Rev. Port. Obstet.* 5:363, 1952.

79. Marchac, D., and Olarte, G. de. Reduction mammaplasty and correction of ptosis with a short inframammary scar. *Plast. Reconstr. Surg.* 69:45, 1982.

80. Marino, H. Glandular mastectomy: Immediate reconstruction. *Plast. Reconstr. Surg.* 10:204, 1952.

81. Marino, H. *Plasticas Mamarias.* Buenos Aires: Ed. Cient. Arg., 1958.

82. McIndoe, A.H. Review of 80 cases of mammaplasty. *Rev. Cir. Struct.* 8:39, 1938.

83. McKissock, P.K. Reduction mammaplasty with a vertical dermal flap. *Plast. Reconstr. Surg.* 49:245, 1972.

84. Meyer, R., and Kesserling, U.K. Reduction mammaplasty with an L-shaped suture line. *Plast. Reconstr. Surg.* 55:139, 1975.

85. Mir y Mir, L. Reduction mammaplasty. *Plast. Reconstr. Surg.* 41:352, 1968.

86. Monard, P. La mastopexie esthetique par la transplantation du mamelon. *Pratique Chir. Illustree* (Pauchet.) Paris, G. Doin, 1926.

87. Montant, C., and Dubois, F. *Chirurgie Plastique De Seins.* Paris: Maloine, 1933.

88. Morestin, H. Hypertrophie mammaire. *Bull. Mem. Soc. Anat. (Paris)* 80:682, 1905.

89. Morestin, H. Hypertrophie mammaire traite par la resection discoide. *Bull. Chir. (Paris)* 33:649, 1907.

90. Nedkoff, N. Fine neue Schmittmethode der Brustkorrektur. *Zeutr. Chir.* 27:1503, 1930.

91. Nitter, H. Hyperplasia of the mamma. *Norsk Wag. Laegevid* 83:673, 1922.

92. Noel, S., and Martinez, L. La chirurgie esthetique, nouveaux procedes de correction du prolapses mammaire. *Le Concour Med. No.* 46:1928.

93. Passot, R. La correction esthétique du prolapsus mammaire par le procédé de la transposition du mamelon. *Presse Méd.* 33:317, 1925.

94. Peixoto, G. The infraareolar longitudinal incision in reduction mammaplasty. *Aesthetic Plast. Surg.* 9:1, 1985.

95. Peixoto, G. Reduction mammaplasty: A personal technique. *Plast. Reconstr. Surg.* 65:217, 1980.

96. Penn, J. Breast reduction. *Br. J. Plast. Surg.* 7:357, 1955.

97. Perel, L. A propos de la plastie mammaire par la methode oblique. *Ann. Chir. Plast.* 7:77, 1962.

98. Pitanguy, I. Breast hypertrophy. *Translations of the Second International Congress of Plastic and Reconstructive Surgery.* London, 1960. Edinburgh: Livingstone Ed., 1960. Pp. 509–522.

99. Pitanguy, I. Contribuicao a tecnica do enxerto livre para a correcao das grandes hipertrofias mamarias. *Rev. Lat. Am. Cir. Plast.* 7:75, 1963.

100. Pitanguy, I. Mamaplastias estudo de 245 casos consecutivos e apresentacao de tecnica pessoal. *Rev. Bras. Cir.* 42:201, 1961.

101. Pontes, R. A technique of reduction mammaplasty. *Br. J. Plast. Surg.* 26:365, 1973.

102. Pousson, M. De la mastopexie. *Bull. Mem. Soc. Chir. (Paris)* 23:507, 1897.

103. Pousson, M., and Michel. Sur un cas de mastopexie. *J. Med. Bordeaux* 27:495, 1897.

104. Prudente, A. Amputacao plastica da mama na mastopatia fibrosa cistica: Regeneracao glandular. *Arg. Cir. Clin. Exp.* 6:670, 1942.

105. Prudente, A. *Contribuicao ao estudo da plastica mamaria. Cirurgia esthetica dos seios.* Publicitas Ed., 1936.

106. Ragnell, A. Operative correction of hypertrophy and ptosis of the female breast. *Acta. Chir. Scand.* (Suppl) 113:13, 1946.

107. Regnault, P. Breast reduction: B technique. *Plast. Reconstr. Surg.* 65:840, 1980.

108. Regnault, P. Reduction mammaplasty by the "B" technique. *Plast. Reconstr. Surg.* 53:19, 1974.

109. Ribeiro, L. A new technique for reduction mammaplasty. *Plast. Reconstr. Surg.* 55:330, 1975.

110. Robbins, T.H. A reduction mammaplasty with the areola-nipple based on an inferior dermal pedicle. *Plast. Reconstr. Surg.* 59:64, 1977.

111. Schatten, W.E., Hartley, J.H., and Hamm, W.B. Reduction mammaplasty by the Dufourmentel-Mouly method. *Plast. Reconstr. Surg.* 48:306, 1971.

112. Schreiber, F. Operation der Hangebrust. *Beitr. Klin. Chir.* 147:59, 1929.

113. Schultz, R.C., and Markus, N.J. Platform for nipple projection: Modification of the inferior pedicle technique for breast reduction. *Plast. Reconstr. Surg.* 68:108, 1981.

114. Schurter, M., and Letterman, G. Amputation mammaplasty with free nipple grafts. *J. Am. Med. Wom. Assoc.* 16:854, 1961.

115. Schwarzmann, E. Beitrag zur Vermeidng von Mammillennekrose bei einzeitiger Mammaplastik schewerer Falle. *Rev. Chir. Strut.* 7:206, 1937.

116. Schwarzmann, E. Die technik der Mammaplastik. *Chirurg.* 2:943, 1930.

117. Sepulveda, A. Tratamento das assimetrias mamarias. *Rev. Bras. Cir.* 71:11, 1981.

118. Serafin, D. History of Breast Reconstruction. In N.D. Georgiade (ed.), *Reconstructive Breast Surgery.* St. Louis: Mosby, 1976. Pp. 1–17.

119. Skoog, T. A technique of breast reduction. *Acta Chir. Scand.* 126:453, 1963.

120. Smith, G.A., and Schmidt, G.H. Experience with the Ribeiro reduction mammaplasty technique. *Ann. Plast. Surg.* 3:260, 1979.

121. Strombeck, J.O. Mammaplasty: Report of a new technique based on the two pedicle procedure. *Br. J.*

Plast. Surg. 13:79, 1960.

122. Tamerin, J.A. A mammaplastic procedure. *Plast. Reconstr. Surg.* 7:288, 1951.

123. Tamerin, J.A. The Lexer-Kraske mammaplasty: A reaffirmation. *Plast. Reconstr. Surg.* 31:442, 1963.

124. Thomas, T.G. On the removal of benign tumors of the mamma without mutilation of the organ. *N.Y. Med. J. Obstet. Rev.* 35:337, 1982.

125. Thorek, M. Esthetic surgery of the pendulous breast, abdomen and arms in the female. *Ill. Med. J.* 58:48, 1930.

126. Thorek, M. Histological verification of efficacy of free transplantation of nipple. *Med. J. Rec.* 134:474, 1931.

127. Thorek, M. Plastic reconstruction of the breast and free transplantation of the nipple. *J. Int. Coll. Surg.* IX (2):194, 1946.

128. Thorek, M. Plastic reconstruction on the female breasts and abdomen. *Am. J. Surg.* 43:268, 1939.

129. Thorek, M. *Plastic Surgery of the Breast and Abdominal Wall.* Springfield, Illinois: Thomas, 1942. Pp. 1–356.

130. Thorek, M. *Plastic Surgery of the Breast and Abdominal Wall*, Springfield, Illinois: Thomas, 1942.

131. Thorek, M. Possibilities in the reconstruction of the human form. *Med. J. Rec.* 116:572, 1922.

132. Thorek, M. Twenty-five years' experience with plastic reconstruction of the breast and transplantation of the nipple. *Am. J. Surg.* 67:445, 1945.

133. Velpeau, A. *Traite des maladies du sein et de la region mammaire.* Masson et Cie., Paris, 1854, London, H. M. (trans.). *A Treatise on the Diseases of the Breast and Mammary Region.* Sindenham Soc., 1856.

134. Verchère, F. Mastopexie lateral contre la mastoptose hypertrophique. *Med. Mod.* 9 (Paris):540, 1898.

135. Villandre, cit Thorek, M. *Plastic Surgery of the Breast and Abdominal Wall.* Springfield, Illinois: Thomas, 1942. Pp. 185–686.

136. Virenque, M. *Chirurgie Esthetique; le Sein.* Paris: Maloine, 1928.

137. Wise, R.J. A preliminary report on a method of planning the mammaplasty. *Plast. Reconstr. Surg.* 17:367, 1956.

138. Zeis, E. *Die Literatur und Geschichte der Plastischen Chirurgie.* Leipsig: Engelmann, 1863–4. In F. McDowell, F. (ed.), *Series of Plastic Surgery Indexes*, Vol. 1. Baltimore: Williams & Wilkins, 1977.

139. Zeis, E. *Handbuch der Plastischen Chirugie.* Berlin: G. Reimer, 1838.

2

Scott L. Spear,
Rondi K. Walker, and
Sharon Romm

Pertinent Anatomy of the Breast

Embryology

The mammary gland develops during the sixth week of fetal life from solid ectodermal projections into the underlying mesenchyme. Development occurs along the mammary ridges — thick strips of ectoderm that extend from the axilla to the inguinal region. Mammary ridges (or "milk lines") appear during the fourth week but atrophy in humans between the sixth and ninth developmental week except in the pectoral region [8]. At this time, a primary mammary papilla or bud forms, then produces several secondary buds and ducts. These ducts canalize, then become the lactiferous ducts and sinuses [9].

In the late fetal period, the mammary gland flattens vertically, creating a shallow mammary pit. The lactiferous sinus opens into the base of this pit or rudimentary nipple. The area surrounding the pit becomes pigmented, forming the areola. Further nipple development occurs in the perinatal period as a result of proliferation of mesenchyme underlying the areola. The nipple, however, often remains depressed and poorly formed at birth.

Only the main mammary ducts are present at parturition, and the breast remains underdeveloped until puberty. The female breast then rapidly enlarges due to the increase in connective tissue and fat. The ductal system further develops under the influence of ovarian hormones [14]. The glandular tissue remains incompletely developed until pregnancy, when the intralobular ducts undergo rapid evolution forming buds that become alveoli. The male breast undergoes little postnatal development unless estrogens are present.

Topography

The volume of the female breast extends vertically from the second or third to the sixth or seventh ribs, while its medial border is the sternum and its lateral margin lies in a variable position along the anterior axillary line [9]. The inframammary fold, found between the fifth and eighth ribs, marks the inferior extent of the well-developed breast. The fold does not precisely follow any one rib or intercostal space but courses obliquely across one or more ribs and interspaces as they turn superolaterally around the thorax (Fig. 2-1). The microscopic extent of glandular tissue is greater than the apparent breast as seen on the chest wall. Breast tissue is bound to the clavicle and upper abdomen and beyond the axillary fascia to the anterior edges of the latissmus dorsi muscle [4]. The upper lateral quadrant of the breast is most dense and also has the highest incidence of neoplasm, both benign and malignant [3].

Breasts vary in weight and size. The average nonlactating breast weighs approximately 200 gm, whereas the average lactating breast may approach 500 gm*. The normal female breast averages 11 cm in craniocaudal length and 4 cm in depth [2]. Most breasts are distinctly conical, although any pair of breasts, even in women with no endocrine abnormality, may be unequal in size or contour.

Fascia

The mammary gland is enclosed between the superficial and deep layers of the superficial fascia. The superficial layer is a thin and delicate structure that is thicker at the inferior portion of the

---

* This figure for average weight of the female breast appears in several editions of *Gray's Anatomy of the Human Body*, the most recent being the 30th American edition, edited by C.D. Clemente (Philadelphia: Lea & Febiger, 1985, P. 1582). No mention, however, is made in that edition or in others concerning how the value was obtained.

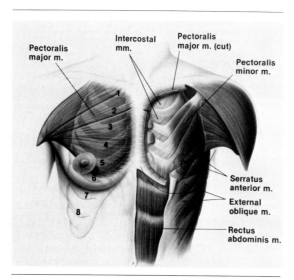

Fig. 2-1. *Topographic and muscular anatomy of the female thorax. An adult woman's breast most often overlies all or some portion of the pectoralis major, serratus anterior, rectus abdominis, and external oblique muscles. The inframammary fold is commonly centered near the sixth intercostal space with the nipple at some varying height depending on the size of the breast and the degree of nipple ptosis.*

mammary gland and becomes thinner as it approaches the clavicle [9]. The deeper layer splits off the superficial fascia and passes deep to the mammary gland. Between this deep layer and the fascia of the pectoralis major, there is a well-defined space, the retromammary space [3]. The retromammary space contains loose areolar tissue and allows the breast to glide freely over the chest wall [3]. Portions of the deep layer of the superficial fascia form connective tissue extensions that pass through the retromammary space and join with the fascia of the pectoralis major [9]. These extensions help support the breast.

The breast is firmly fixed to the skin in the area of the areola, and the remainder of the lobules are attached to the skin by dense fibrous bands termed *Cooper's ligaments* [1]. These ligaments are clinically significant because the connection they provide to the underlying stroma may result in skin retraction in certain disease states, such as carcinoma and fibrous breast lesions [14]. The axillary fascia is composed of two layers: the superficial pectoral fascia, surrounding the pectoralis major muscle, and a deeper costocoracoid fascia covering the pectoralis minor muscle [3]. The costocoracoid

fascia, whose inner portion spans the axilla between the pectoralis minor and the clavicle, conducts the cephalic vein, thoracoacromial vessels, and anterior thoracic nerves [3]. The outer portion of the costocoracoid fascia is triangular and stretches from the lateral edge of the pectoralis major muscle to the coracobrachialis muscle. The base of the triangular fascia fuses with the superficial fascia of the axillary skin and forms the hollow of the axilla [3].

Glandular Elements

The breast is composed of alveoli, small sac-like dilatations, that lead into the lactiferous ducts. The alveoli are lined by a layer of cuboid epithelial cells and a second layer of myoepithelial cells [3]. Myoepithelial cells are also found in the lactiferous ducts and provide a muscular mechanism for ejecting milk [2, 3].

A lobule is composed of 10 to 100 alveoli in the lactating glands, and many lobules form a single lobe that is drained by 15 to 20 lactiferous ducts [9]. The terminal portion of the lactiferous duct dilates, forming the lactiferous sinus before it empties into the nipple. The breast is further compartmentalized by blood vessels, nerves, lymphatics, and Cooper's ligaments.

The nipple contains sebaceous glands that are located around the opening of the lactiferous sinuses. The areola has three types of glands: sweat glands, occasional accessory mammary glands, and specialized sebaceous or Montgomery glands [2]. The glands of Montgomery are small nodules projecting from the surface of the areola. The nipple is composed of two layers of circular and longitudinal smooth muscle. Contracture of the musculature makes the nipple firm and erect and allows milk to be emptied from the lactiferous sinuses [2, 3].

Associated Musculature

The breast has an intimate association with the pectoralis major and minor, serratus anterior, latissimus dorsi, subscapularis, external oblique abdominis, and rectus abdominus muscles. Portions of these muscles form the posterior breast border (see Fig. 2-1) [9]. The pectoralis major and minor muscles overlie and protect the brachial plexus and other axillary structures. The origin of the external oblique abdominis is located between the

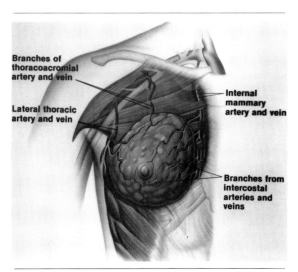

Fig. 2-2. Arterial and venous anatomy of the breast. The female breasts are beneficiaries of a generous and overlapping blood supply provided primarily by the internal mammary, lateral thoracic, and intercostal arteries. The generous capacity of this arterial system has allowed the design of a variety of different skin patterns and nutrient pathways for performing breast reduction and reconstruction. There exists both a substantial superficial and deep venous drainage network of the female breast. The superficial system overlies the breast itself and, although quite variable, usually drains collaterally. The deep system drains primarily through the internal mammary vein (to the innominate), the axillary vein (to the subclavian), and the intercostal veins (through the azygous, vertebral, and superior vena cava).

serratus anterior laterally and the rectus sheath and the rectus abdominus medially. The nerve innervators of the serratus anterior are carried within its fascia. Damage to this nerve with denervation of the serratus produces winging of the scapula [14]. The thoracodorsal vessels and nerve enter the latissimus dorsi muscle along its anterior border after passing through the axillary fat pad and fascia at the posterior axillary line. The fascia on the deep surface of the latissimus dorsi continues as the axillary fascia.

Vascular Supply
The arteries supplying the breast are derived from the thoracic branches of the internal mammary artery, the axillary artery, and the intercostal arteries (Fig. 2-2). The chief blood supply to the breast is from perforating branches of the internal mam-

mary artery. These vessels are branches from the first, second, third, or fourth perforators in the lateral margin of the sternum and traverse and penetrate the pectoralis major muscle to the medial edge of the mammary gland. The first and second perforating branches run above and below the second costal cartilage. The branches of the second, third, and fourth intercostal vessels are large and supply the superior medial quadrant of the breast [6]. Of these penetrating branches, the second intercostal branch is the largest and usually directly supplies the mammary gland [6]. The deep portion of the mammary gland and skin over the inner third are supplied by the internal mammary artery.

The superior lateral quadrant of the breast is supplied by means of the pectoral branch of the thoracoacromial artery. Lying between the pectoralis major and minor muscles, it supplies these muscles as well as the deep surface of the gland [5, 6]. The lateral thoracic artery, a branch of the second part of the axillary artery, also feeds the superior lateral quadrant [5, 6]. It lies lateral to the pectoralis major muscle in the anterior axillary line.

Branches of the intercostal arteries supply a small region of the posterior aspect of the breast. Maliniac's dissection and roentgenographic studies of 103 injected female cadavar breasts reveal that the intercostal arteries play a minor role [6]. He reported that the internal mammary artery in combination with the lateral thoracic artery supplies 50 percent of the breast [6]. The lateral thoracic and internal mammary artery are generally responsible for blood supply to the nipple [6, 9].

The veins of the breast are superficial and subcutaneous, traveling deep to the superficial layer of the superficial fascia. The veins receive circumareolar tributaries, pass across the midline, and drain primarily medially and superiorly to the upper quadrants [7]. Three systems supply deep venous drainage of the breast (see Fig. 2-2):

1. Internal mammary vein to the innominate vein.
2. Axillary vein to the subclavian vein to the innominate vein [9].
3. Intercostal veins to the azygos and vertebral veins and ending in the superior vena cava [9]. There is free communication between the vertebral venous plexus and the intercostal veins [9].

The cephalic vein terminates in the axillary and

may act as a collateral drainage pathway if the axillary vein is blocked.

Innervation

The skin of the upper quadrants of the breast is innervated by the supraclavicular branch of the cervical plexus, derived from C3 and C4. The skin of the lower quadrants is innervated by the lateral cutaneous branches of the thoracic intercostal nerves [3, 9]. Most authors agree that the nipple's sensibility is derived from the lateral cutaneous branch of the fourth intercostal nerve. The area of the medial aspect of the breast is also innervated by the intercostal nerves by means of the anterior perforating cutaneous branches [9].

Lymphatics

Superficially, the breast and overlying skin are drained radially by multiple lymphatic pathways,

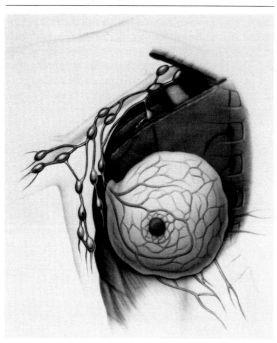

Fig. 2-3. Lymphatic drainage of the breast. The surface of the breast has lymphatic drainage via multiple radial channels radiating from the nipple. The deeper lymphatic system that drains the lobules drains primarily to the axilla and on to the subclavian and jugular systems. A lesser amount of lymphatic drainage from the medial breast occurs along the internal mammary chain.

whereas its deep surface and parenchyma are drained by underlying channels (Fig. 2-3) [3, 5, 9, 12]. The pathways draining the right breast form a single trunk that empties into the junction of the internal jugular and the subclavian vein on the right side, or it separately joins the subclavian vein, internal jugular, and nearby veins. The left breast lymphatics usually terminate in the thoracic duct but may drain into the internal jugular and subclavian vein [3, 5, 9, 12]. Lymphatics accompany the internal mammary artery and the trachea, empty into the thoracic duct, or drain toward the upper and anterior surfaces of the diaphragm.

Lymphatic drainage of the breast can be divided into a superficial system draining the skin and a deeper system draining the lobules [3, 5, 9, 12]. The drainage from the upper quadrants passes to the axilla, as does drainage from the lower medial quadrant and adjacent abdominal wall [3, 5, 9, 12].

Whereas lymphatic communication occurs between the breast and the inferior medial quadrant of the liver, diaphragm, and peritoneal cavity by way of the internal mammary chain of lymphatics, drainage across the midline to the breast of the opposite side has not been demonstrated [12]. In summary, the breast's lymphatic drainage is primarily to the axilla, with lesser drainage occurring along the internal mammary chain.

Anatomic Variation

Anomalies of the human breast include absence of one or both breasts, accessory nipples, accessory breasts and major breast, or underlying chest wall asymmetry.

Absence of one or both breasts, or "amastia," is rare [3]. It may occur bilaterally, but usually it is unilateral and may be associated with absence or underdevelopment of pectoral girdle, chest wall, or arm [3, 10].

Accessory breasts and nipples, termed *hyperthelia*, are the most common breast anomalies and are said to occur often in a rudimentary form in 1 to 2 percent of individuals [11]. They appear twice as frequently in females as in males and are often hereditary [3]. Accessory breasts may contain all or some components of the normal breast. They usually occur in a curved line extending from the groin to the axilla, corresponding to the "milk line" of embryos, but have been reported in the cheek and neck and also on the medial aspect of the thigh [13].

Absence of the nipple and polythelia, in which the single breast has more than one nipple, have been observed [3]. Some breasts may have two or more nipples within one areola or may have several separate areola-nipple complexes on one breast [3].

Although the breast can be described simply as a sweat gland encased in a skin envelope lying on the thoracic wall, a more detailed picture reveals quite a complex structure. A thorough understanding and appreciation of the anatomic relations of this highly symbolic appendage are necessary for optimal surgical results.

References

1. Cooper, A.P. *The Anatomy and Diseases of the Breasts.* Philadelphia: Lee & Blanchard, 1845.
2. Gray H. Urogenital System. In *Gray's Anatomy* (28 ed.). Philadelphia: Lea & Febiger, 1966.
3. Haagensen, C.D. *Anatomy of the Mammary Gland, Diseases of the Breast* (2nd ed.). Philadelphia: Saunders, 1971. Pp. 4–28.
4. Hicken, N.F. Mastectomy: A clinical pathologic study demonstrating why most mastectomies result in incomplete removal of the mammary glands. *Arch. Surg.* 40:6, 1940.
5. Hollinshead, W.H.: The Thorax, Abdomen and Pelvis. In *Anatomy for Surgeons*, Vol. II. New York: Harper & Row, 1968. Pp. 11–18.
6. Maliniac, J.W. Arterial blood supply to the breast: Revised anatomic data relating to reconstructive surgery. *Arch. Surg.* 47:329, 1943.
7. Massuopust, L.C., and Gardner, W.D. Infrared photographic studies of the superficial thoracic veins in the female: Anatomical consideration. *Surg. Gynecol. Obstet.* 91:717, 1950.
8. Moore, K.L. *The Developing Human. Clinically Oriented Embryology* (2nd ed.). Philadelphia: Saunders, 1977. Pp. 379–380.
9. Rehman, I. Embryology and Anatomy of the Breast. In H.S. Gallager, H.P. Leis, R.V. Snyderman, and J.A. Urban (eds.), *The Breast.* St. Louis: Mosby, 1978. Pp. 3–21.
10. Spear, S.L., Romm, S., Hakki, A., and Little, J.W. Costal cartilage sculpturing as an adjunct to augmentation mammoplasty. *Plast. Reconstr. Surg.* 79:921, 1987.
11. Speert, H. Supernumerary mammae, with special reference to the rhesus monkey. *Quart. Rev. Biol.* 17:59, 1942.
12. Turner-Warwick, R.T. Lympatics of the breast. *Br. J. Surg.* 46:574, 1959.
13. Weinshel, L.R., and Demakopoulous, N. Supranumary breasts with special reference to the pseudomammae type. *Am. J. Surg.* 60:76, 1943.
14. Wilson, R.E. The Breast. In D.C. Sabiston (ed.), *Textbook of Surgery, The Biologic Basis of Modern Surgical Practice* (11th ed.). Philadelphia: Saunders, 1977. Pp. 623–666.

COMMENTS ON CHAPTER 2   *Robert M. Goldwyn*

In thinking of the anatomy of the breast, we plastic surgeons are concerned particularly, and appropriately so, with the blood supply of the nipple-areola. While it is obviously true that every anatomic aspect of the breast, especially its sensation, should be important to us, necrosis of the nipple is the catastrophe that we most dread. That devastation is immediate and visible, unlike numbness of the nipple, whose consequences are invisible and realized by the patient with certainty only later. The paradox is that plastic surgeons fear most necrosis of the nipples, yet building a new one is an established procedure, whereas an asensate nipple is irrevocable.

The nipple-areola seems to survive under a multitude of different and even adverse circumstances. As we know from our own experience and from that of others who have contributed to this book, the nipple-areola has a 98 percent chance of remaining viable when transplanted as a free graft or left attached to a central mound, or to the skin and subcutaneous tissue only, as after subcutaneous mastectomy, or when it is based on any single quadrant of the breast, or on various pedicles — even more imaginative.

Spear, Walker, and Romm have clearly described the blood supply to the breast from its three principal sources: the internal thoracic, axillary, and aortic intercostal arteries. The medial lateral mammary arteries are the major arterial sources and pass close beneath the skin on the anterior surface of the breast. Supplementing these in the lower half of the gland are small posterior mammary arteries from the intercostals laterally and the interior thoracic medially, which gives off several perforating arteries, the largest being through the second and third intercostal spaces. Edholm and Strombeck [4] performed angiography in 12 patients with breast hypertrophy and concluded that the internal thoracic and axillary arteries are the major suppliers and the intercostal arteries are the minor suppliers.

What does this all mean in terms of the strategic nipple-areola? Edwards has written:

The medial and lateral mammary arteries course toward the center of the breast more or less embedded in the subcutaneous fat. Small branches supply the overlying skin; larger branches penetrate the gland. Their terminal portions surround the nipple and areola and anastomose with each other, most often in an anastomotic circumareolar ring, from which the nipple is supplied. Secondary arcades peripheral to the areola may also be seen. The anastomoses may form only a semicircular arcade. Infrequently, the mammary arteries send only radiating branches to the areola and nipple without any conspicuous anastomoses. In an average case Marcus found the medial arteries lined within the subcutaneous fat of the periphery of the gland at a depth of 0.5 to 1.5 cm., the lateral somewhat deeper 1.0 to 2.5 cm. As they near the areola, the arteries lie immediately beneath the dermis but somewhat deeper than the veins [5].

These comments of Edwards are based not only on the findings of Marcus [11], but also on those of Salmon and Carr et al [2]. Vesalius [18], about 400 years ago, and Cooper [3], about 150 years ago, demonstrated a clearly defined superficial vascular system related to the nipple and areola (Figs. 2-4 and 2-5). Cooper found that in a lactating breast, the largest veins lie superficial to the arteries, some of which are accompanied by additional veins. The vessels may form incomplete circumareolar rings, with secondary, more peripheral arcades. This cutaneous supply to the nipple and areola is related embryologically to the fact that the breast, including the pectoral skin, is of ectodermal origin.

Marcus [11] classified areola-nipple circulation into three types: the circular type (Fig. 2-6A), about 70 percent of instances, in which the medial lateral arteries anastomose in a typical circumareolar ring to supply the nipple; the loop type (Fig. 2-6B), which can be found in 20 percent of female breasts, characterized by branches anastomosing above and below the nipple, forming a loop; and finally, the most tenuous vascular supply, the radial type (Fig. 2-6C), in which strong anastomosis is lacking and the branches to the nipple are in the less frequent radial pattern, occurring in 6 percent of female breasts.

Lalardrie and Jouglard [10], in their concise and thoughtful book, classified techniques of breast reduction into those whose vascular safety of the nipple and areola depend on glandular vessels, glandular and cutaneous vessels, and cutaneous vessels only. Examples of methods of breast reduction using a single pedicle and based on glandular vessels would be the techniques of Biesenberger [1], Joseph (1931) [8], Penn [12], and Dufourmentel

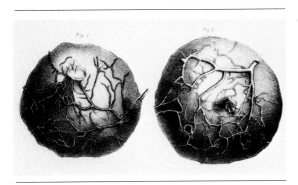

Fig. 2-4. Left. *Arteries going to the breast and nipple.* Right. *Veins returning blood from the nipple and breast. The veins on the left pass to the internal mammary arteries; those on the right pass to the axillary vein. The posterior or axillary branch forms a circle around the nipple and a network with frequent communications on the surface of the breast. (From A. Cooper.* The Anatomy and Diseases of the Breasts, *plate IX. Philadelphia: Lea & Blanchard, 1845.)*

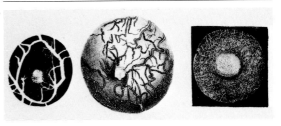

Fig. 2-5. Left. *Vein injected around the nipple (from a dry preparation). Radial branches proceed from the circle to the nipple, where they divide.* Middle. *Distribution of the arteries on the breast and nipple.* Right. *Preparation of the veins injected in the areola nipple, showing the capillary branches of the vein in the papillae and exhibiting erectile tissue of these vessels. The arteries form a tree; the veins form a network. (From A. Cooper.* The Anatomy and Diseases of the Breasts, *plate X. Philadelphia: Lea & Blanchard, 1845.)*

and Mouly (see Chap. 13). Those using a double pedicle but depending on glandular vessels are the techniques of Gillies and McIndoe [6], Ragnell [14], and Pitanguy [13]. Those methods whose glandular and cutaneous vessels account for the blood supply to the nipple and areola are the earlier method of Joseph [7] and the techniques of Schwartzmann [15] and Strombeck [17]. Finally, those methods wherein the cutaneous blood supply of the nipple and areola constitutes the only nutrition are the techniques of Lalardrie [9] and Skoog [16] as well as those of Weiner and Hauben (see Chapters 16 and 17).

Lalardrie and Jouglard [10] have written:

With cutaneo-glandular undermining, we must count on the principal glandular pedicles alone. The external pedicle may be sacrificed, but in exceptional cases the anatomical disposition does not permit the internal pedicle to vascularise by itself the remaining gland of the areola and nipple.

If all cutaneo-glandular undermining is to be avoided we must:

—either retain one peripheral glandular thickness protecting the preglandular vessels, if the cutaneous vascularisation around the areola and nipple is to be wholly or partly sacrificed.

—or preserve, wholly or partly, the continuity of the subcutaneous vascularisation around the areola and nipple. This is sufficient to ensure the complete viability of the areola and nipple and of the remaining glandular stump.

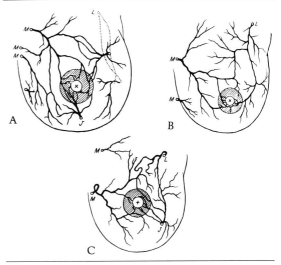

Fig. 2-6. *Types of periareolar plexuses.* A. *Circular plexus, in which branches of main arteries form a complete ring around the nipple. This ensures maximum blood supply and is present in 70 to 74 percent of cases.* B. *Loop type of plexus, occurring when the lateral thoracic artery predominates. Branches anastomose above and below the nipple, forming a loop. This type is present in 20 percent of cases.* C. *Radial type of plexus, without an anastomosing ring around the nipple. This type has the least blood supply to nipple and is present in 6 percent of cases. (Key: M = internal mammary artery; L = lateral thoracic artery; J = intercostal artery.) (From G.H. Marcus. Untersuchungen uper die arterielle Blutversorgung der Mamilla. Arch. f. klin. Chir. 179:361, 1934. Reproduced in J.W. Maliniac.* Breast Deformities and Their Repair. *Baltimore: Waverly, 1950.)*

In this case the function of the recurrent glandular vessels behind the areola and nipple indicates that it is advisable to retain for them a dermo-glandular support rather than a purely dermal one.

The venous glandular vascularisation of the breast is mostly on the surface or is superficially drained. It must be respected in operations with cutaneo-glandular undermining, and any glandular manoeuvre which may constitute a hindrance to venous blood flow is to be avoided.

The anatomical disposition of the mammary nerves accounts for the fact that, in large glandular resections, particularly behind the areola and nipple, there is a temporary or sometimes permanent reduction in nipple sensitivity.

Perhaps those patients, the unfortunate 6 percent, who lack a vigorous anatomosis around the areola and nipple and have only the radial pattern are the ones who develop nipple necrosis when seemingly the operation for reduction has proceeded normally. Perhaps additional factors, such as a history of smoking or inadvertent cutting or torsion of the pedicle decreases further their already diminished blood supply.

Most of us who have had the unfortunate experience of witnessing nipple necrosis in one of our patients have a difficult time in understanding the cause, let alone in finding a successful treatment. Arterial and/or venous insufficiency of the nipple-areola can occur, from either venous engorgement (hence, the sometimes successful use of leeches) or from arterial insufficiency, for which, as yet, there is no immediate remedy. We are also ignorant about the specific nipple-areola vascular pattern for the individual patient whose breasts we happen to be reducing.

Perhaps as techniques for assessing microcirculation become more advanced and less invasive, we may some day know the blood supply to the nipple and areola, not just from a textbook, but from the actual pattern of the patient. We could then design our pedicle accordingly. As matters now stand, we have to be content with being either fortunate or skillful since, in 98 percent of instances in which we do a breast reduction, we do not produce significant nipple-areola necrosis.

REFERENCES

1. Biesenberger, H. Eine neue methode der mammaplastik. *Zentralbl. Chir.* 55:2382, 1928.
2. Carr, B.W., Bishop, W.I., and Anson, B.J. Mammary arteries. *Q. Bull. Northwest* 16:150, 1942.
3. Cooper, A. *The Anatomy and Diseases of the Breast.* Philadelphia: Lea & Blanchard, 1845. Plates IX and X.
4. Edholm, P., and Strombeck, J.O. Influence of Mammaplasty on the Arterial Supply to the Hypertrophic Breast: Angiographic Studies Before and After Operation. *Acta. Chir. Scand.* 341[Suppl.], 1965.
5. Edwards, E.A. Surgical Anatomy of the Breast. In R.M. Goldwyn (ed.), *Plastic and Reconstructive Surgery of the Breast.* Boston: Little, Brown, 1976. Pp. 37–57.
6. Gillies, H., and McIndoe, A.H. The technique of mammaplasty in conditions of hypertrophy of the breast. *Surg. Gynecol. Obstet.* 68:658, 1939.
7. Joseph, J. Zur Operation der hyperetrophischen Hangebrüst. *Dtsch. Med. Wochenschr.* 51:1103, 1925.
8. Joseph, J. Nasenplastik und sonstige Gesichtsplastik nebst Mammaplastik. Leipzig: Verlag Curt Kabitzsch, 1931. P. 770.
9. Lalardrie, J.-P. "The dermal vault" technique. Reduction mammaplasty for hypertrophy with ptosis. In *Transacta der III Tagund der Vereinigund der Deutschen plastichen.* Chirurgen: Köln, 1972. Pp. 105–108.
10. Lalardrie, J.-P., and Jouglard, J.-P. *Chirurgie Plastique du Sein.* Paris: Masson et Cie, 1974. Pp. 19–26.
11. Marcus, G.H. Untersuhchungen uber die arterielle Blutversorgung der Mamilla. *Arch. Klin. Chir.* 179:361, 1934.
12. Penn, J. Breast reduction II. Transactions of the International Society of Plastic Surgeons, Second Congress, 1959. Edinburgh and London: E. & S. Livingstone, Ltd., 1960. P. 502.
13. Pitanguy, I. Une nouvelle technique de plastic mammaire. *Ann. Chir. Plast.* 7:199, 1962.
14. Ragnell, A. Operative correction of hypertrophy and ptosis of the female breast. *Acta Chir. Scand.* 113[Suppl.], 1946.
15. Schwartzmann, E. Die Technik der Mammaplastik. *Chirurgie* 2:932, 1930.
16. Skoog, T. A technique of breast reduction. *Acta Chir. Scand.* 126:1, 1963.
17. Strombeck, J.O. Macromastia in women and its surgical treatment. *Acta Chir. Scand.* 341[Suppl.], 1964.
18. Vesalius, A. De humani corporis fabrica. Venetiis: F.F. Senesis & J. Criegher, 1568. P. 368.

3

Melvin Spira

Pathology of the Hypertrophic Breast

The surgeon might appropriately ask whether there are any anatomic variations peculiar only to the large breast or whether the large breast is merely "more of the same." Is there a difference in the breasts of a young adult as opposed to those of an aged patient when both types of patient exhibit classic ptosis and breast enlargement and are to undergo the same operative procedure, reduction mammaplasty? What is the relationship of height, weight, and age to the large breast? Can a nomogram be constructed? Is the fat content of the breast in direct proportion to the degree of overall obesity? Is there a difference in the skin of the breast in patients undergoing reduction mammaplasty versus the skin of the mature patient with a normal-sized breast?

The breasts are composed of glandular tissue interspersed with and supported by fibrous tissue and fat and are covered with skin overlying a layer of subcutaneous tissue. In general, the more glandular and fibrous tissue present, the firmer the breast will be, and vice versa.

Smith et al [2], in evaluating breast size, form, and position in 55 female volunteers varying in age from 18 to 31 years, found remarkable variations in volume and only a general correlation between volume and brassiere size. Of note was the lack of relationship between measured breast volume, chest wall circumference, and brassiere cup size in many patients. Although there was a volumetric difference between left and right breasts (left larger than right), the difference was not statistically significant. They did find statistically significant differences between left and right breasts in axilla-nipple distance, in nipple-midline measurements, and in the distance from the lowest point of the breast to the nipple with the patient in an upright position.

Regnault and Daniel [1] divided the female population seeking breast reduction into two principal groups. The younger women exhibit developmental hypertrophy secondary to obesity, virginal hypertrophy, or, rarely, endocrine abnormalities. Those with virginal hypertrophy and endocrine abnormalities present with glandular enlargement and minimal ptosis. True virginal hypertrophy is a relatively uncommon condition occurring soon after the onset of normal puberty and is characterized by massive unilateral or bilateral breast enlargement. It results from an abnormal organ response and not elevated hormonal levels. Greatly increased fibrous connective tissue and moderate ductal proliferation are seen on histopathologic examination. Although progesterone therapy may arrest hypertrophy, surgery is usually necessary to reduce the volume. Hypertrophy owing to endocrine abnormalities is diagnosed by a history of precocious puberty and requires evaluation by an endocrinologist. Those with hypertrophy secondary to exogenous obesity exhibit a primary increase in breast size with subcutaneous and interglandular deposition of fat and usually demonstrate greater ptosis. The older group of patients tends to be seen postmenopause. These women present with sagging breasts that are enlarged to varying degrees and are symptomatic; the breasts of this second group are characterized by lobular atrophy and replacement with fat tissue.

Surprisingly, some plastic surgeons do not understand the correlation between chest wall measurement and brassiere size (see Table 19-1, in which Regnault and Daniel describe the relationship between breast measurement in terms of volume and chest size to brassiere size). Note that a 36A cup has the same basic volume as a 32C cup, with breast volume dependent on both the actual cup measurement and chest size. Body circumference, or actual brassiere band size (34, 36, and so on), is measured with tape around the trunk under the arms and across the sternum above the breast.

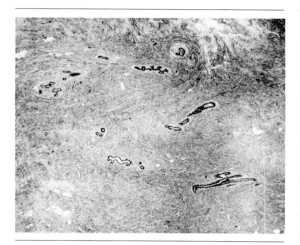

Fig. 3-1. Representative field of tissue removed from a 19-year-old woman with purported "virginal hypertrophy." It was impossible to distinguish on an objective basis from other 19-year-old breast tissue (hematoxylin and eosin stain, ×10).

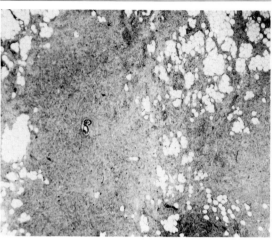

Fig. 3-2. Representative field from a 53-year-old woman's left breast reduced following contralateral mastectomy for carcinoma (hematoxylin and eosin stain, ×10).

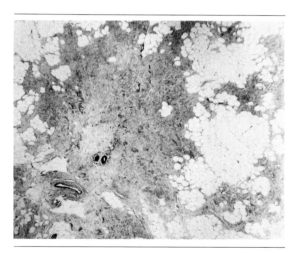

Fig. 3-3. Representative field from a 70-year-old woman having bilateral reduction mammoplasty (hematoxylin and eosin stain, ×10).

The measurement around the trunk across the fullest part of the breast mound at the nipple determines cup size. Each 1-in. difference is equal to a cup size. For example, if the first measurement is 36 in. and the second is 39 in., brassiere size would be 36C. When ptosis accompanies enlargement, these measurements can be made with the patient wearing light brassiere support.

Analysis of the last 100 breast reductions performed by the author in which an attempt was made to relate the histopathologic diagnosis to the age of the patient and the amount of breast tissue removed revealed no statistically significant relationship between these factors. Interestingly, 63 of the patients (ages 15 through 76) exhibited normal breast tissue according to the pathologist reports, and 13 were found to have normal breast tissue with fibrosis (ages 16 through 39). Fifteen patients (ages 17 through 30) were diagnosed as having fibrocystic disease. Three patients, all older than 35 years, exhibited fibroadenomas. One patient, age 52, showed benign ductal hypertrophy. Three specimens (ages 19 through 40) were labeled by the pathologist as simply "hypertrophy," and one 30-year-old patient exhibited "lipohyperplasia." There was one case (age 55) of focal apocrine metaplasia.

In a limited quantitative study of the proportionality of epithelial, stromal, and fatty components of breast tissue from women having reduction mammaplasties and age-matched controls (samples of tissue from uninvolved quadrants in cases of mastectomy for carcinoma), no significant differences were found (Figs. 3-1 through 3-3). Control samples for comparison with teenage "virginal hypertrophy" were not available.

The inherent variability from individual to individual and the changing proportionality over the age spectrum makes the answer to what makes some breasts too big problematic. Might it be adipocytic hypertrophy? If so, the answer will require sizing of fat cells not only in the breasts but also in other sites. Relative to the skin of patients with hypertrophic breasts, no features that might be deemed characteristic or might be associated with the underlying enlargement have been observed. Skin changes are usually secondary to age, number of pregnancies, degree of ptosis, and body weight variations — not to breast size per se.

Although there is considerable variation in size and symmetry of both breasts and nipple-areola complex, the presence of breast tissue in the anterior axillary fold, or axillary breast, does relate to macromastia, or breast hypertrophy. Whereas this is common in the obese patient, axillary breasts are occasionally seen in the individual of normal weight and height and are usually composed of true glandular tissue, which histologically resembles normal breast tissue.

In answer to the questions posed at the beginning of this chapter — whether the condition is called macromastia, macromasia, hypermastia, breast hypertrophy, breast hyperplasia, gigantomastia, or simply large breasts — most patients, in the absence of breast disease, exhibit histopathologic characteristics associated with age and weight rather than with size.

References

1. Regnault, P., and Daniel, R.K. *Aesthetic Plastic Surgery.* Boston: Little, Brown, 1984. Pp. 499–505.
2. Smith, D.J., Jr., Palin, W.E., Jr., Katch, V.L. and Bennett, J.E. Breast volume and anthropomorphic measurements: Normal values. *Plast. Reconstr. Surg.* 78:331, 1986.

COMMENTS ON CHAPTER 3   *Robert M. Goldwyn*

Based on "a limited quantitative study (pathologists' reports) of the proportionality of epithelial, stromal, and fatty components of breast tissue for women having reduction mammaplasties and age-matched controls," Spira has concluded that in the absence of breast disease, most patients "exhibit histopathological characteristics associated with age and weight rather than size." From conversations that I have had with pathologists who have looked at tissue from individual patients following reduction, I am not surprised by this finding. However, it did seem unusual to me that a pathologist could find nothing wrong in the tissue of breasts that were massive.

Thorek [4] reviewed extensively the microscopic findings of tissue from hypertrophic breasts in mostly adult patients as reported by well-known pathologists throughout the world; they were essentially unremarkable. A typical description, quoted by Thorek, is that of LeDouble:

The principal mass of the breast consists of mature connective tissue elements without elastic fibers. In the interior of this tissue some glandular elements are present in the form of numerous tubes with blind ends, which are either single or branching and filled with epithelium.

Velpeau allegedly was the first to describe the pathologic changes taking place in hypertrophic breasts and coined the term *"engorgement-hypostatique."* Microscopic appearance of the breast tissue, however, was far less dramatic than either the gross or clinical appearance.

At the turn of the century, Dietel, also cited by Thorek, gave what he considered to be the histologic characteristics of genuine hypertrophy of the breast: "equal increase in volume of the breast of its components (glandular substance and connective tissue framework), with retention of the normal structure and form." Spira's observations would seem to confirm at least the observation that the "normal structure and form" of the breast have been retained.

The most frequent type of true hypertrophy of the female breast occurs during adolescence following normal puberty. Haagensen [1] stated that microscopic findings in this kind of hypertrophy show "surprisingly little that can be termed abnormal. The epithelial elements are not remarkable.

The excessive growth appears to be on the part of the connective tissue and fat. The relative proportions of these elements and any particular example of breast tissue are difficult to assess from microscopic study." One of the reasons is that the number of lobules and acini vary according to the phase of the menstrual cycle. For example, in the premenstrual stage, the average number of lobules per low-powered field, as studied by Haagensen [2], was 7.2, and the average number of acini per lobule was 30.2; in contrast, in breast tissue from women in menopause, the average number of lobules per low-powered field was 2.3; the average number of acini per lobule was 11.2.

According to Page and Anderson [3]:

Virginal hypertrophy has a *trend* toward fewer lobules than normal breasts, often has a hyperplastic change in epithelium as seen in juvenile fibroadenomas, and has abundant fibrous tissue ranging from cellular to hyalinized areas . . . The differentiation between virginal hypertrophy and juvenile fibroadenoma cannot be made on histological examination. It requires knowledge of the clinical setting. The juvenile fibroadenoma is usually a unilateral lesion resulting in displacement of the nipple. The skin is often stretched, cyanotic and has distended veins. Conversely, virginal hypertrophy is bilateral, does not displace the nipple, and lacks the cutaneous and venous alterations seen in the patient with juvenile fibroadenoma.

In summary, Spira has given us an important observation based on his systematic study of women with hypertrophic breasts — namely, the histologic appearance, contrary to what one might expect, does not correlate with the breast size, even though the clinical appearance of the breasts may be spectacular.

REFERENCES
1. Haagensen, C.D. *Diseases of the Breast* (3rd ed.) Philadelphia: Saunders, 1986. P. 62.
2. Haagensen, C.D. *Diseases of the Breast* (3rd ed.). Philadelphia: Saunders, 1986. P. 50.
3. Page, D.L., and Anderson, T.J. *Diagnostic Histopathology of the Breast.* Edinburgh: Churchill Livingstone, 1987. P. 77.
4. Thorek, M. *Plastic Surgery of the Breast and Abdominal Wall.* Springfield, Illinois: Thomas, 1942. Pp. 105–142.

4

Sharon Romm

Endocrinology and Physiology of the Breast

The breast is a target for almost every body hormone. Working alone, a hormone can exert direct influence, and, when several act in concert, they bring to bear a combined permissive effect. Through all life's stages — childhood, sexual maturation, the reproductive years, and the regressive decline of menopause — hormones, ultimately controlled by the hypothalamus and neurotransmitters, govern breast growth and function.

Breast development requires the coordination of multiple hormones. Some, such as estrogen, progesterone, and prolactin, combine with specific receptors in the gland's cells. They induce increased synthesis of nucleic mRNA and so encourage new protein production. Estrogen promotes duct growth; prolactin and progesterone develop the lobules and alveoli; prolactin is instrumental in milk production [25]; and epithelial stem cell division relies on the presence of growth hormone.

Other substances are less direct in their action. Follicle-stimulating hormone (FSH), luteinizing hormone (LH), adrenocorticotropic hormone (ACTH), and thyroid-stimulating hormone (TSH) affect the breast via hormones secreted from their target glands. Also in this category are steroids from the ovaries, adrenals, and thyroid, and insulin, which enables prolactin to develop mature milk manufacturing cells. Even though this original information was obtained by studying rats surgically deprived of ovaries and pituitary and adrenal glands, the conclusions are also applicable to humans [20].

Fetal Period

Breasts, as part of the integumentary system, originate in the mammary ridge, a structure that appears in the sixth week of fetal life as an epidermal thickening between the limb buds. Each breast is represented by a disk, lens-shaped by the seventh week and globular by the eighth week. Between weeks 15 and 20, the primary milk ducts form, canalizing and branching and eventually finding their way to open onto the nipple's surface [1]. Surrounding the ducts is a crisscrossing mantle of contractile myoepithelial cells, destined to aid in milk expulsion in the adult. In the late weeks of gestation, the blind ends of the ducts bud into alveoli lined with a single layer of milk-secreting cells. Influenced by maternal estrogen, the cells secrete whitish "witches milk" — colostrum — at birth and real milk for several weeks thereafter [10].

Fetal hormones control gland differentiation. In addition to genetic influence, hormones can cause irregularities in adult size or shape. However, once the embryonic stage has passed, hormonal modification is impossible and only surgery can effect change. Exceptions are patients with primary amenorrhea resulting from lack of ovarian estrogens; here, estrogen therapy can promote growth during adult life [26].

Adolescence

Shortly before menarche, estrogen production accelerates, causing breast fat and connective tissue to proliferate. Ducts, previously short and vaguely tubular, begin to lengthen and branch. Their terminal ends bud into alveoli. The pale areola and nipple darken and grow larger as the breasts start to swell to their pubescent shape [26, 30].

Hormones elicit change in the adolescent breast. Estrogen from the ovaries' graafian follicles encourage duct maturation. Progesterone, secreted by the corpora lutea, stimulates alveola growth [11]. Neither of these hormones is totally effective alone or even in combination. Additional hormones, including insulin, cortisol, thyroxin, prolactin, and growth hormone, are needed for full glandular development [26].

Reproductive Years

Cyclical changes occur in the breast of the menstruating female. In the first weeks of the cycle, the parenchyma proliferates, epithelial sprouts form, and cellular RNA replicates — all events induced by rising estrogen. When, in the second half of the cycle, progesterone appears, ducts dilate and cells lining the alveoli turn secretory. DNA synthesis increases as estrogen and progesterone levels rise [25].

During the week preceding menstruation, hormonal changes can bring about breast discomfort. Primed by estrogen and influenced by progesterone, breasts swell and become tender [11]. The sensation of fullness is attributed to the effect of histamine, which, activated by the presence of estrogen, increases vascular permeability so that fluid seeps from vessels into surrounding tissue. Even prolactin, exerting its relatively minimal effects in the nonlactating breast, has been accused of provoking premenstrual discomfort [25].

Pregnancy

During pregnancy, the breasts become large and ready for milk production. Estrogen and progesterone, provided initially by the corpus luteum and placenta, increase. Despite their abundance, however, their effects are only preparatory. They establish the secretory state, but milk production must wait until after parturition [25].

The breast is readied for lactation by complex hormonal interactions. In the nongravid state, a prolactin inhibitory factor (PIF), now known to be the central nervous system neurotransmitter dopamine, is released by the hypothalamus to keep prolactin levels low. During pregnancy, the prolactin-producing cells of the pituitary undergo hyperplasia, and prolactin levels rise as hypothalamic dopamine levels increase.

Prolactin, an anterior pituitary peptide hormone, appears at 8 weeks of gestation, and levels rise from 75 ng/ml to 200 ng/ml by term [25, 30]. This hormone stimulates breast growth and milk production. But, until birth, the milk-producing effect of prolactin is squelched [28]. High levels of estrogen and progesterone permit prolactin to exert its preparatory effect but repress milk production [25].

Additional hormones prepare the breast during pregnancy for milk production. Placental lactogen [4], growth hormone and cortisol and insulin, readily available in pregnancy, enhance the growth of ducts, lobules, and alveoli.

Although all hormones necessary for growth and secretion are already present during pregnancy, the gestational breast produces only colostrum, composed of transudate and desquamated epithelium [26].

Lactation

After parturition, estrogen and progesterone levels quickly decline. In the 3 or 4 days it takes for these hormones to clear the circulation, the breasts engorge. Prolactin can now, unrepressed by estrogen and progesterone, exert its full effect.

Prolactin sustains milk protein, casein, and fatty acids and maintains the volume of secretion. Suckling elicits a transient increase in the hormone, important to initiate milk production. Each nursing episode makes prolactin increase five- to tenfold, but, as weeks go by, prolactin levels gradually return to normal until even the nursing-induced rise is negligible. Yet, for unknown reasons, successful lactation can continue for months [10]. Only when she wants to abort lactation and takes bromergocryptine, a dopamine agonist, or an estrogen-androgen combination, does a woman's milk production cease [29].

Suckling also stimulates the posterior pituitary to release oxytocin, an event often dependent on the mother's reaction to events or environment. Anticipation of nursing can cause milk to spill from the breasts, and fright or stress can instantly inhibit milk release [26].

Menopause

In the years preceding menopause, usually between the ages of 35 and 45, the glandular epithelium gradually begins to disappear and alveoli and lobules shrink. When ovarian steroid production ends, the breasts decidedly involute, and the ducts, alveoli, and lobules degenerate. By the time senile regression is complete, all that remains of the functioning breast are small islands of parenchyma surrounded by fat and leathery connective tissue [25, 31].

In the past, observers linked estrogen replacement to breast cancer, a connection since proved unfounded [13]. But when the correlation between benign breast disease and estrogen replacement was also examined, a higher incidence of this condition was noted in women using estrogen therapy. In premenopausal women, breast symptoms show cyclical variation, suggesting a relationship between hormones and benign breast disease [27].

Breast Cancer

Breast pathology has, in past decades, become linked with breast endocrinology. Quantification of steroid receptors in tumor cells, independent of disease stage or lymph node status in a cancer specimen, is recognized as a reliable prognostic index. Presence or absence of receptors serves as a guide to adjuvant therapy, now generally acknowledged to prolong and improve life [17].

Even though useful clinical advances have been made in the last 20 years, the correlation between breast cancer and hormone shifts can be traced back a century and a half. In 1836, Astley Paston Cooper, British anatomist and surgeon, noted the correlation between breast tumor growth and the menstrual cycle [5]. The finding that cancer growth could be influenced by endocrine manipulation dates to 1896, when George Beatson reported that oophorectomy induced remarkable regression of disease in two premenopausal patients with advanced breast cancer [3].

Observations on the endocrine system and cancer lay dormant until scientists could isolate and identify steroids. Charles Huggins, a Nobel laureate in 1952, made a discovery with long-term therapeutic implications. He recognized that some breast and prostate cancers are sensitive to the influence of hormones [14]. By utilizing total endocrine ablation, he found that remission could be attained in postmenopausal women with advanced breast cancer.

It appeared then that certain women could benefit from endocrine control, but the problem lay in identifying the right patient. More harm than good might result from inappropriate surgical or pharmacologic manipulation. The solution to this problem lay in detecting steroid receptors in tumor cells — first estrogen, then progesterone. By recognizing which patients had receptor-positive tumors, physicians could now, with remarkable accuracy, predict a beneficial course of action.

The era of identifying patients suitable for endocrine therapy was initiated by the discovery that rat mammary tumors avidly absorbed labeled estrogen [23]. Then, in 1961, a labeled synthetic estrogen was given to women with advanced cancer. More of this hormone was retained by the cancerous tissue of women whose disease improved following adrenalectomy than by the tissue of women unresponsive to surgical endocrine ablation [9]. Soon afterward, specific estrogen receptors were found in the cancer cells' cytoplasm [16], and scientists subsequently developed laboratory methods to identify hormone-responsive tumors [15].

Some tumors have estrogen receptors in the form of a single protein located in the tumor cell's cytoplasm. When the tumor cell is exposed to estrogen, the hormone joins with the receptor protein and the complex enters the nucleus. This activated receptor complex can, by a process not yet understood, induce new nucleic acid synthesis, the first step toward production of more tumor. If the estrogen receptors are blocked by a chemical such as tamoxifen, a nontoxic antiestrogen, it is theorized that protein synthesis — and therefore tumor proliferation or replication — is inhibited [6].

The presence of estrogen receptors and, more recently, progesterone receptors [12] is an excellent prognostic indicator, independent of the patient's tumor size and lymph node and menopausal status [6], for the duration of the disease-free interval the patient might enjoy. Breast cancer is more indolent and survival more likely in patients with estrogen-receptor–positive tumors, and, fortunately for women with tumors positive for both estrogen and progesterone receptors, 75 percent are likely to respond to endocrine manipulation.

Benign Breast Disease

"Fibrocystic disease," more appropriately termed *physiologic nodularity* [19], is a common disorder characterized by unprovoked breast pain, tenderness, and palpable irregularities that fluctuate in intensity with the menstrual cycle. Discomfort often begins during the third week of the cycle and subsides with the onset of the menstrual flow. Although many women are prone to this condition, symptoms are less pronounced in those who are multiparous, ovulate with regularity, or take oral contraceptives [8].

The changes of physiologic nodularity are attributed to several causes, the most generally acknowledged of which is hormonal imbalance. More controversial is the role of prolactin excess [7] and nutrition. Methylxanthines found in tea, coffee, chocolates, and soft drinks are said to exacerbate benign disease [22].

Caring for patients with chronic breast pain is trying because this problem affects daily life and sexual image and is emotionally charged. Several treatments have been tried, all with varying success. Diuretics occasionally alleviate pain, as does thyroid hormone, when appropriately given to symptomatic patients with clinical or occult thyroid deficiency. Abstinence from foods containing methylxanthines and vitamin therapy utilizing vitamins A or E has been used with variable success.

Steroids of many kinds, alone or in creative combinations, have been tried: chorionic gonadotrophin, androgens, estrogens, and synthetic and natural progesterone [18]. Excess prolactin is a suspected culprit, so bromocriptine, the prolactin-lowering medication, has been used and shown to relieve some cases of premenstrual mastalgia. But any benefit this drug offers should be weighed against its unpleasant side effects of nausea, dizziness, and nasal congestion [19]. Results of most therapies are discouraging, and even those studies lauding the effectiveness of a particular agent must be viewed somewhat critically, since spontaneous remission is high [18].

Treatment options changed in 1980, when the Federal Drug Administration (FDA) approved the synthetic testosterone derivative danazol, a weak androgen [24]. Danazol suppresses FSH and LH, thereby reducing the stimulus for ovarian steroidogenesis. Stimulation to the breast is, as a result, diminished. As long as the drug is administered in a small enough dose, it can alleviate symptoms without the adverse side effects of hirsutism, weight gain, and amenorrhea [21].

Treatment of symptomatic women athletes differs from that of their sedentary counterparts. Luteal insufficiency and anovulatory cycles are common in this group of women, and breast pain and tenderness often accompany these menstrual irregularities. Danazol is not, however, the appropriate medication for relief. The anabolic effects of this drug are undesirable; in the case of competitive athletes, progesterone is therefore the treatment of choice [2].

Acknowledgment. The expert comments of Mona M. Shangold, M.D., Associate Professor of Obstetrics and Gynecology, Georgetown University Hospital, Washington, D.C., are sincerely appreciated.

References

1. Arey, L.B. *Developmental Anatomy* (6th ed.). Philadelphia: Saunders, 1960. P. 450.
2. Baeyens, L. Breast problems in athletes. *Physician and Sports Medicine* 15:25, 1987.
3. Beatson, G.T. On the treatment of inoperable cases of carcinoma of the mamma: Suggestions for a new method of treatment, with illustrative cases. *Lancet* 2:104, 1896.
4. Botella-Llusia, J. *Endocrinology of Woman.* Philadelphia: Saunders, 1973. P. 469.
5. Cooper, A.P. *The Principles and Practice of Surgery.* London: Cox, 1836. P. 333.
6. Desombre, E.R., Holt, J.A., and Herbst, A.L. Steroid Receptors in Breast, Uterine, and Ovarian Malignancy. In J.J. Gold and J.B. Josimovich (eds.), *Gynecologic Endocrinology* (4th ed.). New York: Plenum, 1987. P. 511.
7. Dogliotti, L., Mussa, A., and Sandrucci, S. Prolactin and Benign Breast Disease. In A. Angeli, et al (eds.), *Endocrinology of Cystic Breast Disease.* New York: Raven, 1983. P. 273.
8. Drucker, B.H., and deMendonca, W.C. Fibrocystic change and fibrocystic disease of the breast. *Clin. Obstet. Gynecol.* 14:685, 1987.
9. Folca, P.J., Glascock, R.F., and Irvine, W.T. Studies with tritium labeled hexoestrol in advanced breast cancer. *Lancet* 2:796, 1961.
10. Frantz, A.G., and Wilson, J.D. Endocrine Disorders of the Breast. In J.D. Wilson and D.W. Foster (eds.), *Williams' Textbook of Endocrinology.* Philadelphia: Saunders, 1985. P. 402.
11. Harley, J.M.G. The endocrine control of the breasts. *Practitioner* 203:153, 1969.
12. Horwitz, K.B., and McGuire, W.L. Specific progesterone receptors in human breast cancer. *Steroids* 25:497, 1975.
13. Horwitz, R.I., and Stewart, K.R. Effect of clinical features on the association of estrogens and breast cancer. *Am. J. Med.* 76:192, 1984.
14. Huggins, C., and Bergenstal, D.M. Inhibition of human mammary and prostate cancers by adrenalectomy. *Cancer Res.* 12:134, 1952.
15. Jensen, E.V., Block, G.E., Smith, S., et al. Estrogen receptors and breast cancer response to adrenalectomy. *Natl. Cancer Inst. Monog.* 34:55, 1971.
16. Jensen, E.V., Desombre, E.R., and Jungblut, P.W. Estrogen Receptors in Hormone-Responsive Tissues and Tumors. In R.W. Wissler, T.L. Dao, and S. Wood (eds.), *Endogenous Factors Influencing Host-Tumor Balance.* Chicago: University of Chicago Press, 1967. P. 15.

17. Kiang, D.T. The Importance of Hormone Receptors and Markers in Breast Cancer. In J.S. Najarian and J.P. Delaney (eds.), *Advances in Breast and Endocrine Surgery.* Chicago: Year Book, 1986. P. 175.

18. London, R.S., Sundaram, G.S., and Goldstein, P.S. Medical management of mammary dysplasia. *Obstet. Gynecol.* 59:519, 1982.

19. Love, S.M., Gilman, R.S., and Silen, W. Fibrocystic "disease" of the breast—a nondisease? *N. Engl. J. Med.* 307:1010, 1982.

20. Lyons, W.R., Li, C.H., and Johnson, R.E. The hormonal control of mammary growth and lactation. *Recent Prog. Horm. Res.* 14:219, 1958.

21. Mansel, R.E., Wibey, J.R., and Hughes, L.E. Controlled trial of the antigonadotropin danazol in painful nodular benign breast disease. *Lancet* 1:928, 1982.

22. Minton, J.P., Foecking, M.K., Webster, D.J., et al. Response of fibrocystic disease to caffeine withdrawal and correlation of cyclic nucleotides with breast disease. *Am. J. Obstet. Gynecol.* 135:157, 1979.

23. Mobbs, B.G. The uptake of tritiated oestradiol by dimethyl-benzanthracene-induced mammary tumors of the rat. *J. Endocrinol.* 36:406, 1966.

24. Nezhat, C., Asch, R.H., and Greenblatt, R.B. Danazol for benign breast disease. *Am. J. Obstet. Gynecol.* 137:604, 1980.

25. Reyniak, J.V. Endocrine physiology of the breast. *J. Reprod. Med.* 22:303, 1979.

26. Speroff, L., Glass, R.H., and Kase, N.G. *Clinical Gynecologic Endocrinology and Infertility* (2nd ed.). Baltimore: Williams & Wilkins, 1978. P. 167.

27. Trapido, E.J., Brinton, L.A., Schaiarer, C., et al. Estrogen replacement therapy and benign breast disease. *J. Natl. Cancer Inst.* 73:1101, 1984.

28. Tyson, J.E., and Friesen, H.G. Factors influencing the secretion of human prolactin and growth hormone in menstrual and gestational women. *Am. J. Obstet. Gynecol.* 116:377, 1973.

29. Varga, L., Latterbach, P.M., Pryor, J.S., et al. Suppression of puerperal lactation with an ergo alkaloid. A double blind study. *Br. Med. J.* 2:273, 1972.

30. Vogel, P.M., Georgiade, N.G., Fetter, B.F., et al. The correlation of histologic changes of the human breast with the menstrual cycle. *Am. J. Pathol.* 104:23, 1981.

31. Vorherr, H. *The Breast: Morphology, Physiology, Lactation.* New York: Academic, 1974.

5

Forst E. Brown and
Steven K. Sargent

Mammographic Changes After Reduction Mammaplasty

Breast cancer strikes approximately one in ten women in the United States and is the second leading cause of cancer deaths among American women. Its incidence appears to be increasing; in 1987, there were 130,000 cases diagnosed, with an estimated 41,000 deaths [1]. Earlier diagnosis means an increased cure rate. Women with small tumors that have not metastasized to the regional lymph nodes have a 90 percent 5-year survival rate. Generally, the smaller the tumor at the time of detection, the less likely that the spread to regional nodes has occurred and the higher the cure rate. Mammography has been shown to be the most effective technique in detecting small nonpalpable breast cancers. In the Breast Cancer Detection Demonstration Project (BCDDP), 42 percent of neoplasms were detected by mammography alone, and 9 percent were detected by physical examination alone [2]. The key to decreasing breast cancer mortality is early detection.

Women who have had reduction mammaplasty continue to carry a risk of breast cancer comparable to that of the general population and related to the same risk factors. Therefore, these patients should have periodic screening no less carefully than others. However, reduction mammaplasty alters the breast contour and produces parenchymal scarring. Such changes can interfere with periodic breast examination and mammography. Therefore, it is important to define the mammographic alterations occurring after reduction mammaplasty to determine their frequency and progression over time and to decide on a program of postoperative management that is consistent with good cancer screening [6].

Mammographic Technique
There are two principal radiographic techniques for imaging the breast: xeromammography and film-screen mammography. Although each technique has its advocates, there does not appear to be a significant difference in the ability to detect cancer.

XEROMAMMOGRAPHY
This technique was first introduced by Wolfe in 1976 [27]. It uses a photoconductive plate of selenium-coated aluminum as the image receptor. The plate is charged with positive ions, and the breast is x-rayed using the plate (instead of x-ray film) to record a latent electrostatic pattern corresponding to areas of different density within the breast. The Xerox processing equipment converts the electrostatic pattern to a blue and white image on paper. Most xeromammography units give a slightly higher radiation dose to the breast than a similar quality film-screen unit. In our experience, xeromammography demonstrates the periareolar skin changes after reduction mammaplasty to better advantage than film-screen studies.

FILM-SCREEN MAMMOGRAPHY
Film-screen mammography uses a high-definition screen in close contact with x-ray film. The x-ray beam is passed through the breast to create an image on the film. Two views of each breast, a craniocaudal and an oblique-lateral, should be obtained, as in xeromammography. Breast compression is essential to achieve maximum image sharpness and contrast, to minimize x-ray dose, to achieve homogeneous film density, and to spread the breast tissue and reduce superimposition of glandular tissue and masses. A dedicated mammographic unit should be used, and careful attention to quality control is mandatory. Film-screen units produce images of higher contrast and give somewhat lower radiation doses to the breast than xeromammography. Film processing with film-screen units is generally more reliable (less "down time").

35

Table 5-1. *Breast examinations with mammographic changes (44 patients)*

	Postoperative time interval (months)			
	0–6	6–12	12–24	>24
Number of breast examinations	38	32	23	50
Periareolar changes	28	18	9	35
Inferior pole alterations	35	28	19	43
Asymmetric densities	17	15	13	21
Fat necrosis	1	2	2	4
Calcification	1	1	4	21

Source: Adapted from F.E. Brown, S.K. Sargent, S.R. Cohen, and W.D. Morain. Mammographic changes following reduction mammaplasty. *Plast. Reconstr. Surg.* 80 : 691, 1987.

Risks After Mammography

There are no precise data on the risk of breast cancer induction from mammography. All information has come from extrapolation of data from those groups of women exposed to high doses of radiation and from high-dose animal experiments. The former include two groups: Japanese women exposed to gamma and neutron radiation in Hiroshima and Nagasaki following the atomic bombings [12, 16, 26], and those women who received repeated chest fluoroscopy to monitor their pneumothorax therapy for tuberculosis prior to the awareness of the potential carcinogenesis of radiation [5, 14, 18, 19]. These groups of women, who were exposed to radiation doses hundreds and thousands of times greater than exposure from routine mammography, experienced an increased incidence of breast cancer. This was especially true for younger women (younger than age 30). It also appears clear that there was a 10- to 20-year latent period for the development of radiation-induced breast cancer.

It is uncertain whether the very low doses of radiation from current mammographic units can cause breast cancer. If a risk exists, it is too small to be measured experimentally. The best estimates of the theoretical risk obtained by extrapolating from the data on women exposed to high-dose radiation are as follows: In women older than 30 years, after a minimum latent period of 10 years, the increased incidence of breast cancer from a single mammographic examination on modern equipment would be 1 case of cancer per 2 million women per year [9]. The natural breast cancer occurrence rate is 800 cases per million women per year at age 40; 1,800 cases per million women per year at age 50; and 2,500 cases per million women

per year at age 65. A recent review suggested a risk of 1 case in 25,000 for women aged 40 to 49 after 10 years of screening with mammography, compared with a natural risk of breast cancer development of 128 in 10,000 [7].

The bottom line is clear: A theoretical risk of breast cancer induction by mammography does exist. The exact risk is unknown but is so small that it cannot be measured experimentally. Compared with the rate of "natural" occurrence of breast cancer, the added risk of mammographic induction seems very small compared with the potential benefit of early detection.

Mammographic Changes After Surgery

Reduction mammaplasty involves resection of breast tissue, reshaping of the remaining breast, and repositioning of the nipple-areolar complex. The latter is most frequently supported by a de-epithelialized pedicle. This surgical procedure produces changes in the breast that can be observed on mammography and may be difficult to distinguish from cancer. These changes are described in the three series reported by Brown et al. [6] (Table 5-1), Swann et al. [24], and Miller et al. [17].

There is an *alteration in the contour of the breast*, seen particularly on the mediolateral view. The contour of the upper and lower halves of the breast may become more symmetric after surgery. There is a *downward shift of the ductal and fibroglandular tissue*, best seen on the mediolateral view. In the normal breast, most of the ductal and fibroglandular tissue is concentrated in the outer quadrants; after surgery, the majority lies below the nipple level. This surgical repositioning of the

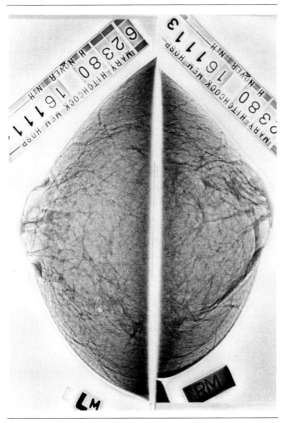

Fig. 5-1. Craniocaudal view of both breasts 2 months after reduction mammaplasty showing periareolar and medial scarring.

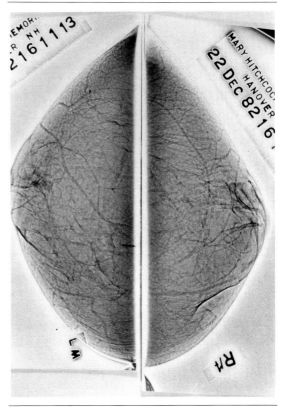

Fig. 5-2. Same patient as in Fig. 5-1. Craniocaudal view of both breasts 2½ years after reduction mammaplasty reveals a marked interval decrease in scarring.

breast can produce a non-anatomic orientation of the fibro-glandular tissue.

There is an *elevation of the nipple* with respect to the skin circumference of the breast. In contrast to the normal breast, there is more skin below and less skin above the nipple.

Thickening of the areolar skin (62% in Miller et al.'s series [17]) or *periareolar contour changes* or both, are seen frequently. These findings are related to the postsurgical scarring after repositioning of the nipple and circumferential suturing; they are most marked on the first postoperative mammogram and usually diminish with time (Figs. 5-1 and 5-2).

Scarring of the inferior pole is a common finding (90%). In some patients who have had pedicle transposition of the nipple, a *retroareolar fibrotic band* may be present. Such mammographic changes are related both to the subcutaneous de-

epithelialized pedicle flap and to the vertical scar lying between the areola and the inframammary fold (Fig. 5-3). *Distorted architecture* is common. Thirty-one of 33 patients in Swann's series demonstrated a characteristic *swirled pattern* [24]. Surgery interferes with the normal flow of structures toward the nipple.

Disruption of the areolar ducts is a variable finding. Nipple grafting results in the division of all ducts. Nipple transposition may preserve some of the connections of the nipple ductules with the underlying parenchyma. In Miller et al.'s series [17], 11 of 14 patients who had had nipple transposition showed continuity of some of the ducts, and 2 patients had a typical convergence of all ducts leading into the nipple.

Areas of *fat necrosis* may occur. The mammographic appearance of fat necrosis varies, ranging from a well-circumscribed round or ovoid area of decreased density (traumatic oil cyst) to an irregular area of increased density with or without calci-

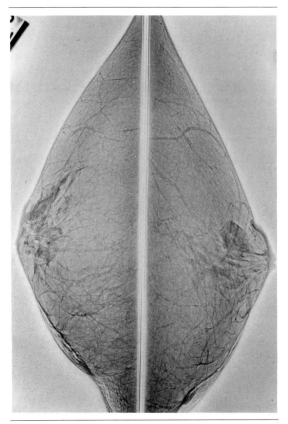

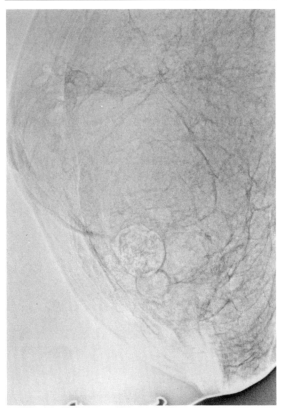

Fig. 5-3. Xeroradiograph demonstrating periareolar and inferior pole changes 8 months after reduction mammaplasty.

Fig. 5-4. Fat necrosis is demonstrated in a mammogram 6 months after surgery.

fications, mimicking cancer [4]. Fat necrosis was not reported in the series by Miller et al. and was identified in approximately 10 percent of the patients described by Brown et al. [6] (Fig. 5-4).

Asymmetric densities are present in approximately 50 percent of patients [6] (Fig. 5-5) and are apparently a manifestation of differing degrees of postoperative scarring between the two breasts. Such asymmetric findings can be of concern to the mammographer looking for early signs of malignancy. When they occur in areas of surgical trauma, and, most important, if they decrease in size with time, these densities are less likely to indicate cancer.

The occurrence of *calcifications* is unusual in the first year after reduction mammaplasty but is present in greater than 40 percent of patients after 2 years [6]. These calcifications are often coarser than the typical malignant calcifications and usu-

ally occur in the periareolar and inferior portions of the breast along suture lines (Fig. 5-6).

SERIAL MAMMOGRAPHIC CHANGES

Serial mammograms were obtained on 25 of our patients for at least 2 years after reduction mammaplasty. These provided an excellent documentation of the natural course of the radiologic changes after this surgery. The changes were fairly predictable. Architectural changes such as periareolar and inferior pole alterations were most marked on the first postoperative mammogram and usually decreased with time (Figs. 5-7 and 5-8). In none of the 25 patients did these changes become more pronounced with time. Asymmetric densities were present in 50 percent of patients in the first year but in less than 25 percent after 2 years. In patients in whom they persisted, the densities did not enlarge and usually decreased in size and prominence. This interval improvement seen

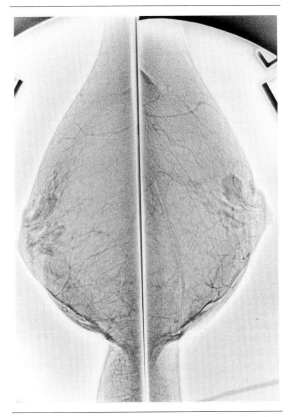

Fig. 5-5. Asymmetrical density in breast 4 months after surgery.

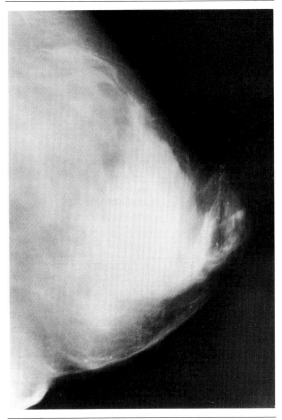

Fig. 5-6. Mediolateral views taken 2 years after reduction mammaplasty showing development of calcifications along suture lines.

with benign postoperative changes, as opposed to the expected interval progression with breast carcinoma, was extremely helpful in distinguishing between postoperative changes and malignancy.

Calcification tended to develop later, however, and thus may present a diagnostic problem. Approximately 3 percent (1 of 38) of our patients developed calcifications in the first year after surgery. By the second year, 20 percent of examinations demonstrated calcifications; after 2 years, this rate was greater than 40 percent. The number and extent of the calcifications also increased with time (Figs. 5-9 and 5-10). Postoperative calcifications were frequently coarser than those typically seen with malignancy (Fig. 5-11). They occurred in the periareolar and inferior portions of the breast, the sites of greatest surgical trauma. The appearance of the calcifications, their location, and the time interval usually allowed for a fairly confident differentiation between benign calcification and carcinoma.

In summary, the mammographic changes following reduction mammaplasty are predictable. Initially, there will be areolar, periareolar, and inferior skin changes that become less pronounced over time. Focal abnormalities consistent with scarring or fat necrosis may develop but do not progress and, in fact, tend to decrease with time. Calcifications are common and tend to develop in the second and third year. They are often coarser than typical malignant calcifications and occur in the periareolar and inferior portions of the breast, usually along suture lines. Knowledge of these expected mammographic alterations and their time course may help distinguish between postoperative change and carcinoma.

Cancer Screening for the Post-Reduction Mammaplasty Patient

Optimal care of women who have had reduction

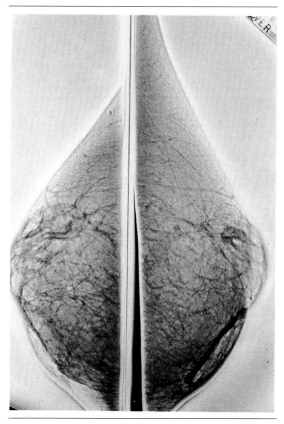

Fig. 5-7. Lateral view of breast demonstrates scarring several months after surgery.

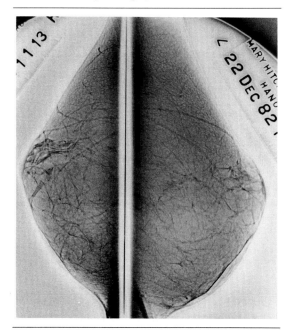

Fig. 5-8. Same patient as in Fig. 5-7. A comparable view 1 year after surgery shows a significant decrease in scarring.

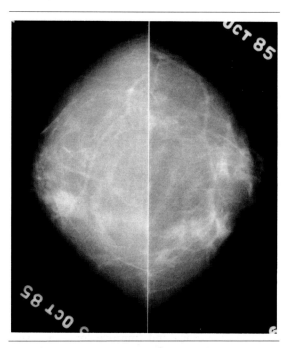

Fig. 5-9. Mammogram 1 year after surgery demonstrates minimal postoperative scarring but no calcifications.

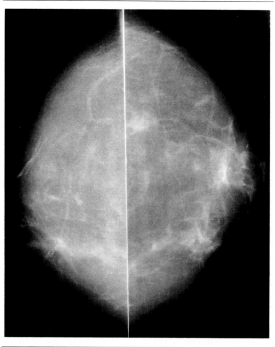

Fig. 5-10. Same patient as in Fig. 5-9. Two years after surgery, calcifications begin to appear.

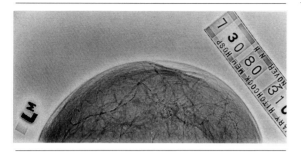

Fig. 5-11. Clustered microcalcifications typical of carcinoma.

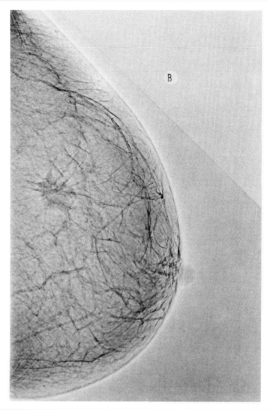

Fig. 5-12. Mass with spiculated margins typical of carcinoma. This should not be mistaken for postoperative change.

mammaplasty requires periodic examination [10]. These patients have a risk of developing breast cancer comparable to that in the general population. The BCDDP reported an annual detection rate of 3 cases per 1,000 women screened [3]. Periodic mammography and physical examination of the breast will provide the best opportunity to discover early lesions and improve long-term survival. Shapiro et al. [21], in the Health Insurance Plan of New York breast cancer screening program, demonstrated a 30 percent decrease in mortality in women older than 50 years who had annual physical and radiologic examinations. Adding annual mammograms to annual breast examinations every year for 10 years for women aged 40 to 49 years might decrease the probability of death from breast cancer by 26 percent [7]. Tabar et al. [25] reported a 31 percent decrease in mortality in Swedish women offered screening mammography every 2 to 3 years.

The perceived value of mammography in identifying obscure breast cancers must be tempered by an appreciation of the frequency of false-negative readings. The rate reported in the literature ranges from a low of 5 percent to a high, in a select group of patients, of 69 percent [20]. In a breast cancer detection center with dedicated equipment and experienced radiologists, the false-negative rate should not exceed 10 percent [20].

Clinical evaluation of the postoperative patient may be difficult. Palpable masses may be due to scarring, deep-seated hematoma, cysts, or fat necrosis. Isaacs et al. [11] reported the diagnostic problems in seven post-reduction mammaplasty patients who developed such masses. Mammography was helpful in the evaluation of these patients. However, intramammary scar tissue after surgery may mimic the mammographic appearance of car-

cinoma (Fig. 5-12) [22, 23]. Correlation of the findings with the physical examination is important. The appearance of the scarring and the relationship with the overlying skin may also be helpful in the differential. The most important factor in the evaluation is the change with time.

There are radiographic characteristics of breast calcifications that provide clues in estimating the risk of carcinoma [8]. Yet clusters of stippled calcifications in the nonoperated breast require histopathologic study of the involved tissue. This need not be so in the post-reduction breast, since the calcifications seen after surgery show a distinct pattern and location.

Mammographic changes after reduction mammaplasty show a predictable evolution with time. Despite the difficulties that may arise in the interpretation of a single mammographic examination, serial studies will provide screening that should be

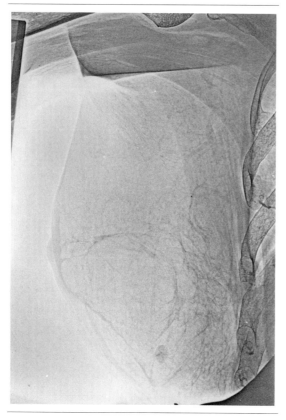

Fig. 5-13. Patient 1. Nodule "suspicious for malignancy" is seen in mammogram 9 months after surgery. Biopsy showed chronic inflammation associated with ruptured inclusion cyst.

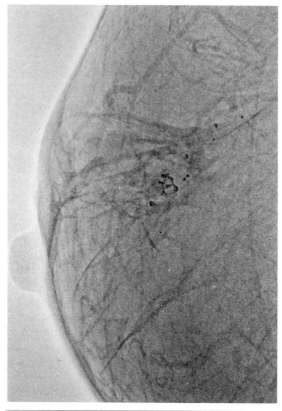

Fig. 5-14. Patient 2. Calcifications are shown to have developed in mammogram 13 months after surgery. Biopsy showed chronic inflammation consistent with granuloma.

comparable to that in the general population. We recommend that patients having reduction mammaplasty who are 35 years of age or older and those with a history of breast cancer in first-degree relatives have preoperative mammograms. Such screening studies can locate an obscure cancer. Kallen et al. [13] reported three patients with breast cancer from a group of 273 undergoing mammaplasty; one cancer was identified in the preoperative mammogram. Postoperative mammograms should be repeated between 3 and 6 months. This time interval between the pre- and postoperative mammograms should delineate those x-ray changes caused by surgery alone. There is little likelihood that the interim development of carcinoma would be responsible for the mammographic changes [23]. This early postoperative study will also provide a baseline for later compar-

ison. Mammographic examination thereafter should follow the guidelines of the American Cancer Society and the American College of Radiology (i.e., a mammogram every 1 or 2 years from age 40 to 49, and annually thereafter) unless the findings on a particular examination necessitate more frequent follow-up [2, 15]. Since there are some investigators who believe that there is a reduced benefit for routine mammography for women aged 40 to 49 years, a patient in this age group should participate in the decision of whether to have annual or biannual examinations [7]. Breast examination should be coordinated with the mammographic studies, and the operating surgeon should be willing to take responsibility for coordinating these examinations.

As in the general population, surgical biopsies should be performed when there are clinically suspicious masses or lesions seen on mammography that are suspicious for cancer. These would include later-developing or enlarging masses or areas of clustered microcalcifications geographically removed from the sites of greatest surgical trauma. In our series, four lesions fell into this category; they appeared late and did not regress as expected. All were benign lesions with chronic inflammation or cyst formation or both [6]. Two examples are shown in Figs. 5-13 and 5-14.

This program of perioperative and postoperative monitoring of the patient having reduction mammaplasty should provide an excellent cancer screen. Breast cancer will eventually develop in some postoperative patients but should be detected earlier, decreasing the mortality rate from this disease.

Portions of this chapter and Figs. 5-1, 5-2, 5-3, 5-4, 5-11, 5-12, 5-13, and 5-14 are reprinted with permission from F. E. Brown, et al. Mammographic changes following reduction mammaplasty. *Plast. Reconstr. Surg.* 80:691, November 1987.

References

1. *Cancer Society Facts and Figures–1987.* New York: American Cancer Society, 1987. P. 10.
2. New American College of Radiology Guidelines on mammography. *ACR Bull.* 38:6, 1982.
3. Baker, L.H. Breast Cancer Detection Demonstration Project: Five-year summary report. *CA* 32:194, 1982.
4. Bassett, L.W., Gold, R.H., and Cove, H.C. Mammographic spectrum of traumatic fat necrosis: The fallibility of "pathognomonic" signs of carcinoma. *Am. J. Roentgenol.* 130:119, 1978.
5. Boice, J.D., and Monson, R.B. Breast cancer following repeated fluoroscopic examinations of the chest. *J. Natl. Cancer Inst.* 59:823, 1977.
6. Brown, F.E., Sargent, S.K., Cohen, S.R., and Morain, W.D. Mammographic changes following reduction mammaplasty. *Plast. Reconstr. Surg.* 80:691, 1987.
7. Eddy, D.M., Hasselblad, V., McGiveny, W., et al. The value of mammography screening in women under age 50 years. *J.A.M.A.* 259:1512, 1988.
8. Egan, R.L., McSweeney, M.B., and Sewell, C.W. Intramammary calcifications without an associated mass in benign and malignant diseases. *Radiology* 137:1, 1980.
9. Gohagen, J.K., Darby, W.P., Spitznagel, E.L., et al. Radiogenic breast cancer effects of mammographic screening. *J. Natl. Cancer Inst.* 77:71, 1986.
10. Greenberg, G. (ed.). Rising number of suits allege delay and incorrect diagnosis of breast cancer. Plastic Surgery News Supplement (American Society of Plastic and Reconstructive Surgeons, Inc.), August 25, 1986.
11. Isaacs, G., Rozner, L., and Tudball, C. Breast lumps after reduction mammaplasty. *Ann. Plast. Surg.* 15:394, 1985.
12. Jablon, S., and Kato, H. Studies of the mortality of A-bomb survivors. V. Radiation dose and mortality, 1950–1970. *Radiat. Res.* 50:649, 1972.
13. Kallen, R., Broome, A., Muhlow, A., and Forsby, N. Reduction mammaplasty: Results of preoperative mammography and patient inquiry. *Scand. J. Plast. Reconstr. Surg.* 20(3):303, 1986.
14. MacKenzie, I. Breast cancer following multiple fluoroscopies. *Br. J. Cancer* 19:1, 1965.
15. Mammography guidelines 1983: Background statement and update of cancer-related checkup guidelines for breast cancer detection in asymptomatic women age 40 to 49. *CA* 33:255, 1983.
16. McGregor, D.H., Land, C.E., Choi, K., et al. Breast cancer incidence among atomic bomb survivors, Hiroshima and Nagasaki, 1950–1969. *J. Natl. Cancer Inst.* 59:799, 1977.
17. Miller, C.L., Feig, S.A., and Fox J.W., IV. Mammographic changes after reduction mammoplasty. *Am. J. Roentgenol.* 149:35, 1987.
18. Myrden, J.A., and Quinlan, J.J. Breast cancer following multiple fluoroscopies during artificial pneumothorax treatment of pulmonary tuberculosis. *Can. Med. Assoc. J.* 100:1032, 1969.
19. Myrden, J.A., and Quinlan, J.J. Breast carcinoma following multiple fluoroscopies with pneumothorax treatment of pulmonary tuberculosis. *Ann. R. Coll. Phys. Can.* 7:45, 1974.
20. Newsome, J.F., and McLelland, R. A word of caution concerning mammography. *J.A.M.A.* 255:528, 1986.
21. Shapiro, S., Strax, P., and Venet, L. Periodic breast cancer screening in reducing mortality from breast cancer. *J.A.M.A.* 215:1777, 1971.
22. Sickles, E.A., and Herzog, K.A. Intramammary scar tissue: A mimic of the mammographic appearance of carcinoma. *Am. J. Roentgenol.* 135:349, 1980.
23. Sickles, E.A., and Herzog, K.A. Mammography of the postsurgical breast. *Am. J. Roentgenol.* 136:585, 1981.
24. Swann, C.A., Kopans, D.B., White, G., et al. Observations on the postreduction mammoplasty mammogram. *Breast Dis.* 1:261, 1989.
25. Tabar, L., Fagerberg, C.J.G., Gad, A., et al. Reduction in mortality from breast cancer after mass screening with mammography: Randomized trial from the Breast Cancer Screening Working Group of the Swedish National Board of Health and Welfare. *Lancet* 1:829, 1985.
26. Tokunaga, M., Norman, J.E., Asano, M., et al. Malignant breast tumors among atomic bomb survivors, Hiroshima and Nagasaki, 1950–1974. *J. Natl. Cancer Inst.* 62:1347, 1979.
27. Wolfe, J.N. Breast patterns as an index of risk for developing breast cancer. *Am. J. Roentgenol.* 126:1130, 1976.

6

Carolyn J. Cline

Psychological Aspects of Breast Reduction Surgery

This chapter represents what I have learned from several hundred breast reduction patients with whom I have worked during the last 9 years. Most of them have taught me something — either painstakingly or abruptly — about the psychological significance of the breast, the psychodynamics of breast reduction surgery, preoperative psychological evaluation, and intraoperative and postoperative psychological processes. I was able to learn from them because my previous training as a professional clinical psychologist had prepared me to look for and listen to both conscious and unconscious messages.

When we speak, we use words both as a description of concrete reality and as metaphors for our psychological reality. One patient, Nancy, said, "I'm afraid to go without a bra. I need the support." Here the word "support" has two meanings: one, on the descriptive level, is the physical reality of supporting her breasts; the second, on the metaphorical level, is the psychological support she needs. Another patient, Jennifer, used words that are also both descriptive and metaphorical: "Otherwise I'll end up just like my mother," she said. On the descriptive level, she meant with the low back pain, poor posture, and sore shoulders that her mother had. On a metaphorical level, Jennifer meant "like her mother" and therefore not who she is in her own right. By tuning in to language at both levels, one can understand both what is being said consciously as well as the unconscious message. A few guidelines will be given at the end of this chapter to facilitate learning this skill, which we can all master if we are attuned to it.*

---

* For those who wish to pursue this subject in depth, I strongly recommend Theodore Reich, Listening with the Third Ear. New York: Farrar, Straus & Giroux, 1948.

No Patient Exists in a Vacuum

Most breast reduction patients are reasonably well adjusted. They are prepared for and capable of dealing with the surgery they undergo. Gifford [4] has insightfully described some of the underlying psychological dynamics at work in our patients. Occasionally, the nature or intensity of these psychological processes can cause significant problems in the perioperative period. Few patients will need to see a psychotherapist or counselor, but, as plastic surgeons, it is imperative that we are able to recognize those patients for whom surgery at the time is psychologically contraindicated or who need referral in addition to surgery.

It is increasingly evident that in plastic surgery — and in medicine in general — we must view patients not as isolated entities but as persons intrinsically and inextricably entwined with the perceptions, needs, and demands of others. Spouses, parents (living and deceased), children, even society at large, all play a role in determining a patient's needs and behavior.

I would like to propose a field theory of psychological evaluation and treatment for our patients. In physical science, field theory states that the objects of the world are a series of electromagnetic particles defined fully only in the context of their entire environment; their behavior can be predicted only by knowing the characteristics of the objects around them. As physicians, we must recognize that our patients, too, can be understood only in relation to dynamic processes — both the processes within the individual (intrapersonal phenomena) and those that occur between the individual and significant others (interpersonal phenomena).

Such an understanding is essential to our work because when we alter the body, we alter the mind — the psyche. Each part of the body has symbolic meaning for each individual, meaning that is often laden with emotion. This symbolism stems from both childhood development and the current interpersonal environment. As we discuss the intrapersonal phenomena relevant to breast reduction, the depth of the interactive process between soma and psyche will become clear. If we define "successful" plastic surgery as that which truly enhances the life of the patient, a plastic surgeon must be able to view the world (and the body) through the eyes of the patient and discuss relevant surgical issues in that light. To do otherwise is perilous and ultimately less rewarding professionally. Furthermore, it has become clear that the majority of medicolegal altercations arise from faulty communication between the physician and the patient. The refrains "I didn't want to end up looking like *this*" or "I didn't know it would be like *this*" can begin a series of emotionally draining consultations, surgeries, and potential legal hassles. This is at best an inefficient mode of practice and at worst a tragedy for both patient and plastic surgeon. In evaluating a patient for breast reduction surgery, the plastic surgeon should be aware of the following:

I. Intrapersonal phenomena
  A. The meaning of "the breast" and breast reduction surgery for that patient based on:
    1. Her childhood development
    2. Her current identity and maturation dilemmas
II. Interpersonal phenomena
  A. The meaning of her breast and breast reduction surgery to significant others, including parents, where appropriate, spouses or boyfriends, and children
  B. The meaning of her breast within the context of societal pressures

Intrapersonal Issues: A Breast is a Breast is a Breast

Most of us, plastic surgeons and patients alike, cannot fully comprehend the profound psychological processes with which we deal when we alter body parts. When we plan changes to the breast, we are tampering with one of the most emotionally laden parts of the body. Our feelings about the breast stem from our earliest experiences and form the bedrock of our personalities. Slight shifts in this bedrock can lead to major readjustments in the personality and body image, much as an earthquake can make a building move by shifting the ground beneath its foundation. (Those of us in California may find this analogy more compelling.)

The breast attains such deeply rooted significance because it is at the center of our very first, regular experience with the outside world: the suckling experience. Whether a baby is male or female, whether breast- or bottlefed, the suckling experience has tremendous impact, either negative or positive. To the infant, the breast is associated either with warm cuddling and sumptuous sufficiency or, in its absence, cold rejection and hunger.

Anyone observing a baby feverishly suckling will also notice that after a few minutes, the infant will chew and pull on the nipple. This is not to obtain nourishment, but to express "aggression" and relieve tension. Thus, the suckling experience is also a means of discharging energies that later will be identified as aggression, anxiety, and hostility. In this manner, the breast becomes an object on which much frustration and hostility are projected [3, 6].

Shortly after birth, depending on the circumstances surrounding suckling, the infant regularly experiences the world as soft and satisfying with adequate relief of aggression and tension, or uncomfortable, dissatisfying, and tension-provoking. These experiences are symbolized as either the "good" breast or the "bad" breast, respectively. However, the infant cannot distinguish self from nonself. An infant cannot, for example, judge whether an intestinal cramp is coming from its own body or the outside world. Indeed, the concept of "me" versus "them" is not even present. The world/self is amorphous and global. Only what feels good or does not feel good can be sensed, and, since the infant cannot distinguish itself from the mother's breast, the positive or negative feelings aroused by the breast come to be associated with its own body.

In this manner, our primitive early experiences form the basis of our feelings about our bodies and the world around us. We are either basically satisfied and comfortable or vaguely uncomfortable and dissatisfied. This entire preverbal bedrock of feelings lying deep below the personality surface is symbolized by the breast. Laid upon this primitive foundation are the later developmental experiences of self [6, 8]. Thus, when a woman presents in the office for "breast surgery," she is also talking about her basic view of self and of the world, either to a great or small degree, depending on personality structure. Is it any wonder then that breast surgery has such a profoundly positive effect on psychologically and physically well-suited candidates? Change the problematic breast and you have changed their world.

Fortunately, most of our patients are essentially healthy, "well-built" personalities who can adjust to the shifts we create with our handiwork. But knowing the depths of what we are dealing with argues strongly for us to attend very carefully to what the patient *says*, how the patient *thinks*, and what the patient *wants*. For some patients, changing "the breast" (read: self, world) is enough to overcome the negative feelings about "the breast" (read: self, world) with which she has been living.

For other patients, however, the specifics of the aesthetic results may be fraught with meaning. Size, for example, may not merely be a matter of being able to buy one type of dress as opposed to another but may represent a dynamic psychological need that *we* cannot fathom and the patient cannot even verbalize (so basic and preverbal is the phenomenon). The patient has intuitive knowledge of the true source of the problem and will try, unconsciously, to communicate it to us.

Apart from the infantile experience and its intrapersonal ramifications for breast surgery, there are numerous other developmental phenomena along the way that contribute psychological baggage. As we grow through our developmental childhood stages, a girl's feelings about her body —positive or negative—are continually being formed by identifying with her mother. She notes how her mother views her own body, as well as her father's attitude toward her mother's body. She also senses how each of her parents feels about *her* body. If she hears words of endearment and respect regarding her body and receives loving, gentle physical handling, she will develop a more positive image of her body. The opposite treatment results in her dissatisfaction with, and even rejection of, her own body. This normal process of taking in the views of others about both the female body and her own body is termed *internalization*.

Long after the death of our parents, their attitudes toward us live on in the way *we* feel about our bodies. As one divorced middle-aged woman put it, "Daddy was always complimenting mom on what great breasts she had, and they *were* perfect—small, pointy. I can't remember *ever*

being that small . . . I've just always had these big, ugly things . . . (I got) from my grandmother." No matter what physical problems her mammary hypertrophy had caused her, this patient's breast ideal was rooted in her relationships with her mother and father and that parental relationship. Is this comment coming from a person who has felt unloved by her father and is now saying, "Maybe if my breasts looked like my mother's, my father would finally love me?" Perhaps. Is this a way of saying, "My problems attracting men would be over if I had the kind of breasts men (my father) like?" Perhaps. In any case, statements like these are a tip-off that further exploration of this patient's expectations may be necessary to avoid disappointment and possible depression. A psychological referral may be advisable, both for evaluation purposes and to give the patient the opportunity for psychological or other practical interventions to help her realize all she is striving to become.

Jennifer, 24, a graduate student still living at home, described a litany of physical complaints related to her evident gigantomastia, then said casually, "My breasts are just like my mother's . . . big and ugly. She'd kill me if she knew I was here talking to you . . . ," she continued, only half jokingly, " . . . but I want these things off. Otherwise I'll end up just like her." Upon further discussion, it came out that this young woman was struggling with a hostile yet dependent relationship with her mother. Changing her breasts was a desperate attempt to separate from her mother psychologically and to address her fear that she would become "just like mother" psychologically, thereby failing to develop fully her own potential as a unique individual. Jennifer did undergo surgery for massive hypertrophy, but later she also entered psychotherapy to learn how to become effectively independent.

In Jennifer's case, the mother was still alive; Anne came to my office 4 years after her mother's death. Anne, a 54-year-old unmarried secretary, suffered from severe degenerative spinal arthritis. She became overwhelmingly anxious a few days prior to her breast reduction surgery. She experienced sleep disturbances—insomnia alternating with violent nightmares of imminent danger. Terrified, she was convinced that she was going to die from anesthetic complications. We talked, and she told me of her close relationship with her mother, who had also been large-breasted. Anne, an only child, had devoted her life to her mother's well-being. Her mother had been a subtly domineering woman, and Anne mentioned that her mother had taken great pride in pointing out to Anne and others the physical resemblance between mother and daughter. According to the patient, she did not resemble her mother at all except for breast size.

At one point in this discussion, Anne sobbed, "I'm all Mother has. She's had a tough life and now I'm taking away one of her few pleasures." The patient's use of the present tense signified that although her mother was dead, her internalized "mother," very much alive within her, was arguing unconsciously and violently against the anticipated change. Her terror of dying during surgery symbolized the punishment she feared she deserved and would receive from her internalized "mother." To Anne, changing her breasts symbolized betraying her mother, who had communicated to her daughter a lasting message: If you love me, you'll be like me. Anne's breasts symbolized her mother's gratification and were proof of the daughter's love and obedience.

Anne's surgery was canceled; she was referred for psychotherapy to help resolve this conflict prior to attempting surgery again. Her terror, insomnia, and nightmares were signals that her psyche was not yet ready to handle the imminent body change necessary to treat her progressive spinal disease. Eleven months after her original surgery date, Anne underwent successful breast reduction without fear of anesthesia and without regret.

These patients exemplify how changing the breast can be laden with psychodynamic significance, based on the unique intrapsychic meaning that the breast symbolizes. Each patient unconsciously communicated the need for careful evaluation and subsequent psychotherapeutic intervention. Jennifer's use of violent, graphic language — "she'd kill me if she knew" — and Anne's expression of conflict and anxiety through insomnia, nightmares, and terror of anesthesia presented to the surgeon the signs that for these patients, breast reduction surgery was psychologically problematic. Some have said that hemorrhage is the only defense of the anesthetized patient; so may it be said that the presentation of unconscious material through unusual language and behavior and through the development of "neurotic" symptoms may be the best defense of the psychologically troubled patient. We must learn to give these signals equal respect and attention.

Interpersonal Issues: Whose Breast Is It, Anyway?

When evaluating breast reduction surgery patients, it is my belief that the significant others in the patient's life should be strongly encouraged to participate in at least one of the preoperative consultation sessions. I see patients at least twice preoperatively excluding the preoperative marking session. I believe it prudent to see the people with whom the patient will interact in the immediate and long-term postoperative period because they will either support or sabotage the patient's efforts toward change. How others respond will depend on their general anxiety level regarding operations, the role of the patient in their relationship, and the significance to them of the patient's breast.

In regard to general anxiety about "operations," in my experience it is amazingly reassuring for parents and spouses simply to meet the surgeon. Establishing physical contact and giving information can often turn resolute obstinancy into supportive, intelligent concern. This is because much resistance, particularly on the part of fathers and husbands, is based on fear that "something bad" will happen to their loved one. Rather than taking the time out of a busy life and hectic schedule to find out what the surgery is all about, many fathers and husbands may take the position that "it's not necessary and I don't want you to do it." If they can be brought into the situation and educated, much of the resistance will subside. I remember a gentleman approaching me after a lecture on a cruise for which I was the ship's doctor. This fellow asked if I would mind talking to his wife, who, interestingly, had missed the lecture. As she approached, he called out "Emily, you don't need a breast reduction, you need a breast lift."

"But Carl," she murmured, both embarrassed and amazed by his boisterous enthusiasm, "You said you wouldn't let me do anything."

"That's because I didn't know anything about it!"

Emily smiled happily. We discussed a few issues, and I left wondering if the tables had not been turned — perhaps he was comfortable now, but having "permission" forced her to face her own ambivalence and fears about the procedure.

Meeting the surgeon also allows the parents and spouses to discuss their apprehension, thus lessening its impact. People often associate operations with unfortunate experiences of others — for example, anesthetic deaths or anoxic brain damage. If they have the opportunity to bring these fears out in the open, they can be reassured by valid information.

Daughters and Mothers

For the young virginal hypertrophy patient, the most significant family member to assess is mother. Even in apparently straightforward cases, breast reduction surgery can further complicate the ordinarily tempestuous and emotional relationship between mother and daughter during adolescence. In addition, it is important to be aware that whereas her daughter's breast surgery makes a mother anxious about her child's physical well-being, it may also lead her to reflect on her feelings about her own breasts. Just whose breasts are being operated on gets confused at times. In situations like this, mothers' comments range from "I want to spare her the agony of big breasts, whether she likes it or not," to "I've lived with them, why can't she?"

With all virginal hypertrophy patients, to be sure that no harm is unwittingly done, it behooves the plastic surgeon to get an idea of the mother's attitude toward the surgery. In my experience, the problematic emotional issues of mother-daughter relationships that can surface during evaluation for breast reduction are competition, separation, and vicarious fulfillment.

Competition between mother and daughter—specifically a mother's envy of the younger and possibly more beautiful daughter—can complicate the issue of breast reduction surgery. This confusion of the physical and emotional realities can lead to pressure on the patient either for or against surgery. Linda's mother, a 38-year-old, 5' 6" buxom, mini-skirted, blond bombshell, pressed her daughter *and* the surgeon for Linda's breast reduction. "She doesn't need breasts that size," exclaimed Alexandra. "All they'll do is make her a target for every oversexed man on the street. Besides, she's too small to have to carry that load around." Linda was only about an inch shorter than her mother. Further exploration revealed that calling her daughter "small" was Alexandra's way of expressing her need to have Linda be "less than" herself. Similarly, Alexandra's clothing accentuated her own voluptuousness, whereas her daughter was apparently to be denied this option.

Psychoanalytic literature equates the breast in women with the penis in men; in my experience, this, to a large degree, is accurate, given the increase in self-esteem and emboldened behavior seen in postoperative breast augmentation pa-

tients.* These women often take more initiative in sexual behavior and in social and professional matters than they did prior to surgery. From this standpoint, Linda's mother's overwhelming vehemence regarding her daughter's "need" for breast reduction can be seen as an attempt to castrate her daughter, to keep her "smaller" or "less than" she. Even gentle attempts to enlighten this mother failed. Her largely unconscious but powerful needs overshadowed her capacity to see the inappropriateness of her behavior. She left in a huff, dragging a beleaguered Linda behind.

The opposite attitude surfaced in a similar dilemma involving Lisa, a 19-year-old girl, and her mother, Jill. Jill was the small-breasted woman in the family who, Lisa informed me, was admired for her "perfect" breasts. Jill resisted the idea of her daughter's breast reduction lest Lisa rival her position as "the beautiful one" in the family. "I think she's fine just the way she is . . . lots of girls are a little large-breasted, and they do just fine," she said, in the presence of her uncomfortably massive daughter.

"But Lisa doesn't feel fine either physically or emotionally," I interjected.

"We can't have everything in this life, you know, dear," she replied sprightly to her daughter's pleading look. Lisa became helplessly dejected. Only by continually reassuring mother that Lisa would not have "everything" by undergoing breast reduction (implying indirectly it would not jeopardize Jill's position as "the beautiful one" in the family) was it possible to enlist her mother's support. Lisa underwent her much needed surgery without undue commotion.

The separation of a grown daughter from her mother can be a difficult and painful process, particularly for the mother. Breast reduction surgery on girls in late adolescence can trigger separation issues. Monica, 18, made an appropriate request for breast reduction surgery that provoked great anxiety in her large-breasted mother, Doris. Doris's fear that her daughter would later regret her action seemed reasonable. But during thorough discussions with both Monica and Doris, separately as well as together, Doris's anxiety and hostility became more intense. Finally, with great

---

* Although one may argue against this analogy by pointing out that men do not seek penis *reduction* surgery, I would emphasize that if men with large penises suffered the physical and social liabilities that mammary hypertrophy patients do, they, too, might seek relief.

frustration, she exclaimed, "If she does this, things will never be the same." Upon further inquiry, it became clear that making Monica's breasts *different* from her own symbolized to Doris her impending separation from her daughter. It was a sign of Monica's progressive *differentiation* of her self from her mother. Monica's desire to make her breasts different (from her mother's and from how they "had always been") signified to Doris not only a permanent change in the breasts but also in the mother-daughter relationship.

When I raised this question, ever so gently, Doris had to face squarely her intense feelings of grief and anxiety about the inevitable loss of "what had been." Once she acknowledged her pain, she was able to separate the very real physical issues of breast reduction surgery from her own emotional issues. Ultimately, this enabled her to be more supportive of her daughter's decision.

In some cases, a mother's wish to have her daughter's breasts operated on represents her desire to repair her own damaged self-image and lack of confidence about her breasts, a kind of vicarious fulfillment. Janet's mother, a large-breasted, 46-year-old, matronly woman named Joyce, started out the consultation by saying, "We're here because I don't want Janet to suffer the way I have all my life. I've had pain all my life in my neck, my back, my shoulders even bleed. I don't want Janet to go through all that."

I turned to Janet, a quiet, passive, obviously buxom 18-year-old, and asked, "How do *you* feel about your breasts?"

"They're okay," she shrugged.

"Do they cause you any pain or discomfort?"

"Not really, 'cept I can't exercise real well 'cause they flop up and down and they hurt."

"Anything else?" I pushed.

"Nope," she replied.

"Do you want to change them?"

"Well, my mother says I should—that I'll be sorry if I don't," she said.

"Janet doesn't know what she wants," Joyce interjected. "—but I do. I know what it's like later on . . ."

After speaking to Janet alone, I ascertained that Janet did have more symptomatology from her massive breasts than she was admitting in her mother's presence, but breast reduction was not high on her list of priorities. I gently explained to Joyce that *her* desire for her daughter's breast re-

duction was not shared by Janet and that Janet needed some time to make her own decision. I went on to say that Joyce seemed to be suffering herself (implying both physically and emotionally) and wondered if *she* had considered breast reduction.

Wife-Husband Issues

In my experience, the majority of husbands support their wives decisions to have breast reduction surgery; however, the operation challenges their capacity for change and adaptation. How husbands react to breast reduction depends, again, on the meaning of the breast to them; after all, they, too, suckled at their mother's breast. Their wives' breasts are fraught with symbolic emotional significance in addition to sexual significance.

One husband, Richard, who initially was overtly supportive of his wife Joan's wish for breast reduction surgery, became increasingly resistant as the operation drew near. He began to worry excessively about how he would run his shop without her for 2 weeks, even though another employee had agreed to take on the extra work. He refused to drive her to the hospital, saying he did not want to fight the traffic into and out of the city. As these signs of anxiety increased, I asked to see husband and wife again.

"I can't get along without her," Richard pleaded. "My business is still shaky and I just can't spare her." Upon further discussion, the symbolic meaning of Richard's words was evident: Richard's confidence was "shaky." He had always liked Joan's large breasts but agreed to go along with breast reduction surgery only because of her complaints of neck and lumbar pain, and the visible welts on her shoulders. His metaphoric language indicated that nestling in Joan's breasts was a source of comfort and security on which he depended. It gave him the confidence to face the world. Thus, "I can't get along without her" translates to "I don't know if I can get along without her big breasts." On an unconscious level, his wife's breasts symbolized the warmth and security of mother's breasts, which as we discussed earlier, are the very source of life for the infant. The imminent change represented a threat to his security and confidence, already shaken by financial and professional instability.

Recognizing the depth of Richard's dependency on his wife's breasts, I suggested that this might not be the best time for the operation. When Richard's business was more stable and he felt more confident about his future, I added, the couple should reschedule the operation. Joan was disappointed, but she concurred; intuitively, she understood his dilemma. It was not that his needs were more important, but his inability to deal with the operation at the time would have threatened a relationship they valued highly, thus jeopardizing Joan's longer-term adjustment and happiness.

Even when there is no overt resistance on the husband's part, the postoperative period calls on his ability to adapt. Men vary in their abilities to tend to the sick; in general, they are less used to the sight of blood than are women, with their monthly menstrual cycles. A husband's care-taking ability should be assessed and another person selected by the patient to assist with postoperative care if necessary.

After all is said and done, however, the couple is alone together in bed. How do the scars, the smaller size, and the different shape affect the man's sexual response? This depends on what associations a man brings to the old breast and the new scars. For some men, scars represent injury or illness; to others, they represent violence and mutilation. Many men are successful at selectively inattending to their wives' scars. "I don't even notice them," said one husband at his wife's 6-week postoperative visit. Their sexual life had resumed unchanged. In another case, however, Frank, a strong supporter of his wife's decision to have breast reduction, became impotent at the sight of the scars. They stirred up in him fantasies of violent mutilation, and, with images of blood and guts running through his head, he could not perform. Even when hidden in nightgowns or camisole tops, the scars bothered him. He became extremely agitated, as did his wife. Over time, however, the violent fantasies diminished in frequency and intensity, finally ceasing altogether. His sexual responsiveness returned within a 6-month period. Prolonged sexual dysfunction would have indicated the need for psychotherapeutic intervention.

Other reactions have been milder but constitute variations on a theme. Even as late as 6 months postoperatively, some partners still fear that touching the postoperative breast will hurt the woman, despite reassurances to the contrary. These men taught me to warn other spouses that after breast reduction surgery, their sexual respon-

siveness or the nature of the sexual experience may change but will usually return to normal over time.

Mothers and Children

Breast reduction surgery can also affect the patient's children, particularly those ages 1 to 6 years, prior to latency age. Children at this age tend to see themselves as the cause of all parental behavior; if the parent leaves or becomes unhappy, it is their fault. So, if a mother must leave home, go to a hospital — where sick people go — and then cannot hug or pick up the child during the early postoperative period, the child personalizes the problem. "Mommy went away because I did something bad; she went to a scary place and maybe she won't come back," says the child's mind. When the mother returns, the child thinks "Mommy isn't hugging me because I'm bad." Children need to be reassured from the outset that Mommy loves them very much, and that yes, she will go away for a few days but she will be back soon. After surgery, the child needs to know that Mommy wants to hug them more than anything, but her doctor said she cannot while she has a "boo-boo" on her breast.

In my opinion, young children should not be exposed to the sight of bloody dressings and early wound care changes because they already have mutilation fears regarding their own breasts — and this is true of boys and girls. One youngster ran crying and screaming from his mother's room. "A monster! A monster! A monster stabbed my mommy!" Pre- and postoperative instructions should include a few sentences of parental guidance about preparing children for the recovery period.

Societal Pressures

American society seems more obsessed with the breast than is any other culture. In the United States, the breast is the primary focus of a woman's feminine identification. The American media emphasizes the female breasts as symbols of sexuality and eroticism, often to the exclusion of other attributes. This breast mania encourages women to assess their desirability by the appearance of their breasts. Thus, the developing girl, no matter what her actual breast size and shape, interprets her own development also in terms of societal expectations. Generally, larger breasts are equated with greater femininity and greater sexual prowess. This perception is reflected in the "joking" comments of a colleague of mine, a male general surgeon who assists at breast reduction surgery. "Tsk, tsk, tsk—" he's quipped before many a case, "—another travesty."

Thus, to request breast reduction surgery is a courageous act, contraindicated by deeply ingrained societal admonitions. Since the need for physical and psychological relief is so great in good candidates for breast reduction, most patients do not have much internal struggle related to society's wishes and expectations. By the time they have made and *kept* a consultation appointment, pressure to remain large-breasted is usually a nonissue.

All plastic surgeons are well aware of the disagreeable social reactions experienced by large-breasted women. The most obvious is a lifetime of enduring obscene gestures and comments from strange men in the street. From an early age, there are subtle and not-so-subtle advances by "friends" of the family, relatives (including fathers), and fathers of peers. There is the embarrassment of undressing in front of other girls and feelings of inferiority stemming from being different. One patient, now a psychologist, remembers failing English in high school because she preferred to say she had not read the book rather than get up in front of the class to read a book report.

The majority of these women feel undervalued as people and resentful that they are admired more for the breasts that they bear than for any other characteristics they possess. TV star Loni Anderson once said, "Before my breast reduction, nobody ever talked to my face." Indeed, a well-controlled experimental study confirms that compared to small-breasted women, large-breasted women are perceived as being "relatively unintelligent, incompetent, immoral and immodest" [7]. Large-breasted women come to resent their breasts and dissociate from them. They perceive their breasts as separate entities that are the source of all their psychological pain. The attribution of all social and professional failure to their breasts is dangerous, because it can prevent a woman from addressing other weaknesses or developing her intellectual and personality strengths. They believe, instead, that all would be fine if it were not for their breasts. Although Goin et al [5] report that all three women in their study

who viewed their breasts as obstacles and handicaps external to themselves had no difficulty with postoperative adjustment, a number of these patients within my practice have experienced an initial euphoria followed gradually by disappointment and depression when all in their lives does not change. Interestingly, however, none of them has expressed regret about the operation. Still, it is prudent to point out gently to these patients that their change in breast size may reveal aspects of their physical selves that they had not expected to see (like a large abdomen previously hidden by the pendulous breasts), as well as aspects of their personalities unrelated to their breasts that may have been contributing to their unhappiness.

Although breast reduction patients are often the happiest patients postoperatively, there are psychological sequelae which, although transient, should be described to the patient *and family* preoperatively. In my opinion, they should be part of the preoperative and postoperative information and instructions given to the patient. The common postoperative sequelae that occur immediately after surgery have been eloquently described by Goin et al. [5]. Mourning for the lost body part is not uncommon. One of my patients, Rita, who was of native American origin, requested that she be given the resected breast tissue for proper burial. Body image disturbances also occur. In my patients, these have been manifested by phantom sensations of the breasts as they were previously, or feelings of transient depersonalization ("I'm not me anymore").

One interesting case involves a patient who at first seemed to me to be describing body image disturbance. As I discovered, she was using the same words to describe a problem of a different nature. Nancy told me 3 months after surgery that she had been wearing her bra all the time, even to bed. "I'm afraid to go without a bra," she said. "I need the support." On the face of it, this statement would seem to require only an explanation and reassurance regarding her fear of the original ptosis returning. However, the question "Support in what way?" offered a glimpse of a deeper anxiety.

"I'm afraid I'll fall apart," she said.

Again, there is a tendency to interpret these words to mean "I'm afraid my incisions will open up," but, refusing to *assume* anything, I asked, "Fall apart how?"

With this question she dissolved in tears. "My

husband and my brother had a bad fight 3 weeks ago and I haven't seen my brother since then. He's always been my closest friend — my biggest supporter." Finally, everything was clear. The support of the bra was being used symbolically as a substitute for the lost psychological support from her brother. Without "support," she feared all would "fall apart." Interestingly, if we further recognize that the bra supports the breast — the primitive symbol of life and the world to the infant, then the bra is capable of supporting her life or her world. Having gotten to the bottom of this anxiety, which anyone can do by being sensitive and keeping certain interview guidelines in mind, I could empathize with her dilemma and suggest ways for her to deal with it. Undoubtedly, her breast surgery made her feel more vulnerable to the impact of the loss, but the precipitating factor behind her compulsive need for the bra was an interpersonal one. Only when Nancy addressed the interpersonal problem would her emotional pressure be relieved.

Practical Suggestions: The Interview

Because of time and financial pressure and a desire for action rather than talk, many plastic surgeons have reduced the amount of time reserved for evaluation and postoperative attention. Most of us have become proficient in describing the appropriate technical details together with the risks and benefits in a very short period of time. Many of us believe that the rest is the patient's concern. This attitude arises in part from the fact that we have been trained as authorities who know what is best; therefore, we do not have to listen to the patient. We see ourselves as specialists in our technical field, and indeed, this is our only domain of professionally acknowledged expertise.

This tendency to focus on the technical details of an operation to the exclusion of the life context in which it will occur also reflects the personality and perceptual style of the surgeon — his or her way of viewing the world [2, 9]. There are two major types of perceptual style: the field-*independent* style and the field-*dependent* style. The field-independent style, most characteristic of the male in Western society, tends to focus on the small details of a complex configuration, as though the meaning of each object is *independent* of the context. The field-dependent style, more frequently characteristic of women, focuses on taking in and understanding the entire configuration and the relationship of its parts. The unconscious assumption is that the meaning of a part is *dependent* on its relationship to other parts and to the whole. The field-independent person would be exceedingly effective finding the needle in the haystack; the field-dependent person might wonder if it is worth looking for it at all.

This difference in perceptual style between the sexes can lead to confusion and misunderstanding. Because each may focus on different aspects of a shared experience, either person may become frustrated with the other's style. To many men, women are "diffuse," "scatter-brained," or "spacy," while many women find men "unaware," "narrow-minded," or "incapable of understanding."

What does this all have to do with breast reduction surgery? The characteristically field-independent male plastic surgeon, sitting across the desk from the primarily field-dependent patient, has a different view of the reality of the situation before a word has been spoken. He will focus on the risks and benefits of the procedure, the technical details, and the size and shape of the breast. If well trained, he will extend attention to total body habitus, balance, and proportion. She, on the other hand, may be viewing the issue of breast reduction within the larger context of her life situation. To her, the discrete detail — the breast — has its meaning in the context of an entire constellation of intrapersonal and interpersonal relationships; its meaning depends on her entire field of related physical and emotional experiences. The focusing only on the discrete detail (the breast) by the surgeon, to the exclusion of the relational/emotional meaning of that detail, can be interpreted by the patient as a failure to "understand."

Another factor contributing to unsatisfactory communication is that most plastic surgeons, male and female, have not been trained to deal with emotional issues in either their personal or professional lives. They are natural action-oriented rescuers. At the site of a damsel in distress — crying, angry, or disappointed, either pre- or postoperatively — they feel helpless. For most, this is an uncomfortable and often-denied reaction. There are several ineffective defensive responses in these situations: The physician may attempt to placate or console the patient by mainly irrelevant expressions of reassurance, such as "there, there." He or she may play the white knight and jump to action with an attempt at reoperation "to make everything OK." Or, the surgeon may adopt a totally defensive posture, implying or stating that the problem comes from the patient's healing, and not the doctor's handiwork. Because of the fear of eliciting emotional reactions, many surgeons stick to details, leaving contextual issues untouched.

We have all experienced unsatisfactory and frustrating patient-doctor interactions. It seems to me that there are some steps that can be taken to use the interview time efficiently while also improving communications. I do not suggest that we intrude recklessly into patient's lives as voyeurs; I do suggest that we take a few moments to determine carefully whether operation is in the patient's best interest from the standpoint of his or her life.

I believe it is wise to listen carefully to the patient's verbal messages on both the descriptive and metaphorical level, and to note body language. There are often key words that tip us off to strongly affective unconscious ties; these can vary from the joltingly harsh to the slightly inappropriate. Phrases such as "I *hate* my breasts," "I want these things *hacked* off," or "She would *kill* me if she knew" invite cautious and gentle further inquiry. The question "In what way do you hate your breasts?" or "*How* do you hate your breasts?" elicits much more information than "*Why* do you hate your breasts?" or "*Why* do you want to hack them off?" The term *why* suggests that you are judging the patient's point of view or asking her to justify her point of view rather than explicate it. Never assume that you already know the answer. You do not. The famous psychologist Gordon Allport [1] once gave this simple but profound advice to his students: "If you want to know how a patient feels about something, ask him."

If a woman with massive, pendulous breasts were sitting in front of you (the plastic surgeon) and she said, "I hate my breasts," you might think, "Yeah, I can understand that. I'd hate to have those ugly, heavy things on my chest." Upon further inquiry, you might be surprised to find out that the woman hates them because her husband taunts her about them. She may actually accept and even like her breasts and is turning to surgery to solve a marital problem — not a sound expectation for breast reduction surgery.

I act ignorant when first interviewing a patient because I really do not know anything consequential about a patient at an initial interview. It is interesting how we as surgeons learn quickly not to assume anything during operations; we learn immediately the dire consequences. There is nothing like the sudden surge of arterial blood flooding the surgical field to teach us not to *assume*. Our general surgery and plastic surgery training have effectively disciplined us to probe carefully and dissect gently to learn the whereabouts of a structure. Yet, we often cavalierly interpret the words of a patient, spouse, or friend to fit our preconceived ideas instead of probing to learn what the speaker means. Patients do say what they mean and usually mean what they say; our mistake is often not encouraging them to say more so that *we* can understand what they mean.

In many instances, a quick, simple question has saved the day — for example, Nancy, who "needed the support" of her bra and was afraid she'd "fall apart." My impulse to interpret on the descriptive level — that Nancy was concerned about her incisions coming apart without a bra — "made sense"; however, had I taken her assertions at face value I would have missed the point. I never would have been able to help the patient relieve her tension and the compulsive behavior driven by it. The simple questions "Support in what way?" and "How do you feel you're going to fall apart?" elicited the deeper meaning of what the patient was saying. It took all of 3 minutes. In the case of Richard, who pleaded "I can't get along without her," at face value his words referred to his need for help in the shop; again, this misses the point. When I asked, "In what way can't you get along without her?" his answer revealed the depth and extent of his current dependency on her and the meaning of her large breasts to him. Within the context of their relationship, his psychological need contraindicated the surgery at that time. Again, our discussion took all of 5 minutes to arrive at this conclusion. Playing dumb, as we plastic surgeons are about the patient's life, and phrasing follow-up questions with "In what way do you . . ." or "how do you mean . . ." often rapidly sheds light on the dynamic process behind the emotionally loaded words or statement.

Establishing Rapport

The essence of rapport is the feeling of being heard, understood, and taken seriously. Rapport can rapidly be established by inviting the patient into the consultation with a question such as "Tell me about what you don't like about your breasts." Listen astutely; I *look* at the patient while she is talking: this reflects attentiveness. Even if I do not absolutely need to, I take a few notes so that she knows that she is being taken seriously. Then, I generally ask, "What do you know about breast reduction?" This allows me to begin the interview at the patient's level of knowledge and sophistication. This saves time, but more important, the patient realizes I am tailoring the consultation to her — another way of letting her know I respect her and her needs. This allows the patient and significant others, if present, to become gradually more comfortable, which in turn makes them more likely to be open in answering further questions.

I notice the patient's nonverbal or body language: How is she presenting herself to me? Is she sitting with arms defensively crossed in front of her, or partially turned away from me, or squarely in front of me, arms at the side, "open?" Does she shake her head "no" while answering "yes" to a question? If so, I feed that information back to the patient by saying something like "You seem unsure about that — at the same time you were saying you wanted it, you were shaking your head 'no.'" The patient may agree, or she may be totally surprised; she may even become argumentative. In either case, she will be gratified that you took the time and care to notice such details of communication. For you, the surgeon, her response — whether open, defensive, or belligerent — will be a tip-off to the presence of potential area of conflict for the patient and will give you information about how she will or will not work with you.

After explaining risks, I ask the patient and others how they feel about what they have heard and inquire what fears they have about the operation. I follow up their responses with questions designed to get to the real meaning of their words, questions such as "In what way . . . " or "How do you imagine . . . " For example, a patient says, "I'm afraid I'll die." I say, "Die? In what way?" Granted, I feel like an idiot; after all, dying is dying. Yet, I have heard a wide range of responses to such a question: "My father died during an operation when I was 10 and I've been terrified ever since" (anxiety based on history); or "My mother always said she would kill me if I got rid of the family chest" (intrapersonal conflict); or "My husband threatened to divorce me if I do this, and I'd die without him" (interpersonal conflict). The

anxiety based on history is the only case in which standard statistical-type reassurance may be helpful; the other answers require empathy and referral to a competent counselor for conflict resolution prior to surgery.

Preparing the Patient for Psychological Sequelae of Operations

Goin et al. [5] emphasize how helpful it is to advise patients in advance of the kinds of psychological phenomena they may experience after operations. This will smooth the postoperative experience and reduce anxiety and consequent pain. It will also reduce the number of postoperative telephone calls to the office. It is helpful to repeat these advisories throughout the pre- and postoperative sessions, because patients often do not hear them the first or even the second time. The following is a list of psychological sequelae I advise patients about:

1. Prior to your operation, you may feel increasingly apprehensive about the aesthetics of the result, about pain, and even about the risk of dying. This is normal, but if you or your spouse (or parents) become overly anxious about these issues, please make an appointment to discuss these matters.
2. After the operation, you need not look at your breasts until you are ready. You have permission to look without seeing. Your breasts will be swollen, black and blue, and sometimes misshapen. Do not spend a moment worrying about size or shape issues; the swelling, bleeding and discoloration go away with time. Only at the end of 3 to 6 weeks will you have some idea of what the final result will look like.*
3. After the operation, it is normal to experience depression and mourning for the part of your body that is gone. Some people have periods of depression alternating with elation. Sometimes you may feel, "Where have I gone? I'm not me anymore." This, too, is normal. Both mourning and depression may last several days, or inter-

---

* I advise patients to remove dressings and bra and shower 1 to 2 days after surgery, then replace a few 4 × 4 dressings as needed, and the bra. Follow-up examinations are frequent enough that I can determine whether complications are occurring.

mittently for a few weeks. Gradually, you will feel better and more like your old self.

4. You will have some pain, but you will also have as much pain medication as you need. Please take them liberally, as directed; that is what pain pills are for. You will not become addicted to them during the short period that you will need them.

5. You may experience strange sensations in your breasts. You may become anxious either that they are completely gone or that they are still overly large. This is normal and these sensations will subside in a short period of time as your body adjusts.

6. You may feel apprehension about how you will react and feel during your first postoperative sexual encounter. You may be worried about change of sensation and ability to be aroused. I suggest that you refrain from sexual manipulation of your breasts for at least 6 weeks; at that time, all usually goes well and improves as time goes on. The most important sexual organ lies between your ears — the brain. It will function well — trust it.

7. You may worry about your partner's sexual response. Rarely is this a problem. Sometimes men can experience impotence or relative impotence; sometimes they are fearful of touching your breasts lest they hurt you. These transient problems are *theirs*, not *yours*. With tenderness, communication, and understanding, they usually resolve themselves over time.

8. If you have children, tell them beforehand what will be happening. They do not need the exact surgical details, but young children need assurances that you will be fine and that you love them. They need to know that your disappearance for a few days and your subsequent inability to pick them up or hug them has nothing to do with a change in feeling toward them. A good way to put this is, "I have a little problem" — or "boo-boo" or whatever language you use for injury — "and the doctor says I have to be in the hospital Monday, Tuesday, and Wednesday,"

for example. "I'll be back to love you just like I do now, but the doctor says I won't be able to hug you close or pick you up right away because of the boo-boo. But I'll still love you and think you're the best girl or boy, and soon we'll be able to play and hug again." Repeat these assurances several times before your surgery and many times during the early postoperative period.

Young children should not be exposed to bloody dressings or dressing changes. This can only add to the anxieties they already have.

The psychological impact of what we as plastic surgeons do more often than not is positive, both for the patient and the surgeon. Focusing further on the intrapersonal and interpersonal issues of our patients and learning more about the interactive process between us and our patients can only enhance our effectiveness.

References

1. Allport, G.H. Personal communication, 1965.
2. Elkind, D., Koegler, R., and Go, E. Field independence and concept formation. *Percept. Mot. Skills* 17:383, 1963.
3. Elmhurst, S.I. The Early Stages of Female Psychosexual Development. In M. Kirkpatrick (ed.), *Women's Sexual Development.* New York: Plenum, 1980. Pp. 107–126.
4. Gifford, S. Emotional Attitudes Toward Cosmetic Breast Surgery: Loss and Restitution of the "Ideal Self." In R.M. Goldwyn (ed.), *Plastic and Reconstructive Surgery of the Breast.* Boston: Little, Brown, 1976. Pp. 103–122.
5. Goin, K., Goin, J., and Gianini, H. The psychic consequences of a reduction mammoplasty. *Plast. Reconst. Surg.* 59:533, 1977.
6. Klein, M. The Oedipus Complex in the Light of Early Anxieties. In E. Jones (ed.), *Contributions to Psychoanalysis 1921–1945.* London: Hogarth, 1948.
7. Kleinke, C.L., and Staneski, R.A. First impressions of female bust size. *J. Soc. Psych.* 110:123, 1980.
8. LaBarre, W. Personality from a Psychoanalytic Viewpoint. In E. Norbeck, D. Price-Williams, and W. McCord (eds.), *The Study of Personality.* New York: Holt, Rinehart, & Winston, 1968. Pp. 65–87.
9. Shapiro, D. *Neurotic Styles.* New York: Basic Books, 1965.

COMMENTS ON CHAPTER 6   *Robert M. Goldwyn*

Although most plastic surgeons lack the psychological training of Cline and are not likely to possess her insight and sensitivity, all of us can make the attempt to understand the patient as an individual as well as her motivations for seeking reduction mammaplasty. This process takes time, no matter how astute the surgeon. A thorough, satisfying, and successful initial consultation is not apt to take place when the surgeon is rushed and tired or has already decided to operate because of his or her belief that the psyche is an extraneous part of a patient or because his or her reputation, ambition, pride, or financial needs compel an operation on demand. Fortunately for the patient and our specialty, most plastic surgeons are caring doctors and want to know their patients and give them the result that they expect. However, the stresses resulting from an overbooked day can lead to careless shortcuts that ultimately cost the surgeon and the patient more time and aggravation later. Because most patients who come to the plastic surgeon expect an operation and a very high proportion receive it, most plastic surgeons are too treatment-oriented sometimes to the exclusion of larger considerations of personality, interrelationships, and motivation.

My experience jibes with that of Cline: Most women one sees for reduction mammaplasty are stable emotionally. Their large breasts are an encumbrance physically, emotionally, and socially. The large size of their breasts has decreased their self-esteem and has adversely affected their view of themselves as much as it has distorted others' perception of them.

I need not recapitulate what Cline has already written about the initial interview. I would like to add for emphasis, however, that the surgeon and the patient should have discussed in detail the breast size that the woman expects as a result of her operation. At the request of plastic surgeons' attorneys, I have read too many records that lack mention of this discussion and, as a consequence, the surgeon was held responsible for not providing adequate information for a proper informed consent.

Under no circumstances, however, should the surgeon *promise* a specific cup size. I usually tell patients something like: "I know what you want

and I'll do my best to give it to you but it is difficult, if not impossible, to guarantee that your breast size will be a large B and not a small or medium C. At operation, even when we set you up, it is difficult to predict the ultimate size that you will be because of the swelling from the surgery and also because we do not know exactly how you will heal, how your skin and breast tissue will shrink and come together. That is unpredictable."

Immediately prior to operation, with the patient sitting or standing, and *not medicated*, I ask the patient again about the size that she wishes. Frequently the patient has changed her mind. Often, in fact, she may call the office to discuss the matter again or she may write a letter. The surgeon should be more than willing to see the patient once more to resolve any ambiguity that the patient may have or that the surgeon may have about this vital matter.

Cline, being female, is less likely to be accused wrongly of unprofessional conduct in the examination of a female patient than would a male plastic surgeon. For this reason, I, as a male, never examine a patient initially without a female staff member present. It is much easier to have a chaperone present than to protest one's innocence later.

Although most patients for reduction mammaplasty have well-integrated personalities, many of them will experience a transient, mild depression immediately after operation. The change in a patient's body image may be profound as may be also the social consequences of this physical transformation. The once obese, large-breasted woman now realizes that she must lose weight to remain in proportion. Furthermore, she cannot cite her macromastia as an excuse for her unwillingness to exercise. More has happened to her than simply a reduction of her breast size. Her intimates, especially her parents if she is a teenager, have higher expectations of her performance socially and academically. They may wrongly anticipate that she will immediately diet, quickly find new friends, and rapidly become a star student. For most patients, life does improve but certainly not at once and not in every aspect simultaneously.

Cline has given excellent advice about warning some patients concerning the possible dip in their emotions postoperatively. The important point is that the surgeon has spent the time with the patient prior to operation, has gotten to know her, and, after operation, must be available and not regard the patient's depression along with her tears as a lack of appreciation for his or her surgical efforts that might have been splendid, indeed. The problem is a personal one — more so for the patient and much less so for the surgeon. The worst reaction on the part of the surgeon is to become angry at what he or she perceives to be ingratitude or to become distant, either not returning a telephone call or not seeing the patient frequently in the office or by handing off the patient to one of the office staff to manage the psychological problems. It is not necessary in most instances to resort to a psychotherapist. The surgeon can usually do the job, but if the patient is not responding, one should not avoid a consultation with a psychiatrist. The most difficult part but the most simple for the surgeon is simply spending more time with the patient, being empathetic with her, giving her reassurance by saying that this type of depression is well known and almost always passes in a few weeks. Both the patient and the surgeon will do better if the surgeon and the patient have established good rapport prior to the operation. "Getting to know you" is best done leisurely at the initial consultation and not urgently after the operation.

7

Saul Hoffman

Medicolegal Aspects of Reduction Mammaplasty

"The nature of surgery for breast reduction, with all its attendant risks, makes it a fertile field for complications, beyond which, moreover, there lies a vast minefield of potential errors that are hazards to the unwary surgeon"[15].

Paul K. McKissock

Approximately 40,000 reduction mammaplasties are done in the United States every year. Although the majority of these patients appear to be satisfied with the results, many are not, and some are unhappy enough to begin a malpractice suit against the plastic surgeon (Fig. 7-1)[10, 11].

Most publications on reduction mammaplasty have dealt with technical details. This chapter addresses the medicolegal problems that may result from this operation. Risk management, including the issue of informed consent, is discussed.

Survey of the American Society of Plastic and Reconstructive Surgeons

To determine the extent of the problem, a questionnaire was sent to all members of the American Society of Plastic and Reconstructive Surgeons (ASPRS) (Fig. 7-2). Thirty-eight percent of the members responded. Since a 10 percent sample is normally a valid statistical indication for the total population sampled, it can be concluded that the 38 percent response rate for the survey is both valid and representative of the total ASPRS membership. In addition, the records of 50 cases of reduction mammaplasties involved in litigation were reviewed and analyzed (Table 7-1).

Eleven percent of the responding surgeons stated that a malpractice suit had been precipitated by a reduction mammaplasty patient. As expected, the majority of the dissatisfied patients were unhappy with their scars. Other less common sources of dissatisfaction were asymmetry, nipple position, loss of sensation, and pain (Table 7-1).

The following are some representative comments from the plastic surgeons responding to the questionnaire.

"Scar hypertrophy remains a problem."

"This has been the surgical procedure I have seen most often in malpractice medical review panel proceedings against plastic surgeons."

"No patients dissatisfied."

"I know of no other procedure which results in as many pleased patients."

"Happiest patients in my practice."

"I do many scar revisions in these patients."

"As a lawyer, I see ten or more bad results per month."

"I only do patients with real macromastia — watch out for mastopexy patients."

"I have had fewer complications and much improved patient satisfaction since performing this procedure by a free nipple graft technique."

"I do a two-stage reduction to reduce the medial extension of the scars."

"I use very detailed consent forms."

"Proper patient selection and counselling is important for a good result."

"One case with nipples too close together postoperatively. The nipples were repositioned, scars resulted, and the patient sued."

"Patient wanted me to pay for her revision by another surgeon."

"This is a lousy operation with predictable complications."

"High satisfaction rate. I let them see scars of previous

Fig. 7-1. Letter from a plastic surgeon.

18 Jan 88

Dear Dr. Hoffman

Would you please send me a reprint of Reduction Mammoplasty: A Medicolegal Hazard?

I performed 3 yrs ago a reduction on a 18 girl (w). First visit, I told her and her mother I wouldn't do a reduction on a young female because of the large scars it left on the breasts, etc. They came back a few weeks later and begged for the surgery — she said she couldn't live with the huge breasts anymore. I performed the surgery with a good result; with wider horizontal and end hypertrophied scars. I advised revision, etc; but, saw a lawyer and started a suit.

In your research — any advice for defense? Thanking you in advance.

Yours truly,

patients. I turn down 30 – 35% of these patients because of obesity or poor expectations."

"I have revised several cases where the nipples were too high."

"One lawsuit from a cautery burn which resulted in hypertrophic scarring."

"One suit after nipple loss."

"I tell patients they will probably need a touch-up procedure, for which I do not charge them."

"100% satisfaction."

"Two preoperative visits include husband or boyfriend — extensive informed consent."

"I have more trials and tribulations with this operation than any other."

"Beware the young single patient."

"I do not do reduction mammaplasties any longer! I think they are the leading cause of malpractice suits. I review three to four cases per year for defense attorneys."

"Best operation I do."

"I think this procedure is intrinsically incapable of producing the results many patients expect. They are regarded as a cosmetic procedure despite any explanation to the contrary. Given the present liability climate, it is a very risky procedure and I avoid doing it whenever possible."

"Biggest problem is in doing it at too early an age."

"I am surprised that reduction mammaplasty is a source of litigation for other surgeons. These are my happiest group of patients."

"I have seen several patients who are suing other doctors because of malpositioned nipples."

"One suit based on loss of sensation, the other on scarring."

"Avoid operating on smokers."

"I won't do this procedure."

"Best procedure I do."

Risk Management

In spite of good medical care, complications and unsatisfactory results will occur and may lead to a lawsuit. Risk management involves an awareness of the potential medicolegal problems and taking steps to prevent them.

INFORMED CONSENT

A patient has the right to be fully informed about the realities, risks, complications, and alternatives to a proposed treatment or surgical procedure before deciding whether or not to submit to it [20]. Although few plastic surgeons would disagree with this statement, there are many issues regarding informed consent that remain unsettled [2].

Many of the respondents to the questionnaire mentioned that they were careful to inform their patients about the scars and other problems that might occur. Seventy-six percent of them used a standard consent form (Fig. 7-3). It is important to realize that these forms by themselves, however, are almost useless since they do not inform (patients usually claim not to have understood or read them). When used, they must be supplemented with an in-depth discussion of the operation, attendant risks, and possible complications. The surgeon must open up a line of communication with his or her patient by spending adequate time with her and making certain that she understands the procedure. Although proper informed consent is important in prophylaxis against a malpractice action, it should not be viewed as a means of protecting oneself but as an opportunity to establish rapport with the patient. "Ethically valid consent is a process of shared decision making (between physician and patient), based on mutual respect

Dear Colleague:

We are attempting to obtain information on the frequency of malpractice actions by patients who have undergone reduction mammaplasty. By analyzing this data it may be possible to reduce the risk of being sued for this procedure. Please take a moment to answer the enclosed questionnaire as accurately as possible.

Thank you.
Saul Hoffman, MD
New York, NY

This independent survey is being printed, mailed and tabulated by Plastic Surgery Management Services, Inc., a subsidary of the American Society of Plastic and Reconstructive Surgeons, 233 N. Michigan Avenue, Suite 1900, Chicago, Illinois 60601.

Questionnaire (Note: Numbers in parenthesis are for tabulating purposes only).

1. How many reduction mammaplasties do you perform (10) annually? _____

2. Reduction mammaplasty cases account for approximately (20) _____ % of the surgical procedures I perform annually.

3. What procedure do you prefer?   (30) _____

4. Do you show photographs to your patients preoperatively?
   (40) _____ no   (50) _____ Yes

5. If yes, do you show photographs
   (60) _____   a) of your own patients
   (70) _____   b) from journals, textbooks
   (80) _____   c) other _____

6. Do you use the Breast Reduction brochure published by ASPRS to explain the surgery to patients?
   (90) _____ yes   (100) _____ no

7. Do you use a standard informed consent form?
   (110) _____ yes   (120) _____ no

8. Have any cases of reduction mammaplasty precipitated a malpractice action against you?
   (130) _____ yes   (140) _____ no
   If yes, how many?   (150) _____

9. Please estimate the total percentage of patients who were dissatisfied with their results compared to the total number of reduction mammaplasties you have ever performed.
   (160) _____ %

10. Of those patients who were dissatisfied, what was the source of dissatisfaction? Please give percentages.
    (170) _____ % a) scars
    (180) _____ % b) asymmetry
    (190) _____ % c) nipple position
    (200) _____ % d) sensation
    (210) _____ % e) other _____

11. Of those patients who were dissatisfied, how many have you revised?   (220) _____

Comments _____ _____

_____

_____

(230)

Please refold this questionnaire with Plastic Surgery Management Services as return addresse, staple, stamp and mail. Thank you.

Fig. 7-2. Questionnaire.

Table 7-1. Complaints (50 patients)

Scars	43
Asymmetry	11
Size — 2 too small	5
— 3 too large	
Nipple loss — 2 complete	8
— 6 partial	
Nipple sensation	3
Nipples "too high"	6
Inverted nipples	2

and participation, not a ritual to be equated with reciting the contents of a form that details the risk of particular treatments" [25]. In addition, patients who are well informed experience less anxiety and show greater satisfaction with the results of their surgery [1, 4, 5, 14, 21] and even less pain [6].

Several studies have shown, however, that patients do not retain most of the information given to them [12, 22]. Leeb et al [12] found an overall retention rate of 25 percent in a series of 100 patients in the general plastic surgery population. Many surgeons reinforce their verbal discussions with written materials, such as photographs and videotapes, to improve patient recall and enhance understanding. It is a mistake, however, to depend solely on these materials to inform the patient. Goldwyn [9] believes that printed information helps to educate the patient and helps her to remember things discussed during the consultation. Medicolegally, it may prove to be helpful since the surgeon can record what information was given. Goldwyn shows several examples of patient information sheets in his book *The Patient and the Plastic Surgeon.*

Many patients deny the possibility of complications, even when told repeatedly [8]. We must therefore document what the patient has been told. If a lawsuit should occur, written documentation will support the surgeon's testimony that proper informed consent was given. Some surgeons will use audiotapes or videotapes to document informed consent. This may be good protection but is probably not necessary in all but the most complex cases. Also, it may undermine the doctor-patient relationship.

The courts have agreed that it is not necessary to spell out every possible complication; only those that are common or serious should be mentioned. There may be some disagreement as to which com-

plications should be discussed. Is it necessary, for instance, to discuss the possible loss of a nipple? This complication occurs rarely, and mentioning it might discourage a patient who otherwise would benefit from this procedure. Personally, although I discuss possible problems with wound healing, in general I do not specifically mention possible loss of a nipple.

Since scarring is the most significant sequela that affects the aesthetics of our final result, it is imperative that patients understand the nature of the scars. Photographs that demonstrate a range of results can be helpful since most women are not aware of the appearance of mammaplasty scars. Goin [7] states that showing photographs to patients in a preoperative consultation can be useful to diminish, rather than enhance, the patient's expectations. Some patients will accept the scarring more readily than others. In general, as would be expected, younger single women are the least tolerant. Most women would gladly trade markedly enlarged, symptomatic breasts for smaller and more shapely ones, even though scarred. With a clear understanding of the procedure and realistic expectations, they will be happy.

Financial considerations are important to most patients, who should also know exactly how much the operation will cost. Any unexpected charges might produce a hardship that could lead to dissatisfaction, finding fault with the surgery, and even consultation with an attorney. It is imperative, therefore, to discuss costs, including those incurred when revisions are necessary. There must be a clear understanding of the policy for charging for secondary surgery.

When Complications Occur

Preparing a patient for possible complications should begin with the initial discussion. Those who are properly informed cope better with complications [6]. The common complications should be mentioned as part of the informed consent, including what to expect if a complication occurs, how it will be managed, and how it will limit the final result. Patients with hypertrophic scars have told me that although they were disappointed, they had been warned of the possibility of such scars and were willing to accept them. Others have said that their surgeons told them that the scars would be "practically invisible" or "a thin white line." These women tend to be angry at their surgeons. Several patients have stated that if they had

Procedure: REDUCTION MAMMAPLASTY

You and your doctor are considering an operation on one or both of your breasts to alter the size, position, and appearance of the breast(s). The operation is called a reduction mammaplasty and involves surgical cuts on one or both breasts. The operation is not an emergency, nor is it usually necessary to improve or protect the physical health of the patient. Although complications from this type of surgery are uncommon, they do sometimes occur. It is possible that this operation will not help you. It is even possible that you will be worse after the operation than you are now. Your doctor can make no guarantee as to the results that might be obtained from this surgery.

Some of the possible complications of reduction mammaplasty are:

Bleeding; infection; fluid collections in the breasts; erosion, sloughing, and damage to the skin and nipples of the breasts; alterations in the milk production of the breasts; lack of symmetry of the breasts (they don't look alike); swelling and congestion of the breasts; decreased nipple sensation; personality changes and mental difficulties following the surgery, sometimes occurring even when there is a good cosmetic result; and allergic or other bad reactions to one or more of the substances used during the course of the procedure.

Some of the complications of reduction mammaplasty can cause the need for further surgery; some of the complications can cause permanent deformity, unsightly and painful scarring, and prolonged illness; very rarely, some of the complications can even cause death. Furthermore, there are alternatives to this surgery available to you, such as merely accepting your present status of losing weight.

ADDITIONAL RISKS AND ALTERNATIVES: _____
(To be filled in here and on reverse side
by doctor as necessary)   _____

                                       _____

I CERTIFY: I have read or had read to me the contents of this form; I understand the risks and alternatives involved in this procedure; I have had the opportunity to ask any questions which I had and all of my questions have been answered.

DATE: _____ TIME: _____ SIGNED:_____
                                                          (Signed by patient or person legally
                                                          authorized to consent for patient)

WITNESS: _____ PHYSICIAN: _____
(A GENERAL CONSENT FORM MUST ALSO BE SIGNED BY THE PATIENT.)   (Signed by physician)

Prepared by In-Forms No. 1123

Fig. 7-3. Typical consent form. (Published by and used with permission of In-Forms, Albuquerque, NM.)

known what the scars would look like, they would not have had the operation (Figs. 7-4 and 7-5).

Fifty unhappy patients were questioned about the reason for their complaints (Table 7-1). Forty-three of them were concerned with their scars. The next most common complaint was asymmetry, which occurred in 11 cases. Most women do have some asymmetry, which should be brought to their attention preoperatively. It should be made clear that symmetry is often not possible to obtain. Careful preoperative evaluation and marking will avoid gross asymmetry and malpositioned nipples (see Case 1). A 20 percent solution of silver nitrate will leave a mark for up to 10 days that cannot be washed off. Markings can therefore be applied prior to admission to the hospital. Photographs should be available for viewing in the operating room to remind the surgeon of the preoperative appearance. The amounts to be resected from each breast are estimated, and the specimens are weighed in the operating room to ensure adequate reduction. When the resection has been completed, temporary sutures or staples approximate the wound edges, and the patient is placed in a sitting position [13, 24]. This allows the surgeon to evaluate the size, symmetry, and nipple position.

Loss of nipple sensation was a complaint in 3 of the 50 cases. If the patients are warned about this possibility preoperatively, it does not usually present a problem. Sensation can usually be preserved by avoiding the transection of the third and fourth intercostal nerves. The inferior pedicle technique preserves sensation in the majority of cases.

Nipple inversion was a more common complaint with the lateral pedicle technique (Strömbeck), occurring when there is too much pull on the pedicle. Supporting the nipple with dermis peripherally will usually prevent this problem. Secondary correction by releasing the pedicle may be necessary.

A common problem that is difficult to correct and can occur with all types of reduction mammaplasties is "bottoming out" (Fig. 7-6) [18, 23]. This places the nipple too high in relation to the breast mound. Several important steps in the procedure will help to prevent this problem: (1) Careful preoperative marking and location of the new nipple position (at the inframammary fold or slightly lower in markedly pendulous breasts) (Fig. 7-7A,B); (2) sitting the patient up in the operating room before determining the final nipple position

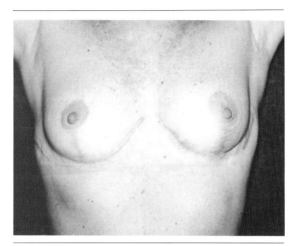

Fig. 7-4. A 39-year-old woman 2 years following mammaplasty. Several steroid injections had been administered. This patient was upset by the medial and lateral extensions of the scars, which were visible in a bathing suit.

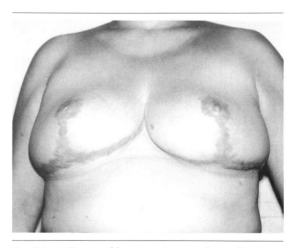

Fig. 7-5. A 50-year-old woman 5 years after reduction mammaplasty. Three thousand grams of tissue was removed. She was relieved of her symptoms and satisfied with the results of the operation.

(Fig. 7-7C); (3) keeping the nipple to inframammary fold distance less than 7 cm; and (4) adequate reduction. McKissock [16] states that the most effective prophylactic maneuver to combat loss of shape is to reduce the breast adequately.

We have found the inferior pedicle and the McKissock procedures to be the most versatile and complication-free. Eighty percent of the people responding to the questionnaire used one of these techniques. A surgeon should not be a slave to one method, however. Amputation and free grafting is an excellent technique to reduce large breasts in older women (Fig. 7-8). Nipple loss is rare, and some sensation usually returns with time.

Several procedures to shorten the inframammary scar have recently been reported and seem effective for slight to moderate hypertrophy [3, 17, 19]. Reducing the length of the inframammary fold scar will be helpful in preventing patient dissatisfaction.

Case Reports

CASE 1

A 22-year-old woman consulted a plastic surgeon complaining of excessively large breasts since the age of 15. Her breasts became even larger after a pregnancy; she began to experience back and shoulder pain. A reduction mammaplasty was recommended and she was scheduled for surgery.

Postoperatively, she was pleased with the size and shape of her breasts and expressed gratitude in a note to her surgeon. Subsequently, it was observed that her nipples were too high and could be seen above her brassiere.

Corrective surgery was performed to lower the nipples, but this process resulted in considerable scarring of the upper portion of the breasts. Scar revisions were carried out on two occasions by another surgeon, with some improvement (Fig. 7-9).

The patient was unhappy about the need for two additional operations and the resultant scars, which were visible when she wore a bathing suit or low-cut dress. A settlement of $25,000 was offered but refused, and the plaintiff eventually lost the case.

The patient expected to have inconspicuous scars on the undersurface of her breasts but instead ended up with severe scarring above the nipples. This case does not involve informed consent because in the normal course of events, one would not expect scarring above the nipples. Excess or unusual scarring will lead to an unhappy patient. If the scarring occurs as a result of a complication, such as infection or hematoma, it would not be considered malpractice. In this case, however, a technical error was probably responsible for the poor result.

The patient stated that preoperative marking was not done. The surgeon claimed that the breasts were marked preoperatively in the operating room. Attempting to mark a patient in the operating room while she is under sedation and propped up does not allow for accuracy. It is preferable to do the marking with the patient in the standing or sitting position with her full cooperation. There is no substitute for careful, unhurried preoperative planning.

In the past, it was not uncommon to see the nipples located too high after a reduction mammaplasty. This result was due in part to insufficient consideration of postoperative changes that cause the mammary gland to descend so that the nipple assumes a high position relative to the breast. In addition, placing the nipple at a given distance from the clavicle without considering the position of the inframammary fold can result in malposition of the nipple.

Allowances must be made in the overly large breast for the elasticity of the remaining skin, which causes a shortening effect after the excess weight is removed. The nipple in these cases should be placed slightly lower than the inframammary fold. Despite all of these precautions, the nipples may still be somewhat higher than one would like. When the nipples are so high that secondary surgery is necessary to lower them, which usually leaves scars above the areola, the treatment can be considered a departure from the acceptable practice of plastic surgery.

CASE 2

A patient was entitled to a new trial on the issue of damages in her malpractice action against a physician who performed breast reduction surgery on her, a Connecticut appellate court ruled.

The patient sought a breast reduction operation after losing approximately 70 lb. Her breasts, even after the weight loss, remained heavy and pendulous. She suffered pain and had deep ridges on her back where her brassiere straps cut into her shoulders.

She consulted a plastic surgeon. He told her that an operation was medically indicated but recommended that she see her regular physician before going forward with the operation. Her regular physician then recommended a local physician to perform the operation.

He told her he had performed the operation many times, that her breasts would be "contoured fine," and that her nipples would be reduced in

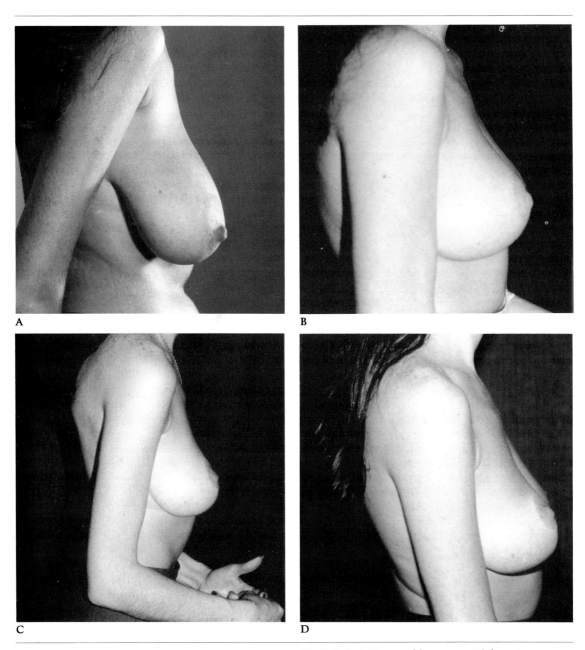

Fig. 7-6. A. A 25-year-old woman with breast hypertrophy. B. Three months post–reduction mammaplasty. Note satisfactory nipple position. C. 1.5 years postoperatively. D. 2.5 years postoperatively. Note change in nipple positioning with tendency to bottom out.

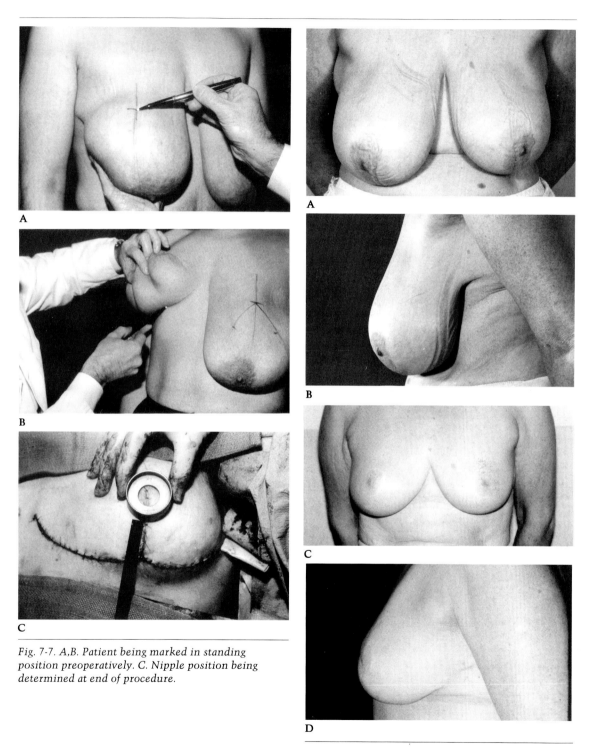

Fig. 7-7. A,B. Patient being marked in standing
position preoperatively. C. Nipple position being
determined at end of procedure.

Fig. 7-8. A. A 65-year-old woman with large, pendulous
breasts. B. Lateral view. C. 5 years post–reduction
mammaplasty with free nipple grafting. D. Lateral
view. Note satisfactory contour and nipple position.

68

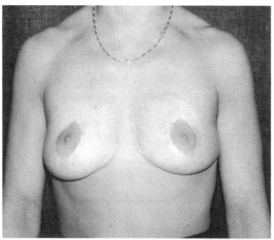

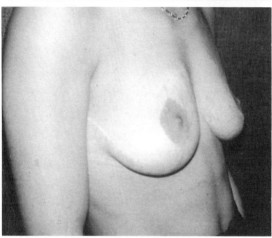

Fig. 7-9. A 22-year-old woman post–reduction mammaplasty; a procedure to lower the nipples and two scar revisions.

size to conform to the new size of her breasts. He performed a bilateral reduction mammaplasty using a Conway-type procedure. The operation resulted in visible welt-like scars above the inframammary crease, flat and misshapen breasts, and overly-large nipples that were insensate and misplaced. The patient suffered adverse psychological reactions to these physical conditions and on one occasion attempted suicide.

She filed an action against the hospital and the surgeon. A trial court directed a verdict for the hospital, but a jury returned a verdict of $30,000 in favor of the patient against the physician.

On appeal, the appellate court said that the directed verdict in favor of the hospital was correctly granted. The patient presented no expert testimony to establish the standard of care applicable to the hospital or to establish that any such standard had been violated. Furthermore, the claim that the hospital had been negligent in granting surgical privileges to the physician that permitted him to perform a breast reduction procedure for which he was unqualified was not established by evidence, the appellate court said.

Two plastic surgeons testified in the patient's favor. They said that the procedure the operating surgeon used was the incorrect one and that the patient did not fall into the category of women who required a Conway-type operation. The appellate court said the trial court had erred in excluding a psychiatrist's testimony.

The trial court also erred in instructing the jury to apply a stricter standard to the patient's claim of mental suffering than it did to those of physical suffering. The court remanded the decision to the trial court for a new trial on the issue of damages only (Buckley v. Lovallo, 481 A.2d 1286 [Conn. App. Ct., Sept. 18, 1984]).

References

1. Andrew, J.M. Recovery from surgery with and without preparatory instruction for three coping styles. *J. Pers. Soc. Psychol.* 15:223, 1970.
2. Barber, B.B. *Informed Consent in Medical Therapy and Research.* New Brunswick: Rutgers University Press, 1980.
3. Basile, D.O. Mammaplasty: Large reduction with short inframammary scars. *Plast. Reconstr. Surg.* 76:130, 1988.
4. Bertakis, K.D. The communication of information from physician to patient. A method for increasing patient retention and satisfaction. *J. Fam. Pract.* 5:217, 1977.
5. Denney, M.K., Williamson, D., and Penn, R. Informed consent: Emotional responses of patients. *Postgrad. Med.* 60:205, 1976.
6. Egbert, L.D., Battit, G.E., Welch C.E., et al. Reduction of postoperative pain by encouragement and instruction of patients. *N. Engl. J. Med.* 270:825, 1964.
7. Goin, J.M. On showing photographs preoperatively to patients (letter). *Plast. Reconstr. Surg.* 54:90, 1974.
8. Goin, M.K., Burgoyne, R.W., and Goin, J.M. Facelift operations—the patient's secret motivations and reactions to "informed consent." *Plast. Reconstr. Surg.* 58:272, 1976.
9. Goldwyn, R. *The Patient and the Plastic Surgeon.* Boston: Little, Brown, 1981. Pp. 223–246.
10. Hoffman, S. Reduction mammaplasty: A medicolegal hazard? *Aesth. Plast. Surg.* 11:113, 1987.
11. Hoffman, S., and Schiavetti, A. A reduction mammaplasty with legal implications. *Ann. Plast. Surg.* 9:506, 1982.

12. Leeb, D., Bowers, D.G., and Lynch, J.B. Observations on the myth of "informed consent." *Plast. Reconstr. Surg.* 58:280, 1976.
13. Letterman, G., and Schurter, M. A sitting position for mammaplasty with general anesthesia. *Ann. Plast. Surg.* 20:522, 1988.
14. Leydhecker, W., Gramer, E., and Krieglstein, G.K. Patient information before cataract surgery. *Ophthalmologica* 180:241, 1980.
15. McKissock, P.K. Complications and Undesirable Results with Reduction Mammaplasty. In R.M. Goldwyn (ed.), *The Unfavorable Result in Plastic Surgery*. Boston: Little, Brown, 1972. P. 739.
16. McKissock, P.K. Complications and Undesirable Results with Reduction Mammaplasty. In R.M. Goldwyn (ed.), *The Unfavorable Result in Plastic Surgery*. Boston: Little, Brown, 1972. P. 746.
17. Marchac, D., and DeOlarte, G. Reduction mammaplasty and correction of ptosis with a short inframammary scar. *Plast. Reconstr. Surg.* 69:45, 1982.
18. Millard, D.R., Mullin, W.R., and Lesavory, M.A. Secondary correction of the too-high areola and nipple after mammaplasty. *Plast. Reconstr. Surg.* 58:568, 1976.
19. Peixoto, G. Reduction mammaplasty: A personal technique. *Plast. Reconstr. Surg.* 65:217, 1980.
20. Redden, E.M., Baker, D.C., Meisel, A. The patient, the plastic surgeon and informed consent: New insights into old problems. *Plast. Reconstr. Surg.* 75:270, 1985.
21. Rittersma, J., Casparie, A.F., and Reerink, E. Patient information and patient preparation in orthognathic surgery: A medical audit study. *J. Maxillofac. Surg.* 8:206, 1980.
22. Robinson, G., and Merav, A. Recall by patients tested postoperatively. *Ann. Thorac. Surg.* 22:209, 1976.
23. Smith, J.W., and Gillen, F.J. Repairing errors of nipple-areolar placement following reduction mammaplasty. *Aesth. Plast. Surg.* 4:179, 1980.
24. Smoot, E.C., Ross, D., Silverberg, B., et al. The sit-up position for breast reconstruction. *Plast. Reconstr. Surg.* 77:60, 1986.
25. The President's Commission for the Study of Ethical Problems in Medicine and Biomedical and Behavioral Research. Making Health Care Decisions. Vol. 1 Report. Washington: U.S. Government Printing Office, 1982.

COMMENTS ON CHAPTER 7   *Robert M. Goldwyn*

Hoffman's chapter confirms the fact that reduction mammaplasty can be either a gratifying operation or a gruesome one for the patient as well as the surgeon. Of those surveyed, about one in ten surgeons who responded stated that they had been involved in a lawsuit because of this procedure.

The polarity of comments is striking: from the joyous "no patients dissatisfied" (one wonders whether the surgeon carefully followed his or her patients) to the anguished "I have more trials and tribulations with this operation than any other." I would hope that by now the latter surgeon has either improved his or her patient selection and/or operative technique or has ceased doing reduction mammaplasty, an alternative that under the circumstances would be more indicative of wisdom than of cowardice, just as persisting in performing a procedure that has given predictably poor results is more an indication of stupidity than of bravery.

In Chapter 8, I have given an overview of the patient's passage from the initial consultation to the last postoperative visit. In this sequence, every patient and every surgeon can experience an event that might lead to a malpractice suit. From having reviewed many cases for attorneys defending plastic surgeons, I can state that the most common causes of dissatisfaction on the part of patients were poor placement or numbness of the nipple; incorrect breast size, as judged by the patient; partial or total nipple-areola necrosis; undesirable prominent scars, sometimes secondary to infection and/or dehiscence; and, in most instances, allegedly inadequate informed consent.

Hoffman has noted, as have other surgeons, that patients recall poorly what they hear from their surgeon or any physician and also what they have read. For this reason alone, proper documentation of the information given to patients is mandatory. In many attempts to help other surgeons facing a legal battle, I have found that inadequate records have been the chief reason for the plastic surgeon's losing a case or settling it before it went to court.

Even a thorough record and a meticulous effort in the informed consent process will not prevent a suit, but they may win it for the beleaguered surgeon when the plaintiff claims that she did not understand what she had heard and what she had signed, despite having been given the opportunity to take the form home for study and discussion with friends or family (Figs. 7-10 and 7-11).

Unlike Hoffman, however, I do warn each patient specifically and bluntly about possible nipple necrosis. I also show every prospective patient for reduction mammaplasty slides of other patient's results, but not just excellent outcomes. My emphasis is on the average and the poor result, particularly with regard to scarring, because many patients believe that plastic surgeons are invisible menders. In my experience, nothing surpasses a slide of a thick, ugly scar for conveying vividly to the patient the possibility that she could have the same misfortune, since, indeed, it did happen to someone else. Even then, however, one must contend with the seemingly indestructible force of human beings to deny reality in the face of all facts.

Not every frank complication or unfavorable result necessarily leads to the courtroom. The surgeon who properly manages an unpleasant outcome cannot only avert a suit but can sometimes have a pleased patient despite her initial misery and anger (see Chap. 8). The stronger the bond between the surgeon and the patient, the less likely the recourse to the legal arena. However,

ROBERT M. GOLDWYN, M.D.

Because insurance coverage varies with different companies, I understand that I may be responsible for the hospital costs associated with any surgery undertaken to improve a result or to treat a complication.

_____
Date

_____
Signature

_____
Witness

Fig. 7-10. Form making patient responsible for hospital costs associated with possible additional operative procedures.

ROBERT M. GOLDWYN, M. D., INC.
– AUTHORIZATION –
REDUCTION MAMMAPLASTY

Patient's name _____

1. I authorize Robert M. Goldwyn, M.D. (the "Doctor"), and his assistants to perform upon me (or my _____) the operation known as reduction mammaplasty (breast reduction).

2. The nature and effects of the operation, the risks and complications involved, as well as alternative methods of treatment, have been fully explained to me by the Doctor and I understand them.

   The following points, among others, have been specifically made clear:

   a. The scars are permanent.
   b. Although having the breasts match is the surgical objective, perfect symmetry of nipples, areolae, and breasts cannot be achieved.
   c. Complications after reduction mammaplasty can be those after any surgical procedure.
   d. Bleeding and infection following breast reduction may occur and may require an additional procedure(s) for treatment.
   e. There is a possibility that the blood supply to one or both nipples and areolae and skin of the breasts may become impaired and necrosis (death of tissue) may result. This complication may require later reconstruction.
   f. There is a decreased likelihood of breast nursing after reduction mammaplasty.
   g. As far as now known, this operation does not influence the later development of breast cancer.
   h. Swelling and ecchymosis (black and blue marks) takes several weeks to disappear; several months are necessary for the breasts to assume their final shape.
   i. While every attempt will be made to make each breast, including nipple and areola, as normal and pleasing in appearance as possible, the objective cannot always be attained.
   j. Sensation to the breast, including nipple and areola, is usually altered and may be decreased permanently.

3. I authorize the Doctor to perform any other procedure which he may deem desirable in attempting to improve the condition stated in Paragraph 1 or any unhealthy or unforeseen condition that may be encountered during the operation.

4. I consent to the administration of anesthetics by the Doctor or under the direction of the physician responsible for this service.

5. I understand that the practice of medicine and surgery is not an exact science and that reputable practitioners cannot guarantee results. No guarantee or assurance has been given by the Doctor or anyone else as to the results that may be obtained.

6. I understand that the two sides of the human body are not the same and can never be made the same.

7. For the purpose of advancing medical education, I consent to the admittance of authorized observers to the operating room.

8. I give permission to Robert M. Goldwyn, M. D., Inc., to take still or motion clinical photographs with the understanding that such photographs remain the property of the corporation.

9. I am not known to be allergic to anything except: (list) _____

I certify that I have read the above authorization, that the explanations referred to therein were made to my satisfaction, and that I fully understand such explanations and the above authorization.

Signed _____
(Patient or person authorized to consent for patient)

Witness _____   Date _____

Fig. 7-11. Form for authorization to perform reduction
mammaplasty.

occasionally not even a relationship that might have pleased Sir William Osler can thwart a patient bent on revenge and compensation, especially if urged by a well-meaning but destructive friend or family and a willing contingency-fee attorney.

When this galling situation arises, the surgeon's record, as mentioned, can be either a strong ally or a Benedict Arnold. Failure to record in detail not only the content of office consultations but also that of telephone calls may be the deciding factor. A few minutes spent in dictating into the record will save hours — verily days — of self-recrimination.

As Hoffman has correctly stated, the form used for "informed consent" does not alone suffice. The patient's chart must contain in full what the surgeon told the patient regarding the nature of the procedure, alternative treatments (rarely any with significant mammary hypertrophy), the likely outcome (in particular with regard to scarring), and possible complications. If all this is in the record, the plastic surgeon (like the one whose cry for help to Hoffman we see in Fig. 7-1) will already have in his or her possession the best "advice for defense," to use that unhappy surgeon's term.

The two other cases that Hoffman presented illustrate not only how plastic surgeons can err (placing nipples too high and guaranteeing a result: "contoured fine") but also the intricacies of the legal system in the United States.

Of particular interest was the testimony for the defense of two plastic surgeons who stated that another surgeon had used the "wrong" technique — the Conway procedure (reduction with nipple grafting). Without more knowledge of that case, I cannot judge whether the patient's unwanted outcome was a result of the method itself or its execution. I am not championing the Conway procedure, but I hope that we plastic surgeons would not condemn a colleague for using a technique for reduction mammaplasty because it is not popular. The Thorek prototype of reduction utilizing nipple-areola grafting is still useful for certain patients and, as demonstrated by Gradinger in Chapter 31, can give excellent results.

A few years ago, a plaintiff's attorney tried unsuccessfully to enlist me to testify that a plastic surgeon who had used the Strömbeck method had used an "inappropriate, incorrect, and discarded procedure." These are strong adjectives to describe a method that is still reliable although not currently the most popular one used.

8

Robert M. Goldwyn

Reduction Mammaplasty: A Personal Overview

The primary objectives of reduction mammaplasty, whose evolution is well documented in Chapter 1, are to reduce the weight of the breast as well as to create a more pleasing shape and maintain the safety of the nipple-areola as well as that of the patient. The ideal operation would be simple, speedy, safe, scarless, and bloodless. The ideal result would be breasts of the contour and volume desired by the patient, breasts that are symmetric with the nipples everted, breasts with normal or unchanged sensation and potential for lactation, and breasts with absent or minimal scarring.

Without such a utopian procedure, we must care for today's patient with today's knowledge. This book shows that various surgeons using different techniques can obtain excellent results. We also know that a good technique in the hands of a poor surgeon can produce a bad outcome.

When is a Breast Large?

Deciding when a breast is large is not always easy. More than 100 years ago, Velpeau [33] wrote:

It is . . . difficult to say exactly where hypertrophy ceases to be natural and becomes morbid. However, when in a woman, who does not increase in other parts of her body, in an adult whose growth has ceased, and who is neither pregnant nor suckling, we observe one or both the mammae increasing in size, insensibly but markedly and permanently, without the patient appearing to be ill in other respects, we may conclude that she is the subject of hypertrophy of the breast.

For the patient, the breast is large or too large when she thinks it is. For the surgeon, it is large depending on his or her bias and assessment of the breast in relation to the age and build of the patient. For the insurance company, the breast is judged large depending on the amount of tissue removed, which might have to be from 300 to 750 gm, depending on the criteria used for third-party payment. Since the volume of the breast determines its size, it would be more logical to give measurements in cubic centimeters instead of grams. However, since most plastic surgeons (and all insurance companies) think in terms of weight, no attempt has been made in this book to change an author's unit of measurement.

Lalardrie and Jouglard [15] concluded that a desirable breast volume is around 275 cm³, but this magic number varies with the patient's physique and preferences. Using measurements of height and frontal projection of the breast, Lalardrie and Jouglard [15] found that when the breast volume exceeded 50 percent of the "normal" or "ideal" breast volume, some degree of hypertrophy existed. They had five categories:

Ideal	250–300 cm³ (volume)
Moderate hypertrophy	400–600 cm³
Rather significant	600–800 cm³
Significant	800–1000 cm³
Gigantomastia	>1500 cm³

Although writers, including myself, use the term *hypertrophy* to refer to large breasts, *macromastia* is probably a better word because it is nonspecific with respect to etiology and histology. Hypertrophy is really an increase in the volume of cells, whereas hyperplasia is an increase in the number of cells. The microscopic findings of the tissue removed in the course of breast reduction are discussed in Chapter 3.

The Patient and the Result

INITIAL CONSULTATION

The operation of reduction mammaplasty begins when the surgeon first sees the patient. However, because of its elective nature, it may also end with this visit if the patient or the surgeon or both decide that the procedure is not indicated or if each or both are dissatisfied with the other. The patient, of course, may choose to go to someone else.

The age of patients wanting reduction mammaplasty ranges from prepubital to postmenopausal. My experience includes patients 12 to 78 years of age. Why some defer operation for so long is worthy of a study by itself. Some of the reasons are discussed by Dr. Cline in Chapter 6.

One of my patients, in her late 50s, planned a reduction on the first anniversary of the death of her husband, who had forbade her to have the procedure. In a curious way, even though she was showing her independence, her timing was evidence that her husband was still a controlling force.

Whatever the patient's age, the basic complaint is usually the same: The size of the breasts interferes with her leading what she considers a normal life. For some women, it is an encumbrance to exercise; for others, it complicates buying clothes or attending social functions, especially in the summer when she may develop intertrigo (Fig. 8-1). The feelings of these women toward their breasts usually have lowered their self-esteem and may have hampered heterosexual relationships. The majority of women with macromastia consider themselves deformed, feel conspicuous and embarrassed, and resent being noted for this aspect of their body, over which they have had no control. They will complain that men fixate on their breasts to the exclusion of their personality or intellect. Unlike patients with small breasts who may be able to hide their problem with a padded bra, patients with extremely large breasts, even with the most ingenious brassieres, may remain an object of unwanted scrutiny.

In addition to these psychological and social problems, large breasts may have physical consequences: poor posture or frank kyphosis; intertrigo; pain in the back, neck, and shoulder-strap areas, with deep grooving; pain in the upper extremity; and occasionally decreased sensation and strength in the ulnar distribution of the hand [14].

Although some patients may complain that the large breasts interfere with exercise, it is seldom

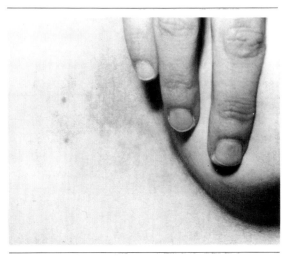

Fig. 8-1. Intertrigo in a 23-year-old woman.

on the basis of compromised pulmonary function [12], as once was thought [6]. More often, the encumbrance of their hypertrophied breasts make some women reluctant to exercise, and, as a consequence, their tolerance for physical exertion is low.

Many patients with large breasts are obese. Some are overweight because of their genetic predisposition and habitus. Others gain weight as a conscious or unconscious effort to make their breasts appear smaller by comparison to the rest of their body. For many, obesity is a manifestation of their depression because of self-imposed social isolation in response to their feelings of inferiority. Obesity becomes one means of keeping men at bay in order to avoid an intimacy that they fear might lead to subsequent exposure of their breasts.

For younger patients who have these psychological and physical problems, one would think that in our society today, obtaining surgical relief would not be difficult. Often, however, it is. Many patients relate their embarrassment over discussing their condition with either parent, even their mother, especially if their mother has normal-sized breasts. Although fathers in our culture may dote on their daughters, they often present the greatest obstacle to their child's seeking a reduction mammaplasty. These fathers do not simply fear that the operation has an inherent danger; they also regard large breasts as an asset, not an affliction. Some patients have told me that their male pediatrician or male family doctor explicitly warned them to avoid a procedure that would eliminate a feature that might later attract men. However, the large-breasted woman is becoming less a victim of male ignorance and chauvinism as more women enter the practice of medicine and as public understanding of this condition increases because of the informative and sympathetic accounts of the procedure in women's magazines and on television programs.

At the time of the initial consultation with the patient for reduction mammaplasty, the surgeon would be wise to inquire why someone important in that person's life is *not* present with her. Why is the father, for example, or husband or boyfriend absent? That individual may be the key to the patient's happiness or unhappiness with the surgical result. If, for example, a husband is opposed to his wife's having a reduction mammaplasty, I would not schedule her until I had a discussion with him. If he was adamantly against the procedure, I would not do it. Although I recognize that the patient has her rights, I also have mine and do not wish to become enmeshed in a marital battle with both sides possibly united against me.

The preoperative appraisal of a patient with large breasts requires a thorough history, including personal, familial, and social aspects, and a careful physical examination. All drug sensitivities must be known. Any aspirin-containing medicines should be identified, because they should be discontinued at least 10 days prior to operation to reduce hazard of bleeding from their anticoagulating effect. Some drugs, such as reserpine and certain oral contraceptives, promote breast engorgement. In addition, birth control pills may increase the incidence of thrombophlebitis. Oral contraceptives, interestingly, have been shown to produce lobular hypertrophy with true acinus formation. The surgeon must find out the patient's previous operations or illnesses, because they may be pertinent to the planned reduction mammaplasty. For example, a previous episode of hepatitis would influence the anesthetic agent chosen for the procedure. The patient's smoking status must also be known. All cigarettes should be stopped at least 2 weeks prior to operation. Some patients who are heavy smokers might need pulmonary function studies.

Every surgeon who treats the female breast is dealing not only with an organ of appearance, function, and sexuality but also with one of carcinogenesis. No surgeon should forget that the patient may have a breast malignancy, and every means must be taken to rule out its presence. A careful family history in this regard is important. A significant history would include premenopausal breast cancer in a mother or sister. It is also important to remember that breast cancer is more common in nulliparous women or those who have had their first child after the age of 33 years.

The surgeon should also determine whether the patient forms cysts or has had "lumps" that required aspiration or biopsy.

It is also critical to know whether the patient is receiving therapy for any condition, physical or emotional. It is not enough to ask the patient whether she is going to a psychiatrist. She may honestly say that she is not when, in fact, she is in treatment with a social worker, psychologist, or pastoral counselor. It is unwise to embark on reduction mammaplasty without conferring with the therapist to determine whether the operation performed at this time is in the patient's best interests. Many patients surprisingly have considered breast reduction for years and may have made the appointment with the plastic surgeon without ever having discussed the matter with their therapist. I prefer writing a letter rather than calling the therapist so that I am more likely to receive a thoughtful reply. A letter from the therapist is good documentation for the record. A harried practitioner receiving a telephone call is less likely to give as careful an appraisal as he or she would in response to a letter that requests one in return. If the therapist believes that the reduction mammaplasty should not be undertaken, I would not be enthusiastic about proceeding. If, however, I thought that the patient seemed unstable emotionally and should not have the operation even though the therapist approved, I would request her therapist to arrange a consultation with another psychiatrist or psychologist. I do not like to assume sole responsibility for the patient's psyche in the event the patient in therapy develops a postoperative depression. More now than in the past, psychiatrists are less opposed to the procedure and less liable to tell the patient to adapt to her condition. However, some of these patients have significant emotional problems other than those generated by the size of their breasts; the surgeon should be aware of them.

During the consultation with the patient, the surgeon should note the interaction not only between himself or herself and the patient but also between the patient and whoever has accompanied her (e.g., mother, husband, boyfriend, girlfriend), since these dynamics may affect the patient's reaction to her surgical result.

Physical Examination

Even though we live in an age where bodies are exposed and the female is supposedly more at ease with a member of the opposite sex, I prefer that the patient undress by herself, retaining her clothes from the waist down, and put on an examination gown. I examine her in the presence of one of my female secretaries. This era of the body revealed is also one of the physician sued. The patient should not be given any opportunity to misinterpret a careful breast examination for something else.

Before focusing on the breasts, the surgeon should make a general appraisal of the patient in order to assess her height, build, and weight. It is important to look for asymmetry of the breast or of the body and for axillary breast tissue, scoliosis, pectus excavatum, and carinatum. If present, these conditions must be pointed out to the patient and taken into account while planning the operation. To detect curvature of the spine, the patient should bend forward and flex laterally while the surgeon stands behind.

With regard to each breast, the surgeon should note whether the primary problem is one of ptosis with excess skin or excess weight or both. The examination of the breast must be as careful as that done by a good general surgeon. Is there skin retraction that might indicate an underlying carcinoma or ulceration of the nipple-areola that might signify Paget's disease? One should remember that the upper outer quadrant of the breast is the most common location for carcinoma. A systematic breast examination should include palpating for cervical, axillary, and supraclavicular nodes, the last being a frequent sign of metastasis from primary breast cancer, which might arise from a nonpalpable, microscopic focus of malignancy.

The examination of a large breast is difficult but should nevertheless be performed systematically and as thoroughly as possible. Each breast should be inspected with the patient's arms at her sides, the arms elevated and then placed behind her head with her sitting and supine.

In a study of the volumes of the right and left breast of 248 women, Loughry et al [17] found no significant relationship between the handedness of the patient and the larger breast volume. More-

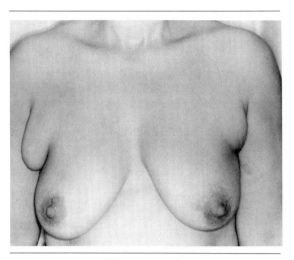

Fig. 8-2. A 38-year-old woman with prominent bilateral axillary breast tissue.

over, their biostereometric analysis did not confirm the generally accepted clinical impression that the left breast volume dominated. Although a size difference in breast pairs was documented, neither breast was significantly larger statistically.

One should note grooving and irritation of the shoulders from brassiere strap pressure. Sometimes, as previously mentioned, sensation and motor power in the ulnar nerve distribution to the hand is decreased [14], and this should be tested. Although this condition is relatively uncommon, it is important to record the patient prior to operation to forestall the allegation that nerve damage occurred during the procedure.

I measure the distance of the nipples from the sternal notch on the midclavicular line and in relation to the inframammary fold. This gives me an idea of how pendulous the breast is and how much nipple transposition will be necessary. The surgeon should examine the breast with the operation of reduction mammaplasty in mind. For example, where is the patient's fullness — laterally, medially, superiorly, inferiorly, or throughout? Any asymmetry, as mentioned, must be described to the patient. If the patient has nipple inversion, she should be told so.

Does the patient have axillary breast tissue, and, if so, to what degree (Fig. 8-2)? Does its presence concern her? Some patients may not notice axillary breast tissue until after reduction has removed their major problem. In those situations, both the patient and the surgeon might regret not removing the tissue at operation. If excision of the axillary breast tissue will involve another incision in each axilla, the patient should be told about it. Sensation of the nipple and areola must be assessed not only by asking the patient about her sensibility there but also by testing: Light touch can be evaluated with one's finger or a piece of cotton, but a more objective means is pain perception ascertained with the instrument the dentist uses to determine pulp viability [7]. Since this method is quantitative, preoperative measurements can be compared to postoperative measurements.

Taking Photographs

Pre- and postoperative photographs — front, side, oblique, and occasionally, if scoliosis is present, from the back views — should be obtained with the patient undressed to the waist. One must include the area between the mid neck and interiliac line, extending always well below the lowest point of the breasts. Although it is comforting for the patient to be told that her face will not be photographed, omission might have medicolegal repercussions. Recently I became aware of two instances where photographs that failed to show the patient's face were not admissible in court in the defense of the doctor.

For photographing breasts, it is important to use standard conditions both before and after the operation.

While the patient is undressed, I demonstrate the incisions I plan so that she has an idea of where the scars will be. My secretary and I leave the room while she dresses. Discussing the procedure in detail with the patient half dressed is poor manners and certainly will not facilitate her recall.

Informing the Patient

The objective of informing the patient is literally to inform the patient so that she can make an intelligent decision concerning the proposed procedure, its advantages, its risks, and alternatives of treatment, if any. Too often the process of informing the patient degenerates into a litany whose purpose is to defend the doctor if a suit arises at a later time. Some surgeons impart information verbally only or in combination with written and visual material.

However the surgeon informs the patient, it should be done with care and not with such rapidity that it leaves her bewildered and uninformed. Reciting complications like Hail Marys will not help the patient's comprehension and recall of what the surgeon has discussed.

What one tells the patient about reduction mammaplasty varies with the patient, her condition, the proposed treatment, and the idiosyncrasies of the surgeon. In general, I begin by first saying to the patient whether or not I believe she should have the operation. Are her breasts large enough to benefit anatomically from a reduction mammaplasty? Is she physically and emotionally suitable for the procedure? Does she have ptosis primarily requiring mostly skin resection? This distinction is critical in planning the procedure as well as in securing insurance coverage, which usually is determined by weight of tissue removed, being less, of course, if only skin is excised than if both skin and breast tissue are removed.

While talking to the patient, I also study her reactions and those of anyone with her. When I detect anxiety, I stop to determine its cause and to relieve it, I hope, as far as reality permits.

I have found that the easiest way for me to inform the patient about reduction mammaplasty is to take her through the operation sequentially, telling her that she will be admitted to the hospital on the day of operation and that a couple of hours later she will be put to sleep for a procedure that lasts about three and one-half hours (bilateral reduction). Most patients fear anesthesia (i.e., relinquishing control), but, if the patient's dread is extreme, a consultation with the anesthesiologist well before hospitalization is helpful. Anesthesia rather than the operation itself frightens most people. The reality is that it would be extremely unusual for surgeons through a technical mistake to cause a patient's death, but cardiac arrest, although rare, does occur, even in young, healthy patients. Furthermore, most patients have heard about such a catastrophe. In the United States, the patient has usually chosen a surgeon because of his or her reputation and possibly on the advice of friends, family, or another physician. She has established a bond with that surgeon and knows who will be doing her operation. She will likely not know her anesthesiologist until the hour of operation, although she may have met a representative of the anesthesia department a few days prior to her hospital admission, during the course of her preoperative assessment.

Informing the patient about reduction mammaplasty includes talking about pain. Although surgeons may rightly consider pain not a major feature of the postoperative course, the patient, not the surgeon, experiences it. The first 12 hours are the worst, and I tell the patient that she will likely receive morphine (if she is not allergic to it) or its equivalent. I also mention that when she leaves the hospital, usually 2 days afterward, her pain will not be acute and she will be given medication, such as codeine or phenacetin, to control it.

Patients also want to know the type of dressing they will have when they go home. Whatever the surgeon's routine, the patient should be familiar with it. I prefer using the patient's old brassiere, without the wires, because it easily holds the dressings. I tell them to plan being out of school or work for about 2 weeks, not to drive for about 1 week, and to avoid exercise, other than walking, for about 3 weeks. I also tell them that I will remove the stitches around the twelfth day after operation. To plan their schedules, patients want an idea of how frequently they must return for follow-up visits.

An extremely important part of the consultation is telling the patient about possible complications. I first begin with the worst: death. Although this disaster is possible, I also state that is rare. I do not think it is fair or advisable to frighten a patient; I also believe it is important not to hide reality. By bringing up what the patient herself likely fears but may be afraid to articulate helps to lessen anxiety, not to increase it. The patient thereby realizes the surgeon has empathy and is aware of her worst fear.

I next discuss other complications along with their incidence, for example, infection (incidence of less than 5%), postoperative bleeding (less than 1%), and loss of the nipple and areola from decreased vascularity (less than 5%). With regard to nipple necrosis, one should not use the term *losing the nipple;* otherwise, the patient will conclude that somehow during operation the surgeon or one of the team has carelessly mislaid it.

Every patient must understand that reduction mammaplasty can result in altered sensation of the nipple and areola in particular, but also to the skin of the rest of the breast. She must also appreciate that sensation may be *permanently* changed or even absent, the latter having a probability of less than 5 percent. If the surgeon is planning to transplant the nipple and areola, some sensation may return but less than after nipple transposition [30].

I inform patients in the childbearing age that their ability to lactate will decrease. That information is of little interest to someone 60 years of age

or even to most teenagers, but it is of concern to a young woman's mother. For patients who may be considering becoming pregnant in the immediate future, I advise deferring the reduction until after delivery and 6 months after nursing.

To every patient, I say that reduction mammaplasty does not increase the likelihood of breast cancer since some patients may have that misconception.

Blood transfusion is also important to discuss, especially in this era of acquired immunodeficiency syndrome (AIDS) phobia. Although most patients undergoing reduction mammaplasty will not require a transfusion, a few will. It is sometimes difficult to predict these patients but they are usually those with gigantomastia. Occasionally, a patient may be anemic prior to operation. If so, the cause of that anemia should be investigated if it has not already been. If, at operation, the surgeon finds that the patient requires blood, it would have been wiser to have planned preoperatively for autologous blood, which can safely be stored for 6 months. Blood donation should not be done within 3 weeks of the planned reduction mammaplasty; otherwise, the patient might be anemic and weak at operation. Most hospitals in the United States have made autologous blood transfusion extremely easy for the patient and the surgeon [25, 31].

Showing Photographs

When informing patients about reduction mammaplasty, I also show them photographs of others who have had the procedure. I realize that many surgeons oppose this idea. My aim, however, is not to sell the patient on the operation or a specific result but to give a realistic idea of what she is likely to experience as an outcome, particularly with regard to scars. I carefully present a spectrum of results: poor, average, and superior (Figs. 8-3 through 8-5). If what I consider an excellent result causes the patient to look disappointed or even horrified, I would be reluctant to operate on her because I fear that she will be dissatisfied with the result. Sometimes this type of patient will become more realistic if seen on another visit after she has had the opportunity to digest the information given. But a few patients remain poor candidates from the surgeon's standpoint because of their unrealistic expectations. In the patient's record, I

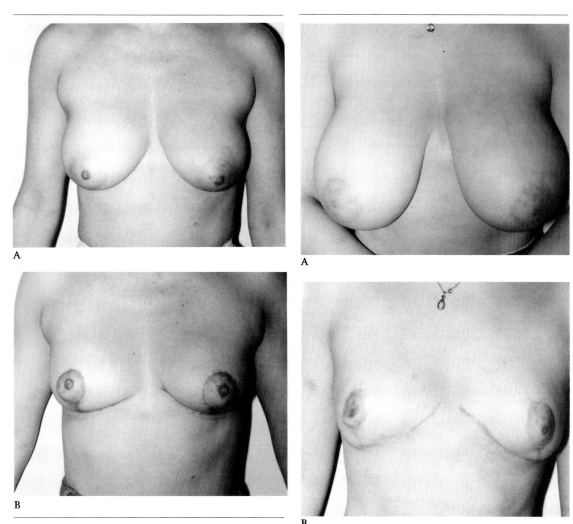

Fig. 8-3. "Superior result." I show the prospective patient on slide-viewer a fifty-two-year-old woman preoperative (A) and postoperative, 3 months (B). Photographs were deliberately taken early to show scars.

Fig. 8-4. "Poor result." I show the prospective patient a 21-year-old woman preoperative (A) and postoperative, 1 year (B). I point out asymmetry of the breast and areola and hypertrophy of scars.

state that I have shown photographs in order to present a "realistic picture" of the various kinds of results that the patient is likely to obtain. I also state clearly that I guarantee no result either explicitly or implicitly.

Fees
After leaving the surgeon's office, the patient should have a precise idea about her financial responsibility. As mentioned previously, most in-

surance companies determine coverage on the basis of the weight of the tissue removed.

For patients with massive hypertrophy, no ambiguity exists about coverage. For other patients, however, it may be necessary to write to the insurance company and to send along photographs (with the patient's written permission or, if she is a minor, with the permission of her parents) before the insurance company decides. Most insurance companies want to know the patient's height and

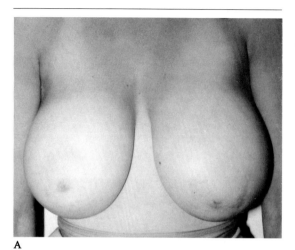

A

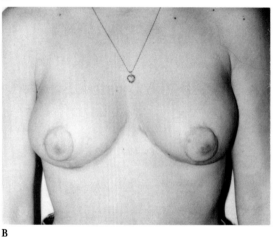

B

Fig. 8-5. "Average result." I show a prospective patient an 18-year-old woman preoperative (A) and postoperative, at 11 months (B).

weight before they give prior approval. It is preferable to receive a written statements affirming coverage from the insurance company rather than a telephone permission, which the insurance company may later deny granting.

I regret having to state here that no surgeon should make fraudulent statements to the insurance company (or to anyone). Unfortunately, a few surgeons, misguided in the belief that they are helping the patient to secure coverage, may exaggerate the weight of tissue removed or may actually increase the weight by injecting saline. These surgeons are committing an unlawful act. Furthermore, if the patient is displeased with the result, she can blackmail the surgeon to refund money or,

as in one instance I know about, demand additional money. The surgeon is not an exception to the legal codes of society.

Mammograms

Every patient 30 years of age or older should have a mammogram prior to reduction mammaplasty. Some oncologists but few radiologists advise mammograms at an earlier age as a routine and especially in patients with a mother or sister who has had breast cancer. Since the breasts of those who come for reduction are not always easy to palpate, mammograms are helpful. In those patients who have had mammograms, I request another set about a year after operation as a baseline for the possible detection of a later breast abnormality.

Size

The surgeon should know the breast size that the patient wants. Some women wish to be "slinky"; others wish to remain buxom. The patient's desires should be followed as much as possible unless they are unrealistic. My observation is that many women are left with breasts still too large even when the surgeon believes that he or she has performed a generous reduction. However, it is better to underdo than over resect, because revision of the former problem is much simpler than dealing with a breast that has been made too small.

As mentioned previously, the surgeon should never promise the patient a specific bra size [28]. Not only do bras labeled the same size vary in capacity depending on the manufacturer and style, but the surgeon may not be able to achieve the size that the patient requests. Instead of promising a patient a certain size, it is better to tell her that an attempt will be made to give her what she wants. This distinction is not just semantic but is medicolegally important.

The New Nipple Site

A myriad of techniques exists to determine the new nipple site (Table 8-1); subsequent chapters will illustrate how various surgeons choose its location. Some surgeons prefer the security of preoperatively determining it [10, 34]; others prefer the latitude of making the final decision during operation [4, 8]. Whatever method the surgeon uses, one fact is clear: A nipple that is excessively low, although not ideal, is not so catastrophic as

Table 8-1. Determination of the new nipple site in patients having reduction mammaplasty

New site of nipple	Year	Author
SITE DETERMINED BEFORE OPERATION WITH PATIENT SITTING		
1. 18–21 cm from sternal notch.	1946	Ragnell
2. Level of midhumerus in midclavicular line.	1949	Maliniac
3. 21 cm from sternal notch and midclavicular point and between the nipples. Nipple plane is 3.75 cm below midhumerus.	1955	Penn
4. Intersection of a circle with center at sternal notch and radius of 19–24 cm with another circle with its center at the xiphoid and a radius of 12.5–17.0 cm. Internipple distance is at least 25.0–27.5 cm.	1958	McIndoe and Rees
5. 22 cm from sternal notch on midclavicular–nipple line. In large hypertrophics, the skin is stretched, thus 23–24 cm from sternal notch. In very short patients, 21 cm is the minimum distance.	1964	Strömbeck
6. 20 cm from sternal notch is average distance, with 10.5 cm from the midline. For shorter women, 18 cm from sternal notch is shortest distance.	1966	Regnault
7. Sixth rib or interspace and 1 cm lateral to the midclavicular line.	1969	Pennisi, Klabunde, Pletch
8. Elevate arms and mark level of new nipple site in nondistensible sternal skin (for patients with small ptotic breasts).	1971	Goulian
9. Same as Strömbeck. In this chapter, Dr. McKissock points out the important relationship with the inframammary fold and stresses the use of "visual approximation" and in the ptotic breast first raising the nipple to the proper level before noting and *then* marking its new position on the midmammary line.	1972	McKissock
10. 11–15 cm from upper border to the middle of the clavicle is the average distance; 8–10 cm is the average distance from the midline.	1974	Meyer and Kesselring
11. On a line from the midclavicular point down through the nipple, the new site of the top of the areola is located 13 cm below the second interspace of the third rib depending on the height of the patient.	1974	Meijer
12. Depending on the patient's build and the amount of reduction desired, the new location of the superior margin of the areola is marked 15–18 cm from the sternal notch.	1974	Regnault
13. Drape cloth tape measure around patient's neck so that it comes down over each nipple. Place fingers in inframammary fold so as to support breast weight. Then place thumb on tape measure in [direct] opposition to fingers, and this will be the new nipple site. It is at least 22 cm from the suprasternal notch with the weight of the breast supported by the hand.	1974	Gerow, Spira, Hardy
SITE DETERMINED DURING OPERATION		
1. Place nipple in desired position at vertex of cone-shaped breast.	1967	Pitanguy
2. 2–3 cm above and medial to present areola as marked preoperatively in sitting position. Final position is chosen a little below and outside the summit of the glandular cone at operation.	1971	Dufourmentel and Mouly

Source: From W.C. Grabb. Comment on P.K. McKissock's Correction of Macromastia by the Bipedicle Vertical Dermal Flap. In R.M. Goldwyn (ed.), *Plastic and Reconstructive Surgery of the Breast.* Boston: Little, Brown, 1976. P. 231.

one that is too high—that is, pops out of the bra, deforms the breast, embarrasses the patient, and does little credit to the surgeon. For that high-riding nipple, remedy is difficult and defense in court is almost impossible. In my opinion, too many techniques and too many surgeons place the nipple too high. A common allegation is that the breast "settles," but, in most instances, the real culprit is not the force of gravity but an error in judgment at the time of marking the breast or during operation. When in doubt, the surgeon should pick a lower site for the nipple.

A common method of locating the new nipple site is to place the index finger in the inframammary fold and transfer by palpation its position onto the anterior aspect of the breast. However, this maneuver is not absolutely precise since the finger has an arc of rotation at the metacarpophalangeal joint so that the nipple placement can vary from 0.5 to 1 cm either higher or lower.

When the surgeon is marking the patient and if she is conscious and unmedicated, one can ask her again about the size she desires. Sometimes a patient may change her mind between the time of the first consultation and the day of operation. Frequently, the patient herself may not have a realistic idea of desirable breast size because of her distorted body image. Although the surgeon may wish to reassure the patient, who is understandably anxious before operation, no promises should be given regarding a specific size.

Antibiotics

The majority of surgeons use pre- or perioperative antibiotics because of the endogenous flora of the breast [29]. The antibiotics should be first administered with the patient awake with all her senses intact to better determine an allergic reaction. Even though one has presumably taken at the initial consultation a careful history concerning allergies, it is advisable again to ask her about drug sensitivities. I recall two patients who between the first office visit and the operation had developed an allergy to penicillin.

In the Operating Room

Most patients will get comfort from having the surgeon at their side during induction. In addition to the psychological benefits, the surgeon should be present for an emergency such as incorrect intubation or cardiac arrest.

With a No. 25 needle, the surgeon can re-mark the previously drawn lines so that subsequent prepping will not erase them.

If antibiotics have been ordered, the surgeon should check that the patient has indeed received them. There is many a slip between the order and its execution.

I find it helpful to have the patient's photographs hanging in the operating room to consult.

It is not necessary here to recapitulate well-known details of prepping and draping except to say that many residents and nurses do not know how to prep correctly, never having learned the

principle of going from the clean area toward the dirty area without returning the sponge to the initial area prepped.

I prefer the patient positioned with her arms on well-padded arm boards and extended at slightly less than right angles from her body. Care must be taken not to hyperabduct the shoulder, not to stretch the brachial plexus, and not to put undue pressure on the ulnar nerve of the elbow or the heels. The surgeon has the responsibility to be sure that no bony prominence is under pressure. I prefer that the patient is wearing alternating pneumatic boots throughout the operation. These have been shown to decrease the incidence of thrombophlebitis [5]. Theoretically, because the tourniquet with its alternating pressure acts on the platelets, the tourniquet can be applied elsewhere, as on the arms. However, tourniquets on the legs are less obtrusive and will not interfere with taking blood pressure readings or administering intravenous solutions and medications. Whether these boots provide more protection if continued in the recovery room and beyond has not yet been documented.

The groundplate to the electrocautery must be properly positioned, and the machine itself should have been tested recently. A distressing complication and a frequent cause of litigation is the inadvertent cautery burn. Sterile plastic drapes on the flanks aid sterility and keep the patient dry from the prep solution and blood.

At some point in the operation, to judge symmetry, the surgeon will want the patient in an almost vertical position. This maneuver should be discussed with the anesthesiologist before the case begins. Some anesthetists dislike having the patient more than 75 degrees upright despite studies that show a 90-degree position will not jeopardize the patient's safety if the patient is raised slowly and carefully.

Some surgeons use a separate instrument table for each breast in the event that if a cancer is encountered either grossly at operation or microscopically later, the cancer would not have been transplanted to the other side. Theoretically, I agree with that recommendation, but since the incidence of cancer found in association with reduction mammaplasty is so small, I do not adhere to it. Over a course of 30 years and 2,000 reduction mammaplasties, I have had only one patient with this unfortunate sequela.

I prefer changing gloves in going from one breast

to the other because glove perforation is more common than we realize.

All tissue removed from each breast must be kept separate and submitted separately to the pathologist. Some surgeons, for symmetry, weigh the tissue of the breast according to the location of the breast from which it has been removed. This method is valid only if the breasts are symmetric.

If any tissue looks suspicious for cancer at the time of reduction, a frozen section is advisable. If a malignancy is found, the surgeon should terminate the procedure and make no attempt to eradicate the cancer. The treatment of breast cancer is controversial, and the patient deserves the opinions of other doctors. Taking matters into one's own hands by embarking on an ablative procedure for which the patient has received no information and has not given permission is bad judgment and may actually be determined to be so by the court.

Drainage

Contrary to what one might expect, the volume of drainage is greater with a Penrose rubber drain [32] than with suction, such as Jackson-Pratt, which, however, is accompanied by a lower rate of infection [2, 16, 22, 32]. Any drain, however, is more likely to predispose to infection [9, 19]. Yet most surgeons doing reduction mammaplasty use drains. Still lacking is a proper randomized study that would answer the question of the value of drainage following reduction mammaplasty. If the surgeon prefers a drain (I do), it should not be brought out at the extreme lateral or medial end of the wound where scarring would be more conspicuous. It is better through a separate stab wound under the breast. There is some evidence that a drain brought out through the incision is associated with a higher infection rate than drains that emerge through another opening [9, 32].

Blood Loss

Careful use of the electrocautery or the injection of epinephrine or norepinephrine [3] will decrease blood loss, but nothing is a substitute for compulsive hemostasis. Some surgeons object to the electrocautery because they believe that it increases serum formation despite the lack of objective evidence. Bilateral breast reduction in most patients can be accomplished with a blood loss of much less than a unit if the surgeon uses the electrocautery.

Judging Symmetry

Symmetry is the ideal, yet absolute symmetry is rarely achieved. Symmetry depends on the relative size and shape of the breast prior to operation, the amount of tissue removed, and, more important, the amount and location of the tissue left. What counts, of course, is the patient's final appearance and getting some idea of what it will be. The patient should be placed as close to a sitting position as possible before the operation is concluded. At this point, the opinions of others are invaluable. Some surgeons create such an ambience of fear in the operating room that no assistant or nurse would dare tell him or her that the patient's breasts are asymmetric. The unintimidated anesthesiologist from his or her perspective can also be helpful in detecting a mismatch.

Being a conservative surgeon, I advise anyone in doubt to remove less tissue rather than more tissue — a maxim that I stated earlier. The dilemma arises if one has resected an appropriate amount on one side but too much on the other side. To make the remaining side too small might displease the patient, but her confronting gross asymmetry would also upset her. If the discrepancy is severe, it is probably a better idea to conclude the operation with that asymmetry and then discuss with the patient an augmentation rather than proceeding on one's own to insert an implant, as happened to one patient whom I saw in consultation. That sequence, not surprisingly, was resolved in court.

Suturing

It is remarkable that despite more than 3,000 years of skin suturing, we are still arguing about the best way to do it and searching for the best material. At present I prefer 3-0 Vicryl interrupted, inverted, intradermal sutures with a running 4-0 Prolene intradermal pull-out. Whereas Nordstrom and Nordstrom [20] believe that nonabsorbable intradermal sutures prevent later stretching of the scar, others disagree. For the surgeon, suturing remains a personal, impressionistic matter that has yet to be scientifically resolved.

Nipple-Areola Viability

Nipple-areola necrosis is, from the point of view of the surgeon, a principal fear. Although relatively low in incidence, severe nipple-areola necrosis with loss of a good portion of the areola as well as the nipple has not only a high impact on the patient but on the surgeon as well. At operation, if the nipple-areola remains decidedly blue or white and is thereby showing signs of vascular impairment, the surgeon should seriously think of grafting it. The use of intravenous fluorescein to determine viability in dubious instances is helpful but involves injection of a substance that might not be available in the operating room. Many surgeons do not use it despite the fact that it would offer guidance. To conclude the operation with a nipple and areola that looks moribund is postponing a problem that will be more difficult to manage later. I admit that it takes a strong-minded surgeon to decide to convert a transposed nipple into a transplanted one, but occasionally it is necessary. Under those circumstances, one should not graft the nipple and areola to a dying pedicle but to a viable substrate, either on a platform of dermis purposely left during the course of the inferior pedicle technique, for example, or onto a place where the flaps have been brought together and deepithelialized for the purpose. In this latter situation, the flaps may be under slightly more tension because the keyhole flap of breast tissue has been taken away owing to the necrosis. It is better to have the nipple and areola survive with slightly more tension on the breast than to terminate the procedure with nothing more than prayer to offer the patient who also needed the nipple-areola graft done.

Dressings

Dressings serve to absorb blood and to provide loose support. They should never be too tight; otherwise, respiration will be constricted and vascularity to the flaps and the nipple-areola will be impeded. Applying the dressing carries the danger of lifting the patient incorrectly, resulting in injury to the shoulder or stretching of the brachial plexus. Unless the patient is still under adequate anesthesia, the change in position that accompanies putting on the dressing can cause laryngospasm.

Dressings should permit easy access for inspection of the nipple and areola postoperatively to assess viability.

Intraoperative Awareness

During the time that the patient is in the operating room, especially when she is being induced or is emerging, she may be capable of hearing what is said [1, 26, 35]. Careless talk sinks surgeons. Intraoperative awareness, in fact, may be more common than thought; thus, at all times, every member of the operating team should heed his or her words; otherwise, the consequences for the patient as well as the surgeon could be unpleasant.

After Operation

The surgeon should be present or immediately available when the patient is extubated and returned to the recovery room in case an emergency arises. The surgeon should also either write or supervise the postoperative orders, which must include instructions regarding vital signs, intravenous fluids, subsequent oral intake, antibiotics, and medications for pain or preexisting conditions. The nurses should also be informed about inspecting the nipple and areola: how often to inspect it, what to look for, and whom to call under what circumstances.

Some surgeons routinely discharge their patients the day after operation; for a minimal reduction, going home the same day may also be possible. My preference is to have the patient remain for 2 days until I remove the drains.

Although ultimately most patients having had reduction mammaplasty will be pleased with the result, not every woman is ecstatic immediately after operation (Fig. 8-6). It is important for the surgeon to perform the first dressing change, not simply because a problem might exist, such as impending necrosis of the nipple and areola, asymmetry, or, rarely, infection, but for psychological support; the patient may have difficulty in adjusting to a new body image. Occasionally, a patient will be traumatized by the change in her appearance even though she eventually will be happy about her decision to have had the reduction [11]. Many patients initially avoid looking at their breasts, or, if they do, it is on the sly, with surprise or dismay. Few patients are indifferent. Some patients become faint and dizzy and have to lie flat in bed; some may say, "These breasts don't look like mine and they don't feel like mine," or, "Will they ever look like breasts?" Rarely, a patient may even say that she no longer looks like a woman. This observation is distressing to hear and may herald a difficult readjustment.

The surgeon who may have expected gratitude for having relieved the patient of a deforming bur-

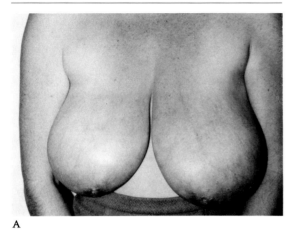

A

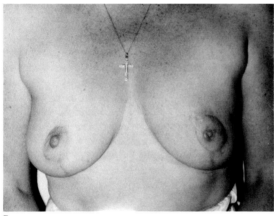

B

Fig. 8-6. A 47-year-old woman preoperative (A) and postoperative at 10 months (B). The patient is now happy with the result but initially, she was very unhappy because she said she looked "too small" and "like a man." Two months later, the patient was pleased with her "feeling of freedom." No psychotherapy was needed — just support and reassurance during frequent visits.

den is now perplexed and disappointed as he or she stands uneasily at the bedside. The emotional response of the patient to this dramatic alteration of her body is well described by Dr. Cline in Chapter 6. Gentleness and understanding, certainly not impatience, are what the patient needs now. She should be reassured that her feelings are not unusual but ordinarily pass in several weeks as she becomes accustomed to her new breasts and body. Rarely is psychotherapy indicated, but, later, if it

seems necessary, the surgeon should not delay suggesting it.

After the drains have been removed, the patient usually goes home in her old bra but without the stays. If this bra is unsatisfactory because it is too large or the patient has neglected to bring it to the hospital, I supply her with one (Sears catalog #78495, cup C-D), which may be larger than she will probably wear but will accommodate the dressings. The patient should know how to change her dressings either by herself or preferably with the aid of a friend or family member. I ask my patients to wear a bra as much as possible, even at night, for the next 4 to 5 weeks. With normal healing, she may resume driving and sex in a week and athletics in 3 weeks.

Many surgeons have someone in the office to remove stitches. I prefer to do it myself because I want to see how the wounds are healing and how the patient is reacting to her operation. For most patients, even a very sympathetic and skillful nurse is no substitute for the surgeon to whom she has gone, in whom she has trust, and who has done her operation. Removing stitches should be done as gently as possible. Nothing disconcerts a patient more than to have her surgeon rush into the room, rip her dressings off, and roughly remove the stitches. The process of suture removal is a modern equivalent of the ancient cure of laying on hands. This can be reassuring to the patient and may strengthen the relationship between herself and her surgeon.

The Unfavorable Result
Elsewhere I have written on how to deal with the patient who has had an unfavorable result [13]. Without repeating the content of those publications, let me emphasize here two cardinal rules: (1) Accept the fact that a problem exists if it does, and (2) be available to remedy it. What justifiably infuriates an aggrieved and grieving patient is the surgeon who tries to talk that person out of a complication or unsatisfactory outcome either by not admitting its presence or by minimizing it, with such ineffectual and infuriating advice as "it's barely noticeable so forget about it," or "learn to live with it." If, for example, a patient perceives her nipples are asymmetric, they probably are. If so, she will resent not only what she considers the surgeon's error but also his or her assumption that she is so stupid as to believe the surgeon's desperate denial of reality.

The patient, if ever she needed a surgeon, needs him or her now when things have gone badly. An understandable but unforgivable reaction is to avoid or flee from an unhappy patient. Nothing is worse ethically and legally. Every physician has the responsibility to see a patient in trouble frequently and not to offer the secretary or nurse as a substitute. Not returning the unhappy patient's telephone calls, for example, is cruel and puerile.

Consider as an example the patient with the infrequent but monumental complication of nipple necrosis. The patient probably left the hospital with her nipple and areola in a state of uncertain viability. At the time of the first dressing change, it might have been apparent that a portion of the areola or nipple was becoming necrotic. The surgeon who should have been there should have told the patient about this possibility. However, now, in the office, the surgeon cannot dodge the issue and must definitely inform the patient about her nipple and areola. The surgeon can also point out the good things, however (it is hoped there are some), about the operation, such as the size and shape of both breasts are excellent (if they are), the nipple-areola on the other side is viable, and, if fate is kind, not all the nipple and areola will be lost (if that is so). The surgeon should let the patient know also that sometimes 10 days will have to pass before the extent of the necrosis is definite. If the surgeon is using the term *necrosis*, he or she should have defined it for the patient.

In another few days, the surgeon should see the patient and begin debridement as soon as the area of necrosis is demarcated. It is hoped that the surgeon will have spoken to the patient's family or a close friend who might have accompanied her to the office. Airing the complication in this way is not only good for the patient's anxiety but is also helpful to the surgeon's anxiety. If another physician has referred the patient, the surgeon would do well to call that doctor and tell him or her about the complication. Often the referring physician can be helpful. It is better for that doctor to hear about this unwanted outcome from the surgeon first rather than from an irate, unhappy patient and family, who might not be able to give a clear account of the event.

To any patient with a significant postoperative complication, I give my telephone number. It is interesting that only rarely does a patient call; the knowledge that I can be easily reached is probably sufficient. Patients dread calling the doctor when he or she is not in the office, especially if the response is one of anger or impatience. Having to endure a complication is sufficient burden for any human being without adding to it the impediment of an unsympathetic and unavailable physician.

With regard to nipple-areola necrosis, I try to have the patient do her dressings as soon as possible. Initially, a family member, a friend, or perhaps a visiting nurse may have to aid her. However, when the patient is able to care for herself, her outlook changes to one of optimism, independence, and less self-pity. The patient will accept the wound better if the surgeon also accepts it as a reality. For the surgeon, necrotic nipple symbolizes failure, and, in fact, it is a failure even though it may not have been the surgeon's fault. To the patient also, the dead nipple-areola is a failure. She had tried to improve her breasts and her body and now she has a festering wound, an unfair mockery of what she had hoped the result would be. The surgeon should remember that if the patient had really expected the complication, despite having been so informed, she would never have had the operation; and, indeed, as the surgeon can point out to the patient, had he or she known that this complication would occur, he or she never would have operated.

If the patient is able to change her dressings herself two or three times a day, usually wet to dry, with saline or even tap water, she will become familiar with the wound and will not treat it as alien to her body.

I usually tell the patient, "We shall see how much tissue will live; if only a small area dies, then it will probably not be necessary to do anything about it. Nature heals things extremely well but you have to help nature by doing your dressings faithfully. Even if a large part of the nipple and areola is gone, we can reconstruct it. This is something we plastic surgeons do when we build a new breast after mastectomy. Fortunately, you do not have that serious a condition, but I know how dreadful this must be for you. I can say that I have not enjoyed it but both of us will get through it together. I have been this way on occasion before."

It is not uncommon that a patient with a serious complication may become the most grateful of all of one's patients. In my experience, a few patients have returned for additional operations, unrelated to the breasts, and have referred other patients.

If during the course of treating a complication, the surgeon senses that a patient would appreciate another consultation, it should be arranged and the patient not put in the difficult position of requesting another surgeon's advice. The patient, however, should have the feeling, based on reality, that the surgeon is not trying to get rid of her but is seeking to reassure her with the advice of someone who is likely to be more objective. Furthermore, the surgeon can tell the patient that if another surgeon thinks of something that is helpful and I have not thought of it, I am grateful for that advice and willingly accept it.

The surgeon who sees another colleague's patient in difficulty should be helpful and not vindictive. Too often, other surgeons, instead of aiding the patient, spend more time in degrading the surgeon, forgetting for the moment that they, too, will also have a complication and, at some point, will need the support of others.

Follow-Up

For a patient 30 years of age or older, I order mammograms about a year after operation to serve as a baseline in case a lesion or mass is detected clinically or radiographically. Many radiologists throw away film after 5 years because of space shortage. Under those circumstances, the patient should request her mammograms in case they are later needed.

The surgeon should pay attention to the findings of the pathologist [18]. The microscopic report should be read thoughtfully, not automatically, and not filed by the secretary without the surgeon's having seen it.

Often, a patient returns within the first 3 months after reduction mammaplasty with a "lump." If the microscopic findings have been benign, without any evidence of a precancerous lesion, the surgeon can be less anxious in following the patient for several weeks more. Any mass, however, that persists for a few months unchanged must be biopsied [23]. A biopsy under local anesthesia is a simple procedure, but refusing to suggest it when indicated can be catastrophic. Rees and Coburn [23] reported a patient who, a few weeks after reduction mammaplasty, had axillary node involvement by the cancer despite the fact that microscopic examination of the tissue removed at the time of reduction showed no evidence of malignancy. Although that report is unusual, it does emphasize the basic tenet of any

physician or surgeon caring for a patient with a mass in the breast or in the axilla: Be quick to biopsy. Every surgeon should remember what almost every patient knows: Only the pathologist can make the definitive diagnosis.

I have found it instructive to follow patients after reduction mammaplasty for at least 2 years. This enables me to see the results of my work. When I discharge a patient from my care, I make certain that she will be receiving regular breast examinations. To ensure continuity, I write the surgeon or internist who is looking after the patient to say that I will not be seeing her unless needed.

Lactation

Despite the fact that hundreds of thousands of women have had breast reductions and have later become pregnant, few studies have been done about the long-term results, and in particular, the ability to lactate. Ragnell [21], in a series of 12 patients, found that 9 were able to lactate; of Strömbeck's patients [27], 50% lactated. Zacher [36] found that 16 of 20 women who had reduction mammaplasties could nurse even when more than 500 gm were resected per side. She detected no relationship between the ability to nurse and the type of transposition technique used (McKissock or inferior pedicle).

Reduction Mammaplasty as a Combined Procedure

Reduction of large breasts is a 3-hour or longer procedure, a sufficient stress for the patient, and enough of a challenge for the surgeon so that combining it with another major operation is unwise. Performing limited liposuction of the abdomen, let us say, would likely be well tolerated and is reasonable, but embarking on extensive liposuction with turning the patient over or doing a face lift in addition to the reduction mammaplasty is inadvisable, in my judgment. I admit that I base this on intuition, conservatism, and perhaps, common sense, in the absence of good data concerning the incidence of complications, such as pulmonary embolism, atelectasis, pneumonia, and infection when reduction mammaplasty is part of a combined venture compared to when it is the sole procedure.

Conclusion

Reduction mammaplasty, if properly performed and with correctly selected patients, can significantly improve a patient's life. Its popularity attests to the need that it answers and the satisfaction that it provides. However, not every woman will be content with the result. Complications can occur. Reduction mammaplasty is by no means a cut-on-the-line operation. A happy patient is the outcome of the fortunate interdigitation of many factors, most of which, but not all, are within the surgeon's control. If, indeed, reduction mammaplasty were simple and an excellent result were automatic, the need for this book detailing various concepts and techniques would not have been necessary. Although a surgeon may believe that one method fits every patient, the reality is that the surgeon may be trying to fit every patient to a single procedure. The surgeon's mind should be sufficiently flexible in order to try to give optimal care to each woman with breast hypertrophy. While not flitting from one technique to another like a butterfly, the surgeon would be wise to have in his or her repertoire two or three procedures along with variations in their execution. The surgeon should also be willing to improve procedures as new knowledge arises, but only after judicious evaluation and not impetuous acceptance.

References

1. Blacher, R.S. Awareness during surgery. *Anesthesiology* 61:1, 1984.
2. Bourke, J.B., Balfour, T.W., Hardcastle, J.D., et al. A comparison between suction and corrugated drainage after simple mastectomy; the report of a control trial. *Br. J. Surg.* 63:67, 1976.
3. Bretteville-Jensen, G. Mammaplasty with reduced blood loss: Effect of noradrenalin. *Br. J. Plast. Surg.* 27:31, 1974.
4. deCastro, C.C., Coelho, R.F., and Cintra, H.P.L.C. The value of nonprefixed marking in reduction mammoplasty. *Aesth. Plast. Surg.* 8:237, 1984.
5. Clagett, G.P., and Reisch, J.S. Prevention of venous thromboembolism in general surgical patients. Results of meta-analysis. *Ann. Surg.* 208:227, 1988.
6. Conway, H. Weight of breasts as handicap to respiration. Argument for reduction mammaplasty. *Am. J. Surg.* 103:674, 1962.
7. Courtiss, E., and Goldwyn, R.M. Sensation in the breast before and after plastic surgery. Unpublished data. 1975.
8. Crow, R.W. Refinements of reduction mammaplasty. *Plast. Reconstr. Surg.* 71:205, 1983.
9. Cruse, P.J.E., and Foord, R. A five year prospective study of 23,649 surgical wounds. *Arch. Surg.* 107:206, 1973
10. Gasperoni, C., and Salgarello, M. Preoperative breast marking in reduction mammaplasty. *Ann. Plast. Surg.* 19:306, 1987.
11. Goin, M.K., Goin, J.H., and Gianni, M. The psychic consequences of a reduction mammaplasty. *Plast. Reconstr. Surg.* 59:530, 1977.
12. Goldwyn, R.M. Pulmonary function and bilateral reduction mammaplasty. *Plast. Reconstr. Surg.* 53:84, 1974.
13. Goldwyn, R.M. *The Patient and the Plastic Surgeon.* Boston: Little, Brown, 1981. Pp. 121–127.
14. Kaye, B.L. Neurologic changes with excessively large breasts. *South. Med. J.* 65:177, 1972.
15. Lalardrie, J.-P., and Jouglard, J.-P. *Plasties Mammaires pour Hypertrophie et Ptose.* Paris: Masson, 1973.
16. Leissner, K.H. Postoperative wound infections in 32,000 clean operations. *Acta. Chir. Scand.* 142:433, 1976.
17. Loughry, W., Sheffer, D.B., Price, T.E., Jr., et al. Breast volume measurement of 248 women using biostereometric analysis. *Plast. Reconstr. Surg.* 80:553, 1987.
18. Lund, K., Ewertz, M., and Schou, G. Breast cancer incidence subsequent to surgical reduction of the female breast. *Scand. J. Plast. Reconstr.* 21:209, 1987.
19. Morris, A.M. A control trial of closed wound suction drainage in radical mastectomy. *Br. J. Surg.* 60:357, 1973.
20. Nordstrom, R.E.A., and Nordstrom, R.M. Absorbable versus nonabsorbable sutures to prevent postoperative stretching of wound area. *Plast. Reconstr. Surg.* 78:186, 1986.
21. Ragnell, A. Breast reduction and lactation. *Br. J. Plast. Surg.* 1:99, 1948.
22. Raves, J.J., Silfkin, M., and Diamond, D.L. A bacteriologic study comparing closed suction and simple conduit drainage. *Am. J. Surg.* 148:618, 1984.
23. Rees, T.D., and Coburn, R. Breast reduction: Is it an aid to cancer detection? *Br. J. Plast. Surg.* 25:144, 1972.
24. Sarr, M.G., Parikh, K.J., Minkem, S.L., et al. Closed-suction versus Penrose drainage after cholecystomy. A prospective randomized evaluation. *Am. J. Surg.* 153:394, 1987.
25. Schifman, R.B., and Steinbronn, K.K. Estimating intraoperative blood loss: When to transfuse autologous units—questions and answers. *JAMA* 260:704, 1988.
26. Schultetus, R.R. Intraoperative awareness. *Today's OR Nurse* 9:22, 1988.
27. Strömbeck, J.O. Late Results after Reduction Mammaplasty. In R.M. Goldwyn (ed.), *Long-Term Results in Plastic and Reconstructive Surgery.* Boston: Little, Brown, 1980. Pp. 722–732.
28. Tegtmeier, R.E. Doctor, I want to be able to wear a 'C' cup. *Aesth. Plast. Surg.* 6:57, 1982.
29. Thornton, J.W., Argenta, L.C., McClatchey, K.D., and Marks, M.W. Studies on the endogenous flora of the human breast. *Ann. Plast. Surg.* 20:39, 1988.
30. Townsend, P.L.G. Nipple sensation following breast reduction and free nipple transplantation. *Br. J. Plast. Surg.* 27:308, 1974.
31. Toy, PTCY, Strauss, R.G., Stehling, L.C., et al. Pre-

disposed autologous blood for elective surgery: A national multicentric study. *N. Engl. J. Med.* 316:517, 1987.

32. Van der Linden, W., Gedda, S., and Edlund, G. Randomized trial of drainage after cholecystectomy. Suction versus static drainage through a main wound versus a stab incision. *Am. J. Surg.* 141:288, 1981.

33. Velpeau, A. *A Treatise on the Diseases of the Breast and Mammary Region.* Trans. by M. Henry. London: Cydenham Society, 1956. P. 176.

34. Violante, M.A. Un metodo presiso para la colocacion del complejo areola pezon. *Circ. Plast. Ibero-Latinoam.* 13:219, 1987.

35. Wilson, S.L., Vaughan, R.W., and Stephen, C.R. Awareness, dreams, and hallucinations associated with general anesthesia. *Anesth. Analg.* 54:609, 1975.

36. Zacher, J.B. Pregnancy and nursing following reduction mammoplasty. Presented at the 55th Annual Meeting of the American Society of Plastic and Reconstructive Surgeons, New Orleans, April 14–17, 1986.

9

Robert M. Goldwyn

Classification of the Breast and the Hypertrophic Breast and Note on Arrangement of Chapters

The Breast

Female breasts, which over millennia have attracted lovers, artists, and poets, have also intrigued classifiers. Despite many efforts, however, a consensus classification remains to be done for the normal-sized as well as the oversized breast.

Anthropologists were among the first to try categorizing the human breast [4]. They concluded that in the Caucasian race, the female breast is usually hemispheric; in what they call the "Negro" race, it is conical or pointed and pendulous. Allegedly, they reasoned that the breast's pendulosity is convenient for nursing and can be increased by compressing the upper chest with a band as in the Loango women. In this way, the mother can place her enlarged breast over her shoulder or under her axilla to nurse her infant on her back.

Thorek [4] claimed that toward the end of the nineteenth century and the beginning of this century, French anthropologists used detailed verbal description in the hope "that a clear and concise picture of a particular contour could be visualized without the addition of pictorial illustrations "e.g., the breasts (negroid) are almost hemispherical in shape, more or less conical, full or voluptuous and hanging."

Ploss and Bartels, anthropologists whom Thorek [4] cited, classified breasts according to size (i.e., large and voluptuous, full, medium, small, or slight); consistency (i.e., erect, sagging, or pendant); and form (i.e., cup-shaped, hemispheric, conical, or udder-shaped).

With Teutonic thoroughness, anthropologists of that era seemed to go everywhere recording types of breasts. Some of these observations may or may not be true but were at least intriguing: "the Javanese have erect breasts"; the Croatians have breasts "which excel in form and solidity, while the breasts of Serbian girls are softer in consistency" [4]. As a final example of that type of pseudoscience, "in dry mountainous countries the female breast does not attain the size which it does in damp and marshy regions" [4].

In their zeal to classify, anthropologists did not neglect the nipple-areola, which they categorized according to size, form, and color.

It is fortunate for those anthropologists of yore that they did not have to have their study approved by the institution in which they taught. For example, Hoerschelmann wrote: ". . . on the whole, the conical nipple is rather rare. Among the nulliparous Estonians there are about 10% with this sort of nipple. The percentage increased decidedly when selected individuals were placed under observation. Of 20 of the prettiest and best formed girls chosen for observation in one year the conical nipple was found 15 times. Among prostitutes, however, distinct conical nipples never occurred" [3]. Another classification, longstanding, is to compare the size and shape of breasts according to fruit: apples, pears, melons, and watermelons [1]. Although convenient, this sort of categorization belongs in the barracks, if even there.

Hypertrophic Breast

Maliniac [2] used three major types of classification for the hypertrophic breast: (1) physiologic

Table 9-1. Classification of breast hypertrophy

I. Consistency
   A. Hypertrophic
      1. Limited ptosis, upper quadrants full
      2. Predominence of glandular tissue
      3. Tight skin brassiere
   B. Pendulous
      1. Significant ptosis, upper quadrants flat
      2. Predominance of fat
      3. Loose, sagging skin brassiere
II. Volume in excess
      0–200 minor
      200–500 moderate
      500–1500 major
      over 1500 gigantomastia

Source: From P. Regnault and R.K. Daniel (eds.). *Aesthetic Plastic Surgery.* Boston: Little, Brown, 1984. P. 500.

(infantile, pubertal, gravid, general adult, atrophied breast of old age), (2) histologic (epithelial hypertrophy, fatty hypertrophy, hypertrophy with cystic disease or other tumor formation), and (3) morphologic (ptosis with an atrophic, normal, or slightly enlarged gland, ptosis with moderate hypertrophy, ptosis with massive hypertrophy, asymmetry).

A contemporary classification is that of Regnault and Daniel (Table 9-1) [3] based on shape, consistency, and predicted volume of excision.

Although not usually considered a coward, I admit that I have run away from imposing on every author a classification for the hypertrophic breast so that every patient discussed and photographed could be viewed and analyzed according to a single system of categorization. A few authors of subsequent chapters have offered their own conceptualization. Although a couple of these, as well as the classification of Regnault and Daniel (see Table 9-1) [3], seem logical and useful to me and obviously are for those authors, it would have been a futile task for me and a ridiculous one for every contributor to this book to classify their patients according to criteria that might not have been their own. What is important, however, and what most authors have stressed, as I have also done in Chapter 8, is to study and examine the patient's breast in order to know its characteristics before seeking to reduce it. An intelligent assessment must include more than the obvious fact that the breast for reduction is too large. Although not all of us have evolved a classification that we could

immediately put into a table, we do have a mental checklist as we appraise a patient for reduction. Only by knowing what should be changed or should not be changed can we perform the appropriate operation.

Classification of Techniques and a Note on the Arrangement of Chapters

Most editors have an urge to classify and organize. This editor is no exception. A significant problem for me, however, was how to arrange logically the chapters describing the various techniques of breast reduction for this book. Some possibilities —not all—were to classify according to:

Chronology of description (e.g., Biesenberger 1928; Arie 1957)
Incision (e.g., inverted "T," "L" [vertical])
Location of pedicle base (e.g., superior, lateral)
Blood supply through pedicle to nipple-areola (e.g., glandular, cutaneous, both)
Undermining (e.g., between skin and gland, none)
Sector of breast from which tissue is excised (e.g., posterior, medial)
Tissue removed (e.g., gland, skin, both)
Effect on inframammary fold (e.g., higher, lower, none)
Marking new nipple-areola site (e.g., preoperative-fixed, intraoperative)
Combination of any, several, or all of the above.

Remembering and taking solace from Emerson's view that "a foolish consistency is the hobgoblin of little minds," my organization is inconsistent and personal. The fact is, however, that many procedures for reduction share similarities, and, in some instances, one may be the progenitor of another or several. Paternity and maternity are definitely ambiguous but familial resemblance is strong.

Personal chronology rather than historical led me to place the chapters in much the same sequence that I had learned and performed the techniques described. Chapter 10, however, is that of Dr. Pitanguy, whose modification of Arie's technique is historically important. The next is the technique described by Dr. Strömbeck, and, in fact, it was the first transposition procedure I had ever done in private practice. The sequence continues with the vertical by pedicle flap (McKissock), lateral approaches (Mouly, Schatten), the superior pedicle (Skoog, Weiner, and Hauben), the inferior pedicle, the B technique (Regnault), and the "dermal vault" (Lalardrie). The next grouping, continuing from the methods of Dr. Regnault and Dr. Lalardrie, represent further attempts, in addition to those of Dr. Pitanguy and Drs. Dufourmentel and Mouly, in reducing the large breast via minimal incisions, in particular trying to shorten or eliminate the horizontal scar. Thus, the reader will find chapters describing the methods of Drs. Kesselring and Meyer, Dr. Marchac, Dr. Peixoto, Dr. Ribeiro, Dr. Pontes, Dr. Bozola, Dr. Lassus, and Dr. Maillard.

Next in line is the volume reduction method (Cloutier), which is distinguished by its use of only the horizontal scar.

Completing the rest of the book is a chapter on reduction with nipple grafting and then special subject chapters: unilateral reduction, reduction in gender dysphoria and, not surprisingly, since I am the editor, a final chapter on complications and unfavorable results following reduction mammaplasty.

I hope that the reader will now realize that a skein of rationality runs through what may have initially seemed a hodge-podge. I hope also that any author who thinks that he or she has been unfairly displaced or misplaced will now accept my apologies.

References

1. Lalardrie, J.-P., and Jouglard, J.-P. *Chirurgie Plastique du Sein.* Paris: Masson et Cie, 1974. Pp. 2–3.
2. Maliniac, J.W. *Breast Deformities and their Repair.* Baltimore: Waverly, 1950. Pp. 39–47.
3. Regnault, P., Daniel, R.K. (eds.). *Aesthetic Plastic Surgery.* Boston: Little, Brown, 1984. Pp. 500–501.
4. Thorek, M. *Plastic Surgery of the Breast and Abdominal Wall.* Springfield, Illinois: Thomas, 1942. Pp. 73–91.

10

Ivo Pitanguy

Reduction Mammaplasty: A Personal Odyssey

Over the centuries the breast has been viewed as the main characteristic of femininity, being glorified in art, literature, and fashion. The concept of the beautiful breast in terms of size and shape has changed considerably through time. In the past, full breasts and exuberant bodies were very much in vogue. Today, we are witnessing a new idea of body harmony, represented by slimmer figures that reflect the dynamic pace of modern living and the preoccupation with healthier habits, balanced diets, and exercising.

These factors, along with the influence of advertising and fashion media, which nowadays calls for a greater exposure of the body, led women to a deeper consciousness of body contouring and, consequently, of breast imperfections.

In cases of mammary hypertrophy, the patient often experiences a rapid change in body image during the difficult teenage years. In areas of warmer climate, such as Rio de Janeiro and California, some of these young women change their social habits and behaviors because they are embarrassed to expose their large breasts. The unfortunate consequence is the development of an inferiority complex, which later becomes compounded by physiologic problems.

Therefore, a surgical procedure that aims at the treatment of this condition should correct the deformity and afford a functional result that does not disrupt secondary sexual functions, while providing a longlasting and gratifying aesthetic result.

Through the experience of more than 2822 patients, the Arié-Pitanguy and classic Pitanguy reduction mammaplasty techniques have survived the test of time because of their simplicity, flexibility, and consistency.

Historical Evolution

The first description of breast surgery dates back to 400 B.C., when Hippocrates wrote about the amputation of a breast in a Scythian woman [17]. By 1669, Durston [8] reported the first attempt of reduction mammaplasty by partially amputating a ptotic breast. Attention was focused on the anatomy of the breast in the eighteenth and nineteenth centuries, following the previous studies of Leonardo da Vinci in the sixteenth century.

More than 200 years elapsed until Czerny [4] presented a study on breast surgery that approached the defects "in a plastic manner." Pousson [18], in 1897, reduced a hypertrophic breast by excising a crescent-shaped piece of skin and gland from the upper pole, while securing the remaining tissue to the pectoralis fascia for support. Several years later, Guinard [10] in 1903 and Morestin [14] in 1909 resected the skin and gland from the lower pole of the breast in patients with macromastia. Following this, numerous contributions were made by Dehner [5] in 1908, Girard [9] in 1910, Lexer [13] in 1912, Auber [2] in 1923, Dufourmentel [6] in 1939, and Kausch [11], in 1916.

By 1922, Thorek [19] had successfully preserved the nipple-areolar complex by performing a mammaplasty using a free graft. Two years later, the first deepithelialized nipple-areolar pedicle was decribed by Lexer [13] and Kraske [12]. However, it was the Biesenberger [3] technique of 1928 that remained the treatment of choice for reduction mammaplasty for almost 30 years and was my preference prior to 1959 [15]. This procedure essentially separated the gland from the skin and removed tissue laterally while rotating the remaining portion of the gland medially to maintain some form of shape.

My experiences using the Biesenberger technique were quite satisfactory in the immediate postoperative period. Initially, the breasts presented a good shape and aesthetic appearance; however, some patients developed complications, and the long-term results were not as satisfactory as expected. One problem inherent to this technique dealt with the wide skin undermining.

This maneuver is contrary to one principle of breast surgery that I believe to be very important. The breast is like a pseudosuspensory organ, and by separating the skin from the gland, one is separating the breast from its embryologic origin. If the proportional separation of the "contents from the container" is too great, in time the breast will have a greater tendency to ptose. Additionally, a certain degree of skin suffering is likely to occur, even if one is careful not to traumatize the skin.

Other procedures used prior to 1959 required larger resections and a certain amount of undermining that often resulted in large dead spaces, hematomas, seromas, infections, and skin necrosis. Resections that involved the upper pole had tendencies to flatten superiorly and sag, with the nipple being projected upward instead of outward. These types of complications were more frequent with procedures that required fixed nipple placement and rigid patterns.

These pitfalls were the primary stimulating factors that forced me to look for an alternate procedure in the late 1950s — one that could maintain a balance between the skin and the gland without undermining, so that the weight of the breast could be supported in a natural brassiere-like fashion.

At that time, Prudente, a surgeon from São Paulo, and Arié [1] developed a technique following the principles of Kraske that created an almond-shaped, subareolar, vertical incision. By 1957–1958, I realized that a reduction could be done without undermining. But there were still some problems with the shapes of these breasts, which were occasionally quite conicle or even projectile.

In 1959, at the British International Society of Plastic Surgeons, my modification of the Prudente-Arié technique was presented. When I elaborated on this paper, which compared my modification of the technique with their technique, I realized that my evolution had been the gaining of skin from the upper pole — not by starting the incision below the nipple, but, rather, by moving the incision above the areola to the place where the new nipple would be naturally located (point A), at the level of the projection of the inframammary sulcus on the midclavicular line [15]. This led to the rhomboid or losangular incision, which came directly or slightly obliquely to the inframammary line (Fig. 10-1), unlike the incision of Dufourmentel and Mouly [7], which extended laterally and medially, giving a type of visual stigmatism when looking at the breasts. This point A was the first step in the evolution of the classic Pitanguy technique, which ultimately evolved into a triangle. However, when treating larger breasts, the resection required removal of more than just a wedge of tissue, such as taken with the rhomboid incision. So, in 1960, I began to excise substantial amounts of gland from the lower hemisphere, in what I called a "keel-like" fashion. In fact, it was not exactly a "keel shape," as I called it, owing to a misunderstanding of the English language at that time, but in the approximate shape of a keel, done in a step-like manner and with variations in size according to each case. This resection worked through the triangle A, B, and C and allowed for treatment of the axillary prolongation and medial extension by creating two pillars of tissue. When approximated, these columns would come together in a stepladder fashion, obliterating any dead space while projecting the nipple outward, through the adipose capsule, to point A. Resection of the inferior pole allowed for access to the superior pole from below. This would avoid injury to the blood supply and innervation to the nipple, which arise superiorly [16].

Creation of this triangle enables the performance of many different types of resections with ease, with consistency, and without being inhibited by fixed measurements or predetermined nipple placements. Most important, shape and long-term reliability are maintained because the gland is not separated from its adipose capsule and overlying skin. This enables the breast to support itself while preserving function and sensitivity to the nipple-areolar complex.

Indications for Surgery
AGE
We found that the ideal age to operate is between 16 and 20 years, when the breast is fully developed and before any irreversible psychological changes occur. Patients younger than 16 years should un-

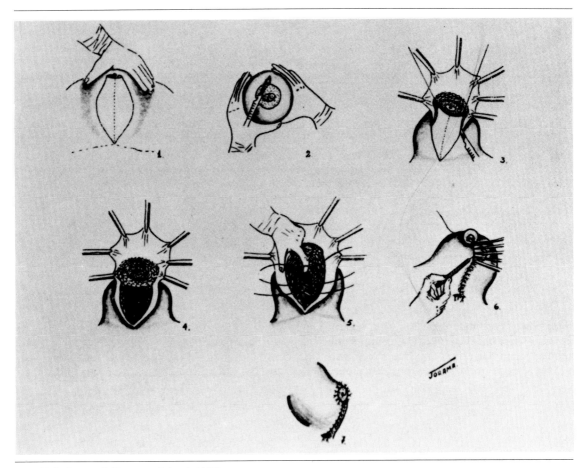

Fig. 10-1. Original diagram of the Arié-Pitanguy technique, published in 1959.

dergo surgery only for severe virginal hypertrophy. The upper age limit depends on the physical condition and unrelated medical problems that would prohibit any major surgical procedure in this age group. Although the benefits in elderly patients are less pronounced aesthetically, the overall improvements in respiration and vertebral problems are most gratifying. The ages of the patients treated at the clinic are summarized in Table 10-1.

PHYSICAL PROBLEMS

The most common complaints experienced by our patients were related to back pain (Table 10-2). The pendulous weight of the breast produces changes in posture, which ultimately may lead to osteoarthrosis and kyphosis with a compensating lordosis in the vertebral bodies (Fig. 10-2). Elderly

Table 10-1. Breast hypertrophy 1959–1987: Distribution by age (2,822 cases)

Age group (yr)	(%)
10–19	6.8
20–29	25.1
30–39	32.2
40–49	19.5
50–59	13.6
60 and over	2.8

Table 10-2. Main complaints in breast hypertrophy 1959–1987 (2,822 cases)

Main complaints	(%)
Physical discomfort	45.1
Bad posture	35.2
Premenstrual pain	35.0
Psychological problems	28.2
Clavicular achromic region deformity	26.8
Backache	26.6

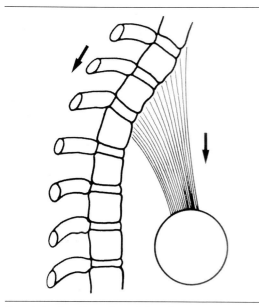

Fig. 10-2. The effect of pendulous breasts on the vertebral column in the cervical area.

patients may experience an increased effort of respiration owing to excessive weight on the secondary inspiratory muscles. The muscles act like a third-degree lever, raising the breasts, which will require an even greater effort to raise the chest wall during inspiration. This may aggravate the condition of those patients with underlying cardiopulmonary problems.

Gravity-dependent lymphatic drainage and venous return are often impeded in large hanging breasts, with a tendency for turgence and edema. This may lead to anterior thoracic pain, which becomes particularly sensitive during the premenstrual period (mastodynia). To support large breasts, heavy brassieres are needed; these can cut deep and painful grooves into the shoulder areas that are virtually impossible to treat surgically. In addition, the submammary fold has a tendency to collect moisture, especially in the summer months or in tropical climates. This becomes an ideal media for fungal infections, which produce difficult to treat intertrigo.

PSYCHOLOGICAL PROBLEMS

The psychological trauma experienced by patients with hypertrophic breasts must not be underestimated. Many patients develop serious complexes that result from the inability to accept their disfigurement. More than one third of our patients openly admitted to psychological problems that were not caused by vanity but rather by the realization of a serious disfigurement in their body contouring.

In the immediate postoperative period, one can already observe a positive behavioral change. The patient's posture becomes more erect, her style of clothing changes, and her social interactions seem to improve almost immediately. Therefore, the psychological profile of a patient should not necessarily be regarded as an absolute contraindication to surgery.

Patient Selection

The ideal patients for the classic Pitanguy technique are those with second- and third-degree hypertrophy and gigantomastia or virginal hypertrophy. When the technique was first being developed, 8 percent of all cases required free nipple grafting. But once the principles of the procedure and its many necessary variations were dominated, the number decreased to 1 percent [16]. After 1961, none of the patients who presented with excessive hypertrophies required free grafting; nevertheless, we do not wish to discard the use of free grafting when necessary.

Patients with mild hypertrophy and pure ptosis are the most suitable for the Arié-Pitanguy technique. The types of incisions should be discussed beforehand with the patient because occasionally the incisions extend below the inframammary sulcus or have to be converted into an L or small T, which may not be appealing to some patients. However, the resulting scars have a tendency to move upward, at least 1 to 2 cm, and are usually

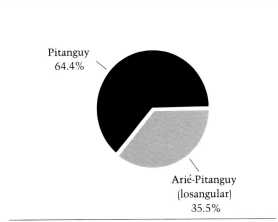

Fig. 10-3. *Graphic representation of 2822 patients undergoing Arié-Pitanguy technique versus classic Pitanguy technique.*

well concealed within 1 to 2 years (see Case 1). The statistics of our clinic are outlined in Figure 10-3.

SPECIAL CONSIDERATIONS

The question often arises about whether to use the classic Pitanguy or the Arié-Pitanguy technique for patients in cases in which either could be used. It has always been my philosophy to minimize scarring, but one must keep in mind two important factors: (1) shape of the breast, and (2) amount of excess skin. For those patients with poor elasticity and much excessive skin, one may try the Arié-Pitanguy technique but will often end up with the incision being converted to a T, having one long arm and one short arm, or to an L, which extends beyond the anterior axillary line. In such patients, it is easier to produce a better shape with more consistent long-term results by using the classic Pitanguy technique (see Case 2).

In the case of a breast with a very heavy lower pole, it is often easier to resect a large amount of tissue through one vertical incision by basing the resection on the center of the gland. Geometrically, this will centralize the breast while allowing the nipple to rise upward and outward in a natural way (see Case 3).

Asymmetric breasts should not be approached with any fixed measures in mind, because both techniques can be applied, depending on the proportions and the adaptations to the contralateral

deformity. With very small breasts, one should try using a single vertical incision and may find it necessary to include a prosthesis on the contralateral side, without having to reduce the larger breast. This may be performed through the transareolar incision described in 1966 or through the submammary sulcus (see Case 4). Under other circumstances, where only one breast needs to be reduced, it can be done by adapting either technique to that side, without touching the opposite breast (see Case 5). This is not often the case though. One breast is usually much larger than the other and will be best suited for the classic Pitanguy technique on both sides (see Case 6).

When one breast has a nice shape with small ptosis, the question always arises whether to include or exclude a prosthesis on one or both sides. In such a situation, one is often better off and has more satisfying long-term results by adapting the contralateral breast to the good one, avoiding the use of a prosthesis whenever possible (see Case 7).

We have encountered an occasional case where the nipple-areolar complex is in good position and may not need to be moved at all. In such cases, one may begin the resection with a rhomboid incision that starts below the areola without touching the periareolar area, or a small periareolar incision may be necessary to move only the nipple-areolar area upward without resecting the gland and skin below the areola.

Preoperative Assessment

All patients should be thoroughly examined for any signs of breast pathology, with a full preoperative radiologic work-up for those older than 35 years of age. Definitive investigations or surgery should be undertaken for any areas of potential pathology. In high-risk patients, the reduction mammaplasty may provide an early diagnosis of carcinoma in areas hidden from the examiners fingers or in radiologic "gray areas" found in large glandular breasts. Of 1,975 cases that underwent pathologic analysis at our clinic, 1,863 presented with benign pathologies, and 21 presented with carcinomas, requiring subsequent surgical intervention. Ninety-one patients were free of pathologies (Table 10-3).

Various other preoperative morphologic factors should be considered when discussing the patient's expectations for the final size and shape of the breasts: (1) height and weight of the patient, (2)

Table 10-3. Histopathologic findings in
breast hypertrophy 1959–1987 (1,975 cases)

Histopathologic findings	No. of cases
Benign pathologies	
Fibroadiposity	1,011
Mammary dysplasia	645
Mammary atrophy	196
Fat necrosis	6
Siliconosis	5
Total	1,863
Malignant pathologies	
Papilliferous carcinoma	14
Adenocarcinoma	5
Fibrosarcoma	1
Paget's disease	1
Total	21
Pathology-free	91

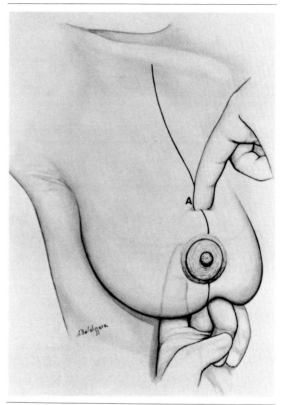

Fig. 10-5

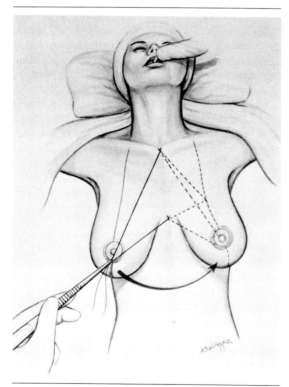

Fig. 10-4

position and size of the nipple-areolar complex, (3)
size and shape of the rib cage, and (4) quality of
skin. Most important, the surgeon should make
sure that the patient clearly understands the limitations of the surgery and should prepare her for
the resultant scarring and any possible complications associated with any procedure.

Surgical Technique: Classic Pitanguy Reduction Mammaplasty

STEP 1: PREPARATION

The patient is placed on the operating room table,
with arms extended at 90 degrees to the axilla,
shoulders perfectly centered, and head elevated to
15 degrees. The back of the table should be elevated to 45 degrees, and demarcation of the skin is
begun. Two sutures are placed for assistance in
marking the skin — one at the suprasternal notch
and a second at the midxyphoid area.

STEP 2: MARKING

1. The midclavicular line is used as the first point

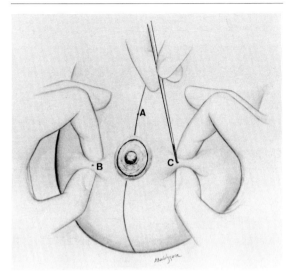

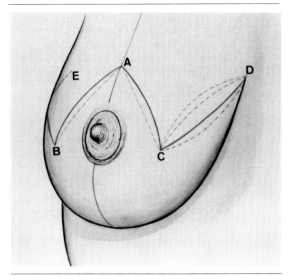

Fig. 10-7

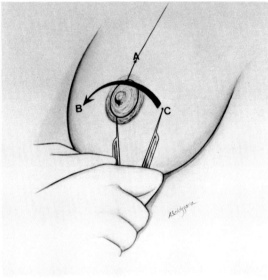

Fig. 10-6

ings should be done on the smaller breast first so the larger breast can be adapted to the smaller. Nevertheless, if the shape of the smaller breast is not good, it should be adapted to the larger breast. With the first two fingers of each hand, the surgeon grasps the breast below a horizontal line drawn through the nipple, at the points where the tissue will be resected. The assistant depresses the midline inferior pole while the surgeon folds the skin in his or her fingers over the clamp. This will allow one to establish points B and C, as well as to determine the amount of potential resection. Points B and C should be equidistant from the nipple on both sides (Fig. 10-6).

4. Points D and E demarcate the limits of the infra-mammary sulcus. Point D is placed medially, being sure not to extend beyond the sulcus, and point E is placed laterally without extending beyond the anterior axillary line. One should try to keep the two points equidistant from the points B and C, while attempting to keep points B-E as short as possible. The points B-E and C-D are connected with a line that should be contoured to the type of resection necessary. With excess skin, the line should be more concave to the sulcus; with more gland and less skin, it should be more convex. The points D and E are connected, and from this point on, one should try to limit the amount of manipulation to the gland by solely using instruments (Fig. 10-7).

of reference. Using a hemostat, the upper suture is placed in the supraclavicular groove and extended through the nipple to arrive below the submammary sulcus. This line is then marked (Fig. 10-4).

2. Placing the fingertips of the dominant hand below the submammary sulcus and pressing slightly upward, one can establish the exact point of the sulcus and mark it: point A. This is placed along the midclavicular line (Fig. 10-5).

3. To establish points B and C, one must first look at both breasts to establish whether or not they are symmetric. If one is larger, the initial mark-

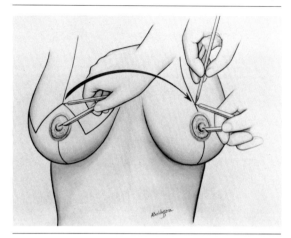

Fig. 10-8

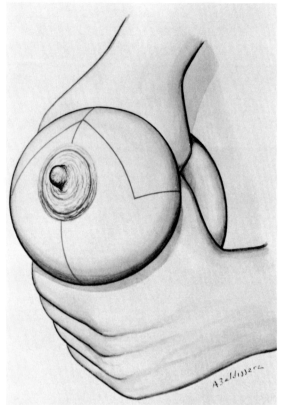

5. Using a compass and marking suture, the exact measurements are transferred to the opposite side. Nipple and areola are then marked on both sides. If the areola is excessively hypertrophic with small breasts, it will be safer to make the areola marking slightly larger so the closure can be done without tension (Fig. 10-8).

STEP 3: SCHWARTZMANN MANEUVER
With the assistant grasping the breast from the axillary base and the medial base, the skin over the areola will become taut and expedite the Schwartzmann maneuver. This is done within the confines of the triangle A, B, C, extending 1 to 2 cm below the areola. Once the proper plane is established here, the dissection will proceed smoothly without injuring the dermis (Fig. 10-9).

The skin is then incised from point A to the areola, and two flaps of tissue are created to aid in retraction once the incisions are extended to points B and C (Fig. 10-10).

STEP 4: RESECTION OF GLAND
A kocher clamp is placed on the skin at point A, and the first assistant elevates the breast off the chest wall exactly perpendicular. The second assistant prepares the cautery to control any major bleeding vessels. This may prevent any break in the surgeon's concentration or avoid disrupting the flow of the resection (Fig. 10-11A).

Using a No. 15 scalpel, a deep incision is made into the gland along the line between C and D. A compress is placed into the wound, and a similar incision is made along the line from B to E. The

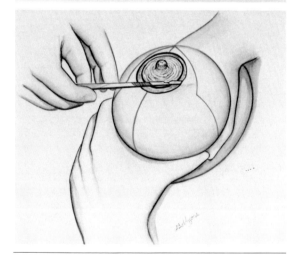

Fig. 10-9

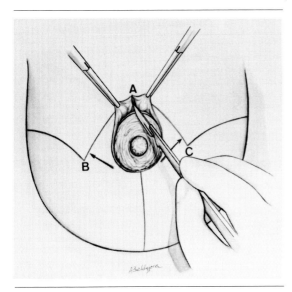

Fig. 10-10

breast is then elevated, and an incision is made between D and E at the inframammary sulcus. One must be sure to bevel the incision upward to leave enough tissue to support the inferior border during closure (Fig. 10-11B).

The gland is again elevated at 90 degrees to the chest wall, and resection is commenced, according to the deformity, commonly in a "keel-like" fashion (which is more like the inner nave of a church) or in a straight amputation fashion. If a keel is desired, the resection is begun from the level of the areola, making incisions first medially, then laterally, and then medially and again laterally, to create a stepladder type of resection that will reapproximate easily and project the nipple upward. The gland is then amputated, weighed, and sent for pathologic sectioning (Fig. 10-11C–G).

One should not attempt to close the breast before going to the opposite side first. When the incision and Schwartzmann maneuver are completed on the other side, the second assistant will raise the first breast for the surgeon to view the necessary amount of tissue to be resected for symmetry.

STEP 5: CLOSURE
The breasts are temporarily closed with a few sutures and compared for size and shape (Fig. 10-12). Once one is satisfied with the outcome, the breasts are closed in two layers. The dermis is approxi-

mated carefully, using 4-0 absorbable sutures for both the horizontal and vertical incisions, in an inverted fashion. One should always suture toward the T, from the medial and lateral edges of the wound. This will help to relieve much of the tension that often develops in this area. The skin is then reapproximated in a running subcuticular fashion using 3-0 monofilament.

STEP 6: NIPPLE-AREOLAR PLACEMENT
One should not suture the skin over the potential nipple-areolar site before marking because when the skin is removed, it tends to open and there may be too much tension when closing the areola. Using the same marker, the surgeon determines the new location of the areola, which should be placed slightly below the optimal site. In almost all cases, there is some degree of rotation upward with the nipple moving into its proper location within the first 4 to 6 months.

After marking the first side, the exact location is transferred to the opposite side using the marking suture. The areola is sutured in a Gillies fashion, by starting at the four quadrants and then circumferencially (Fig. 10-13).

STEP 7: DRESSING
Micropore is placed on the skin in a triangular fashion around the areola, in a perpendicular fashion over the vertical incision, and obliquely directed toward the T, over the horizontal incision, to relieve as much tension as possible. A fluff dressing and plaster cast are applied with a wraparound, stretchable cling.

Arié-Pitanguy Technique
STEP 1: PREPARATION
The preparation of the patient is the same as that described earlier.

STEP 2: MARKING
1. Two marking sutures are placed at the suprasternal notch and midsubxyphoid area. A similar midclavicular line is drawn as in the classic Pitanguy technique.
2. Point A is established as in the classic Pitanguy technique and marked. Point D is placed at the submammary sulcus at or just lateral to the midclavicular line.
3. Points B and C are placed at opposite sides of the areola. The lines are connected to form a losan-

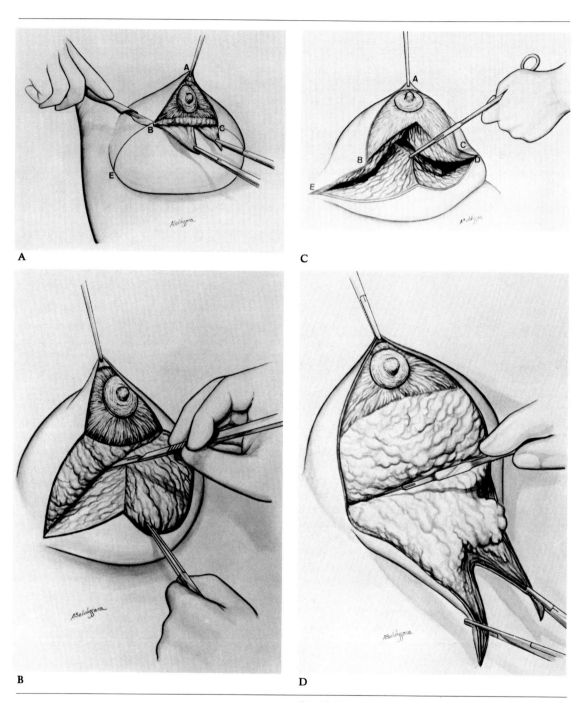

A

C

B

D

Fig. 10-11

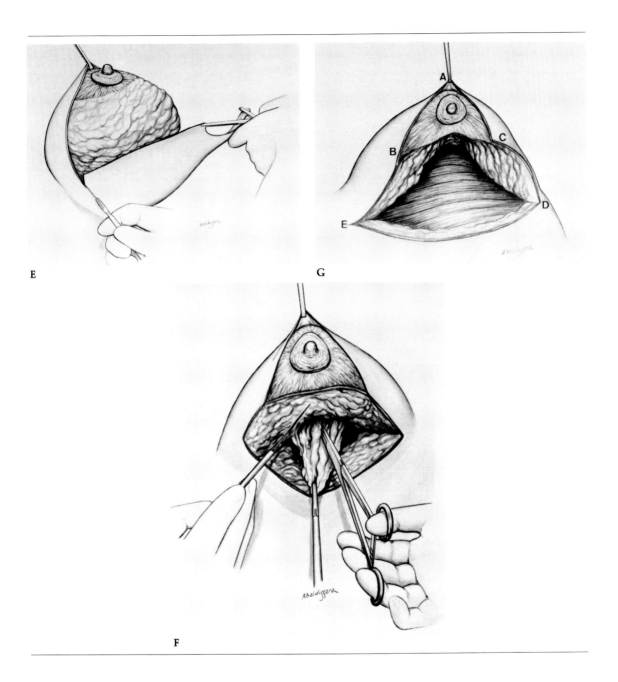

E

G

F

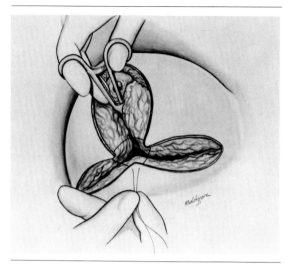

Fig. 10-12

gular or rhomboid-shaped incision (Figs. 10-14 and 10-15).

4. The nipple-areolar complexes are marked as in step 2 of the classic Pitanguy technique. If the breasts are quite small and the areola is hypertrophic, it may be safer to choose a larger template, because there may not be enough skin to close the breast without tension.

One may start with the intention to perform the Arié-Pitanguy technique through a losangular incision but may find that this extends below the inframammary sulcus more than 2 cm and will require conversion to a small L- or T-shaped incision. In other cases, an adequate resection may not be possible with a central wedge of tissue; one then has the option to convert the entire case to the classic Pitanguy technique by creating points D and E. Therefore, it is best to mark the submammary sulcus before beginning if one is not sure.

STEP 3: SCHWARTZMANN MANEUVER
The skin is deepithelialized within the confines of the points A, B, C, and D.

STEP 4: RESECTION OF SKIN AND GLAND
1. Depending on the case, an appropriate wedge of gland may be resected from the central portion of the gland. Unlike the "keel-shape" resection, the excision does not reach the lateral edges of the incision (Fig. 10-16).
2. If only skin resection is sufficient (Fig. 10-17),

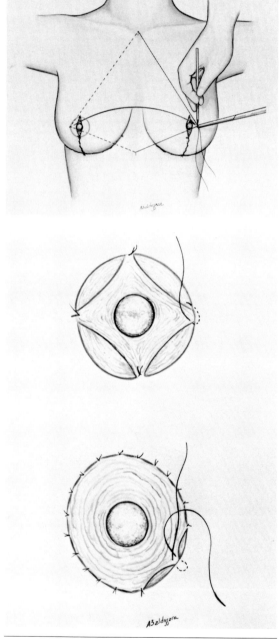

Fig. 10-13

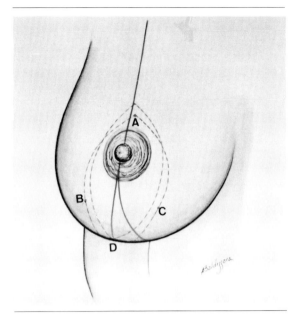

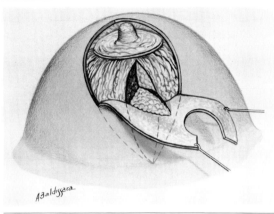

Fig. 10-16

Fig. 10-14

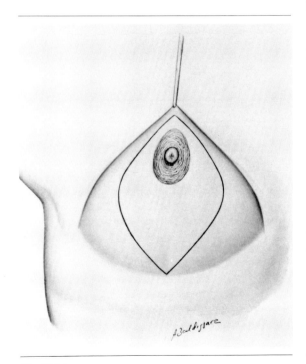

Fig. 10-15

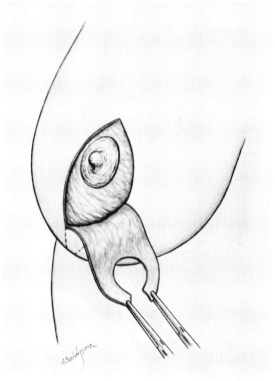

Fig. 10-17

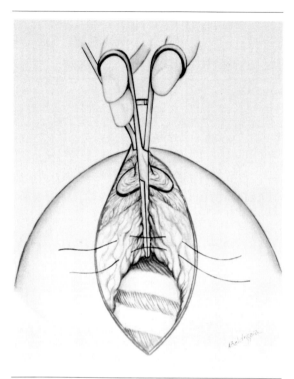

Fig. 10-18

the inferior pole of the gland may be mobilized off the pectoralis fascia by a slight undermining to allow the gland to ride upward freely.

STEP 5: CLOSURE

1. Following glandular resection, the two columns of tissue are reapproximated with several 3-0 long-acting, absorbable sutures. In some cases, the inferior pole will require more bulk. By mobilizing the axillary tail and fixing it to the inferomedial portion of the gland, one can fill this area nicely (Fig. 10-18).

2. When the skin is excessively flaccid, it is often necessary to perform an additional resection of the skin to tighten the skin-envelope over the gland. The excess skin can be undermined and resected with care not to extend beyond the margins of resection and avoid any dead space formation (Fig. 10-19).

3. At this point, the incision may extend below the sulcus. If *greater* than 1.5 to 2.0 cm, it should be converted to a small L or T. If *less than* 1.5 to 2.0 cm, the incisions have a tendency to move upward and give shape to the lower pole through the rotation of the gland in the first 3 to 4 months (Fig. 10-20).

STEP 6: NIPPLE-AREOLAR PLACEMENT

The nipple is placed in a similar fashion to step 6 of the classic Pitanguy technique. When the areola is excessively hypertrophic and the breasts are small, one will be safer and have better long-term results by choosing a larger areolar template because in attempting to make the areola too small, one may not have enough skin to close without tension on the periareolar area.

STEP 7: DRESSING

A dressing similar to that previously described is applied.

Postoperative Care

Antibiotics are routinely given for 5 to 7 days, with parenteral or oral analgesia when necessary. Significant pain in the first 24 hours may be an indication of hematoma formation and warrants removal of the dressing to check the wound. Otherwise, dressings are changed on the first postoperative day and replaced with a soft, elastic, well-fitted brassiere. The following day, patients are discharged with strict instructions to limit all activity during the first week.

Alternate sutures are removed on the seventh postoperative day and the remainder on the tenth day. The running subcuticular sutures are removed in 14 days, with replacement of the micropore. New micropore is used for 7 to 10 more days.

During the first 2 months, the patient is advised to limit all heavy activity and continue to use the compressive brassiere for 6 months. Follow-up checks are done at 3 months and 6 months, when possible. Depending on the case, the patient will be advised to avoid direct exposure to the sun from 3 to 6 months. Breast feeding has been possible as early as 12 to 14 months following the surgery.

Complications

Every plastic surgeon has to work within the limits of the tissues, the different morphologies, and the shortcomings of any surgical specialty. One should select a procedure that is sound, minimizes trauma to the tissues, and affords the least amount of complications.

When we analyzed our series of 245 cases using several different procedures prior to 1961 (group I) and compared them to 2,822 consecutive cases, using the described techniques, from 1961 to the present date (group II), the overall number of com-

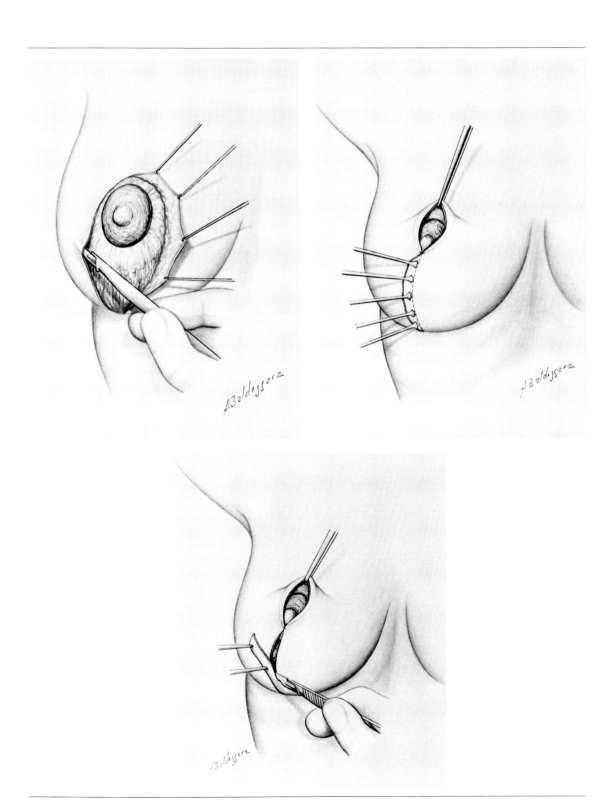

Fig. 10-19

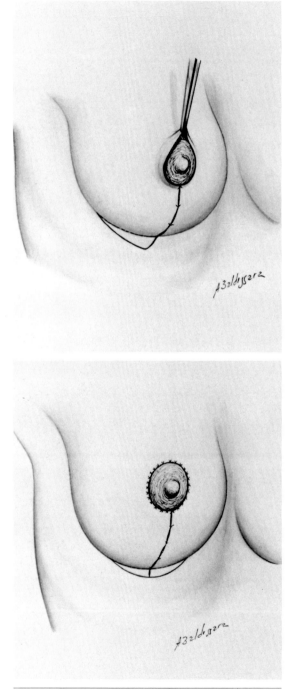

Fig. 10-20

Table 10-4. Complications in breast hypertrophy

Complications	1955–1961 (%)	1962–1987 (%)
Cutaneous problems	3.6	3.8
Areolar problems	1.2	0.9
Hematoma	1.2	0.4
Hypertrophic scar	10.3	1.4
Totals	16.3	6.5

plications decreased significantly (Table 10-4) [19]. The major problems seen in group I were hematoma, nipple and areolar suffering with some complete losses, skin flap necrosis, and hypertrophic scarring. Wide skin undermining and separation of the gland from its natural origin; resection of large amounts of tissue with resultant dead space formation; and disruption of the adipose capsule, which maintains blood supply and sensitivity to the nipple-areolar complex, were the primary problems that resulted in these complications. The long-term results of group I were often much less satisfying than those of group II because of their tendency to ptose, flatten superiorly, and sag inferiorly.

Hypertrophic scarring has always been a problem but tends to flatten if treated with steroids, massage, and compression. There have been a few cases with nipple hypersensitivity and some necrosis of the periareolar skin around sutures that were closed under tension. With time, though, these problems often resolve.

We have not experienced any cases of avascular necrosis of the nipple or major wound infections using the described techniques. Although some small skin infections have been seen, local treatment and routine use of perioperative antibiotics have reduced the incidence of this problem over the years.

One area of particular concern is the periareolar scarring. The areola is one of the most sensitive areas of the breast and should have the least amount of tension on the skin while looking for the best quality scar. In this area, there is a great tendency for opening of the skin, causing widening of these scars. Such problems are often not pleasing to the patient and are quite difficult to treat.

Several new procedures have been developed that reduce the breast through a periareolar incision. Recently, we have seen several patients with very large periareolar scars following these types of procedures. With the advent of any new procedure, there is always much enthusiasm generated. This can create such a momentum that many surgeons do not look closely enough at the potential for complications or poor long-term follow-up. Procedures that avoid scarring the breast must be carefully scrutinized for the proper patient selection and potential for significant scarring. These problems should be well defined before the procedure can be considered a safe and successful mode of therapy.

Conclusion

The two procedures presented herein avoid many of the problems seen with other techniques by going back to the basic principles of breast surgery and respecting the natural embryologic attachment of the skin to the gland while resecting tissue in a geometrically sound fashion that allows for closure without tension. This gives the reduced breast a natural support that will maintain the shape with consistency and longevity (see Cases 8 to 12).

Case Reports

CASE 1

A 31-year-old woman with mild hypertrophy and moderate ptosis is shown in Fig. 10-21. Five weeks following reduction using the Arié-Pitanguy technique, the scar had already begun to move upward, and by the end of 13 months, it was almost completely hidden within the submammary sulcus.

CASE 2

A 36-year-old woman with second- to third-degree hypertrophy, ptosis, and excessive skin in the lower pole is shown in Fig. 10-22. This was reduced using the classic Pitanguy mammaplasty with scars well hidden in the submammary sulcus.

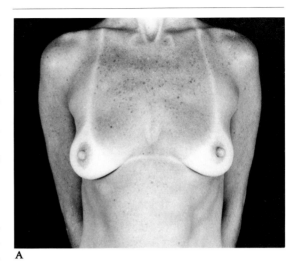
A

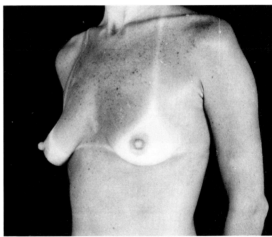
B

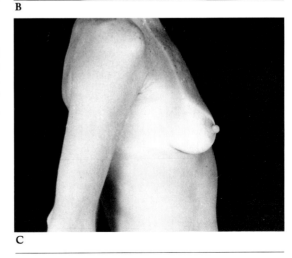
C

Fig. 10-21. A–C. Preoperative.

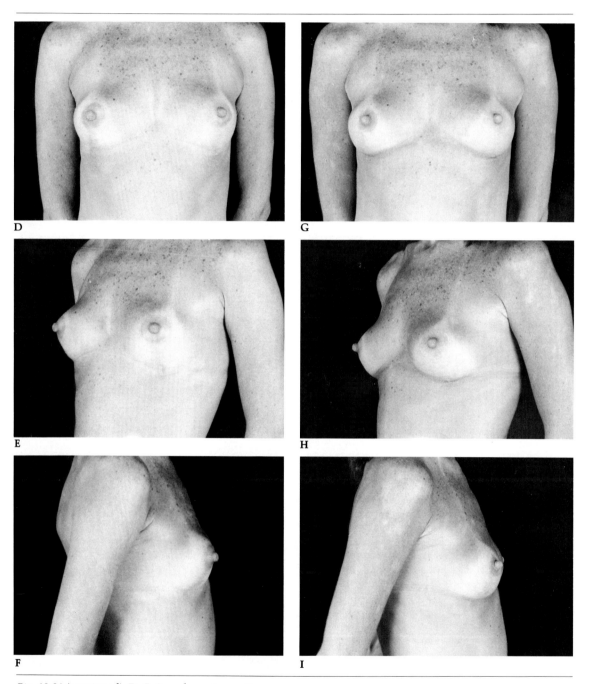

D

G

E

H

F

I

Fig. 10-21 (continued). D–F. 5 weeks postoperative.
G–I. 15 months postoperative.

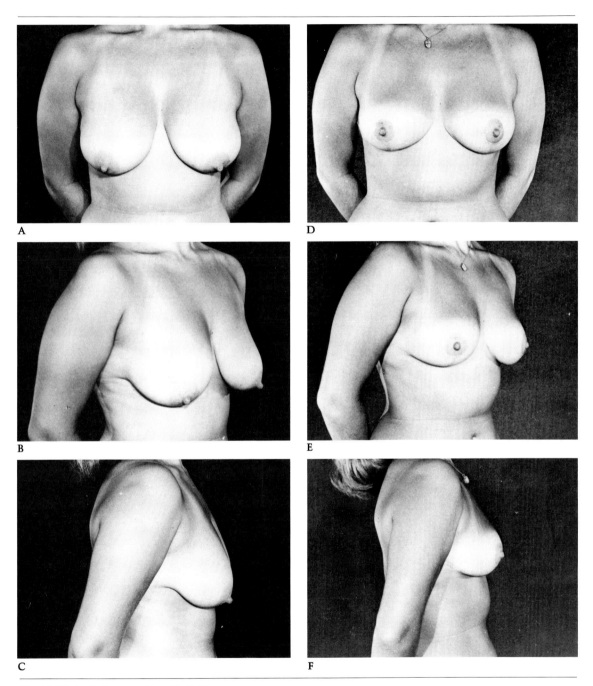

Fig. 10-22. A–C. Preoperative. D–F. 11 years postoperative.

CASE 3

A 23-year-old woman with first- to second-degree hypertrophy and ptosis with areolar hypertrophy is shown in Fig. 10-23. One will have more consistent and reliable results reducing such breasts using the Arié-Pitanguy technique, with a larger areolar template to avoid excessive tension on the periareolar skin.

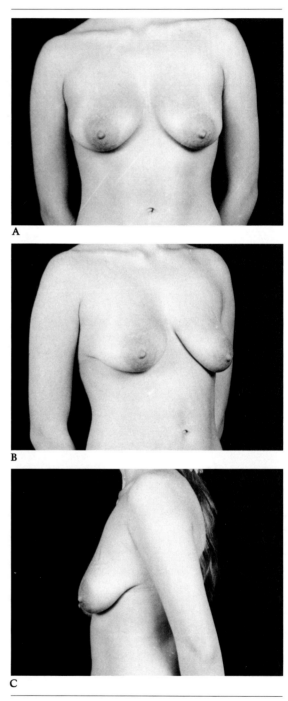

A

B

C

Fig. 10-23. A–C. Preoperative. D–F. 22 days postoperative. G–I. 3 months postoperative.

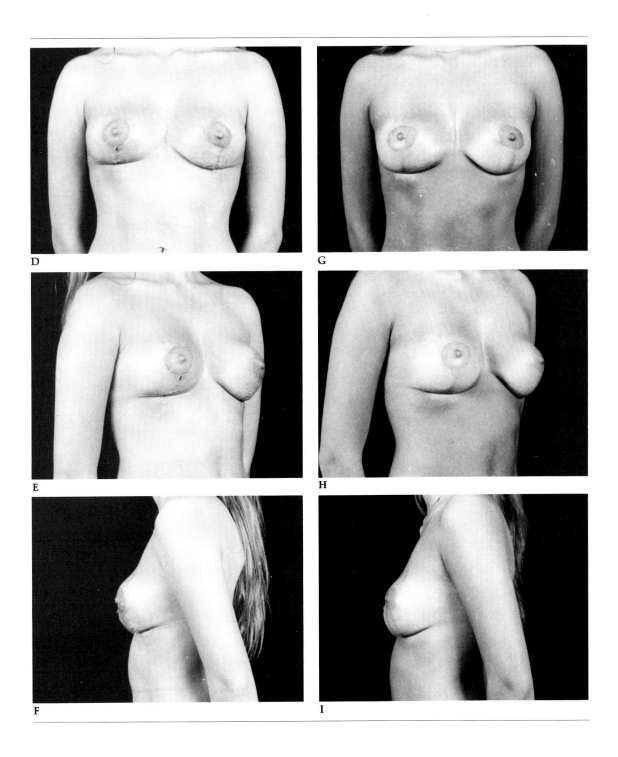

D

G

E

H

F

I

116

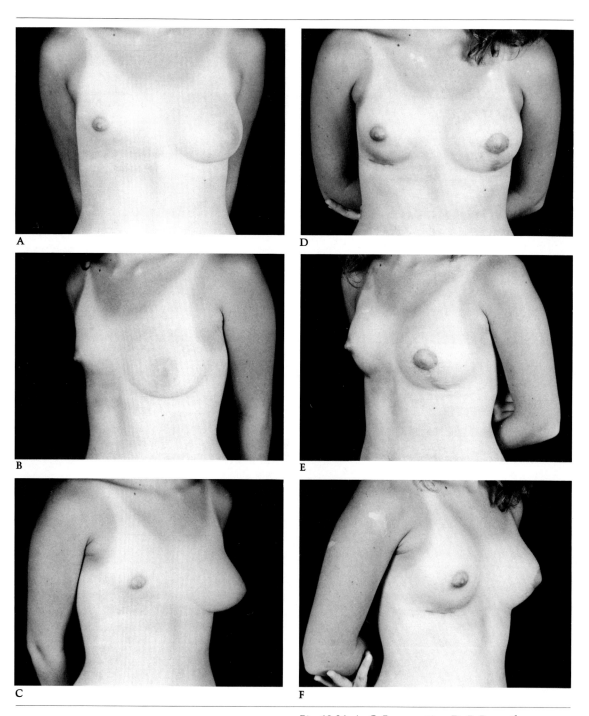

Fig. 10-24. *A–C. Preoperative. D–F. 7 months postoperative.*

CASE 4

A 16-year-old girl with marked asymmetry and hypoplasia of the right breast that would not allow for postoperative symmetry without inclusion of a prosthesis is shown in Fig. 10-24. The left side was quite glandular with a heavy lower pole that was corrected using the Arié-Pitanguy technique and insertion to a submuscular prosthesis in the submammary sulcus.

CASE 5

A 17-year-old girl with marked asymmetry and second-degree hypertrophy on the left side is shown in Fig. 10-25. The right breast had an acceptable size and shape for the patient and did not require surgery. Reduction of the left breast was performed using the classic Pitanguy technique without reducing the right side.

CASE 6

A 28-year-old woman with marked asymmetry and areolar hypertrophy on the left side is shown in Fig. 10-26. Such a case would be most suitable for the classic Pitanguy technique to accommodate both sides with symmetric scars and shapes.

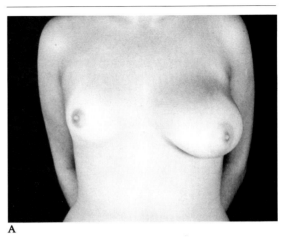

A

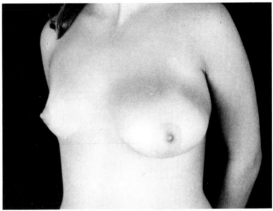

B

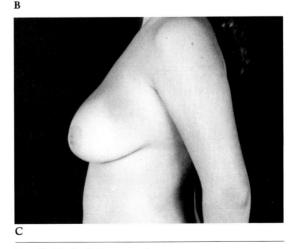

C

Fig. 10-25. A–C. Preoperative.

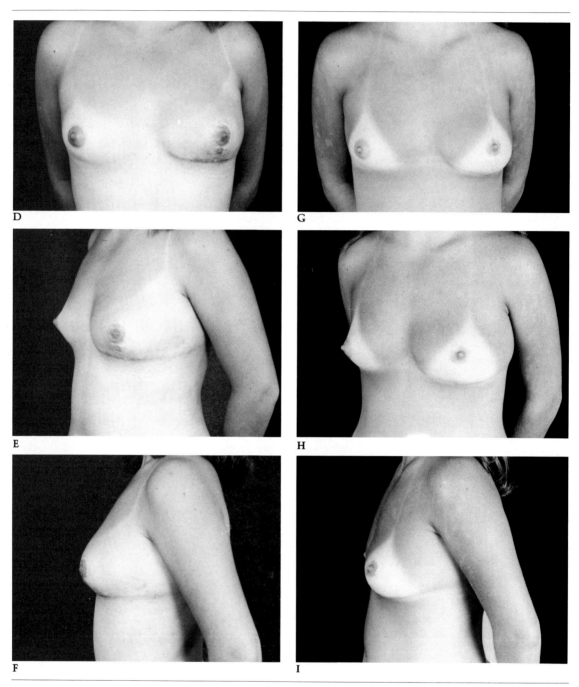

Fig. 10-25 (continued). D–F. 3 months postoperative.
G–I. 2 years postoperative.

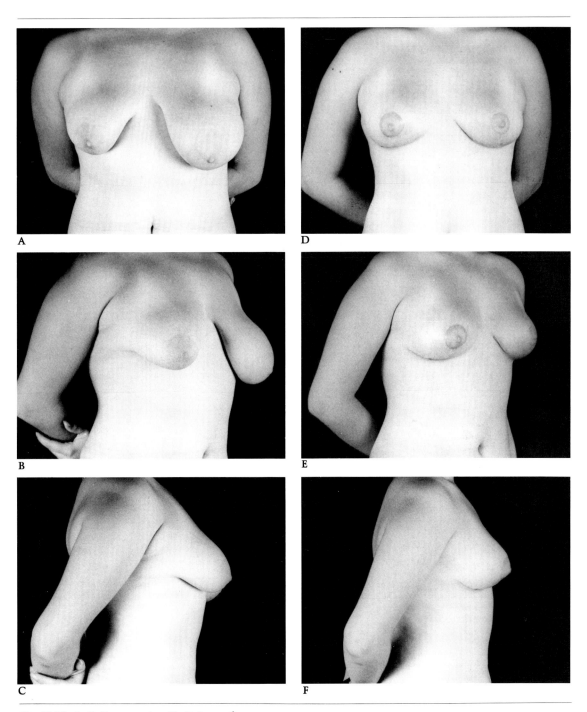

Fig. 10-26. A–C. Preoperative. D–F. 6 months postoperative.

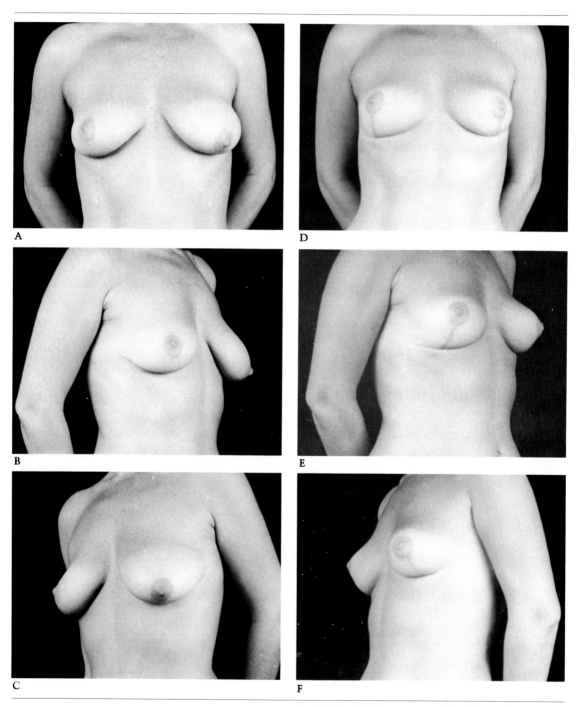

Fig. 10-27. *A–C. Preoperative. D–F. 9 months postoperative.*

CASE 7

A 17-year-old girl with asymmetric breasts and second-degree hypertrophy on the left side but a nicely shaped breast on the right side is shown in Fig. 10-27. Reduction using the Arié-Pitanguy technique allowed for adaptation of the larger, abnormally shaped breast to the better shaped, smaller breast without need for inclusion of a prosthesis.

CASE 8

A 32-year-old woman with mild hypertrophy and moderate ptosis that was corrected using the Arié-Pitanguy technique is shown in Fig. 10-28. Note the movement of the scar and nipple-areolar complex upward with rotation of the gland.

CASE 9

A 21-year-old woman with third-degree hypertrophy that was corrected using the classic Pitanguy technique is shown in Fig. 10-29.

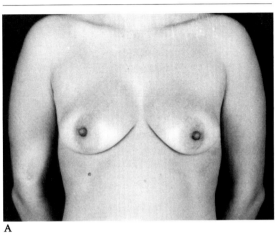

A

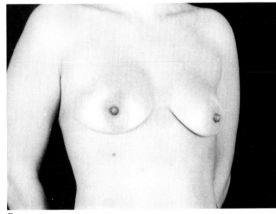

B

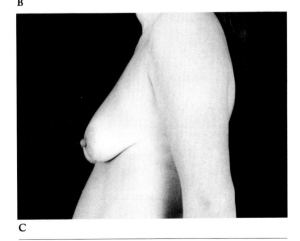

C

Fig. 10-28. A–C. Preoperative.

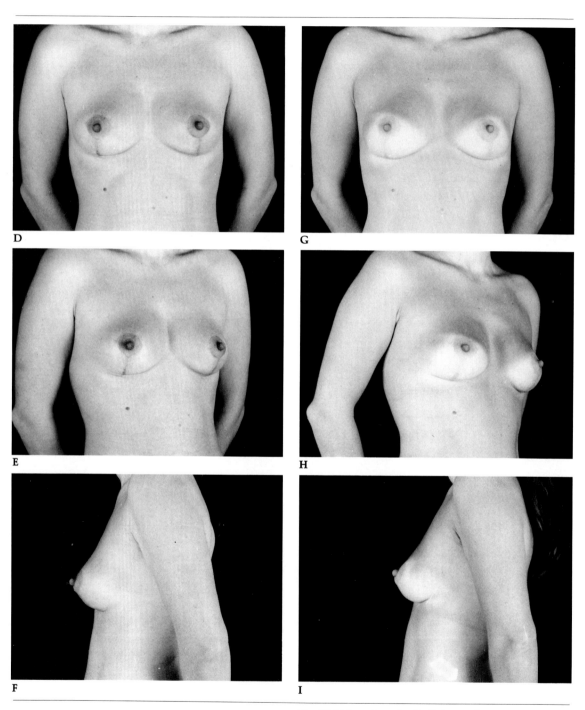

Fig. 10-28 (continued). D–F. 2 months postoperative.
G–I. 22 months postoperative.

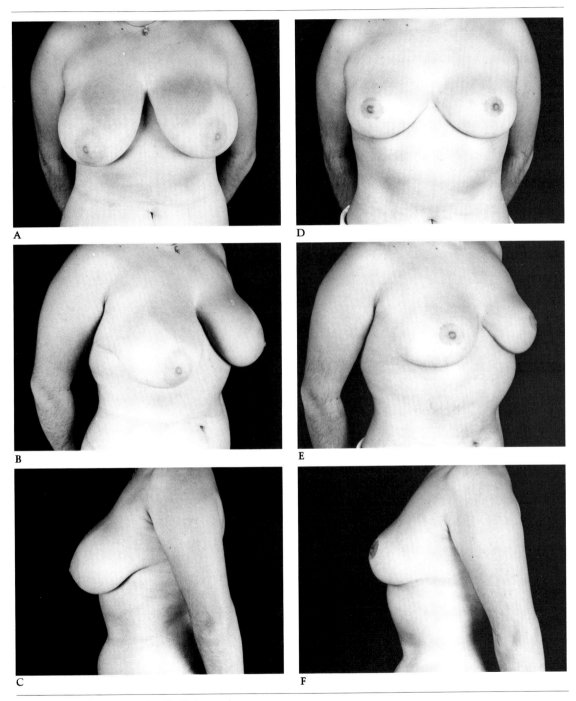

Fig. 10-29. A–C. Preoperative. D–F. 6 months
postoperative.

124

CASE 10

A 39-year-old woman with second-degree hypertrophy and ptosis that was corrected with the classic Pitanguy technique is shown in Fig. 10-30.

CASE 11

A 41-year-old woman with hypertrophy and asymmetric ptosis is shown in Fig. 10-31. Such cases with hanging, protuberous breasts are often more difficult than they appear. However, the classic Pitanguy technique allows one to modify and revise the resections and incisions during the procedure without being inhibited by fixed markings or nipple placement.

CASE 12

A 17-year-old girl with third-degree hypertrophy and mild ptosis is shown in Fig. 10-32. This patient complained of back pain and embarrassment of the large size of her breasts. Note the change in posture following surgery.

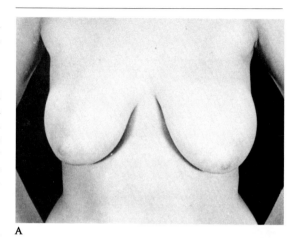

A

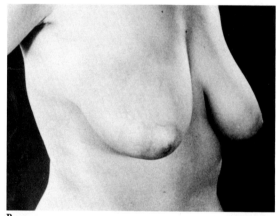

B

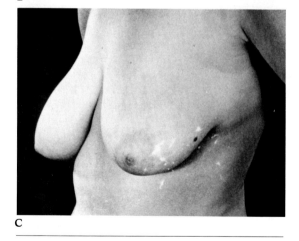

C

Fig. 10-30. A–C. Preoperative. D–F. 6 months postoperative. G–I. 10 years postoperative.

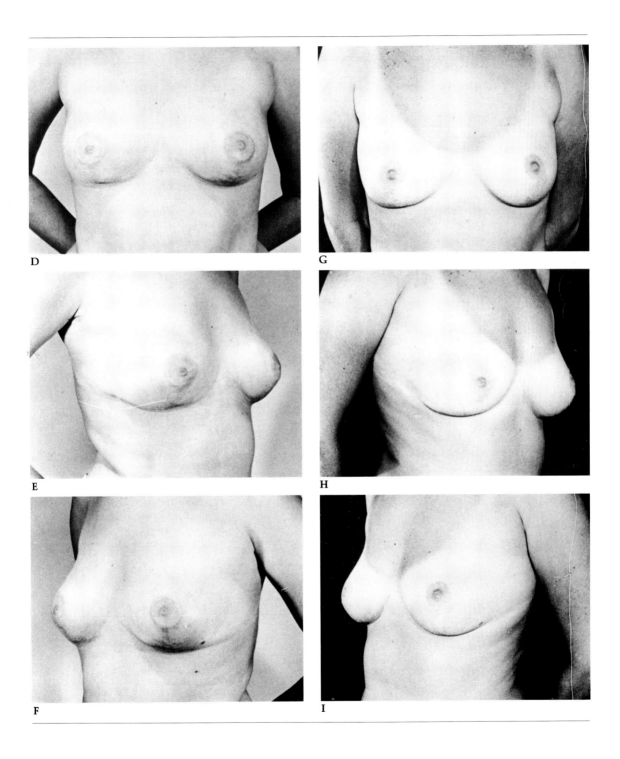

D

E

F

G

H

I

126

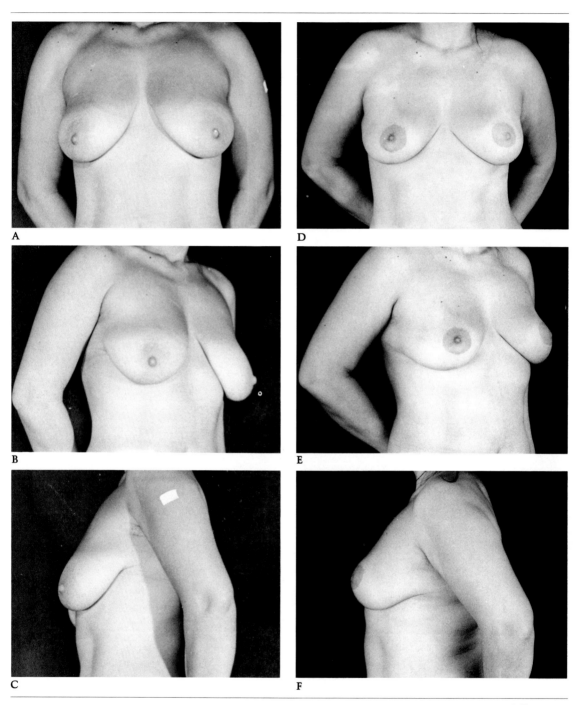

A

D

B

E

C

F

Fig. 10-31. A–C. Preoperative. D–F. 7 years follow-up.

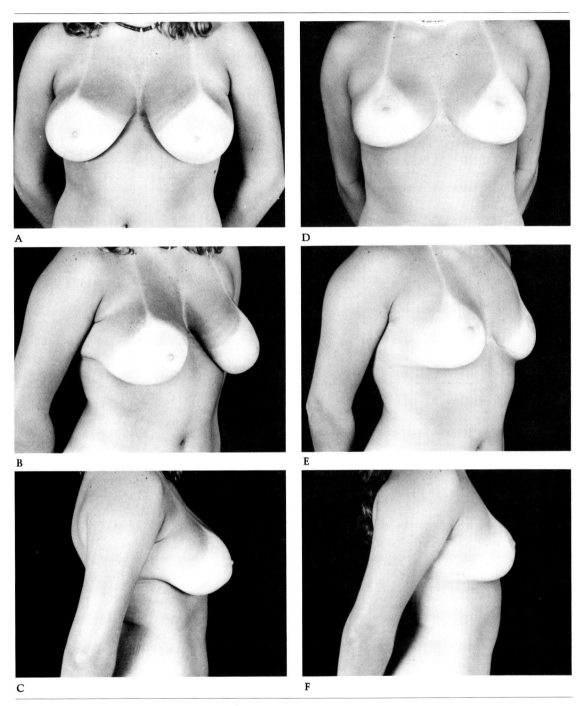

Fig. 10-32. A–C. Preoperative. D–F. 14 months postoperative.

References

1. Arié, G. Una nueva tecnica de mastoplastia. *Rev. Lat. Am. Cir. Plast.* 3:22, 1957.
2. Auber, V. Hypertrophie mammaire de la puberté, résection partielle restauratrice. *Arch. Franco-Belg. Chir.* 3:287, 1923.
3. Biesenberger, H. Blutversorgung und zirkuläre Umschnedung des Warzenhofes. *Zentralbl. Chir.* 55:2385, 1928.
4. Czerny, V. Plastischer Ersatz der Brustdruse durch ein Lipom. *Zentralbl. Chir.* 27:72, 1895.
5. Dehner, J. Mastopexie zur Beseitigung der Hängebrust. *Münch. Med. Wochenschr.* 36:1878, 1908.
6. Dufourmentel, C. *Chirurgie Reparatrice et Correctrice des Formes.* Paris: Masson et Cie, 1939.
7. Dufourmentel, C., and Mouly, R. Plastie mammaire par la méthode oblique. *Ann. Chir. Plast.* 6:1, 1961.
8. Durston, W. Sudden and excessive swelling of a woman's breast. *Phil. Trans. R. Soc.* (4th ed.). London: 1869. P. 78 (cited by Thorek).
9. Girard, C. Ueber Mastoptose und Mastopexie. *Verh. Dtsch. Ges. Chir. Beilage Zentralbl. Chir.* 31:70, 1910.
10. Guinard, A. Cited by Morestin (1903).
11. Kausch, W. Die operation der mammahypertrofie. *Zentralbl. Chir.* 43:713, 1916.
12. Kraske, M. Die operation der atrophischen und hypertrophischen Hängebrust. *Münch. Med. Wochenschr.* 70:672, 1923.
13. Lexer, E. Hypertrophie bei der Mammae. *Münch. Med. Wochenschr.* 59:2702, 1912.
14. Morestin, H. Hypertrophie mammaire traitée par la resection discoide. *Bull. Mem. Soc. Chir. Paris* 33:649, 1909.
15. Pitanguy, I. Breast Hypertrophy. Transactions of International Society of Plastic Surgeons (2nd Congress), London, 1959. Edinburgh: Livingstone, 1960. Pp. 509–517.
16. Pitanguy, I. Mastoplastias. Estudo de 245 casos consecutivos e apresentação de técnica pessoal. *Rev. Bras. Cir.* 42:201, 1961.
17. Pitanguy, I. *Aesthetic Plastic Surgery of Head and Body.* Berlin: Springer-Verlag, 1981. Pp. 3–36.
18. Pousson, M. De la mastopexie. *Bull. Mem. Soc. Chir. Paris* 23:507, 1897.
19. Thorek, M. Possibilities in the reconstruction of the human form. *N.Y. Med. J. Rec.* 116:572, 1922.

COMMENTS ON CHAPTER 10   *Robert M. Goldwyn*

Pitanguy has described as only he could the evolution of the techniques that bear his name and have been germinal to other methods described in this book. The advantages are their simplicity, their preservation of lactation and sensation, their safety in terms of vascular supply to the nipple-areola complex, and their capacity to produce a pleasing breast [2].

I have found Pitanguy's methods useful for breasts that are not enormous or gigantic. With his unique experience, Pitanguy could likely extend his methods to those situations better than I have been able to do. I prefer the inferior pedicle technique for massive macromastia. In using the classic Pitanguy method for those situations, I have found it necessary to resect so much tissue to achieve an adequate reduction and to facilitate upward transposition of the nipple-areola that I have been concerned about the sensation to the nipple as well as the possible jeopardy to blood supply and lactation.

To facilitate transposition of the nipple without tension and to prevent its distortion, Letterman and Schurter [1] described the useful maneuver of making small oblique cuts in the medial and lateral extremes of the dermal pedicle.

The question, therefore, for the surgeon who is planning to reduce a breast that is extremely hypertrophic is whether to use the alternative of the inferior or superior pedicle method, each of which gives the surgeon more latitude. Another alternative to consider with gigantomastia is, of course, free nipple grafting, which, in my experience, is rarely necessary if the inferior pedicle method is used.

In reducing larger breasts with the classic Pitanguy procedure, the inframammary scar lengthens, especially medially, where it might hypertrophy. Therefore, in those situations, one of the advantages of the Pitanguy method — the short scar — is not realized, at least by someone with my experience, although perhaps not with someone of Pitanguy's experience.

REFERENCES

1. Letterman, G., and Schurter, M. Facilitation of the upward advancement of the nipple-areola complex in reduction mammaplasty by Kiel resection. *Plast. Reconstr. Surg.* 67:793, 1981.
2. Marino, H. *Plasticas Mamarias* (2nd ed.). Buenos Aires: Lopez Libreros, 1978. Pp. 97–105.

11

Jan Olof Strömbeck

The Strömbeck Procedure for Reduction Mammaplasty

During my training in plastic surgery in the 1950s, I became familiar with the Ragnell technique for reduction mammaplasty. This technique was presented in Dr. Ragnell's monograph *Operative Correction of Hypertrophy and Ptosis of the Female Breast* published in 1946 [3].

The new position of the nipple was determined preoperatively with the patient in a sitting position on the breast meridian. A horizontal line was assumed drawn from the level of a point marked midway between the acromion and the olecranon process — that is, in the middle of the upper arm to intersect the breast meridian. This point for the nipple was found to be 17 to 20 cm from the upper sternal notch. The operation was done with the patient in a semisitting position and started with circumcision of the areola. The surrounding skin was dissected away as a full-thickness skin graft for about 2 cm around the areola to protect the superficial vessels, nerves, and nonstriated muscle. After that, the remaining skin cover was separated by blunt dissection to the periphery of the gland. A wedge-shaped resection was made from the upper middle part of the gland between the medial and lateral vascular pedicles. After shaping the gland with catgut sutures, the skin cover was shaped according to Biesenberger's method [1], and the suture line takes the form of an inverted T (Fig. 11-1).

In larger breasts, the skin reduction was made differently to give a horizontal skin closure above the submammary groove. An additional resection from the lower part of the breast was made as a second stage. Dr. Ragnell's interest in designing this operation was to preserve a good nursing capacity after the operation. For patients for whom nursing was not a consideration, a subtotal amputation with free nipple grafting could be done.

In my hands, the Ragnell technique did not always give a completely satisfactory result. I found it difficult to achieve full symmetry, and the incidence of circulatory disturbances in the areola, especially in the skin flaps, was rather high.

After having used Wise's pattern [15] to design the skin flaps when doing subtotal amputations with free nipple grafting, I was pleased with the symmetry and shape of the breasts but not always with the appearance of the nipples. It then occurred to me that if the areolar region could be transposed on a glandular pedicle in combination with the use of the pattern, the operation could be made without any undermining of the skin. This would simplify the operation and give safer results.

Dr. Ragnell always stressed the importance of both the medial breast circulation through the internal mammary artery and of the lateral from the lateral thoracic vessels. To me it thus seemed desirable to have one medial and one lateral pedicle, doing the resection of the gland above the areola and from the lower part of the breast. To secure best possible circulation to the areola, I preserved the deep dermis within the pedicles having in mind the buried epithelial flap of Barron (Fig. 11-2). The first operations I did according to this principle turned out quite satisfactorily, and I could publish my experiences with the first 37 patients in 1960 [5].

In this first publication, I listed the advantages to be (1) a one-stage procedure even with large hypertrophies; (2) technically a very simple operation; (3) good circulation in the remaining gland tissue and nipple; (4) no risk of skin necrosis; (5) no stitches in gland or fat, which lessens the risk of necrosis; and (6) cosmetically good and safe results.

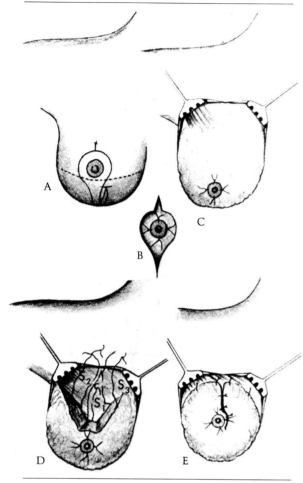

Fig. 11-1. Ragnell's technique for reduction mammaplasty. (From A. Ragnell. Operative correction of hypertrophy and ptosis of the female breast. Acta Chir. Scand.(Suppl.): 113, 1946.)

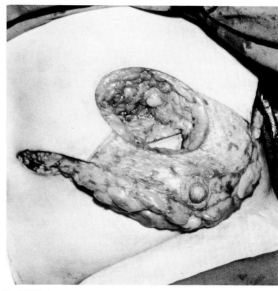

Fig. 11-2. Areola-carrying horizontal pedicle according to Strömbeck's original procedure from 1960.

Development of the Strömbeck Technique

PREOPERATIVE PLANNING

With the patient in a sitting position, the new nipple site is decided by drawing the breast meridian, which divides the breast into two equal halves. On this line, the distance of 19 to 21 cm from the upper sternal notch is marked. The original Wise pattern is placed symmetrically on the breasts and marked on the skin. After having marked the inframammary fold, the lower border lines of the skin flaps are adapted to fit the length. With the use of a standard pattern, the horizontal scar line in large breasts extended very far outside the newly formed breast and in smaller breasts formed a curve below the submammary fold laterally. Sometimes the vertical suture line had to be closed under considerable tension, with a tendency to give wound separation in the T-corner.

The primary shape was most pleasing, but with time, sometimes a sagging of the breast occurred ending up with the nipple position too high [6]. To avoid this, I made two changes in the preoperative planning. First, I decided the new nipple position more individually and used the submammary fold as a guide, marking the projection of the fold on the front side of the breast. Second, I shortened the vertical part of the pattern to 5 cm (Fig. 11-3).

To avoid tension in the vertical suture line, I first used a pattern with a decreased angle between the skin flaps but then found it more convenient to design the size of the skin flaps more individually by merely using the pattern as a guide and changing the angle between the flaps by free hand by testing which length of the skin flaps was necessary for a closure without tension (Fig. 11-4). Another factor to consider in the preoperative planning is the length of the horizontal scar. It should not extend outside the newly shaped breast. The preoperative planning also includes an assessment

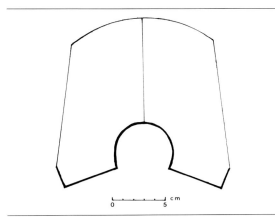

Fig. 11-3. Pattern for preoperative planning of skin flaps.

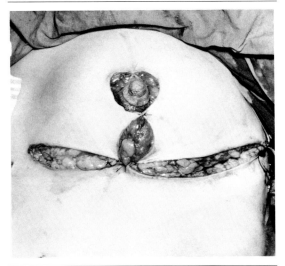

Fig. 11-5. Closure of the skin flaps makes the areola appear in its new position.

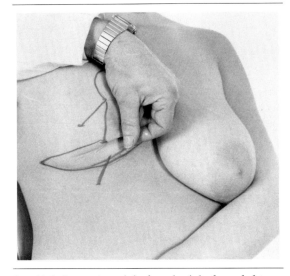

Fig. 11-4. Correction of the length of the lateral skin flap to avoid unnecessary tension.

of the appropriate resection, with special emphasis on side differences and with regard to the patient's wishes.

I have been using different methods for measuring the breast volume [7,14]. With experience, however, resection weight and side differences could be estimated rather accurately by eye.

SURGERY

The operation is made with the patient in the prone position. After circumcision of the areola, the glandular pedicles are designed and the skin

within the pedicles is excised superficially, leaving the deep dermis intact. The resection is made in the keyhole above the areola and horizontally from the lower part of the breast. This leaves the areola on a horizontal glandular bridge between the skin flaps (see Fig. 11-2). When adapting the skin borders to each other, the glandular bridge is folded so that the areola appears in its new position (Fig. 11-5).

It soon became evident that the folding of the glandular bridge was the part of the operation where difficulties could arise, especially in cases where the bridge consisted mostly of fat and dense tissue. And when the pedicles were short, the dermal part of the bridge could not stretch to allow a relaxed transposition of the areola. In those cases, I first divided the dermal part of the shortest pedicle partly or completely. In smaller breasts, I did not make any resection above the areola but divided the dermis with vertical skin incisions and also, if necessary, slightly undermined the skin flaps.

A further development was that I started to sacrifice one of the pedicles, the lateral, relying on the circulation from the medial side. The vessels from the internal mammary artery, judging from earlier experience with the Biesenberger technique, for example, seemed to be sufficient for an adequate circulation to the areola. In these cases, I broadened the base of the glandular pedicle. This made the transposition of the areola much easier and in

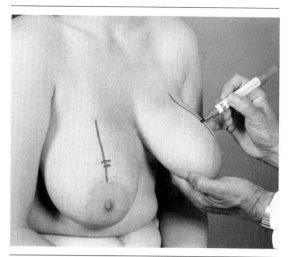

Fig. 11-6. *The projection of the submammary fold is used to determine the new level for the nipple on the breast meridian.*

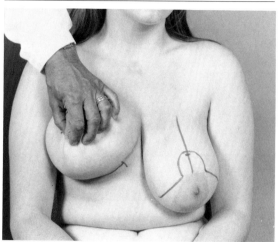

Fig. 11-8. *The length of the submammary incision is marked.*

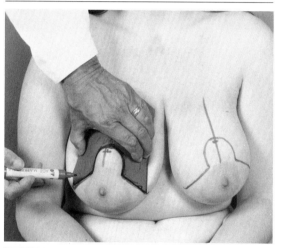

Fig. 11-7. *The pattern is placed on the breast with the upper border of the "keyhole" slightly above the marking for the nipple. The borders of the pattern are marked on the skin.*

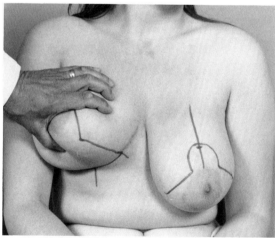

Fig. 11-9. *The point to which the medial skin corner has to be sutured is marked on the submammary fold.*

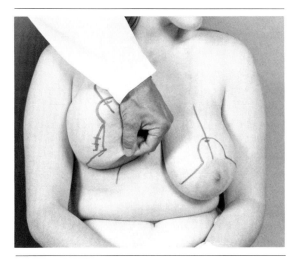

Fig. 11-10. Checking of the length of the lateral skin flap. Often correction has to be made to give an adequate skin cover (see Fig. 11-5).

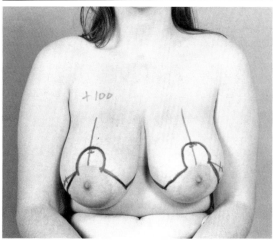

Fig. 11-11. Preoperative planning is completed. Side differences, if any, have to be checked and estimated in volume.

most cases also improved the shape of the breast [8].

With time, I have adopted the technique of using only one medial pedicle and have extended the resection to include even some of the lateral part of the breast gland. This means that instead of starting by creating a horizontal bridge and dividing the lateral pedicle only when it is necessary for getting good transposition of the nipple area, I make one broad medial pedicle from the start.

Present Strömbeck Technique

PREOPERATIVE PLANNING
The patient sits with her arms hanging loosely at each side. The surgeon sits in front of the patient but on a lower stool. The breast meridian is marked to divide the breast into two equal halves. The projection of the inframammary fold is marked on the breast meridian to decide the new nipple position (Fig. 11-6). In patients with very big breasts, the new nipple site should be somewhat medial to the breast meridian to avoid lateralization of the nipple as in those cases in which rather much tissue has to be removed from the lateral part of the breast. Symmetric positioning of the nipples has to be checked. The pattern is placed on the breast so that the center of the upper part of the keyhole for the nipple is slightly above the nip-

ple-marking and turned so that the medial incision line of the pattern will be vertical when the breast is moved laterally (Fig. 11-7). The submammary fold is now marked, and the end points are indicated to make sure that the submammary incision will not extend outside the newly shaped breast (Fig. 11-8). The point to which the lower medial corner of the skin flap arrives when moving the breast laterally is marked on the submammary groove (Fig. 11-9).

The breast is now moved medially, and the length of the lateral skin flap is estimated. In many cases, the necessary length is not in agreement with the length given by the pattern. The lateral vertical incision line has then to be changed, which is easily done by free hand. These end points will now be connected with lower corners of the skin flaps, respectively (Figs. 11-9 and 11-10).

In large breasts, the sum of the upper horizontal incisions might become considerably longer than the incision in the submammary groove to which they are to be sutured, which calls for some gathering when making the suture. In smaller breasts, it sometimes happens that the upper corners of the skin flaps will be within the areola skin when applying the pattern. In such a case, the upper corners have to be transferred outside the areola skin and the vertical part of the skin flap marking has to be drawn by free hand. It is imperative to achieve a full symmetry in the drawings of both

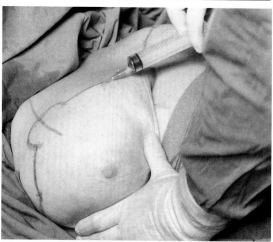

Fig. 11-12. Local anesthesia (0.25% lidocaine with epinephrine 1:400,000) is infiltrated along the incision lines and above the pectoral fascia.

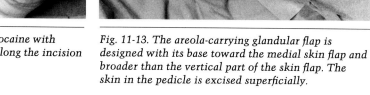

Fig. 11-13. The areola-carrying glandular flap is designed with its base toward the medial skin flap and broader than the vertical part of the skin flap. The skin in the pedicle is excised superficially.

breasts. It is also important to estimate side differences at this time because it is much more difficult to see differences with the patient lying down on the operation table (Fig. 11-11).

ANESTHESIA

The operation is made with the patient in a horizontal position and the arms abducted 90 degrees. General anesthesia is given. In addition, a local anesthetic agent is infiltrated along the incision lines and over the pectoral fascia. A solution of 0.25 percent lidocaine with epinephrine (1:400,000) is used (Fig. 11-12). This decreases the bleeding considerably and also allows for a more superficial general anesthesia. The use of local infiltration of epinephrine does not increase the risk for circulatory disturbances. However, the hemostasis has to be precise. In our experience, hematomas postoperatively have been no problem.

SURGICAL PROCEDURE

To facilitate the first part of the operation, the breast is distended by the application of a tourniquet around the base of the breast. The areola is circumcised superficially, leaving an areola of 4.5 cm in diameter. The areola-carrying glandular pedicle is designed with its base toward the medial skin flap and broader than the vertical part of the skin flap (Fig. 11-13). The base is extended into the "keyhole" and, if necessary, in larger breasts, even below the medial horizontal part of the medial

skin flap. The skin in the pedicle is excised superficially onto the border of the skin flap (see Fig. 11-13).

The resection starts with an incision along the keyhole from the upper lateral corner of the de-epithelialized pedicle, extending laterally along the skin flap all the way to its lateral corner. With the breast stretched in a caudal direction, this incision is carried all the way through the glandular tissue to the muscle fascia (Fig. 11-14). With one hand from beneath supporting the lower part of the breast, the next incision goes along the lateral and lower borders of the pedicle and the medial skin flap to its medial corner. The breast is now divided into two parts (Fig. 11-15), the lower of which is removed after an incision in the submammary groove has been made (Fig. 11-16). If additional resection is necessary, it can be made from the area under the lateral skin flap or above the keyhole. When an adequate resection has been done, the skin is closed (Fig. 11-17). I start with a three-point stitch, joining the two lower corners of the skin flaps to the submammary groove at the point marked preoperatively. The areola is now rotated up to its new position. *The nipple-areola transposition should be made without any traction.* If the pedicle carrying the areola is short and restrains a complete transposition, it is easy to see where the tension lies. Usually this tension is

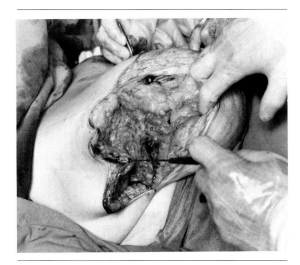

Fig. 11-14. Incision through the glandular tissue along the skin marking from the upper lateral corner of the deepithelialized pedicle to the lateral corner of the marking in the submammary groove.

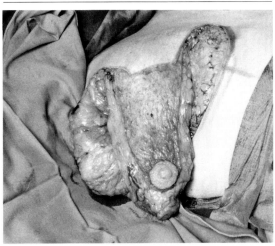

Fig. 11-16. Through an incision in the submammary groove, the resection is completed.

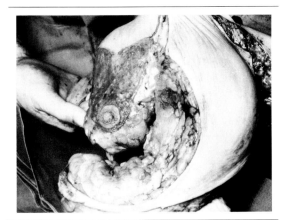

Fig. 11-15. With an incision along the areola-carrying pedicle extended to the medial corner of the submammary marking, the breast is now divided into two parts.

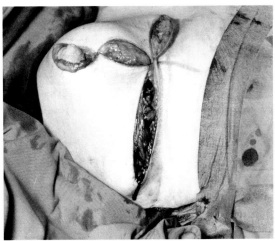

Fig. 11-17. Skin closure starts with joining of the corners of the skin flaps.

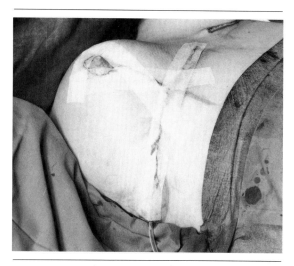

Fig. 11-18. After completed skin closure, the suture lines are taped with micropore.

eliminated by dividing the dermal part of the pedicle partly or totally. Rarely, one has to cut into the fat or pedicle partly or totally to achieve a complete relaxation. When the upper corners of the skin flaps are now joined, the areola should be in the center of the hole designed for it.

Suturing is completed by subcuticular and running intracuticular suturing. The weight of the resected tissue has to be checked carefully to be in accordance with the preoperative estimation to achieve full symmetry in volume. I drain the wound cavity and apply suction. The incision lines are taped with micropore (Fig. 11-18), and a dressing is applied with Surgifix net. Intraoperative bleeding never exceeds 200 ml when using local anesthesia with epinephrine. Blood transfusions do not come into question.

POSTOPERATIVE CARE

The drains can usually be removed the day after surgery but are kept in place for 1 day more if the bleeding has been more than 60 ml. The patients are kept hospitalized for 1 or 2 days after surgery. The stitches are removed after 1 to 2 weeks. When using Dexon intracutaneously, only the ends have to be removed. For young patients, I recommend having the scar lines taped with micropore for at least 3 months. I believe that this reduces the tendency to hypertrophic scarring and, thus, in the long run, gives better scars, even if I have not proved this by randomized studies.

COMPLICATIONS

To evaluate the postoperative complications, I have analyzed the records from my last 323 consecutive cases operated with one medial pedicle.

Hematoma

Small collections are evacuated through the drains. Major hematomas requiring reoperation with evacuation and hemostasis were rare, occurring in only two patients (two breasts) from 323 cases, or 581 operated upon breasts. The hematoma does not influence the final result but may prolong the healing time.

Fat Necrosis

Circulatory disturbances of the fat tissue of the breast may occur in the grossly overweight patient. Minor fat necrosis presents itself after some

Table 11-1. Fat necrosis in relation to obesity and weight of resected tissue in 323 patients (581 breasts) operated with one medial pedicle

	Resection (gm)				Total no. breasts
	<500	500–999	>1000	Total %	
Normal weight <+6 kg	0/221	0/84	0/4	0	309
Fat +6–+15 kg	0/63	3/113	0/10	1.6	186
Very fat >+15 kg	0/17	0/47	4/22	4.7	86
Total %	0.0	1.2	11.1	1.1	
Total no. breasts	301	244	36		581

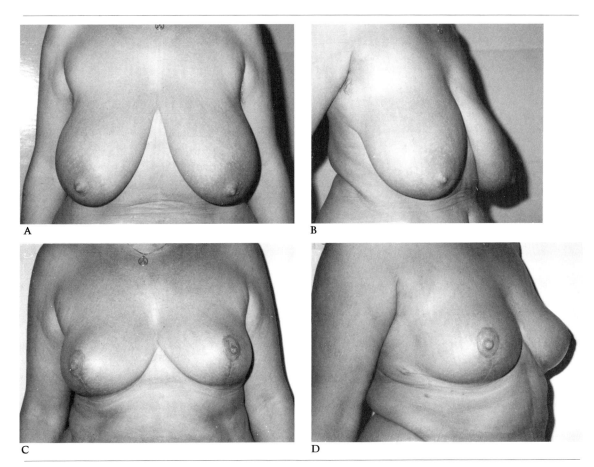

Fig. 11-19. A, B. A 47-year-old patient preoperatively.
C, D. Three months after resection of 860 gm from the
right breast and 850 gm from the left breast.

weeks as hard lumps, which, after considerable time, may soften. They do not require treatment, but if the patient is afraid it might be a malignancy, an excision or needle biopsy may put her mind at rest. A major fat necrosis often advertises its occurrence in the first postoperative days, with a temperature rise to 38.5 to 39° C. The breast is firm, and the skin becomes reddish. It drains spontaneously or after incision and will continue to drain until all necrotic tissue has been expelled, which could take months. In the event of major fat necrosis, it is advisable to reoperate as soon as the necrosis is demarcated (i.e., after 2 to 3 weeks), and excise all necrotic tissue. The frequency of major fat necrosis in my series of 323 consecutive cases can be seen in Table 11-1. Very fat patients with large resections represent the risk group.

The conclusion that the incidence of fat necrosis in a series depends on the weight distribution of the patients has also been drawn from my earlier reports [7,9].

Areola Necrosis

The circulatory disturbance that causes a major fat necrosis may influence the areola circulation, resulting in a total or partial necrosis of areola and nipple. In my series of 323 consecutive cases, partial areola necrosis occurred in three breasts, all in greatly overweight women. The necrotic areas healed spontaneously, leaving somewhat depigmentated areas. No total necrosis of areola and nipple occurred. This complication lengthened the healing time but, in my cases, did not influence the patient's satisfaction with the operation. A tattooing of the pale areas may be done if the patient so wishes.

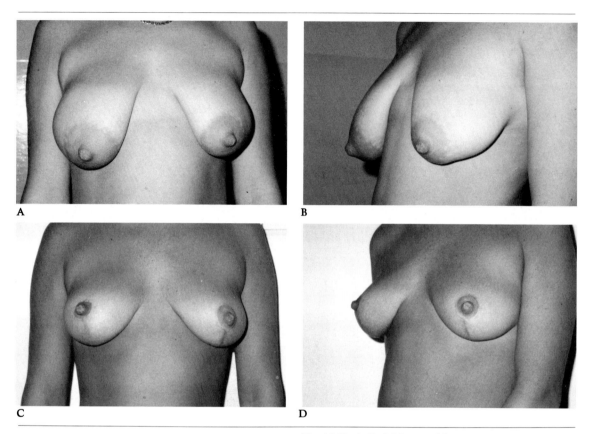

A

B

C

D

Fig. 11-20. A, B. A 24-year-old patient. C, D. One year after resection of 300 gm from the right breast and 200 gm from the left breast.

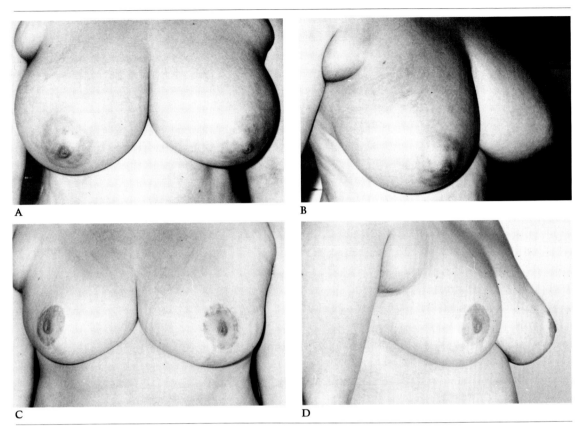

A

B

C

D

Fig. 11-21. A, B. A 27-year-old patient. C, D. Five years
after removal of 1005 gm from the right breast and
1010 gm from the left breast.

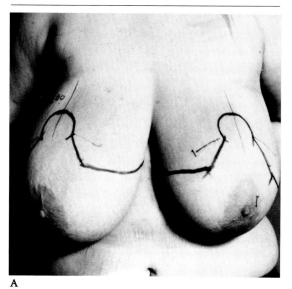

A

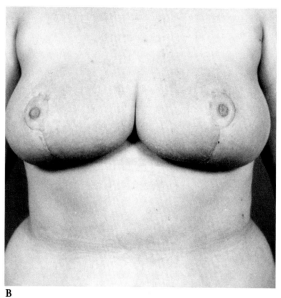

B

Fig. 11-22. A. A 19-year-old patient. B. One month after resection of 2 kg from the right breast and 1.6 kg from the left breast.

RESULTS

The patient's satisfaction with the result depends on whether it is in accordance with her expectations in regard to size, shape, and scars. This calls for an accurate preoperative planning and information to the patient. Especially difficult is the very young patient because she has a tendency to have unrealistic expectations and to form hypertrophic scars. Futhermore, it is more difficult to decide on a proper size. Future pregnancies and weight changes may cause considerable alterations of breast volume. It is good advice to leave the breast in young women somewhat larger than you otherwise would have done [12]. The complication rate of the 323 consecutive patients mentioned previously is based on our clinical records. The patients have not been recalled for examination. Long-term follow-up has been reported earlier [7,9 – 13].

Advantages and Disadvantages of this Technique

This is a simple technique with predictable results. It could be adapted to all types of breasts with hypertrophy or ptosis. The main disadvantage is the rather long incision in the submammary groove. But the submammary scar could and should be kept within the newly shaped breast. As long as this scar does not extend outside the breast medially or laterally, it is of less interest from a cosmetic point of view if the scar is 5 cm or 15 cm in length.

Cases Suitable for this Procedure

It is most easy to use this technique when operating on breasts with moderate hypertrophy and ptosis, but with experience in dealing with the fat and tense breast, it is as easily applied here as well as to all types of breasts (Figs. 11-19 through 11-25). Personally, I alternate with two other techniques. I use the lateral excision with an L-shaped scar, which I prefer to use in younger patients with rather moderate hypertrophy where I want to avoid the medial scar line completely and in cases of mastopexy where no or very small reductions have to be made [10,12]. The inferiorly based pedicle technique [2,4], which I have been using occasionally in very big breasts as an alternative to the very long extended medial pedicle, however, I am using less and less frequently.

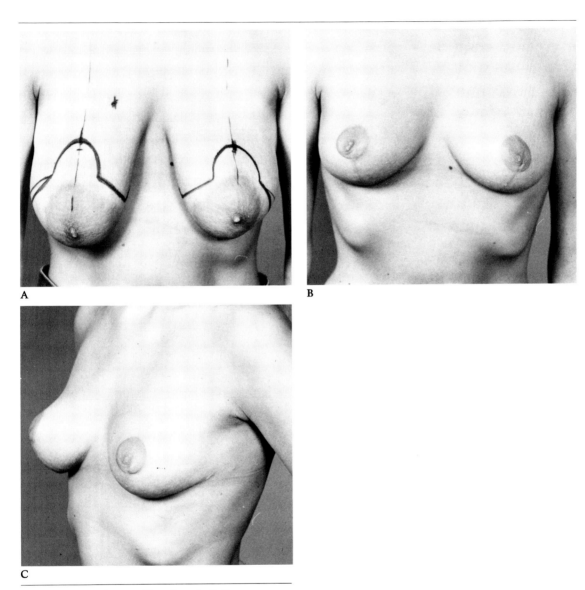

Fig. 11-23. A. A 19-year-old patient. B, C. One year postoperatively; 230 gm were removed from the right breast and 200 gm from the left breast.

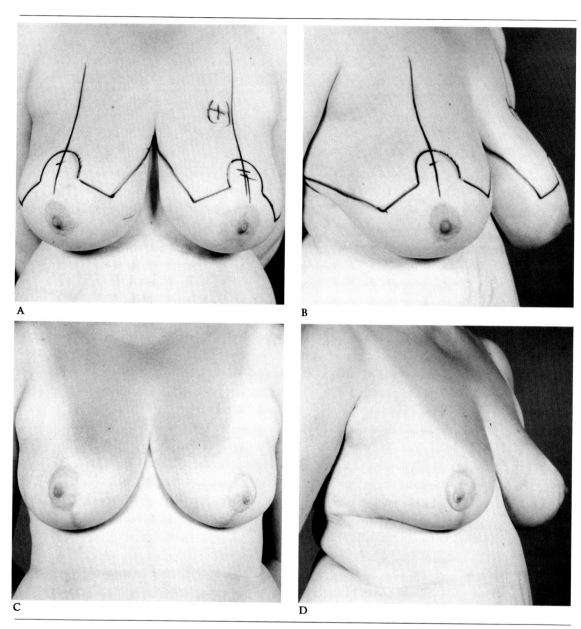

A

B

C

D

Fig. 11-24. A, B. A 40-year-old patient. C, D. Four months postoperatively; 980 gm were removed from the right breast and 1000 gm from the left breast.

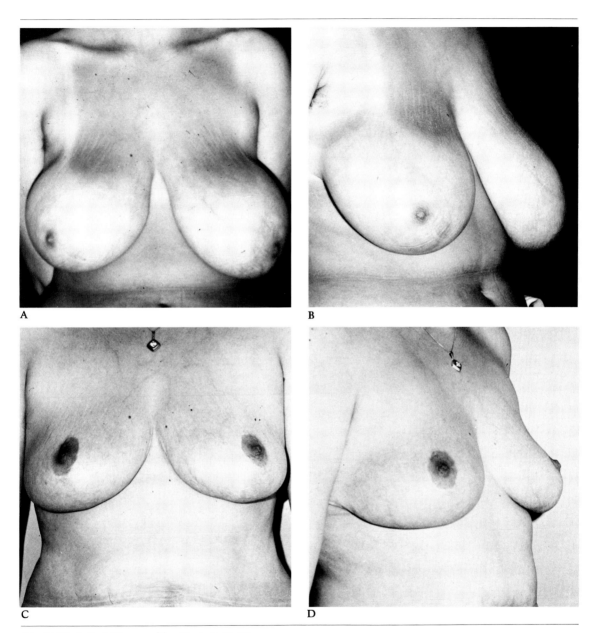

A

B

C

D

Fig. 11-25. A, B. A 21-year-old patient. C, D. Nine years
after removal of 780 gm from the right breast and
885 gm from the left breast.

There are many ways to achieve a good mammaplasty. I have always been of the opinion that an experienced plastic surgeon will have the best results with a technique of which he has a great deal of experience.

References

1. Biesenberger, H. Deformitäten und kosmetischen Operationen der weiblichen Brust. Wien: W. Maudrich, 1931.
2. Courtiss, E.H., and Goldwyn, R.M. Reduction mammaplasty by the inferior pedicle technique. *Plast. Reconstr. Surg.* 59:500, 1977.
3. Ragnell, A. Operative correction of hypertrophy and ptosis of the female breast. *Acta Chir. Scand.* Suppl. 113, 1946.
4. Robbins, T.H. A reduction mammaplasty with the areola nipple based on an inferior dermal pedicle. *Plast. Reconstr. Surg.* 59:64, 1977.
5. Strömbeck, J.O. Mammaplasty: Report of a new technique based on the two-pedicle procedure. *Br. J. Plast. Surg.* 13:79, 1960.
6. Strömbeck, J.O. Reduction Mammaplasty. In T. Gibson (ed.), *Modern Trends in Plastic Surgery.* London: Butterworths, 1964. P. 237.
7. Strömbeck, J.O. Macromastia in women and its surgical treatment. *Acta Chir. Scand.* Suppl. 341, 1964.
8. Strömbeck, J.O. Reduction mammaplasty. *Surg. Clin. North Am.* 51:453, 1971.
9. Strömbeck, J.O. Reduction Mammaplasty by Upper and Lower Glandular Resections. In R.M. Goldwyn (ed.), *Plastic and Reconstructive Surgery of the Breast.* Boston: Little, Brown, 1980. P. 195.
10. Strömbeck, J.O. Benign diseases of the female breast. Surgical treatment and cosmetic aspects. Excerpta Medica International Congress Series 412. Proceedings of the VIII International Congress of Gynecology and Obstetrics, Mexico City, October 17–22, 1976. Amsterdam: Excerpta Medica, 1977. P. 184.
11. Strömbeck, J.O. Late Results after Reduction Mammaplasty. In R.M. Goldwyn (ed.), *Long-term Results in Plastic and Reconstructive Surgery.* Boston: Little, Brown, 1980. P. 722.
12. Strömbeck, J.O. Reduction Mammoplasty. In N.G. Georgiade (ed.), *Aesthetic Breast Surgery.* Baltimore: Williams & Wilkins, 1983. P. 146.
13. Strömbeck, J.O. Reduction Mammaplasty. In J.O. Strömbeck and F.E. Rosato (eds.), *Surgery of the Breast.* Stuttgart–New York: Georg Thieme Verlag, 1986. P. 277.
14. Strömbeck, J.O., and Malm, M. Priority grouping in a waiting list of patients for reduction mammaplasty. *Ann. Plast. Surg.* 17:498, 1986.
15. Wise, R.J. A preliminary report on a method of planning the mammaplasty. *Plast. Reconstr. Surg.* 17:367, 1956.

COMMENTS ON CHAPTER 11   *Robert M. Goldwyn*

For the past three decades, Strömbeck has been a germinal influence in the field of breast reduction. He is one of the few surgeons who not only has contributed new techniques but has objectively analyzed and thoroughly reported his short- and long-term results, the bad with the good. That kind of thoughtful and truthful self-evaluation is unfortunately rarer than it should be, but it has led Strömbeck to evolve better methods for reduction mammaplasty. His chapter records the steps in this quest. The original Strömbeck procedure was the first type of transposition reduction that I ever performed, having learned in my residency only nipple grafting techniques. Early in practice, in 1963, Dr. Eugene Courtiss and I helped each other with our first patients. We had recognized the need for preserving sensation and possibly lactation, two functions that reduction by nipple grafting failed to achieve to a comparable degree.

Strömbeck's original procedure [6], as he has stated, was and is safe in terms of nipple-areola viability because it preserves its principal blood supply within its large medial and lateral flaps. The method, however, has problems, some of which Strömbeck has noted. One disadvantage is the rather long medial scar that has a tendency to become hypertrophic and later, after atrophy, broadens, especially in younger patients whose tendency is to form hypertrophic scars. Another disadvantage is that during the first postoperative year, the areola-nipple complex has a tendency to sink and invert [2]. Strömbeck ascribes this to the fact that the areola-carrying glandular flap sags and pulls the areola with it. Different types of dermal loops have been used to fix the gland and theoretically prevent sagging, but these techniques have not always been successful.

My observation and that of others [2,3] has been that as sagging occurs, the breast descends, the nipple seems to rise, and the breast looks flat and square.

A significant disadvantage of the earlier Strömbeck method was the high frequency of sensory loss in the areola and nipple as a result of damaging branches from the intercostal nerves when excising the lower segment of the breast [7].

Planas and Mosely [5] advised waiting until the time of closure before discarding the inferior dermal fat flap totally so it could be used if desired. In two thirds of their patients, it was excised, but in the remaining group, it was worthwhile in producing symmetry and projection. It may also have resulted in better sensation, but this was not evaluated by those authors.

Elsahy [1], following Pitanguy's principle, modified the technique so that the new nipple site would be selected according to the new shape of the breast during operation rather than according to the predetermined markings prior to reduction.

As Strömbeck has mentioned, in young patients, he utilizes another technique where the resection is done above and lateral to the areola, after which the upper part of the breast is moved laterally and caudally, resulting in an L-formed scar. The resultant breast is rounder medially and flatter laterally, and with time, the contour improves with gravity. He believes that his results with this method are comparable to those achieved by the modified skin excision and L-shaped scar technique of Dufourmentel and Mouly (see Chapter 13), Schatten (see Chapter 4), and Regnault (see Chapter 19). He uses this procedure for young patients whose hypertrophy is moderate and whose breasts are not ptotic. Of the 61 patients he questioned who had this type of procedure, 91 percent thought that they would agree to have the same operation again, and 81 percent believed that their expectations were met [7]. Of those patients, about 20 percent thought that their breast was ptotic, but this group of patients had somewhat better sensations than did those having had the original Strömbeck procedure. Contrary to his expectations, however, the two groups did not differ in their satisfaction with scarring.

Of the 59 patients who were followed, 27 had had the early Strömbeck procedure and 32 had had the L procedure (or as he calls it the L-lateral resection and lateral scar procedure). Of those 59 patients, only 41 had a child after operation, and, of these, 14 nursed for 3 months or longer; 5 nursed for 1 to 2 months, and 22 nursed less than 1 month or not at all.

Perbeck et al undertook a study to measure the skin circulation of the nipple before, during, and after the Strömbeck procedure [4]. In 14 patients, the skin circulation was measured in 25 breasts with laser Doppler flowmetry fluorescein flowmetry. The laser Doppler flowmetry showed that the skin circulation increased after deepithelialization but was reduced about 90 percent (±12%) of the preoperative value. The division of the lateral pedicle did not affect the circulation. After the skin had been sutured, the circulation was about 70 percent of what it had been prior to operation, but by 1 to 4 days postoperatively, the circulation approximated the preoperative value. Their conclusion was that the circulation to the nipple after reduction mammaplasty by the Strömbeck method is adequate and that it is safe to divide the lateral dermal pedicle.

That Strömbeck could amass such an experience is a tribute to his ability and hard work but also to the culture in which he practices, namely, an abundance of large-breasted women, so much so, in fact, that he and Malm [8] described "a model" for giving priority to those patients who needed reduction the most. This ranking was based on various factors such as age, breast volume, weight, ptosis, asymmetry, and psychic or somatic distress.

What does not seem to vary from culture to culture is that patients who initially are pleased with the results of their reduction mammaplasty will remain so 5 or 10 years later. This phenomenon seems to be true in all surgery that attempts to change appearance.

REFERENCES

1. Elsahy, N.I. The modified Strömbeck technique for reduction mammoplasty. *Aesth. Plast. Surg.* 3:135, 1979.
2. Gupta, S.C. A critical review of contemporary procedures for mammary reduction. *Br. J. Plast. Surg.* 18:328, 1965.
3. Muller, E. Late results of Strömbeck's reduction mammaplasty. *Plast. Reconstr. Surg.* 54:664, 1974.
4. Perbeck, L., Alveryd, A., Maattanen, H., and Wallberg, H. Skin circulation in the nipple after reduction mammaplasty by upper and lower glandular resections. *Scand. J. Plast. Reconstr. Surg.* 22:237, 1988.
5. Planas, J., and Mosely, L.H. Improving breast shape and symmetry in reduction mammaplasty. *Ann. Plast. Surg.* 4:297, 1980.
6. Strömbeck, J.O. Macromastia in women and its surgical treatment. *Acta. Chir. Scand. Suppl.* 341:1, 1964.
7. Strömbeck, J.O. Reduction Mammoplasty. In N.G. Georgiade (ed.), *Aesthetic Breast Surgery.* Baltimore: Williams & Wilkins, 1983. Pp. 146–165.
8. Strömbeck, J.O., and Malm, M. Priority grouping and waiting list of patients for reduction mammaplasty. *Ann. Plast. Surg.* 17:498, 1986.

12

Bernard Hirshowitz,
Rony Moscona, and
Yaron Har-Shai

Bipedicle Vertical Dermal Flap Technique for Reduction Mammaplasty: Modifications of the McKissock Operation

To be considered successful, the results of reduction mammaplasty should be both aesthetically and functionally acceptable. The following requirements should be met to achieve these goals.

1. The procedure should be applicable to all cases of large pendulous and ptotic breasts.
2. The operative technique should be relatively simple so that once its broad principles are grasped, senior residents training in plastic surgery can expect to obtain consistently satisfactory results using this operative procedure.
3. The natural adhesion between the skin and the breast proper should be respected and not severed by the raising of skin flaps. The breast is a modified skin gland that develops from an ectodermal ridge and, as such, is a skin appendage.
4. The integrity of the nipple-areolar complex is inviolable, and its blood supply should be maximal. This should be derived from both the cutaneous dermal circulation as well as via the breast proper.
5. The nerve supply to the nipple-areolar complex should be preserved as far as possible. Nipple sensation has much importance for the erotic well-being of a woman.
6. The length of the submammary scar should be limited so that there is no encroachment on the presternal or the axillary areas.
7. Postoperative sagging of the breast should be considered avoidable, and one possibility for preventing it is the retention of a short buried dermal strip extending from the nipple-areolar complex to the inframammary fold.

In 1972, McKissock [12,13] introduced his concept of a bipedicled vertical dermal flap technique (BPVDF) for reduction mammaplasty. The use of a dermal bridge for nipple transposition was popularized by Strömbeck in 1961 [15] and ostensibly considerably influenced McKissock in his design of the BPVDF, which, according to this latter author, has definite advantages over the transverse lying dermal bridge of Strömbeck. With the BPVDF design, the anatomical siting of both the blood and nerve supply to the breast tissue is respected in that the inferior pedicle appears to incorporate many of these structures. In addition, the superior pedicle, by virtue of its continuity with the nipple-areolar complex, acts as a conduit for the subdermal plexus of vessels and nerves to the nipple-areolar complex. Thus, this structure obtains a double blood and nerve supply through both pedicles, ensuring maximal vascularity and innervation.

The wide variety of shapes and sizes of hypertrophic and ptotic breasts can, in our experience, be satisfactorily dealt with [9] using our basic design [10,11], which is a modification of that of McKissock [12,13].

The main points of divergence from the original description are as follows:

1. Limited raising of the new areolar site, together

149

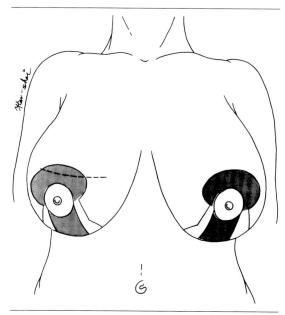

Fig. 12-1. The preoperative designs for reduction mammaplasty illustrate our modifications of the original McKissock concept, which include limited raising of the new areolar site together with a short and broad superior pedicle. The broken line on the left represents the level of the submammary fold.

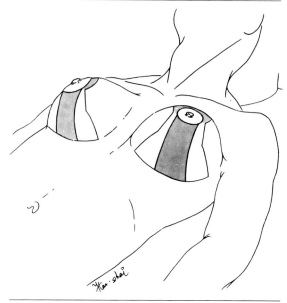

Fig. 12-2. Restricted length of the submammary incision depends on the construction of a narrow-based inferior pedicle.

with a short and broad superior pedicle (Fig. 12-1).
2. Restricted length of the submammary incision (Fig. 12-2).
3. A narrow-based inferior vertical pedicle (Fig. 12-2).
4. Coring out in depth over much of the breast parenchyma (Fig. 12-3).

Limited Raising of the New Areolar Site

There is an intimate correlation between raising the nipple-areola and the extensive coring in depth of the breast parenchyma. The loss of breast mass results in contraction of the remaining superficial breast tissue [2] and skin around the central axis provided by the nipple-areolar complex. The shrinkage of skin may be further explained by the previous stretching of the skin owing to excessive bulk and weight of the underlying breast tissue [2]. When these latter factors are reduced, the natural elasticity of the skin foreshortens the overall dimensions of the breast skin.

As the newly cut nipple-areolar complex is being raised to its new position, the margins of the supe-

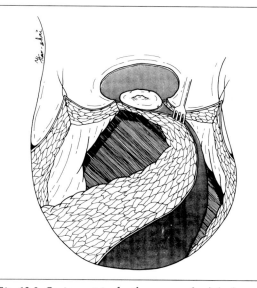

Fig. 12-3. Coring out in depth over much of the breast parenchyma commences with subareolar coring. Special attention is paid to reaching as far out laterally as the axilla. It is here that we effect our main modification of the original McKissock operation. An effort is made not to expose the lateral pectoralis fascia for fear of damage to the lateral cutaneous branch of the fourth intercostal nerve (special nerve to the nipple).

rior pedicle are wrapped around it. This wrapping contributes to the overall elevation of the nipple-areolar complex and also tends to project the nipple forward. In this way, a third dimension is added to the breast reduction.

Restricted Length of the Submammary Incision

Restricting the length of the submammary incision to about 15 cm enables the extremities of this incision to lie within the confines of the newly modeled breast. Medially, this line does not encroach on the sternal area, and laterally, the axilla is "out of bounds." In the erect position, this incision is largely hidden under the breast itself.

The deep coring of the breast parenchyma is done more under the lateral breast flap than under its medial counterpart. This is a result of greater extension of the breast laterally toward the axilla rather than in a parasternal direction. Notwithstanding the limitations imposed by the restricted length of this incision, there is no difficulty in mobilizing the medial and lateral breast flaps. These in turn can be readily brought together along the infra-areolar line.

Narrow-based inferior vertical pedicle. The inferior pedicle markings start on either side of the newly outlined areola and descend by two parallel lines, which widen only slightly as the submammary fold is approached. Accordingly, the base of the inferior pedicle measures not more than 4.5 to 5.0 cm. In constructing the inferior pedicle in depth, both its medial and lateral faces are bevelled outward somewhat as the pectoralis fascia is approached. This, together with the coring under the areola (subareolar), gives the inferior pedicle a truncated pyramidal shape. Bulkwise, the inferior pedicle is adequate for providing the filling necessary to obtain a good contour of the lower half of the breast. If the base of the inferior pedicle is made any wider, there would be a corresponding reduction in the amount of dermoglandular tissue to be excised on either side of the inferior pedicle, since the length of the submammary incision is restricted in advance.

Deep Coring of the Breast Parenchyma

It is here that the main modification of the original McKissock concept is effected. Breast tissue is not only cored out in depth beneath the areola but also upward under the superior half of the breast and sideways under the medial and lateral breast flaps, leaving a 2.0 to 3.0 cm thick layer (see Fig. 12-3) of breast tissue in all directions. Special attention is paid to coring out the lateral breast flap as far out as the axilla. This step enables the breast to be narrow in the transverse dimension and helps to avoid a broad shape to the re-formed breast.

A true bucket handle of the inferior pedicle according to the original McKissock design is not obtained, because the coring out of the inferior pedicle is confined only to where it abuts inferior to the areola.

The thickness of the areola is left at about 1.5 to 2.0 cm, and by so doing, many of the lactiferous ducts to the nipple are divided and their tethering effect is overcome. This permits the nipple-areolar complex to be raised with ease. However, some lactiferous ducts do remain intact; a few patients have been able to breastfeed their babies following this operation.

Blood Supply

The major blood supply of the breast is derived from terminal ramifications of the intercostal and internal mammary systems, with a smaller contribution via the lateral thoracic artery. Skin and gland of the lateral hemisphere of the breast are supplied by anterior cutaneous branches of the intercostals, which perforate the thoracic musculature in the midaxillary line.

The central part of the inframammary area is supplied by the fifth, sixth, and seventh intercostal arteries, which give off numerous branches around the inferior border of the pectoralis major muscle prior to entering the gland. The base of the inferior pedicle, which is located in this area, obtains its nourishment from these vessels; this explains its ample vascularity.

The medial aspect of the breast is supplied by perforating vessels derived from the terminal intercostals and internal mammary artery and that enter the breast parenchyma after piercing the intercostal spaces parasternally. The blood supply to the upper half of the breast is meager and is mainly provided by small branches of the acromiothoracic trunk.

The nipple-areolar complex is supplied by the parenchymal vessels from below via the inferior pedicle and from the subdermal plexus of the surrounding skin, much of which is retained in the

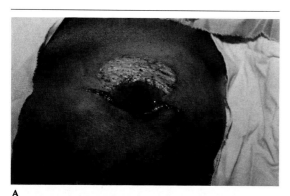

A

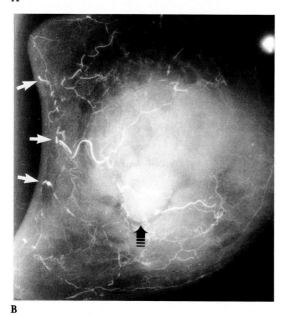

B

Fig. 12-4. A. Photograph of a cadaveric specimen in which the internal mammary artery was cannulated and injected with Microfil. The injection was preceded by deepithelialization of an imaginary superior pedicle and an incision down through to fat on the inferior half of the NAC. Considerable staining of the superior pedicle and the NAC was noted immediately following the injection. B. X-ray of the extirpated cadaveric breast. The internal mammary artery is not seen since it lies too far medial, but its three perforating branches are shown by white arrows. The black arrow indicates where a deep incision was made down through fat on the inferior half of the areolar border. Excellent filling of deep parenchymal vessels by the Microfil can be seen. This, together with the immediate staining of the superior pedicle and NAC by the Microfil, indicate substantial contribution to the blood supply to both superficial and deep breast tissue by the internal mammary artery.

superior pedicle. The wide and broad dimensions of the superior pedicle ensure an adequate amount of vascularity from this source. Thus, much of the blood supply to the breast appears to be contained within the parenchyma of its lower hemisphere, and many of these vessels are retained during the construction of a well-formed inferior pedicle.

A cadaveric anatomical study was performed in which the internal mammary artery was cannulated and injected with Microfil. Its superior epigastric termination was ligated at the level of the costal margin. The injection was preceded by deepithelialization of an imaginary superior pedicle, and a deep incision was made down to fat on the inferior half of the areolar border. Considerable staining of the superior pedicle and the nipple-areolar complex was noted immediately following the injection (Fig. 12-4A).

X-ray examination of the extirpated cadaveric breast shows excellent filling of deep parenchymal vessels by the Microfil (Fig. 12-4B). Both of these observations indicate substantial contribution of the blood supply to both superficial and deep breast tissue by the internal mammary artery.

Innervation

The nerve supply of the mammary gland and its overlying skin is derived from the second through seventh intercostal nerves. Laterally, these nerves appear as the anterior cutaneous nerves and medially as the terminal intercostal branches. The nipple-areolar complex is believed to be innervated from nerve filaments lying superficial to the breast [3]. Other surgeons [1,5] are of the opinion that there is little extension of nerve fibers from the dermal areolar area into the nipple itself and that this structure is supplied mainly from the depth of the breast tissue.

The lateral cutaneous branch of the fourth intercostal nerve is, according to the dissections of Hricko, "a unique nerve to the nipple passing deeply through the breast structure" [7].

Confirmation of this is found in the anatomical cadaver dissections of Farina et al [8], who followed the course of this nerve. Its anterior branch pierces the serratus anterior muscle in the midaxillary line, where it turns anteriorly at a right angle, passing just lateral to the pectoralis major muscle, and enters the mammary gland on its posterior aspect 1.5 to 2 cm from the edges of the gland. This nerve consistently penetrates the left mammary gland at the 4 o'clock position and the right breast at the 8 o'clock position. It maintains the same depth in relation to the surface until midway to the nipple-areolar complex, where it becomes more superficial as it reaches the areola.

By keeping the excision of the lateral breast parenchyma superficial to the deep fascia overlying the pectoralis major muscle, injury to this nerve may be prevented (see Fig. 12-3). This, in addition to the construction of a short and broad superior pedicle, which is likely to leave the superficial nerve filaments intact, are all important factors contributing to normal nipple-areolar sensation. Retention of the BPVDF, we believe, ensures a double nerve supply, and this appears to be borne out by the majority of our patients, who have virtually normal nipple-areolar sensation postoperatively [4].

Changes in Approach in Dealing with Large Pendulous and Ptotic Breasts

The mammary gland extends in its vertical dimension from the second or third to the sixth to eighth ribs, and transversely from the parasternal to anterior axillary lines. Within these boundaries, the shape and size of the breast can vary tremendously. The position of one structure that remains almost constant within the whole gamut of different sizes and shapes of pendulous and ptotic breasts is the submammary fold. It is from this fold that the height of the nipple-areolar complex is determined and the distance of it from the fold is fixed at about 5.5 to 6.0 cm.

These two almost constant features provide the basis of our preoperative markings. Both the outline of the oval-shaped superior pedicle, which is open inferiorly, and the lines of divergence from the extremities of this outline change depending on the degree of breast size and breast ptosis. The range of height and width of the superior pedicle can vary between 2 and 5 to 6 cm and 6 to 10 cm, respectively.

In the small reduction mammaplasties, the extremities of the outline of the superior pedicle converge on the newly marked areolar and may almost abut against it. As the need exists for excision of larger amounts of breast tissue and skin, the separation of the ends of this outline from the margins of the areola are made wider (Fig. 12-5).

As previously stated, the submammary incision is kept as short as possible, to about 15 cm. How-

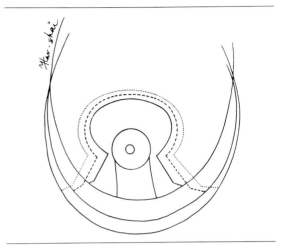

Fig. 12-5. Schematic drawing showing increasing dimensions of the superior pedicle both in height and in width, with increasing degrees of ptosis. By the same token, the angle of divergence of the descending limb becomes more obtuse.

ever, in very large pendulous and ptotic breasts, it is necessary to lengthen these measurements by 1 to 2 cm. In these situations, the descending limbs are correspondingly widely separated from the inferior pedicle. Their ends are joined to those of the submammary incision, and two dermoglandular areas scheduled for excision are outlined on either side of the inferior pedicle.

In the original McKissock operation, these two dermoglandular areas are made much larger than in our modified approach. However, with the addition of breast tissue obtained from deep coring, it is considered that a comparable amount of tissue is excised in both methods.

In the essentially ptotic breast, where the main element for excision is skin, deep coring would be done sparingly.

In the pendulous breast, the weight of the breast tissue contributes to the downward displacement of the nipple-areolar complex. Both this and ptosis influence the distance between the midclavicular point and the nipple. In the almost aesthetically perfect breast, this distance is about 20 cm and is about 3.5 cm below the midhumeral point [14]. Since one is dealing with these two somewhat indeterminate factors, it is difficult to estimate preoperatively the planned postoperative distance of the nipple-areolar complex from the midclavicular point. The implication of this is that when designing the superior pedicle, both breast weight and ptosis must be taken into consideration.

Therefore, in planning the shape of the superior pedicle, the following principle may act as a guideline: The greater the breast weight and degree of ptosis, the greater the height and width of the superior pedicle.

Total Amount of Skin Excised in This Modified Approach

Deepithelialization of both the superior and inferior pedicles yields an amount of skin corresponding to the surface area of each pedicle. To this, the excised skin of the two dermoglandular areas is added. When comparing this total amount with that excised in the McKissock method, it is evident that in this latter method, a larger area of skin is excised.

The obvious question that comes to mind is whether there is any skin redundancy in the modified method. The same rationale that applies to the limited raising of the nipple-areolar complex, concomitant with deep coring of the breast parenchyma, also applies to the need for reduced skin excision. The skin brassiere following these modifications in technique by virtue of natural skin retraction adapts itself to the inside contents of the breast package.

"Dishing-Out" Postoperatively: Is It Preventable?

One of the goals set for a satisfactory outcome following a reduction mammaplasty is the avoidance postoperatively of a forward projection of the inferior hemisphere of the breast and an accompanying upward displacement of the nipple-areolar complex [6].

Following the routine use of our modified BPVDF technique, this deformity seems, in our experience, to be most uncommon. A possible explanation for the preservation of the breast shape in this method is the reining effect of a relatively short continuous sheet of dermis that extends from the superior pedicle to the submammary fold.

The short and broad dimensions to our superior pedicle, in contrast to that in the original McKissock design, permits wide dermal contact with the infolding of the superior pedicle as the nipple-areolar complex takes up its new position. It is very

likely that this contributes an element of strength to the infolding and may be an important factor in preventing postoperative "dishing-out."

It is reasonable to assume that ordinarily the dermis is the main retaining element together with Cooper's ligaments in maintaining breast shape. In our BPVDF technique, both these structures remain intact, and although the dermis strip is narrowed over the inferior pedicle and is buried somewhat in depth, it is sufficient to keep the nipple-areolar complex permanently tethered in its immediate postoperative location.

There is often a relationship between excess weight of the patient and pendulous breasts. In a subconscious effort to conceal the embarrassment caused by oversized breasts, the patient tends to be overweight. Following the operation when breast-size normalcy returns, there is often an accompanying desire to lose body weight. This leads to further reduction in size of the breast. One estimation is that with every kilogram of body weight lost, there is a corresponding 10- to 15-gm loss of breast weight. This point also needs to be considered when planning the extent of reduction mammaplasty to be performed.

Preoperative Markings

Preoperative markings are made while the patient is in both a sitting and reclining position. The nipple-areolar complex is encircled according to its planned new dimensions. The submammary fold is drawn. More or less vertical lines connect the outer limits of the nipple-areolar complex with the submammary fold, creating the inferior pedicle. The base of the inferior pedicle should be between 4.5 and 5.0 cm in width; to obtain this width, it may be necessary to diverge these vertical lines somewhat distally. Only in the very ptotic breast would the base of the inferior pedicle be made 6 cm or more in width.

Depending on the extent of the breast pendulosity and ptosis, the shape of the superior pedicle is delineated. As previously stated, the inferior limits of its outline can abut against the nipple-areolar complex or can be separated from it on both its medial and lateral aspect by 2 cm or more.

From the points where the superior pedicle outline ceases, the descending limbs of 5-cm length begin. The angle of divergence of these limbs from the inferior pedicle will depend on the size of the superior pedicle. The smaller the superior pedicle, the wider is this angle, since the terminating points of the descending limbs are joined to the ends of the submammary fold, which has a fairly constant length of 15 cm. Only in cases of marked ptosis or pendulosity will this length be elongated to 16 to 17 cm. Thus, the size of the superior pedicle will have a direct bearing on the dimensions of the dermoglandular tissue to be excised on either side of the inferior pedicle. The bigger the breast, the larger the superior pedicle and the larger the dermoglandular areas.

Operative Technique

The operation is performed with the patient in the semirecumbent position with a pillow placed under her knees. All the preoperative outlines are revised and are redrawn if necessary. They are incised through to the dermis. Both the superior and inferior pedicles are deepithelialized. Care is taken not to expose the subcutaneous fat, since the integrity of the dermal sheet is considered important in preventing postoperative "dishing-out" of the breast. A strong hook is inserted into the dermis of the upper midpart of the superior pedicle. By applying traction to this hook, the breast is, as it were, suspended in space, enabling all the intramammary excisions to be conducted from the same point of reference. Using either a diathermy cutting current or sharp dissection, both dermoglandular areas are excised. Starting with subareolar coring, the whole extent of the breast is cored out except under the inferior pedicle, which is left intact. An effort is made not to expose the fascia overlying the pectoralis major muscle, for fear of damaging the nerve to the nipple.

Subareolar coring leaves a somewhat thinner layer of tissue than over the rest of the breast itself and is approximately 1.5 to 2.0 cm thick. The retention of breast thickness of between 2 and 3 cm (Fig. 12-6) provides sufficient bulk for a reasonably sized breast, which, together with the inferior pedicle, ensures good breast contour.

It is necessary to incise the dermis of the superior pedicle commencing at the apex of both dermoglandular areas on either side of the nipple-areolar complex to a length of about 1.0 cm. This facilitates the raising of the nipple-areolar complex to its new location and the suturing of the margins of the superior pedicle around it. These incisions do not in any way impair the blood supply of the superior pedicle.

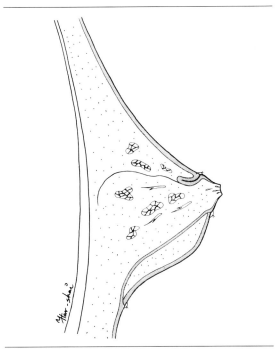

Fig. 12-6. The continuous dermal sheet extending from the superior pedicle to the submammary fold has a reining effect on the NAC preventing "dishing-out" postoperatively. The short and broad dimensions of our superior pedicle, in contrast to that of the original McKissock design, permits wide dermal contact with the infolding of the superior pedicle as the NAC takes up its new position. It is likely that this wide dermal contact contributes an element of strength to the infolding and may be an important factor in preventing postoperative "dishing-out."

Closure of the margins of the two descending vertical limbs is performed using individual catgut or other biodegradable sutures. The skin edges are drawn together along the infra-areolar line, and distally, they meet at about the middle of the base of the inferior pedicle. But this point is not a precise one.

Because of the predetermined length of the descending limbs of 5 cm, the infra-areolar suture line will be of an equal length. However, this can be somewhat adjusted by suturing the margins of the superior pedicle proximal to their terminating points. This will make for tighter closure around the nipple-areolar complex and will elongate the infra-areolar line. The encircling skin margins around the nipple-areolar complex can, if neces-

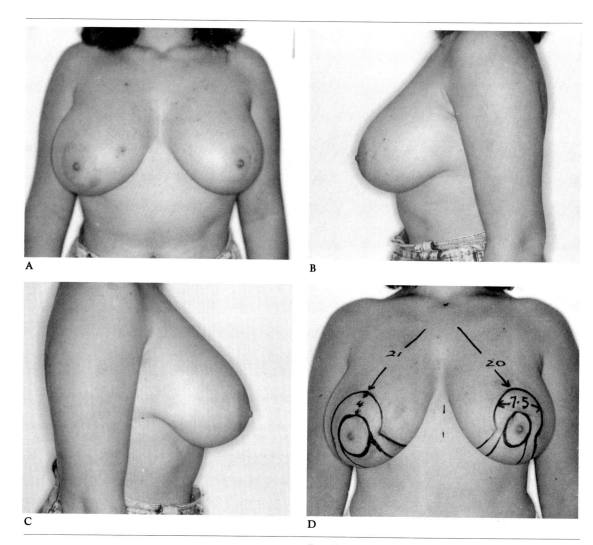

Fig. 12-7. A–C. Preoperative front and side view photographs of large pendulous breasts in a 17-year-old girl. D. Preoperative measurements of same patient, indicating the discrepancy in distance of the MCP from the new upper NAC border to accommodate the extra size of the right breast. The short and broad outline of the superior pedicle is also shown. E. Appearance at the completion of the operation. Six hundred and fifty grams of breast tissue was removed from the right breast, 550 gm from the left breast. F. Front view postoperative photograph of the patient, illustrating that the breast in the upright position effectively hides the submammary scar. G,H. In the postoperative side views of this patient, there is no encroachment of the submammary scar into the axilla.

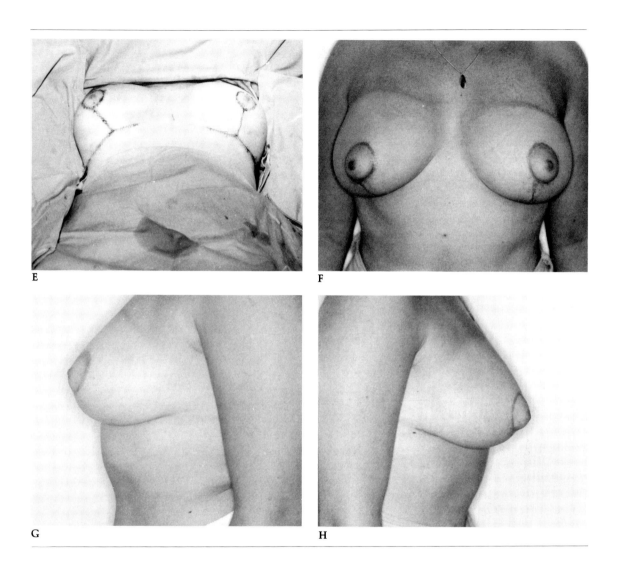

E

F

G

H

158

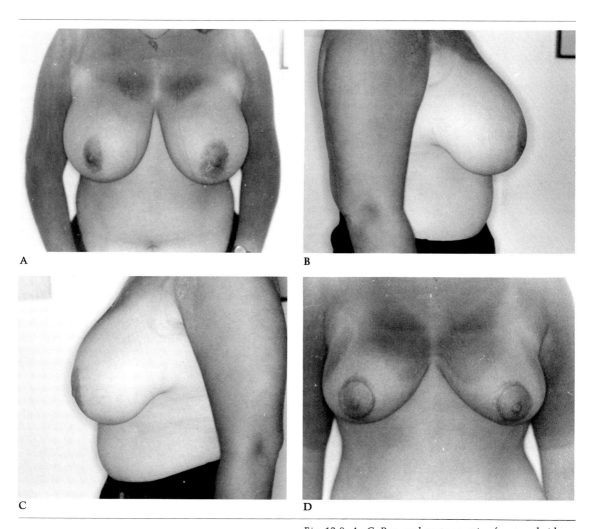

A

B

C

D

Fig. 12-8. A–C. Pre- and postoperative front and side views of large pendulous slightly ptotic breasts in an 18-year-old patient. D–F. Three months postoperative front and side views of the patient. Five hundred and fifty grams of breast tissue was excised from each breast. G. Postoperative view from below shows short submammary scar.

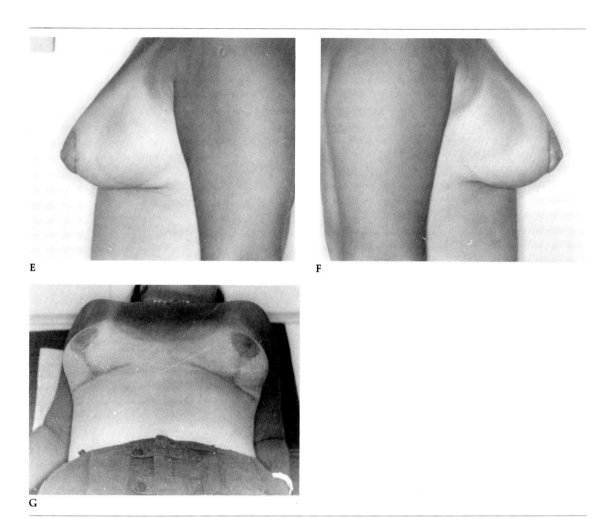

E

F

G

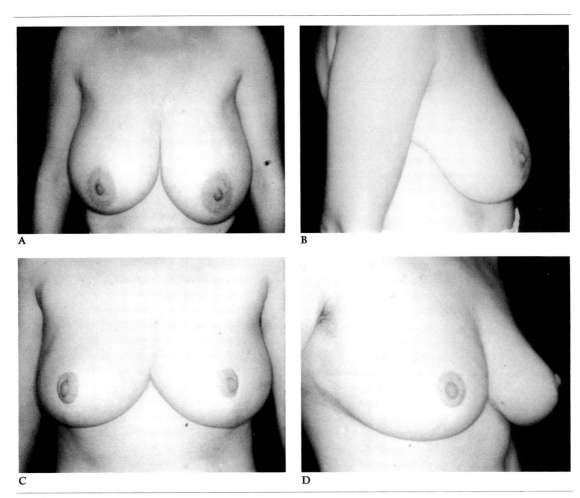

Fig. 12-9. A,B. Preoperative photographs of enlarged and ptotic breasts. C. Postoperative front view of the patient 3 years later. D. Oblique view 3 years postoperatively; good breast contour is retained.

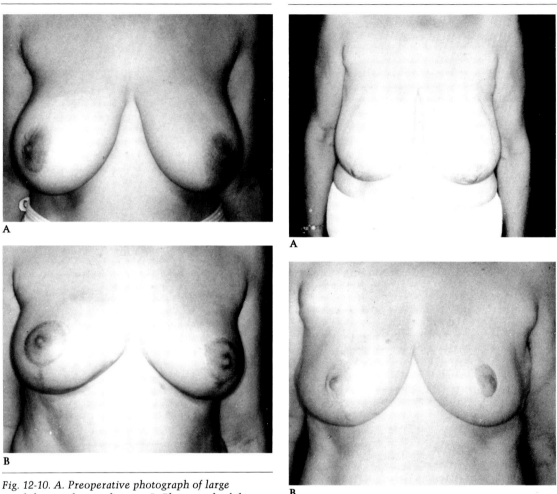

Fig. 12-10. A. Preoperative photograph of large pendulous and ptotic breasts. B. Photograph of the patient 4 months postoperatively.

Fig. 12-11. A. Preoperative photograph of particularly ptotic breasts in a 55-year-old patient. B. Photograph of the patient 4 years postoperatively. Breast shape appears to have been well preserved.

sary, be enlarged by paring away their edges. A certain amount of leeway is therefore provided to arrive at the final closure.

There are instances when, at the termination of the reduction mammaplasty, a depression is noticed above the nipple-areolar complex; this can be a cause for some concern. However, this depression rapidly disappears within a day or two as the breast tissue contracts and obliterates areas of dead space, which account for this depression. An open-ended drain is inserted into the depth of the breast wound. It is usually removed after 24 hours.

Conclusion

These modifications of the original McKissock BPVDF technique for reduction mammaplasty offer both safety and reliability in securing a pleasing operative result. This method appears to be based on sound anatomical principles and also incorporates the natural tendency of tissues to contract.

Senior residents in plastic surgery are generally capable of grasping the broad principles of this operation, which can be performed by them under minimal supervision.

This procedure sets rather definite guidelines in regard to limited submammary incision length. It also allows for considerable freedom in the size of the superior pedicle, which is the focal area for determining the extent of excision of breast parenchyma and skin. These modifications, in our hands, permit breast reduction for almost all shapes and sizes, in the reasonably certain expectation of achieving a satisfactory aesthetic and functional result (Figs. 12-7 through 12-11).

References

1. Cathcart, E.P., Gairnes, F.W., and Garxwen, H.S.D. Innervation of the human quiescent nipple, with notes on pigmentation, erection and hyperneury. *Trans. R. Soc. Edin.* 61:699, 1948.
2. Cloutier, A.M. Volume reduction mammaplasty. *Ann. Plast. Surg.* 2:475, 1979.
3. Cooper, A. *The Anatomy of the Breast.* London: Longman, 1840.
4. Courtiss, E.H., and Goldwyn, R.M. Breast sensation, before and after plastic surgery. *Plast. Reconstr. Surg.* 58:1, 1976.
5. Craig, R.D.P., and Sykes, P.A. Nipple sensitivity following reduction mammaplasty. *Br. J. Plast. Surg.* 23:165, 1970.
6. Dinner, M.I., and Chait, L.A. Preventing the high riding nipple after McKissock breast reduction. *Plast. Reconstr. Surg.* 59:330, 1977.
7. Edwards, E.A. Surgical anatomy of the breast. In R.M. Goldwyn (ed.), *Plastic and Reconstructive Surgery of the Breast.* Boston: Little, Brown, 1976. P. 37.
8. Farina, M.A., Newby, B.G., and Alan, H.M. Innervation of the nipple-areola complex. *Plast. Reconstr. Surg.* 66:497, 1980.
9. Georgiade, N.G., Serafin, D., and Riefkohl, R. Is there a reduction mammaplasty "for all seasons"? *Plast. Reconstr. Surg.* 63:765, 1979.
10. Hirshowitz, B., and Moscona, A.R. Modifications of the bipedicled vertical dermal flap technique in reduction mammaplasty. *Ann. Plast. Surg.* 8:363, 1982.
11. Hirshowitz, B., and Moscona, A.R. Technical variations of the McKissock operation for reduction mammaplasty. *Aesth. Plast. Surg.* 7:149, 1983.
12. McKissock, P.K. Reduction mammaplasty with a vertical dermal flap. *Plast. Reconstr. Surg.* 49:245, 1972.
13. McKissock, P.K. Correction of macromastia by bipedicle vertical dermal flap. In R.M. Goldwyn (ed.), *Plastic and Reconstructive Surgery of the Breast.* Boston: Little, Brown, 1976. P. 215.
14. Penn, J. Breast reduction. *Br. J. Plast. Surg.* 7:357, 1954.
15. Strömbeck, J.O. Mammaplasty, report on a new technique based on the two pedicle procedure. *Br. J. Plast. Surg.* 13:79, 1961.

COMMENTS ON CHAPTER 12   *Robert M. Goldwyn*

When McKissock [5] published his vertical dermal flap technique of breast reduction in 1972, it soon became the favored method [2–4,8,9]; some surgeons still prefer it. It should be noted for historical accuracy that Pers and Bretteville-Jensen [1,7], independent of McKissock, described around the same time their experience with a very similar method that they called *vertical vascular bipedicle* and *tennis ball assembly*.

The reasons for the immediate popularity then of the McKissock operation (as it has come to be called) were several: It lessened but did not eliminate the square look and the almost certain inverted nipples that many of us were getting with the Strömbeck technique; it produced a pleasing breast contour and volume; it maintained rich vascularity to the nipple-areola; it retained nipple-areola sensation as well as most of the other techniques and better than some then used; it was easy to learn and to teach; and it gave a predictable result, especially because the nipple site was predetermined.

Its principal drawbacks then were (and now are) that it produced a long inframammary scar and that it was not an easy method to reduce extremely large breasts. If the nipple transposition is more than 12 cm, in my experience, the infolding of the pedicle makes closure difficult, creates excessive tension on the skin flaps and on the pedicle, and endangers the survival of the nipple-areola.

The inferior pedicle technique, which followed in a few years that of McKissock and Pers-Bretteville-Jensen, proved more suitable for very large breasts, even those that might be termed *gigantomastia*. However, the long inframammary incision still remained.

It was interesting that a few surgeons realized, while they were trying to close the wound after the McKissock procedure had been used for massive breasts, that in order to do so, they had to sacrifice the superior portion of the pedicle beyond the nipple-areola. Miraculously, we thought then, the nipple-areola survived; hence, the evolution of the inferior pedicle technique.

In the modification of the McKissock procedure, Hirshowitz, Moscona, and Har-Shai had, as one of their objectives, the "restricted length of the submammary incision." They accomplished this by excising ". . . more under the lateral breast flap than under its medial counter-part." The authors correctly note that the breast extends laterally toward the axilla more than it does medially toward the sternum. By excising more laterally, the breast is narrowed transversely and thus one avoids a "broad breast shape."

In what the authors call the "decoring," they have made their main modification of the McKissock method. A "true bucket handle," as produced in the classic McKissock procedure, is not what the authors generate by their modification. The reason is that the coring of the inferior pedicle extends upward only to the inferior margin of the areola. By dividing the ducts, tethering is eliminated and the nipple-areola can be easily elevated to its new position.

In large breasts, the authors mention that it is necessary to lengthen the inframammary incision by 1 to 2 cm, to 16 to 17 cm from the usual 15 cm. What they also emphasize is that the greater the weight of the breast and its degree of ptosis, the greater the length and the width of the superior pedicle.

I have used this modified McKissock approach on several occasions, and it successfully reduces the length of the submammary scar so that it does not extend laterally, where most scars then become noticeable and later hypertrophic. It is also true, as the authors claim, that less skin needs to be excised in their method than in the classic McKissock technique. Skin retraction that normally occurs during healing will take care of the modest redundancy that might remain at the conclusion of the operation.

Hirshowitz, Moscona, and Har-Shai have thoughtfully modified the McKissock technique. Indeed, I suspect that anyone using McKissock's original technique or any technique will change it to suit the patient's needs and the surgeon's preferences.

McKissock [6] also has modified his technique, particularly when he advocated the lazy-S type of lateral incision, but then discarded it because closure was under more tension and that would more likely produce hypertrophic scars.

The present authors of this modification have wisely left the McKissock method with its principal advantages, most importantly preoperative marking with predetermination of the new nipple-areola location and the maintaining of the excellent blood supply to the nipple-areola.

For massive breasts — gigantomastia — the McKissock technique in this modification, in my experience, is inadequate. As alternatives, the surgeon has recourse to the inferior pedicle method or to nipple-areola grafting.

REFERENCES

1. Bretteville-Jensen, G. Reduction mammaplasty with a vertical bipedicle and transverse scar: A follow-up. *Br. J. Plast. Surg.* 29:142, 1976.
2. Hoopes, J.E., and Maxwell, G.P. Reduction mammaplasty: A technique to achieve the conical breast. *Ann. Plast. Surg.* 3:106, 1979.
3. Loosli, R.N., Botta, Y., and Maillard, G.F. Plastie mammaire selon McKissock. *Med. et Hyg.* 35:858, 1977.
4. Maillard, G.F., Botta, Y., Dessapt, B., et al. Valoracion de la plastia mamaria de reduccion segon tecnica de McKissock. *Cirug. Plast. Ibero-Latinoam.* 3:327, 1982.
5. McKissock, P.K. Reduction mammaplasty with a vertical dermal flap. *Plast. Reconstr. Surg.* 49:245, 1972.
6. McKissock, P.K. Reduction mammaplasty. *Ann. Plast. Surg.* 2:321, 1979.
7. Pers, N., and Bretteville-Jensen, G. Reduction mammaplasty based on a vertical vascular pedicle "tennis ball" assembly. *Scand. J. Plast. Surg.* 6:61, 1972.
8. Soto-Matos, R., Parejo Gonzalez, L., Colman-Pulgar, E., and Ortega-Gonzalez, E. Mastoplastia de reduccion a pediculo vertical (McKissock) modificaciones y experiences logradas con esta tecnica. *Cirug. Plast. Ibero-Latinoam.* 6:399, 1980.
9. Wexler, Yeschua, R., and Neuman, Z. McKissock breast reduction. *Aesth. Plast. Surg.* 1:229, 1977.

13

Nathalie Bricout* and
Roger Mouly**

Evolution of Ideas in the Lateral Method: The Saint-Louis Technique

The first description of the oblique lateral approach for reduction mammaplasty appeared more than 25 years ago and was described by Dufourmentel and Mouly [4]. This French technique has been used throughout the world and was popularized in the United States by Schatten et al [14]. The initial ideas of the authors were to perform a cutaneous and glandular resection on the lateral aspect of the breast and therefore to leave a single lateral scar without any submammary incision. The same principles are still valid, but, as one can easily understand, modifications have occurred with time.

Since 1961, Dufourmentel, Mouly, and their followers have had only one objective: to improve the quality of the results by (1) reducing the length of the scars, and (2) preserving a satisfactory shape and maintaining a satisfactory volume.

We present the last achievement called the *Saint-Louis technique,* used by one of the authors (Bricout), and which can be applied in any case of hypertrophy and ptosis. This technique is so-called because it has been performed at the Saint-Louis Hospital, in Paris, in the plastic surgery unit headed by P. Banzet and formerly by Cl. Dufourmentel.

This technique will be described in detail, but since its successive modifications reflect the general development of ideas about reduction mammaplasty during the past 25 years, we shall recall these first.

* Department of Plastic Surgery, (Pr.P.BANZET), Hospital Saint-Louis, 1, rue Claude Vellefaux, 75010 Paris, France.
** 97 bis rue Jouffroy, 75017, Paris, France.

History

THE OBLIQUE TECHNIQUE

The oblique technique [4] was conceived to avoid the main failure of Biesenberger's method [1]: the undesirable scars, even though it was the first satisfactory procedure to give a good shape to the breast. As in Biesenberger's method, the oblique technique made use of:

separation of skin from the gland
Schwartzmann's maneuver (i.e., a limited periareolar deepithelialization to preserve vascular supply to the areola and nipple)
external glandular resection

But its originality consisted of (Fig. 13-1):

a lateral approach
a preoperative design, which allowed reduction by lateral resection of excess skin and contents in two planes
a suspension of the residual gland to the axillary region
above all, a *single lateral oblique scar,* which gave this method its name

This single scar (not counting the periareolar one, of course) avoided an inframammary scar. Results were very satisfactory in cases of small or moderate hypertrophy. But when a large glandular resection was indicated, vascular insufficiency — and therefore the risk of necrosis — were identical to those in Biesenberger's technique.

Soon after describing this method, the authors realized that it could be done without any undermining between the skin and the gland, such a modification being safer with respect to the viabil-

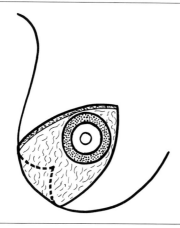

Fig. 13-1. The oblique technique: incisions and periareolar deepithelialization.

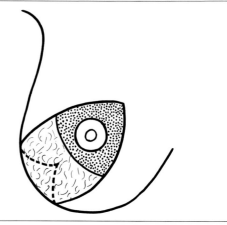

Fig. 13-2. The lateral oblique technique: markings and deepithelialization.

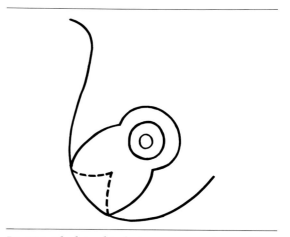

Fig. 13-3. The lateral technique: preoperative markings.

ity of both skin and breast tissue. They were following the same principles of Pitanguy [12,13], Strömbeck [16,17], and Skoog [15]. The oblique technique became the lateral oblique technique.

THE LATERAL OBLIQUE TECHNIQUE
Vascular safety of the nipple-areola complex is preserved by the dermosubdermal flap; cutaneoglandular unity is maintained *without any intercutaneoglandular dissection,* as stressed by Strömbeck in 1960 (double horizontal pedicle), by Pitanguy in 1961 (superior pedicle), and by Skoog in 1964 (external pedicle). In 1965, the oblique technique became the lateral oblique technique [5].

In the lateral oblique technique, the preoperative markings are similar, but the areola is carried by a triangular deepithelialized flap, which has a superomedial apex (Fig. 13-2). Glandular dissection can thus be extended under its posterior aspect, glandular resection is performed in one segment, and the nipple-areola is exteriorized at the end of the operation. Therefore, there is *no intercutaneoglandular dissection,* which is a guarantee of vascular security; resection can be more extensive on the posterior aspect of the breast; and there is still just a single lateral scar.

This technique can also be used in cases of pure ptosis, but in this instance, a dermoglandular flap is rotated under the upper part of the breast at its deep aspect, roughly as in the periwinkle shell operation described by Gillies and Marino [9].

Finally, with a few modifications, this technique became the lateral technique in 1971 [6,7].

THE LATERAL TECHNIQUE
In the basic technique, the final location of the areola is determined at the beginning of the operation, as are the dimensions of the deepithelialized flap, with the aid of a metal ring, which can be opened to define a circle whose diameter is the same as that of the areola (Fig. 13-3).

The dermoglandular flap is used in hypertrophy as well as in ptosis to permit a periwinkle shell-type rotation.

In addition to the basic technique, four variations have been described to treat different types of breast hypertrophy and ptosis: (1) the wedge excision technique for moderate hypertrophy, (2) the modified periwinkle shell operation for the small ptotic breast, (3) the modified skin excision and the L-shaped scar in cases of huge hypertrophy; and (4) the combined operation (periwinkle shell rotation, glandular resection, and L-shaped scar) when there is hypertrophy with significant ptosis inferiorly.

The lateral technique became popular because of its two advantages: (1) safety, because the avoidance of intercutaneoglandular dissection preserved the cutaneoglandular supply, and (2) lateral location of the scar.

The results were very satisfactory in cases of moderate hypertrophy and ptosis, but when it was applied to all cases, its limitations became obvious.

In cases of major hypertrophy, the lateral scar necessarily becomes very long and extends beyond the breast onto the lateral side of the chest. In this subaxillary area, the skin is of a different texture, which is one reason why the scar is often hypertrophic. Furthermore, this external part of the scar also widens because of the tension on it. The scar is also more noticeable because it is no longer hidden by the brassiere.

The problem of skin excess was partially solved by using the artifice of an "L" scar: an external oblique segment and a horizontal segment, almost like the "J" scar described by Elbaz and Verheecke [8]. Still, the excess skin remained difficult to manage.

In cases of major hypertrophy, the other inconvenience is morphologic: It is almost impossible to resect as much glandular tissue under the internal quadrants as under the external ones. This nonhomogeneous glandular resection leaves a breast that is bulky inside and flat outside; this shape becomes worse with time and gravity.

Finally, there is a risk — especially for inexperienced surgeons — of placing the nipple too high and medially, a problem that increases with time and is very difficult to correct.

FURTHER MODIFICATIONS

We have tried to retain the advantages of the lateral technique (a superior pedicle and a rotating flap) while correcting its problems of contour in patients with major hypertrophy and ptosis, which are mainly caused by the nonhomogeneous glandular resection.

The result is the technique we now use: the technique of Saint-Louis [2,3].

The Saint-Louis Technique

The Saint-Louis technique deliberately does not carry anyone's name, because we do not consider it original. As a matter of fact, it directly evolved from the lateral technique utilizing a superior pedicle, and also from the dermal vault technique described by Lalardrie et al [10,11], because of the method of glandular resection and the final location of the scars. The presence of an internally based dermoglandular flap also takes its inspiration from the technique used by Baruch (personal communication, 1969).

Actually, it seems to us that each of these techniques had its limitations and disadvantages, which we tried to avoid. The lateral technique does not reliably give a good shape in cases of major hypertrophy, which is what we most often deal with in young women. The dermal vault, because of its lack of preoperative design, requires adjusting the skin to the residual breast volume as the operation progresses, regardless of how pronounced the hypertrophy and the ptosis may be. This absence of precise initial markings accounts for its adaptability but also the difficulty of this technique, which can be performed only by surgeons already experienced in reduction mammaplasty.

We tried to keep the advantages of these different techniques and to combine them. The preoperative design we use is not a rigid pattern because it must fit each case, and the skin markings act essentially as guidelines.

TECHNIQUE
Preoperative Design

At the beginning, the patient is marked standing upright before she is premedicated (Fig. 13-4A).

A line is first drawn from the upper border of the sternum to the inframammary fold (Fig. 13-4B). This axis crosses the nipple except when it is off-center. In that case, the axis must be adjusted on the breast meridian without deviating from the nipple more than 1.5 cm. The lower part of this line is drawn by lifting the breast upward and inward in relation to the meridian.

A point A is then marked on this line, from 17 to 19 cm from the substernal area. This point depends on the degree of ptosis and cutaneous laxity:

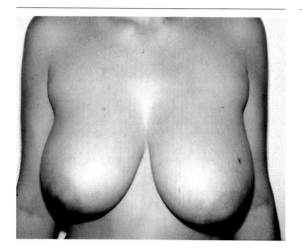

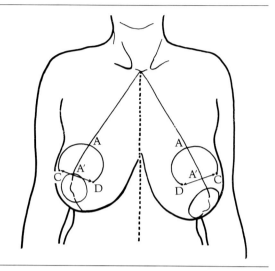

Fig. 13-5. Periareolar markings.

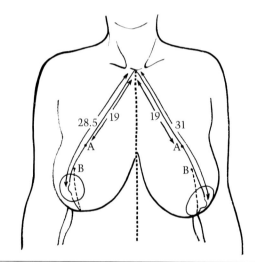

Fig. 13-4. Preoperative aspect.

The more elastic the skin, the taller the woman, and the larger the breast, the lower this point will be on the breast. Indeed, after glandular resection, this point spontaneously comes up because the skin is relieved of the excess glandular tissue. This cutaneous retraction will be more significant if the skin has good elasticity. That is the reason we prefer to operate early in patients with isolated hypertrophy, sometimes when they are 15 years old, before the skin has been stretched excessively.

Then, a point A' is marked, 5 to 6 cm away from point A (Fig. 13-5). We draw a perpendicular line to the axis in A', and mark on this line two points, C and D, each located 4 to 5 cm away from A', C

being on the external side and D on the internal side.

This line C-D will be the anatomical support of the future nipple flap. It can be 8 to 10 cm wide. The more severe the ptosis, the wider it will be, because the nipple-carrying flap will have to be longer. The widening of the flap base increases the vascular safety of the nipple complex.

We then join points A, C, and D with an ellipse, taking care that the lines tangential to the inner side of the ellipse be equidistant to the midline, and no less than 9.5 cm from it (Fig. 13-6). It is only in women less than 5 feet tall that this tangential line can reach to 9 cm from the midline. Less than that, there is the risk of the areola being too medial and the breasts too convergent. This unwanted result is very displeasing and very difficult to correct.

Markings are then finished with the patient in a supine position. We draw the following (Fig. 13-6, a,b):

1. The internal part of the spindle, without pushing the breast beyond the axis. This D-B line, slightly convex inside, is almost parallel to the medial line in its upper two thirds.
2. The external part, C-B, is drawn while gently pulling the breast toward the midline.

If the breasts are not symmetric, neither will the spindles be (the spindle will be wider on the larger side), but the cutaneous segments located between

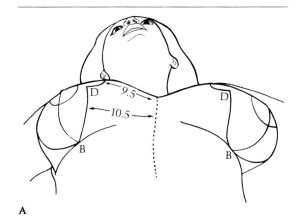

A

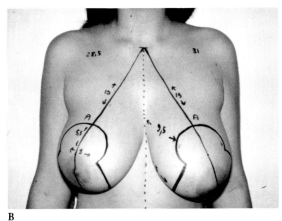

B

Fig. 13-6. In the supine position (A), the internal part of the spindle is almost parallel to the medial line, and the periareolar ellipse is no less than 9.5 cm from it (A, B).

the medial line and the internal edge of the spindle must be equal. The internal edge of the spindle must not be located less than 10 cm from the medial line. The two edges of the spindle must be able to come into contact. This can be checked by pushing the breasts upward and pinching them gently.

At Operation

The patient is placed in a sitting position, arms at the side but slightly away from the body to allow access laterally to the midaxillary region; care is taken that the shoulders are horizontal and the pelvis straight. The head is positioned to avoid cervical hyperextension (Fig. 13-7). The head of the operating table must be moderately raised,

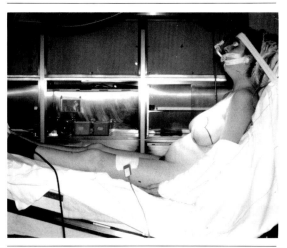

Fig. 13-7. Settling.

with the patient's legs up to prevent her sliding downward. The clavicles and the midaxillary line must be visible after the patient is draped.

The Operation

The markings are completed. The periareolar circular incision is outlined with moderate pressure on the breast; both areolas have a diameter of 4 to 4.5 cm at the beginning of the operation. The dermoglandular flap (Fig. 13-8) is outlined with a medial base D-D' of 6 to 7 cm. (This size decreases spontaneously to 5 cm after breast resection when the skin is no longer overstretched.) D-D' is the anatomical support for the future dermoglandular flap. Its final height of 5 cm is necessary to ensure an adequate size to the breast.

All the hatched area (Fig. 13-9) is deepithelialized.

We then incise the skin and subcutaneous tissue down to the glandular plane from D' to B and C to B to initiate dissection under the subcutaneous fat, and not between skin and fat (Fig. 13-10).

Then we cut along B down to the parietal aponeurotic level and separate almost simultaneously the gland from the deep prethoracic plane, then from the prepectoral one, while not getting into the prepectoral fascia; and the gland as well as all its axillary extension from the skin, while sparing the subcutaneous fat. This deep dissection will be less extensive medially to spare the vascular supply to the future dermoglandular medial flap—

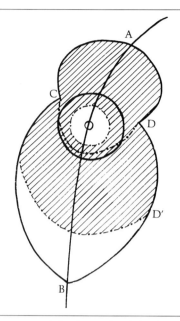

Fig. 13-8. Design of the dermoglandular flap.

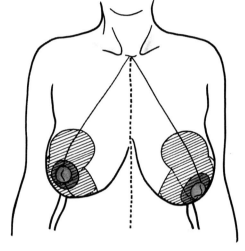

the perforating intercostal vessels that come from the internal mammary vessels.

The gland is also freed from the skin and deep plane from B to D'.

GLANDULAR RESECTION. The nipple-carrying flap is incised 1 cm under the areola, from D to C, then joined to the glandular segment about 1.5 cm thick, held by the assistant with two Kocher clamps pulling upward. The gland is then resected, leaving a layer of uniform thickness attached to the dermis of the skin. The thickness of the layer must be constantly checked during the resection, with the left hand applied to the skin.

The dermoglandular flap is freed, leaving under its two medial thirds a glandular layer a little thicker than under the rest of the glandular segment. The gland left under the flap will serve mainly to give a round shape to the inferoexternal quadrant (Fig. 13-11).

CLOSURE. The areola is closed by eight half-buried stitches through the dermis on the breast skin side to avoid hatch marks and to distribute tension equally on the skin (Fig. 13-12). The dermoglandular flap is located and fixed at its two ends to the

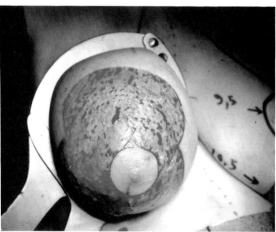

Fig. 13-9. The deepithelialized area.

pectoral muscle, behind the level of the areola, remaining inside the anterior axillary line (Fig. 13-13).

The vertical subareolar incision is then sutured, so that it measures, without tension, 4.5 cm in height. Its lower end is stitched to point B to resect the two large dog-ears (Figs. 13-14 and 13-15).

If at this stage we realize that there is a lack of symmetry because of an unequal amount of skin, it can be corrected in two ways: (1) by removing the skin on the external side of the subareolar incision, or (2) by deepithelializing it on its inner side, which is the origin of the dermoglandular flap.

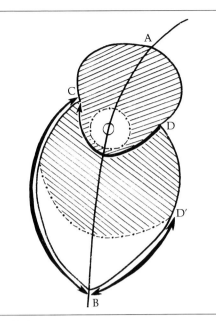

Fig. 13-10. Incisions.

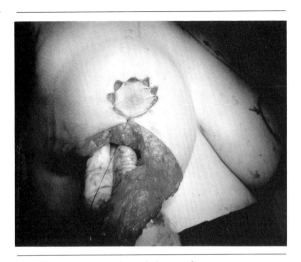

Fig. 13-12. Construction of the areola.

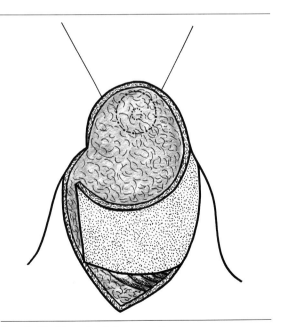

Fig. 13-11. After glandular resection.

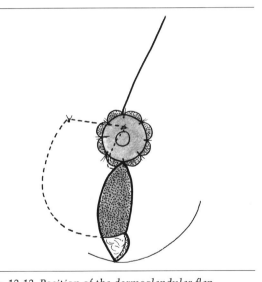

Fig. 13-13. Position of the dermoglandular flap.

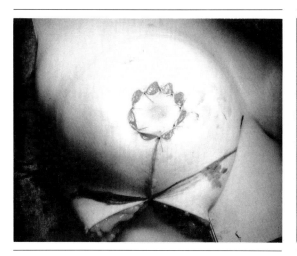

Fig. 13-14. Resection of the dog-ears.

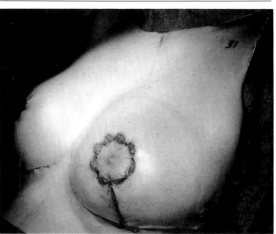

Fig. 13-16. The external part of the inverted T is rather horizontal.

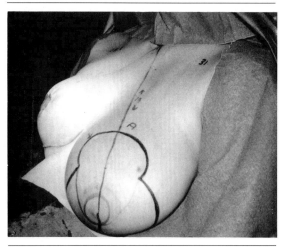

Fig. 13-15. Resection of the internal dog-ear places the scar, slightly curved, in the inframammary fold.

One must be certain that both vertical subareolar incisions are symmetric and equidistant from the sternum. If they are not, the breasts will not look symmetric, even if they have the same volume and had the same shape prior to closure.

Resecting the dog-ear laterally would give a slight curve to the ultimate scar in the inframammary fold.

The lateral dog-ear should be taken out, there-fore, by curving the incision so that the scar will end up horizontal. During this resection, we have to be sure not to pull too much on the upper part of the breast so that the scar does not end up too high (Fig. 13-16).

The sutures are completed: An intradermal stitch closes the areola, a subareolar vertical incision (without any tension), and the horizontal part of the inverted T.

Just prior to closure, a suction drain is placed. The dressing is made with Corticotulle*, sterile gauze, and adhesive elastic bandages.

Final Thoughts
This technique is characterized by:

1. The presence of a spindle that is more vertical than in the oblique technique.
2. A homogeneous glandular resection leaving a glandular layer of regular thickness under the whole cutaneodermal envelope, as in the dermal vault.
3. A flap similar to Gillies' periwinkle shell, but here the flap is dermoglandular instead of glandular and wound on itself as well as attached to the pectoral plane instead of being outside it, as in Baruch's technique.

* Gauze, Vaseline, triamcinolone, neomycin, polymyxin. Laboratoires Sarbach, 42, rue Roget de Lisle, 92151 Suresnes Cedex.

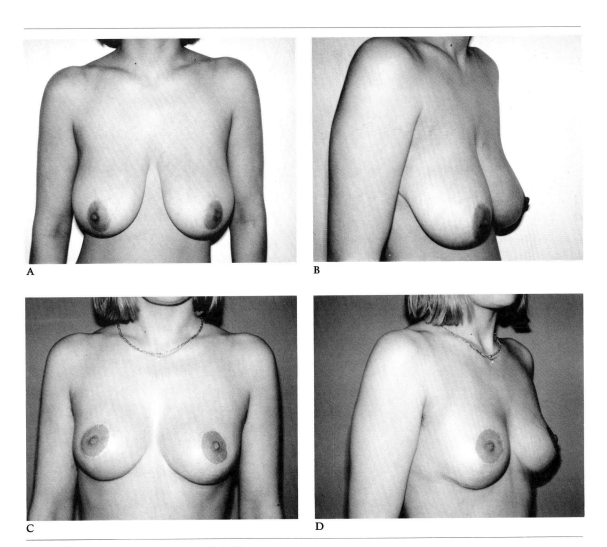

Fig. 13-17. A, B. Preoperative aspect. C, D. Two years postoperatively. Resection included removal of 400 gm from the left breast and 300 gm from the right breast.

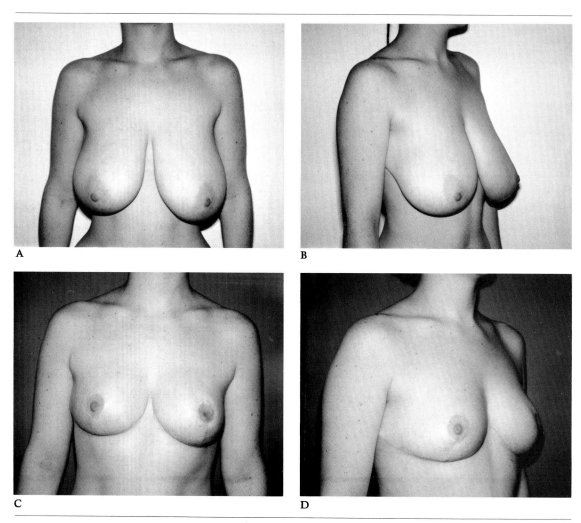

A

B

C

D

Fig. 13-18. A, B. Preoperative aspect. C, D. Two and a half years postoperatively. Resection included removal of 480 gm from the right breast and 620 gm from the left breast.

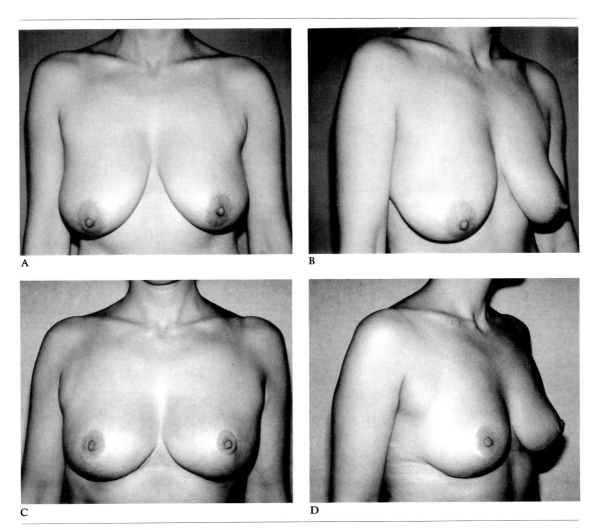

Fig. 13-19. A, B. Preoperative aspect. C, D. Three years postoperatively. Resection included removal of 200 gm from the right breast and 220 gm from the left breast.

176

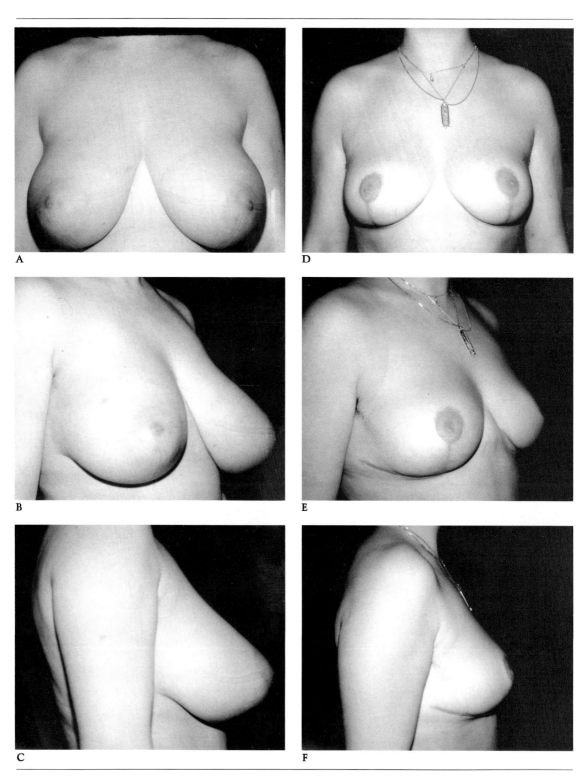

A

D

B

E

C

F

Fig. 13-20. A–C. Preoperative aspect. D–F. Two years postoperatively (hypertrophic scars). Resection included removal of 570 gm from the right breast and 780 gm from the left breast.

As with every method, this technique has advantages, disadvantages, and limitations. Its advantages are its great vascular safety. The only
complication we observed, in that regard, was
hardening of the end of the rotated dermoglandular flap as a result of fat necrosis, and was only in a
few cases. This was likely caused by an extensive
dissection of the gland from the prepectoral plane
medially, injuring the perforating vessels coming
from the intercostal vessels. This extensive dissection is less useful for removing the gland than it is
for shaping the breast and can easily be avoided.

This technique is easy to teach and has been rapidly mastered by our residents. It is well-suited to
breasts with moderate and major hypertrophy,
conditions for which we most often operate (Figs.
13-17 through 13-20). It is also useful for hypertrophy with ptosis and for reducing the opposite
breast after reconstruction.

This technique also has its limitations: It is not
well-suited to cases of pure ptosis because the
spindle is not large enough to provide an adequate
folding of the flap. For the patient with only
ptosis, we use the same design superiorly for the
areola and the area to be deepithelialized, but we
adjust the vertical incision by means of a curved
clamp, as in the dermal vault technique (see
Chap. 20).

Another disadvantage of our method is the
length of the inframammary scar. However, we
have chosen it deliberately. We are well aware of
the fact that at the present time, many surgeons
are trying desperately to develop techniques to reduce or eliminate the horizontal scar, but these
methods also have their problems, especially in
breasts that are severely hypertrophic where the
skin envelope is extremely lax. With time and
gravity, the shape of the breasts will worsen.

Rather than trying to reduce the length of the
inframammary scar, we therefore prefer this
method because it gives an excellent shape to the
breast and maintains the shape over time.

References

1. Biesenberger, H. Eine neue method der mammaplastik. *Zbl. Chir.* 48 : 2971–2975, 1930.
2. Bricout, N. *Chirurgie de Reconstruction du Sein.*
   Paris: Flammarion, 1987.
3. Bricout, N., Grosliere, D., Servant, J.M., and Banzet,
   P. Plastie mammaire, la technique utilisée à Saint-
   Louis. *Ann. Chir. Plast. Esthèt.* 33 : 7, 1988.
4. Dufourmentel, Cl., and Mouly, R. Plastie mammaire
   par la méthode oblique. *Ann. Chir. Plast.* 6 : 45, 1961.
5. Dufourmentel, Cl., and Mouly, R. Dévelopements
   récents de la plastie mammaire par la méthode
   oblique latérale. *Ann. Chir. Plast. Esthèt.* 10 : 227,
   1965.
6. Dufourmentel, Cl., and Mouly, R. Modification of
   "periwinkle shell operation" for small ptotic breast.
   Plast. Reconstr. Surg. 41 : 523, 1968.
7. Dufourmentel, Cl., and Mouly, R. Reduction Mammaplasty by the Lateral Approach. In R. Goldwyn
   (ed.), *Plastic and Reconstructive Surgery of the
   Breast.* Boston: Little, Brown, 1976.
8. Elbaz, J.S., and Verheecke, G. La cicatrice en L dans
   les plasties mammaires. *Ann. Chir. Plast. Esthèt.*
   17 : 283, 1972.
9. Gillies, H., and Marino, H. L'opération en colimaçon
   ou rotation spirale dans les ptôses mammaires mo-
   dérées. *Ann. Chir. Plast. Esthèt.* 3 : 89, 1958.
10. Lalardrie, J.P., Jouglard, J.P., and Morel-Fatio, D.
    Reduction mammaplasty: Our latest experience.
    1st Congress of the International Society of Aes-
    thetic and Plastic Surgery. Rio de Janeiro: February
    1972.
11. Lalardrie, J.P., and Jouglard, J.P. *Chirurgie Plastique
    du Sein.* Paris: Masson, 1974.
12. Pitanguy, I. Aproximâo ecletica ao problema das
    mammaplastia. *Rev. Bras. Cirur.* 41 : 179, 1961.
13. Pitanguy, I. Une nouvelle technique de plastie mam-
    maire. Etude de 245 cas consécutifs et présentation
    d'une technique personnelle. *Ann. Chir. Plast.
    Esthèt.* 7 : 199, 1962.
14. Schatten, W.E., Hartley, J.H., Jr. and Hamm, W.G.
    Reduction mammaplasty by the Dufourmentel-
    Mouly method. *Plast. Reconstr. Surg.* 48 : 306, 1971.
15. Skoog, T. A technique of breast reduction. *Acta Chir.
    Scand.* [Suppl.]341 : 128, 1964.
16. Strömbeck, J.O. Mammaplasty: Report of a new
    technique based on the two pedicles procedure. *Br. J.
    Plast. Surg.* 13 : 79, 1960.
17. Strömbeck, J.O. Macromastia in women and its sur-
    gical treatment. A clinical study based on 1042 cases.
    Acta Chir. Scand. 126 : 453, 1964.

COMMENTS ON CHAPTER 13   *Robert M. Goldwyn*

Bricout and Mouly have given the surgical reader something that he or she seldom gets: an innovator's account of the evolution of a new technique (the Saint-Louis method) based on the shortcomings of that person's old technique. Not every surgeon who is known for a specific procedure is able to recognize its deficiencies, admit them publicly, and then try something new to overcome them.

The authors' mention that a major disadvantage of the previous lateral technique was the hazard of having the nipples too high and too medial, especially if the surgeon was inexperienced. Indeed, as someone not familiar with this method, I did have this problem with the nipples. My reason then for attempting the oblique technique was its chief advantage: only a lateral scar (in addition to the periareolar). However, as the authors correctly state, the lateral technique does not "readily give a good shape" in very hypertrophic breasts, where, unless one takes precautions, the nipple will not be in the correct position and the lateral scar will extend too far on the chest wall. In my experience, the lateral scar is more likely to widen and thicken than are medial scars.

Bricout and Mouly now prefer an eclectic modi-fication that results in the usual horizontal component for the inverted "T." They are willing to accept the disadvantage of a lengthy horizontal scar because of the other advantages of the Saint-Louis method, including vascular safety of the nipple-areola, good breast contour and volume for any kind of hypertrophic breast, and long-term stability of the result with minimal, if any, descent of the breast. Their photographs, indeed, confirm their claims.

A distinguishing feature of their later method is the dermoglandular flap (similar to Gillies' periwinkle glandular shell), turned on itself and attached to the pectoral plane. This may partly account for the fact that the authors have not observed bottoming out of the breast over a long course of time—an observation that has been noted with the inferior pedicle technique if the pedicle's attachment to the chest wall has been interrupted and if the nipple has initially been placed too high.

For the surgeon who has not seen this technique done, he or she may prefer other more familiar methods that accomplish the same results and also give the usual inverted "T" scar.

14

William E. Schatten

Reduction Mammaplasty by the Lateral Approach

In 1965, as an award winner of the Plastic Surgery Educational Foundation, I visited and worked with Dr. Claude Dufourmentel in Paris, France. Dr. Dufourmentel is the quintessential gentleman and surgeon, and we visited several times thereafter. At that time, it was apparent to me that procedures for reduction mammaplasty were more refined in Europe than in the United States. I was particularly impressed with the lateral approach in reduction mammaplasty first described by Dufourmentel and Mouly in 1961 [1] and later modified and described by them in 1965 [2].

I have continued to use and modify the lateral technique since 1965 [3–7]. This has evolved to be a relatively free-form operation. A pattern is not used for preoperative markings, and the nipple site is not tailored according to certain predetermined points; therefore, there is greater latitude in shaping the breast.

The amount, site, and extent of glandular resection is determined by the location and extent of hypertrophied breast tissue and the degree of ptosis. The width of skin to be excised by deepithelialization in the lateral portion of the breast is determined by the degree of ptosis. Hypertrophied glandular tissue in a taut skin envelope requires excision of a relatively larger amount of tissue and a smaller amount of skin (Figs. 14-1 through 14-3).

Hypertrophy and significant ptosis in a breast with most of the tissue in the lower quadrants requires excision of adequate amounts of glandular tissue and skin and different use of the inferiorly based pedicle flap (Figs. 14-4 through 14-6).

Patient Selection

Preoperative factors such as loss of skin elasticity and postoperative factors such as weight of remaining breast tissue affect long-term results regardless of the technique used.

Gigantomastia is difficult to define unless an arbitrary weight or size of breast is used. In general, the lateral approach is ideal for a breast in which no more than 600 to 700 gm of tissue is removed. When a greater amount of tissue should be removed or there is severe ptosis, it is difficult to shape the breast by removing skin only in the lateral quadrants. Here again, the individuality of the breast should be stressed. For example, in a young nulliparous patient with hypertrophied tissue in all quadrants, a greater weight of tissue can be removed by circumferential excision of adequate tissue from the deep aspect of the breast in all quadrants, and a good shape of the breast can be obtained by excision of skin only in the lateral aspect.

The surgeon can decide preoperatively whether or not a good result can be expected using a lateral approach by examining the breasts with the patient in an upright sitting position.

Advantages and Disadvantages of the Lateral Approach

Advantages of the lateral approach are:

1. The location of the lateral scar is good, and there is a minimal amount of scarring. Widening of the scar extending laterally onto the chest wall may occur, but there is no scar in the medial portion of the breast or sternal region.
2. There is good contour of the breast and good nipple projection. The shape is always conical because ptosis is corrected and contour is obtained by rotation of an inferiorly based pedicle

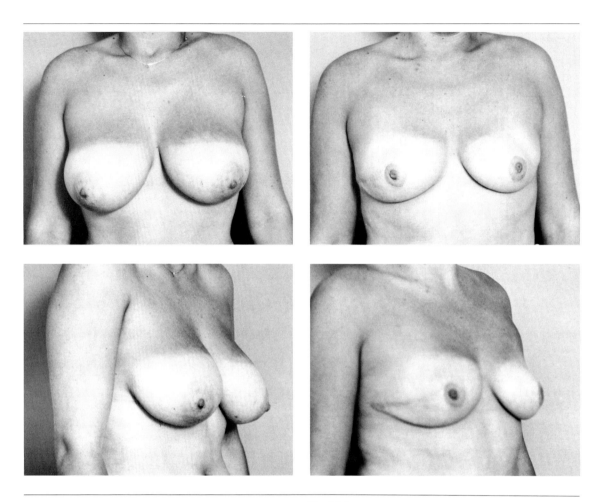

Fig. 14-1.

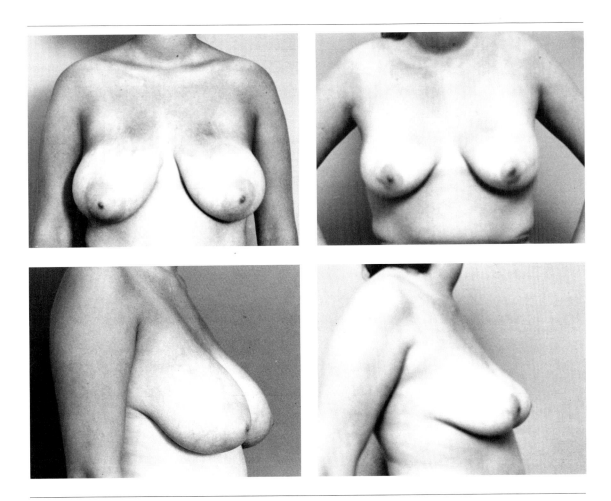

Fig. 14-2.

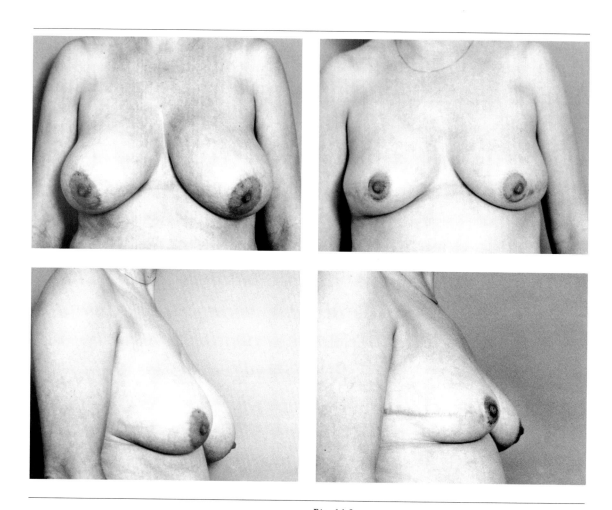

Fig. 14-3.

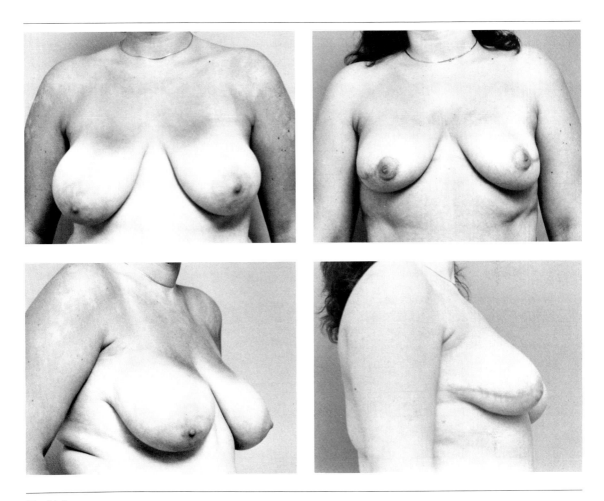

Fig. 14-4.

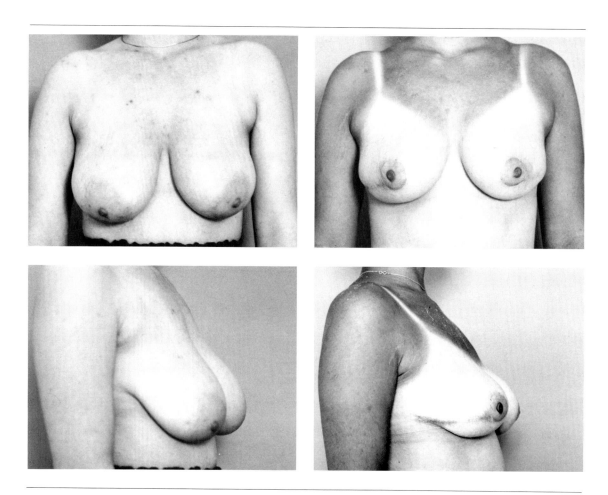

Fig. 14-5.

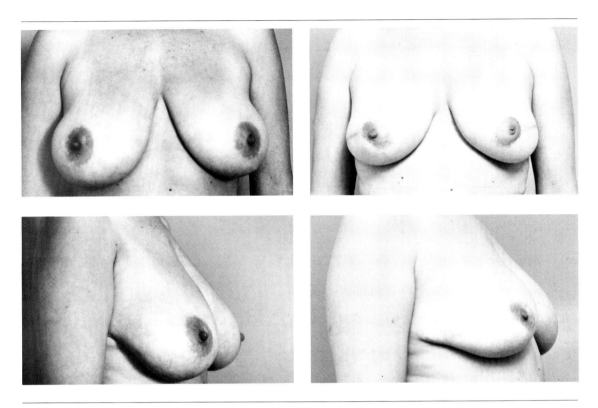

Fig. 14-6.

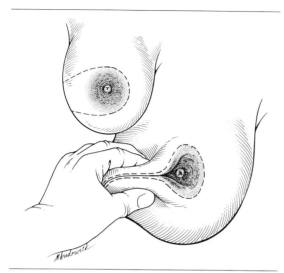

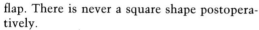

Fig. 14-7. Infolding breast to determine the width of the lateral wedge, ptosis that can be corrected, and primary areas in which resection of tissue will be required.

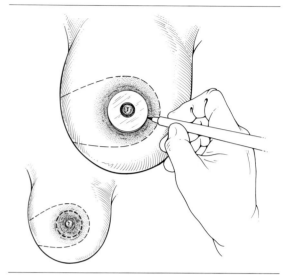

Fig. 14-8. Marking nipple-areola complex that will remain intact.

flap. There is never a square shape postoperatively.

3. Long-term preservation of contour is usual. After resection of glandular tissue, an inferiorly based pedicle is used to reconstruct the breast, and slight overcorrection of ptosis is done to compensate for the effect of gravity postoperatively.

4. There is no danger of necrosis of the nipple-areola complex because it remains on a dermal pedicle and the nipple retains sensation, erectile capacity, and connections with the ductal system. There is no danger of necrosis of skin flaps because skin is not undermined and there is no junction of vertical and horizontal scars.

5. Generous resection of tissue from the deep aspect of the breast can be done without regard to interference with circulation to the remaining gland and skin.

Disadvantages of this technique are:

1. It is difficult to use in reduction of a large breast. As mentioned previously, this can be judged preoperatively by manual examination, and if the breast cannot be fashioned properly, another procedure should be used.

2. A pattern is not used for marking, and this makes the lateral approach somewhat more difficult to understand and to teach.

Technique

My technique of reduction mammaplasty by the lateral approach has come to differ from that of Dufourmentel and Mouly in that I still bury the nipple after glandular resection and exteriorize it after contouring the breast and closing the incision. My technique has changed since my original and subsequent descriptions in that I do not mark any specific points preoperatively. I found these points to be unnecessary and confusing.

With the patient in a semisitting position prior to being anesthetized, I approximate the skin manually along the proposed lines of lateral incisions in order to visualize the reconstructed breast (Fig. 14-7). A marking pen is used to indicate the incisions along the proposed lines. Excessive tension in the lateral closure is undesirable and unnecessary. This can be obviated by marking along lines indicated by pinching the skin. These lines for proposed incisions are checked, measured, and re-checked because the width and location are important. The usual width of the lateral wedge is 7 to 9 cm. The greater the degree of ptosis and the greater degree of skin laxity, the greater the width of the lateral wedge. Medial incisions in the circumareolar area are usually made along the junction of areola and skin, but if the areola is quite distended, these incisions may be within the are-

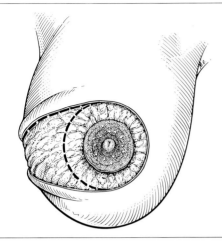

Fig. 14-9. *Outline of incisions of inferiorly based pedicle flap after deepithelialization of the lateral wedge.*

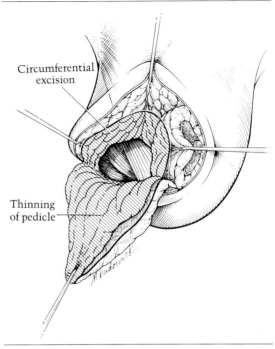

Fig. 14-10. *Inferior pedicle has been reflected, and the entire breast has been undermined by retromammary dissection from the pectoral fascia. The area of tissue to be excised circumferentially from the deep aspect of the gland and pedicle flap is demonstrated.*

ola. The rim of excess areola is excised later when the nipple is exteriorized.

A metal washer 3.5 cm in diameter is used to outline the amount of areola to be saved. The washer is placed on the areola with the nipple in the center of the ring (Fig. 14-8).

Intradermal dissection of skin and glandular resection are done with the patient in a flat position. Skin incisions are made, and intradermal dissection of skin from the entire area between the delineating markings is done (Fig. 14-9). A curving line is marked on the dermis 2 cm lateral to the areola, and this extends across the width of the wedge. The incision along this curving line extends deep to the pectoral fascia; this incision is continued to the superior border of the wedge and then laterally along the entire border to the lateralmost point of the wedge. An inferiorly based dermal-fat-glandular pedicle is then reflected. Retromammary dissection of the entire breast between glandular tissue and pectoral fascia is then done.

It is important to emphasize again that the areas and amounts of glandular resection are determined by the preoperative condition; for example, if there is hypertrophy and ptosis and most of the glandular tissue is in the lower quadrants, resection from the deep aspect of the breast should be primarily from the lower half of the breast. A sufficient bulk should always be left superior to the areola so that this area will be full postoperatively.

It is always necessary to resect an adequate amount of tissue in the upper outer quadrant because lateral closure forces remaining tissue into this area. In a hypertrophic breast, it is always necessary to excise gland and fat from the deep aspect of the inferiorly based pedicle (Fig. 14-10). If there is excess pedicle not required to rotate into the retromammary area of the upper inner quadrant to provide bulk, this excess pedicle is resected at this time (Fig. 14-11).

After complete glandular resection, the patient is placed in a semisitting position so the breast can be contoured properly. It may be superfluous, but it should be emphasized that breasts appear different when a patient is supine than when she is sitting. An assistant then retracts the nipple-areola complex with a large hook and the superior breast with a retractor (Fig. 14-12). Ptosis correction and contouring using the inferiorly based pedicle flap is done by rotating the flap superiorly and laterally. The *undersurface* of the pedicle is fixed to the periosteum of appropriate ribs using 2 or 3 sutures

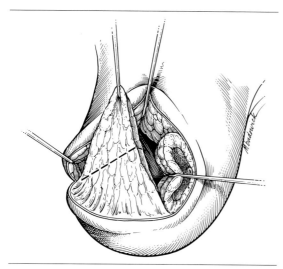

Fig. 14-11. Excess pedicle to be excised in a hypertrophic breast.

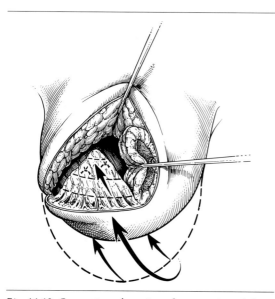

Fig. 14-12. Correction of ptosis and contouring of the breast by fixation of the undersurface of the inferiorly based pedicle flap to periosteum of the ribs.

of 3-0 Surgilon. The sites of fixation are determined by observation of ptosis correction achieved. When the pedicle is rotated and sutured as described, the intramammary fold is elevated and the breast is rotated, and a conical shape results. After fixation of the pedicle, additional excision of tissue is done wherever indicated. Further areas that may require excision become apparent when breast flaps are approximated manually.

Two Penrose drains are placed in the retromammary area and brought out through the lateral pole of the incision. An assistant continues to retract the nipple-areola complex with a large hook in such manner that the nipple can be buried by infolding. Michelle clips are used to approximate skin over this area medially, and this approximation is then continued laterally to close the entire wound.

After this stage in the procedure is completed on one breast, the operating table is flattened and reduction and shaping of the opposite breast is completed to this same stage. A comparison of the breasts is made, and further shaping or contouring is done by further resection of tissue wherever necessary to produce the best symmetry. Michelle clips are removed, and definitive closure of both wounds is done. Care must be taken not to fix the buried nipple-areola pedicle to the skin with sutures used for subcutaneous closure because the buried pedicle must be free for exteriorization. The patient is again placed in a semisitting position so the nipples can be exteriorized. The inframammary fold is the landmark for determining the nipple site. The position of the new nipple is in relation to the newly elevated inframammary fold and newly tailored breast. The inferior border of the new areola is usually 6 to 7 cm above the fold, and the medial border is usually 9 to 11 cm from the midline of the sternum. The 6-cm marking is made, and the metal washer is placed in the correct position to outline the new nipple site (Fig. 14-13). Each nipple should be related to its breast, not to the opposite nipple. The nipples should be placed slightly lateral and lower than desired for final position to accommodate for settling of glandular tissue. The operating table is again flattened, and the nipples are exteriorized. Intradermal dissection of skin is done at the new nipple site. The buried nipple is located behind the new nipple site, a small skin hook is placed along a border of the complex, and the nipple is exteriorized (Fig. 14-14). The pedicle is freed as necessary so that it can be exteriorized easily without tension. If the

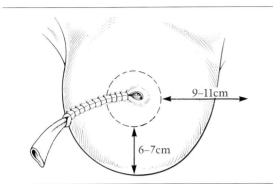

Fig. 14-13. New nipple site is determined in relation to the inframammary fold after ptosis correction.

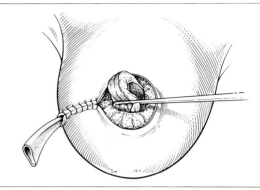

Fig. 14-14. Exteriorization of the nipple after deepithelialization of the new nipple site. The nipple pedicle is freed as much as is necessary so that it can be placed anteriorly without any tendency to retract.

pedicle is not free, the nipple will tend to retract. It is not uncommon to have to free the pedicle by an incision at the dermis–skin junction, and this can be done with impunity. The nipple-areola pedicle is placed anterior to the deepithelialized area, and this increases forward projection. After the nipple lies in position without tension, the areola is sutured to surrounding skin edges at the new nipple site (Fig. 14-15).

It is emphasized that it is important not to deepithelialize too large an area in the nipple region because closure will then result in the medial end being too far medial. If the areola is too large, the area that is deepithelialized should be within distended areola and the remaining rim of areola excised when the nipple is exteriorized at the new nipple site.

The areas for glandular resection are determined by the preoperative situation. For example, in a breast in which there is hypertrophic tissue in all quadrants and there is little ptosis, adequate resection of tissue from the deep aspect in the upper quadrant superior to the nipple is required. On the other hand, in a ptotic breast in which hypertrophic tissue is primarily in the lower quadrants and there is little bulk superior to the nipple, no resection of tissue in the upper inner quadrant should be done.

When the inferiorly based pedicle flap is rotated and fixed to rib periosteum, these fixation sutures should be placed on the deep aspect of the pedicle. This is important to prevent dimpling of skin at the line of closure, that is, if the superior edge of the pedicle is sutured to chest wall tissue instead

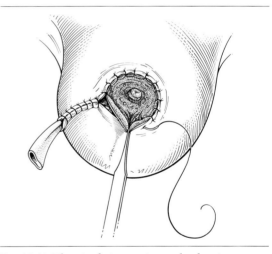

Fig. 14-15. The nipple is anterior to the deepithelialized area, and the areola is sutured to surrounding skin. This increases forward projection of the nipple.

of the undersurface, the skin edge at the inferior border of pedicle will be rolled inward; this results in an unnatural appearance at the time of closure.

In a hypotrophic ptotic breast, the inferiorly based pedicle flap is fixed to obtain maximum correction of ptosis or, in the small ptotic breast, the pedicle is rotated superiorly and medially to obtain maximum bulk without producing undue distortion of the lower outer quadrant (Fig. 14-16).

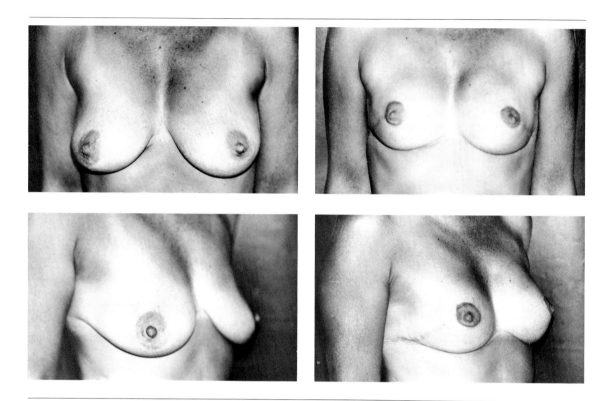

Fig. 14-16.

It has been emphasized that at the time of exteriorization of the nipple at its new site, the nipple pedicle should lie anterior to the newly deepithelialized area without tension so that there will not be nipple retraction postoperatively. To free the nipple pedicle adequately, an incision may be made at the junction of dermal pedicle and skin to free up the pedicle from deep attachments.

References

1. Dufourmentel, C., and Mouly, R. Plastie mammaire par la méthode oblique. *Ann. Chir. Plast. Esthèt.* 6 : 45, 1961.
2. Dufourmental, C., and Mouly, R. Dévelopments ré-cents de la plastie mammaire par la méthode oblique latérale. *Ann. Chir. Plast. Esthèt.* 10 : 227, 1965.
3. Schatten, W.E. Breast Reduction: Lateral Technique Using Inferiorly Based Flap. In *Aesthetic Breast Surgery.* Baltimore: Williams & Wilkins, 1983. Pp. 196–204.
4. Schatten, W.E. Comment. In R.M. Goldwyn (ed.), *Plastic and Reconstructive Surgery of the Breast.* Boston: Little, Brown, 1976. Pp. 250–255.
5. Schatten, W.E. Reduction Mammaplasty by the Lateral Approach. In *Reconstructive Breast Surgery.* St. Louis: Mosby, 1976. Pp. 170–181.
6. Schatten, W.E., Hartley, J.H., Jr., Crow, R.W., and Griffin, J.M. Further experience with lateral wedge resection mammaplasties. *Br. J. Plast. Surg.* 28 : 37, 1975.
7. Schatten, W.E., Hartley, J.H., Jr., and Hamm, W.G. Reduction mammaplasty by the Dufourmentel-Mouly method. *Plast. Reconstr. Surg.* 48 : 306, 1971.

COMMENTS ON CHAPTER 14   *Arnoldo Fournier*

The Dufourmentel-Mouly technique for reduction mammaplasty is one of the best alternatives to obtain a natural conical-shaped breast with well-hidden scars around the areola and on the lateral side of the breast.

Schatten has explained in detail his innovations on this technique and has made interesting observations, on which I have been honored to comment. As Schatten remarks, he carries out generous resection of the breast tissue beneath the nipple-areolar complex and under the medial and the lateral flaps. Most important, no scars are left on the medial or sternal regions.

Since 1974, we (Dr. Claudio Orlich and I) have used the original 1961 Dufourmentel-Mouly technique by the lateral approach on 200 patients. Our approach has been a bit more laborious perhaps in the taking of measurements prior to surgery and with the patient in a semisitting position in order to obtain an exact placement of the new areola and in delineating the new diameter of the nipple-areolar complex. Following the criteria of Dufourmentel-Mouly technique, we make an elliptical marking from the vertex of the new position of the superior border of the new areola to a point where the anterior axillary line crosses the submammary line. A transverse line following the lower border of the areola is then defined.

On resection of the breast tissue from the subareolar triangle, we have excised 3,450 gm (about 8 lb), in the largest breast of our 200 patients with good aesthetic results. The lateral and medial flaps are then approximated with the least amount of tension possible. The dermis is carefully sutured with 4-0 nylon sutures, using inverted U knots every 8 mm. The epidermis is sutured with running 4-0 nylon sutures around the areola and along the incision in the lateral area of the breast.

We have not used Schatten's innovation to improve the contour of the breast by fixing a lateral pedicle to the ribs.

The excellent results obtained by Schatten are shown in a variety of cases, especially in the patient shown in Figure 14-16, with excellent conical, aesthetically pleasing breasts—the goal of breast reduction mammaplasty.

15

Lennart Ohlsén and
Valdemar Skoog

Skoog's Technique of Reduction Mammaplasty

In 1963, Tord Skoog (Fig. 15-1) described his technique of breast reduction, transposing the nipple on a cutaneous vascular pedicle [23]. A very elaborate and instructive chapter on the same subject followed in his book *Plastic Surgery. New Methods and Refinements* published in 1974 [24]. His concept of reduction mammaplasty was prepared with knowledge of the breast being of ectodermal origin and of the arterial and venous vascular supply of the mammary gland.

The vascularization of the female breast was nicely shown by Vesalius [29] in 1568 (Fig. 15-2), and in 1840, Cooper [4] gave a most accurate account of the anatomy of the breast. He emphasized the vascular nature of nipple and areola, describing in detail the principal arteries supplying them. Investigations in autopsy material and in vivo have shown that the mammary gland is supplied by the internal mammary artery, the lateral thoracic artery, and the intercostal arteries [1,6,14,21] and with the subcutaneous vascular system, including the lymphatic network mainly directed toward the axilla.

Skoog considered knowledge of the vascular supply of the female breast necessary for the choice of technique, but various methods of reduction mammaplasty have given rise to different opinions regarding sufficient nutrition of the operated upon breast [3,7,13,20]. The relationship between the mammary gland and the nipple is obvious from an anatomic and functional point of view. The evolution of the breast indicates, however, that the nipple and areola primarily are parts of the pectoral skin that must influence the vascular and nerve supply.

All described methods for transposing the nipple strive to secure an adequate blood supply to the nipple utilizing the glandular or cutaneous vessels, or both. In the majority of procedures, a periareolar incision is made, sacrificing the cutaneous

vessels, with the nipple and areola deriving their blood supply solely from the mammary gland. In some of these methods, the nipple is transposed on a glandular pedicle, singly or doubly based [12]. The glandular resection can then be performed in several ways depending on the method of nipple transposition.

Skoog's technique for transposing the nipple and areola was based on the assumption that the cutaneous vessels alone were sufficient for a viable flap.

Planning the Operation

GENERAL CONSIDERATIONS

The female breast is mobile, and the site of the nipple varies according to age, race, parity, general stature, posture, and the normal asymmetry of the breasts. Estimating the future site of the nipple can therefore seem difficult and may make it impossible to apply a rigid formulation in planning an operation to reduce and reconstruct the breast, because all these variables influence the form of the breast. Skoog, however, found the location of the nipple dependent on two constant coordinates: (1) the central meridian line of the breast, and (2) the level relative to the submammary fold. Relying only on these two coordinates, he found that it was possible to individualize the reconstruction of the breast, creating a breast in shape and size harmonious with the stature of the patient.

Skoog advocated that the central meridian line of the breast had to be outlined with the patient standing or in the sitting position (Fig. 15-3), because the breast in the supine position moves laterally and upward (Fig. 15-4), making fixed skeletal references unreliable. A reduction planned with the breast in this rotated position [24, 27] will result in a medially displaced nipple (Fig. 15-5). The

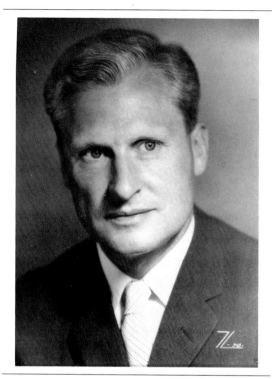

Fig. 15-1. Tord Skoog.

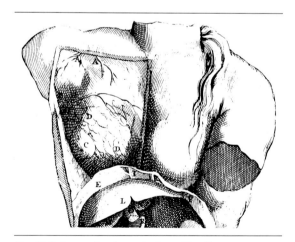

Fig. 15-2. Engraving from Andreas Vesalius.

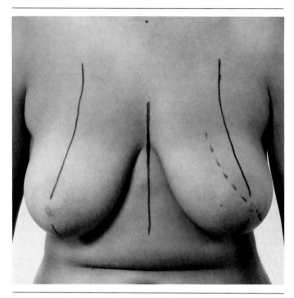

Fig. 15-3. The central meridian line (unbroken line) is outlined, in this case passing through the nipple.

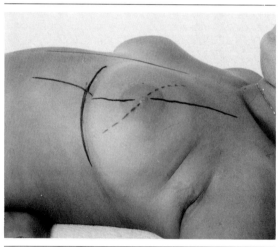

Fig. 15-4. With the patient in the supine position, the breast moves laterally and upward toward the axilla. The central axis of the breast (dotted line) now lies in a different direction.

level of the nipple is decided in relation to the sub-mammary fold, which remains unchanged and in-dependent of the size of the breast. Therefore, Skoog placed the new nipple site on the central meridian line of the breast and at a fixed distance above the level of the submammary fold. In the case of asymmetric breasts, attention must be paid to different degrees of skin retraction when the weight of a hypertrophic breast is taken off the mammary skin.

The reduction of the breast is carried out mainly as a wedge excision.

PREOPERATIVE MARKINGS

In front of the sitting surgeon, the patient is stand-ing or sitting relaxed with her arms hanging down or her hands on her hips. The appropriate mea-surements are drawn on the breast with a marking pencil.

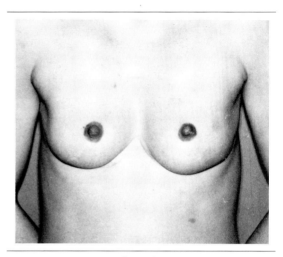

Fig. 15-5. A reduction planned with the patient in the supine position will result in medially displaced areolas, a consequence of poor planning.

Location of the Nipple Site

The sternal notch, the midline, and the central me-ridian line of the breast are outlined (Fig. 15-6). It should be noted that the nipple is not always situ-ated on the central meridian line (Fig. 15-7). The distance from the midline to the central meridian line of the breasts is checked to be certain that it is the same (Fig. 15-8).

The submammary line is drawn (Fig. 15-9).

The meridian line of the breast is continued across the submammary line onto the chest (Fig. 15-10). The level where the breast meridian line crosses the submammary line is marked on the midline (Fig. 15-11).

The level of the submammary fold, now visible between the breasts, is transferred to be marked in the central meridian line of the breast. To be cer-tain that these marks are of the same level, they must be checked with the point at the sternal notch (Fig. 15-12).

The new nipple site is located on the breast me-ridian line 3 to 5 cm above the projected submam-mary line. The distance from the center of the new nipple site to the point of the sternal notch varies but will usually be 21 to 22 cm. The operation with the reduction and the closure will then raise the nipple site 2 to 4 cm, with a final distance of 19 to 20 cm from the sternal notch (Fig. 15-13).

From the marked center of the future nipple, the nipple site is drawn as an oval with a 6-cm diame-ter, in a right angle to the meridian line of the breast, by 4 cm vertically along the meridian line.

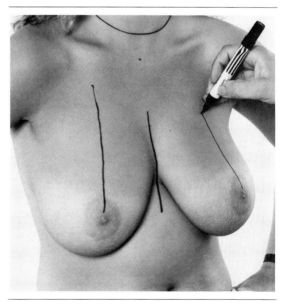

Fig. 15-6. The sternal notch, the midline, and the central meridian line of the breasts are outlined.

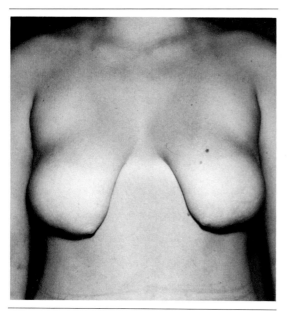

Fig. 15-7. *It should be noted that the nipple is not always situated on the central meridian line of the breast.*

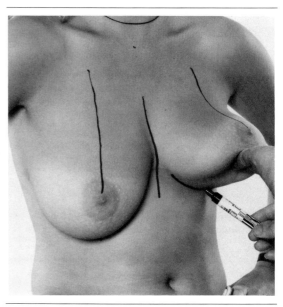

Fig. 15-9. *The submammary line is drawn.*

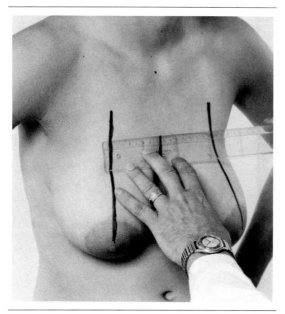

Fig. 15-8. *The distance from the midline to the central meridian line of the breasts is checked to be sure that it is the same.*

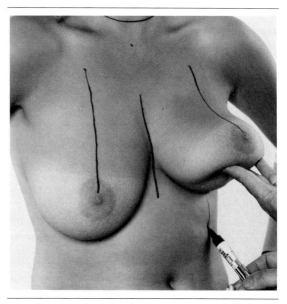

Fig. 15-10. *The meridian line of the breast is continued across the submammary line.*

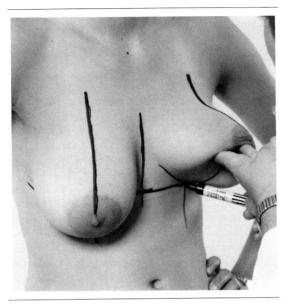

Fig. 15-11. The level where the breast meridian line crosses the submammary line is marked on the midline.

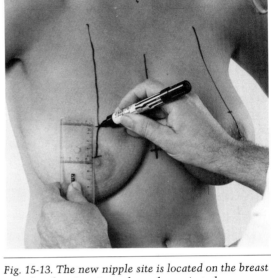

Fig. 15-13. The new nipple site is located on the breast meridian line 3 to 5 cm above the projected submammary line. The distance from the center of the new nipple site to the point of the sternal notch can be between 20 and 23 cm, depending on the weight and stature of the patient, and with the hypertrophy of the breasts, usually the distance will be 21 to 22 cm. The operation with reduction and reconstruction will then raise the nipple site 2 to 4 cm, with a final distance of 19 to 20 cm from the sternal notch.

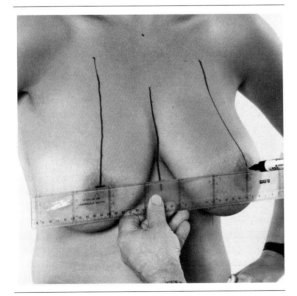

Fig. 15-12. The level of the submammary fold, now visible between the breasts, is transferred to be marked on the central meridian line of the breast, done with the help of a ruler. To be sure that these marks are on the same level, they can be checked toward the point put in the sternal notch.

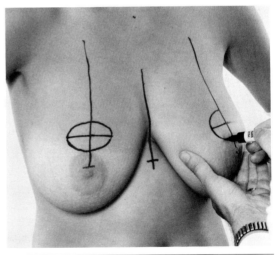

Fig. 15-14. From the marked center of the future nipple, the nipple site is drawn as an oval, measuring 6 cm horizontally, in a right angle to the meridian line of the breast, by 4 cm vertically along the meridian line. When making these markings, the skin has to be flattened and evenly distended.

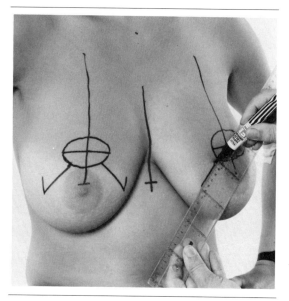

Fig. 15-15. *The wedge to be resected is planned with its apex at the center of the new nipple site. The sides of the wedge measure 5 cm from the oval marking of the new nipple site and at an angle of 110 degrees.*

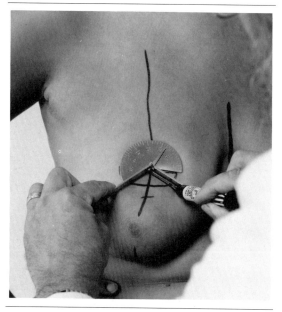

Fig. 15-16. *A goniometer can be used to accurately determine this angle of the wedge resection.*

When making these marks, the skin has to be flattened, with pressure evenly distributed (Fig. 15-14).

Planning the Resection

The wedge to be resected is planned with its apex at the center of the new nipple site. The sides of the wedge measure 5 cm from the oval marking of the new nipple site and at an angle of 110 degrees (Fig. 15-15). Here also, the skin must be evenly distended when these lines are drawn, because there is sometimes a great difference in skin tension both vertically and horizontally, especially in ptotic breasts.

A goniometer can be used to determine accurately this angle of wedge resection (Fig. 15-16). This angle does not change much with the size and shape of the breast and can therefore be used as a standard pattern. However, changing the angle will also give the surgeon the opportunity to change the shape of the reduced breast. If the angle is decreased, the reduced breast will become flatter and more hemispheric, which is more appropriate for older women. If the angle is increased, the result will be a more conical breast, better liked by younger women. The amount of breast tissue resection will, of course, also affect the size and shape of the breast and can be adjusted to the age and stature of the patient.

The end of the medial 5-cm line is drawn to join the medial end of the submammary fold (Fig. 15-17).

The end of the lateral 5-cm line is then drawn to join the lateral end of the submammary line. Incisions for the wedge resection are made along these lines (Fig. 15-18).

When the planning has been completed, the nipple position on each side can be checked, measuring the distance from the center of the new nipple site to the point of the sternal notch. If the breasts are equally large, the distance should be the same. If one breast is larger than the other, the skin above the areola is more distended; this must be taken into consideration. The new nipple site in a heavier breast sometimes has to be placed as much as 1.5 cm below that of a lighter breast (Fig. 15-19).

If the surgeon is not familiar with the technique, we suggest the Skoog device to simplify the design of the resection. It also includes an outline for the oval area to become the new site of the transposed areola (Fig. 15-20).

The site of the new nipple is checked by sup-

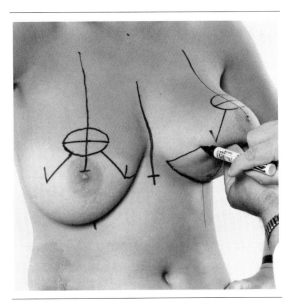

Fig. 15-17. The end of the medial 5-cm line is drawn to join the medial end of the submammary line.

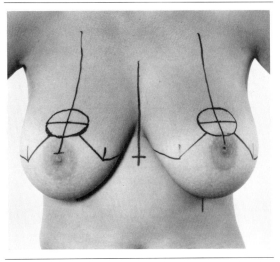

Fig. 15-19. When the planning has been completed, the nipple position on each side can be checked, measuring the distance from the center of the new nipple site to the point of the sternal notch. If the breasts are equally large, the distance should be the same. If one breast is larger than the other, the skin above the areola is more distended; this must be taken into consideration. The new nipple site of a heavier breast sometimes has to be placed as much as 1.5 cm below that of the lighter breast.

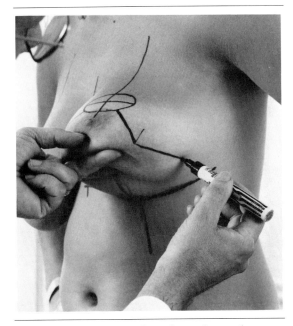

Fig. 15-18. The end of the lateral 5-cm line is then drawn to join the lateral end of the submammary line. The incisions for the wedge resection are made along these lines.

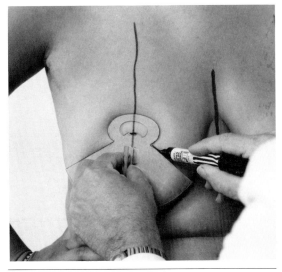

Fig. 15-20. For surgeons not familiar with the technique, Skoog constructed a device to simplify the design of the resection. It also includes an outline for the oval area to become the new site of the transposed areola.

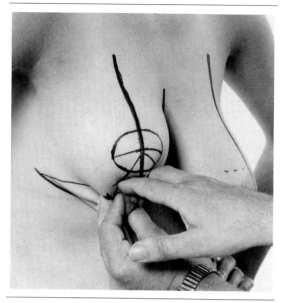

Fig. 15-21. *The site of the new nipple is checked by supporting the breast in its new position. The general appearance of the breast in relation to the woman's torso is appraised to evaluate the amount of tissue to be resected.*

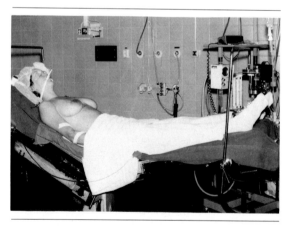

Fig. 15-22. *The operation is preferably performed under general endotracheal anesthesia with assisted ventilation. The head of the operation table is elevated about 30 degrees; this places the patient in a semi-sitting position and aids in the decision of the amount of breast tissue to be removed and in the reconstructive work. The patient's arms are padded and strapped to her sides and her shoulders are leveled with the pectoralis muscle in neutral position, a posture maintained throughout the operation.*

porting the breast in its new position. The general appearance of the breast in relation to the woman's torso is appraised to evaluate the amount of tissue to be resected (Fig. 15-21).

Anesthesia and Operation

The operation is preferably performed under general endotracheal anesthesia with assisted ventilation. The head of the operating table is elevated about 30 degrees; this places the patient in a semi-sitting position and aids in the decision of the amount of breast tissue to be removed. This position also helps to rebuild the breast. The patient's arms are padded and strapped to her sides, and the shoulders are level with the pectoral muscle in neutral position, a posture maintained throughout the operation (Fig. 15-22). The anesthesiologist uses the lower extremities for blood pressure and administration of drugs and fluids (Fig. 15-23). To diminish the blood loss during the operation, the incisions can be infiltrated with 0.25% lidocaine with epinephrine. The patient is draped, and a sheet is arranged to screen off the anesthesiologist (Fig. 15-24). The head end of the operating table is left completely to the surgeon and his or her assistants (Fig. 15-25).

Nipple Flap

The flap containing the nipple is outlined. The skin of the breast is maximally distended by a tight band of gauze around its base (Fig. 15-26). With a flap length estimated at 10 to 12 cm, the base of the flap is placed along the lateral wedge excision line, encircling the nipple and reaching a distance of 3 to 4 cm from the center of the nipple in order to preserve the periareolar vascular plexus.

If the flap length is shorter than 10 cm, the areola may be held back from moving upward to its new position (Fig. 15-27). The base of the flap must then be moved upward.

If the flap is longer than 12 cm, the base of the flap must be extended downward. The base of the nipple flap is thus at least 5 cm, but it can be extended both cranially and caudally to about 7 cm, depending on the length of the flap, since the length of the flap varies with the degree of ptosis (Fig. 15-28).

A superficial circular incision with a diameter of 4 cm is made around the nipple. Another incision is then made along the borders of the outlying flap,

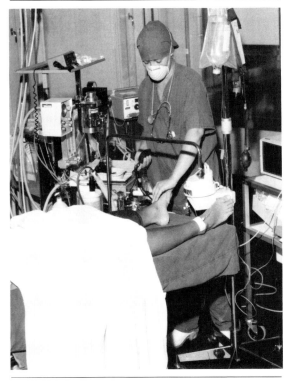

Fig. 15-23. The anesthesiologist uses the lower
extremities for blood pressure and administration of
drugs and fluids. To diminish the blood loss during the
operation, the incision lines can be infiltrated with
0.25% lidocaine with epinephrine.

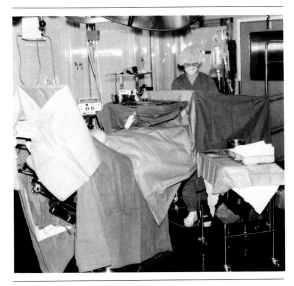

Fig. 15-24. The patient is draped, and a sheet is
arranged to screen off the anesthesiologist.

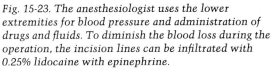

Fig. 15-25. The head end of the operation table is left
completely to the surgeon and his or her assistants.

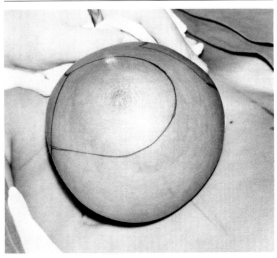

Fig. 15-26. The nipple flap is planned and outlined
with the patient on the operation table. The skin of the
breast is maximally distended by a tight sling of gauze
around the base of the breast. With a flap length
estimated to be 10 to 12 cm, the base of the flap is
placed along the lateral wedge excision line, encircling
the nipple and reaching a distance of 3 to 4 cm from
the center of the nipple in order to preserve the
periareolar vascular plexus.

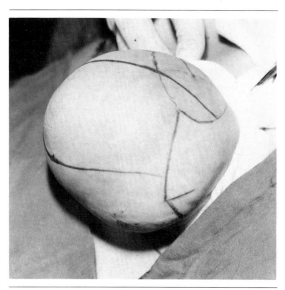

Fig. 15-27. If the flap length is shorter than 10 cm, the areola may be held back and prevented from moving up to its new position. The base of the flap must then be moved upward.

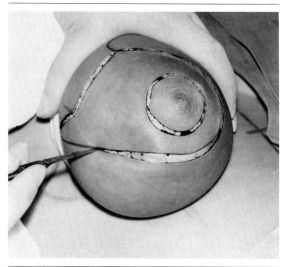

Fig. 15-29. A superficial circular incision with a diameter of 4 cm is made around the nipple. Another incision is then made along the borders of the outlined flap, taking care not to cut through the dermal layer.

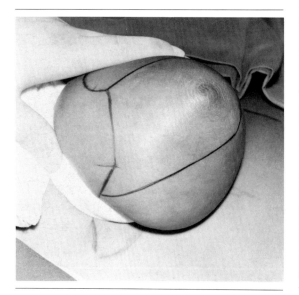

Fig. 15-28. If the flap is longer than 12 cm, the base of the flap must be extended downward. The base of the nipple flap is thus at least 5 cm but can be extended both cranially and caudally to about 7 cm, depending on the length of the flap, as the length of the flap varies according to the degree of the ptosis.

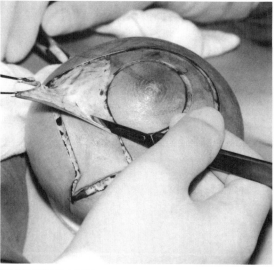

Fig. 15-30. Except for the circumcised areolar area, the flap is denuded by sharp excision with the breast still maximally distended by the tight gauze sling. The deepithelialization is performed in the definite plane where the skin can be removed without difficulty and with almost no bleeding. The deep dermal layer is left intact, protecting the underlying major vessels. The denudation can begin at the base of the flap, especially if the flap is very long.

taking care not to cut through the dermal layer (Fig. 15-29).

Except for the circumcised areolar area, the flap is denuded by sharp excision with the breast still maximally distended by the tight gauze band. The deepithelialization is performed in a definite plane where the skin can be removed without difficulty and with almost no bleeding. The deep dermal layer is left intact, protecting the underlying major vessels. The denudation can begin at the base of the flap, especially if the flap is very long (Fig. 15-30). The denudation of the flap continues around the areola (Fig. 15-31).

The margins of the flap are incised through the subcutaneous tissue, beginning superiorly and continuing distally and then inferiorly (Fig. 15-32).

The tight gauze sling is released, and four towel clips are placed along the borders of the flap for stabilization. The flap is undermined at first distally, giving the flap the thickness of 0.5 to 1.0 cm. Traction is applied to the nipple to increase the tissue under the areola, allowing the nipple to protrude when transposed to its new position (Fig. 15-33).

The lateral part of the flap is then undermined, but with the knife angled to make the lower lateral two thirds of the flap thicker (Fig. 15-34).

By including some glandular tissue in the lower, lateral part, the flap becomes more stable, and it also increases the vascular supply of the flap (Fig. 15-35). Even in flaps of considerable length, 18 – 20 cm, good circulation is apparent.

The Reduction

The skin is removed with the area marked for the new position of the areola (Fig. 15-36).

The nipple flap is held aside, and a central wedge excision of the breast is carried out along the outlined markings (Fig. 15-37). With a towel clip in the center of the new areola position, the breast tissue is brought up and supported into a more normal position, as usually the glandular tissue is displaced inferiorly in relation to the skin.

Excision is carried through the skin and breast tissue from the center of the new areola site to the submammary fold (Fig. 15-38).

Excision extends to the fascia (Fig. 15-39). Laterally, care is taken not to jeopardize the base of the flap bearing the nipple. Because it is the central lower part of the breast, which is resected, the remaining tissue will have sufficient blood supply

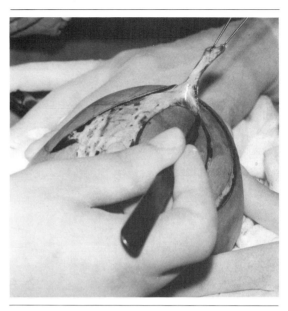

Fig. 15-31. The denudation of the flap continues around the areola.

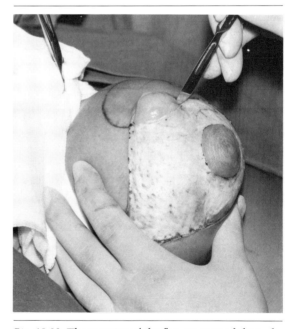

Fig. 15-32. The margins of the flap are incised through the subcutaneous tissue, beginning superiorly and continuing distally and then inferiorly.

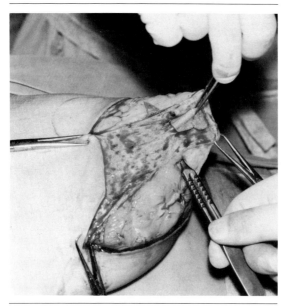

Fig. 15-33. The tight gauze sling is released, and four towel clips are placed along the borders of the flap for stabilization. The flap is undermined at first distally, giving the flap a thickness of 0.5 to 1 cm. Traction is applied to the nipple to increase the tissue under the areola, allowing the nipple to protrude when transposed to its new position.

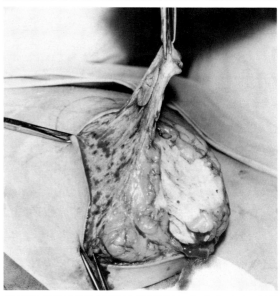

Fig. 15-35. By including some glandular tissue in the lower, lateral part, the flap becomes more stable and it also increases the vascular supply of the flap. Even in flaps of considerable length, 18 to 20 cm, a good circulation is apparent.

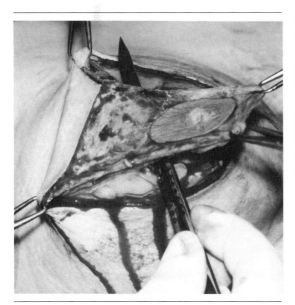

Fig. 15-34. The lateral part of the flap is then undermined, but with the knife angled to make the lower and lateral two thirds of the flap thicker.

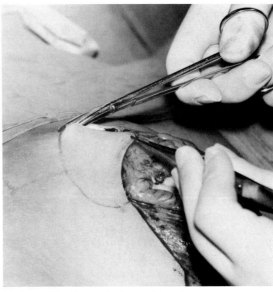

Fig. 15-36. The skin is removed within the area marked for the new position of the areola.

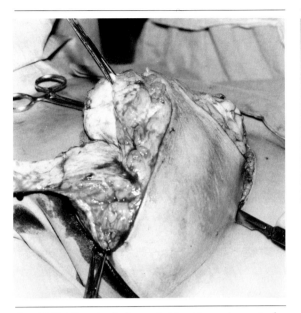

Fig. 15-37. The nipple flap is held aside, and a central wedge excision of the breast is carried out along the outlined markings. With a towel clip in the center of the new areola position, the breast tissue is brought up and supported into a more normal position, as usually the glandular tissue is displaced inferiorly in relation to the skin.

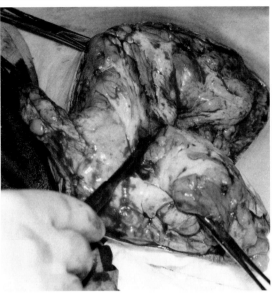

Fig. 15-39. The excision continues down to the pectoral fascia. Laterally, care is taken not to jeopardize the base of the nipple flap. As it is the central lower part of the breast, which is resected, the remaining tissue will have sufficient blood supply from both the medial and lateral mammary arteries, irrespective of the amount reduced.

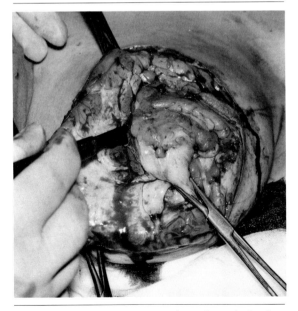

Fig. 15-38. The excision is carried out through the skin and breast tissue from the center of the new areola site to the submammary fold.

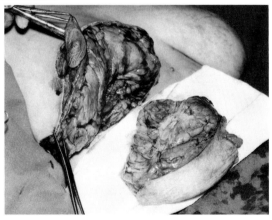

Fig. 15-40. The resection is thus comprised of both skin and breast tissue removed en bloc with clean cuts to avoid traumatizing the poorly vascularized adipose tissue of the hypertrophic breast. If the reduction is found to be insufficient, any excess can be resected from the remaining tissue. The general tendency is to leave too much breast tissue.

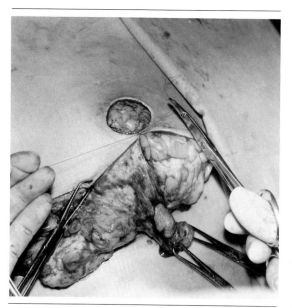

Fig. 15-41. *The reconstruction can now begin, bringing the various components together to form a naturally shaped breast. A temporary suture is placed below the new areola site.*

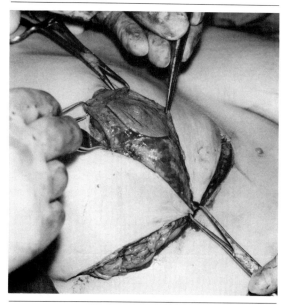

Fig. 15-42. *A towel clip is placed at the corners of the breast segments bringing them together. Tightness in the closure or increased consistency of the breast tissue that now occurs is due to excess of glandular tissue folded and compressed. Such excess has to be excised either superiorly or from the medial or lateral segment of the breast, which are equally well vascularized.*

from both the medial and lateral mammary arteries, irrespective of the amount of reduction.

Thus, skin and breast tissue have been removed en bloc with clean dissection to avoid traumatizing the poorly vascularized adipose tissue of the hypertrophic breast (Fig. 15-40). If the reduction is found to be insufficient, more tissue can be removed. The general tendency is to leave too much breast tissue.

In case of a ptotic breast, care must be taken not to perform the resection too extensively. If too much tissue is resected, the excess tissue available in the submammary region can be used for substitution (see Figs. 15-42 and 15-56).

Positioning the Nipple Flap

The reconstruction of the breast can now begin, bringing the various components together to form a naturally shaped breast. A temporary suture is placed below the new areolar site (Fig. 15-41).

A towel clip is placed at the corners of the breast segments, bringing them together (Fig. 15-42). Tightness in the closure and increased consistency of the breast tissue may now occur, and it is due to excess glandular tissue that has been folded and compressed. Such excess has to be excised either superiorly or from the medial or lateral segments of the breast, which are equally well vascularized.

The nipple flap is shifted to place the areola in its new position, gently draping the flap across the breast (Fig. 15-43). It should be noted that the flap folds at the superior edge of the base, which must be compensated for (see Fig. 15-46).

The extension of the flap is marked on the underlying skin (Fig. 15-44).

The temporary suture is removed, and the bed for the nipple flap is prepared by undermining the area outlined for the flap (Fig. 15-45). This undermining is carried out between the subcutaneous layer and the skin.

A small wedge of tissue is excised at the superior edge of the base of the flap to permit the flap to fold without compression (Fig. 15-46).

The flap is maintained in its new position by a few absorbable 4-0 sutures to keep the flap spread, except for the fold at the superior part of the base, and the flap is kept under normal tension (Fig. 15-47). If, at this stage, the areola becomes cyanotic, it is due to excessive rotation of the flap or the flap has not been spread out sufficiently medially. The flap must then be repositioned to avoid kinking.

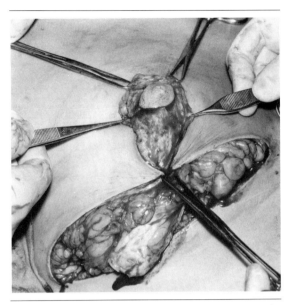

Fig. 15-43. The nipple flap is shifted to place the areola in its new position, gently draping the flap across the breast. It is to be noted that the flap folds at the superior edge of the base, which must be compensated for.

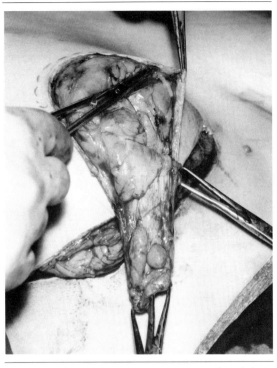

Fig. 15-45. The temporary suture is removed, and the bed for the nipple flap is prepared by undermining the area outlined for the flap. The undermining is carried out between the subcutaneous layer and the skin.

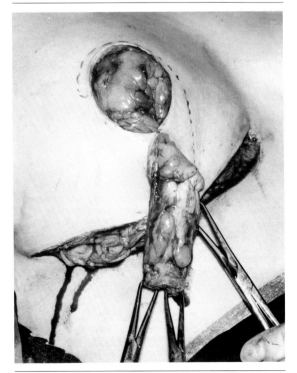

Fig. 15-44. The extension of the flap is marked on the underlying skin.

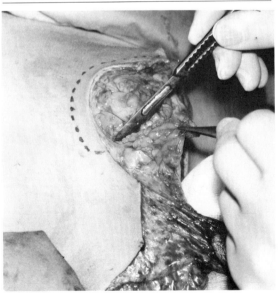

Fig. 15-46. A small wedge of tissue is excised at the superior edge of the flap base to permit the flap to fold without compression.

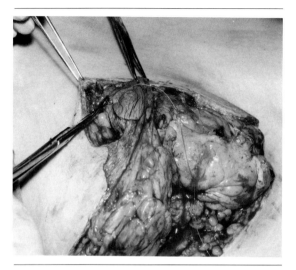

Fig. 15-47. The flap is maintained in its new position by a few absorbable 4-0 sutures to keep the flap spread, except for the fold at the superior part of the base, and under normal tension. If, at this stage, the areola becomes cyanotic, it is due to excessive rotation of the flap or the flap has not been spread sufficiently medially. The flap must then be repositioned to avoid kinking.

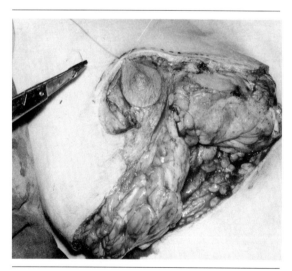

Fig. 15-48. The position of the areola is secured at first by an absorbable 4-0 suture to the skin in the breast meridian line.

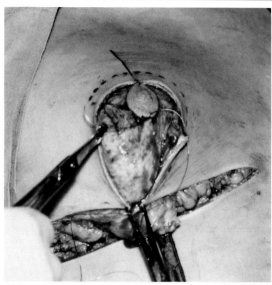

Fig. 15-49. A nonabsorbable 4-0 suture is placed in the skin immediately below the new areola site passing through the areola border diametrically opposite the first suture. The nipple flap is seen nicely spread between the areola and the submammary fold comprising a broad layer of dermal tissue that prevents distention below the nipple and also maintains the conical shape of the breast with the desired convexity above the nipple.

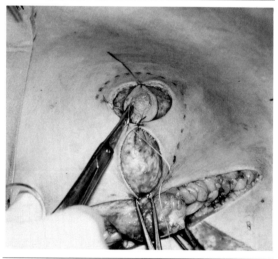

Fig. 15-50. Another two absorbable 4-0 sutures are placed diametrically in a right angle to the previous sutures. To avoid stitch marks in the skin, the sutures are allowed to pass only through the subdermal layer.

The Reconstruction

The position of the areola is secured at first by an absorbable 4-0 suture to the skin in the breast meridian line (Fig. 15-48).

A nonabsorbable 4-0 suture is placed in the skin immediately below the new areolar site and passed through the areolar border diametrically opposite the first suture (Fig. 15-49). The nipple flap is then seen nicely spread out between the areola and the submammary fold, comprising a broad layer of dermal tissue that prevents distention below the nipple and also maintains the conical shape of the breast with the desired convexity above the nipple.

Another two absorbable 4-0 sutures are placed diametrically in a right angle to the previous sutures (Fig. 15-50). To avoid suture marks in the skin, the stitches are allowed to pass only through the subdermal layer.

The two segments forming the lower parts of the breast are easily brought together (Fig. 15-51). They are sutured to each other with a few absorbable sutures (Fig. 15-52). The vascular supply to the main breast has not been impaired. The breast comes together in the meridian line without torsion or tension. Preoperative consistency of the breast thus remains unchanged after the operation, except for the area where the cutaneous flap has been spread out below the areola, where the consistency of the tissue might be firmer. Since the remaining breast tissue used for rebuilding the breast after the reduction is connected to the overlying skin, the possibility of skin necrosis is eliminated. No scarring will occur under the skin; thus, no irregularities in the breast contour will be seen postoperatively.

To stabilize the closure, a resorbable suture with prolonged resorption time (e.g., Maxon 2-0, Davis and Geck) is placed in the meridian line of the submammary excision margin, passing through the underlying fascia and then through the subdermal layers, not too superficially, of the two attached breast segments (Fig. 15-53).

When tightening this suture, new submammary fold is visible both medially and laterally above the original one (Fig. 15-54).

Bringing the breast elements together with a nonabsorbable 3-0 suture, the line of closure will correspond with the central meridian line of the breast (Fig. 15-55).

The tightness of the skin now reveals redundant breast tissue in the submammary region (Fig. 15-56).

The excess tissue is removed and dissection car-

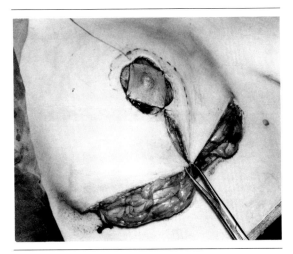

Fig. 15-51. The two segments forming the lower parts of the breast are easily brought together.

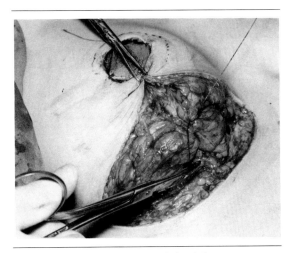

Fig. 15-52. The two segments of glandular tissue are sutured to each other with a few absorbable sutures. The vascular supply to the remaining breast tissue is not impaired by any surgery to the gland and the two parts of the breast tissue are brought together in the breast meridian line without torsion or tension. The preoperative consistency of the breast thus remains unchanged after the operation, except for the area where the cutaneous flap has been spread below the areola, where the consistency might be a little firmer. Since the remaining breast tissue used for rebuilding the breast after the reduction is connected to the overlying skin, the possibility of skin necrosis is eliminated. There will be no scar formation under the skin and thus no irregularities in the breast contour postoperatively.

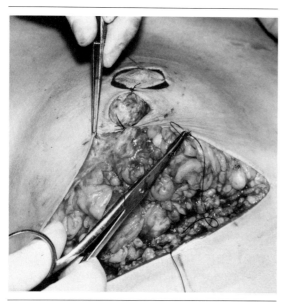

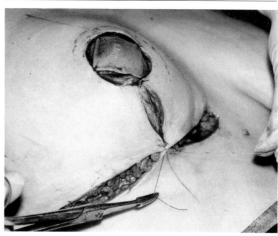

Fig. 15-55. Bringing the breast elements together with a nonabsorbable 3-0 suture, the line of closure will correspond to the central meridian line of the breast.

Fig. 15-53. To stabilize the lines of closure, a resorbable suture with prolonged resorption time (e.g., Maxon 2-0, Davis and Geck) is placed in the meridian line of the submammary excision margin, passing through the underlying fascia and then through the subdermal layers, not too superficially, of the two attached breast segments.

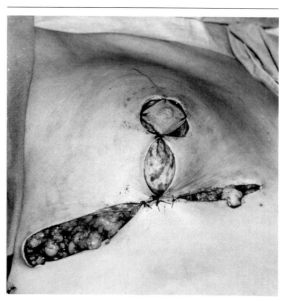

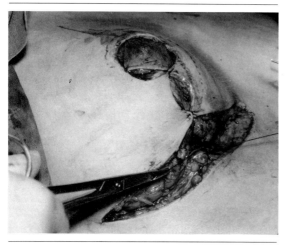

Fig. 15-56. The tightness of the skin now reveals a redundant breast tissue in the submammary region.

Fig. 15-54. When tightening this suture, a new submammary fold is visible, both medially and laterally above the original one.

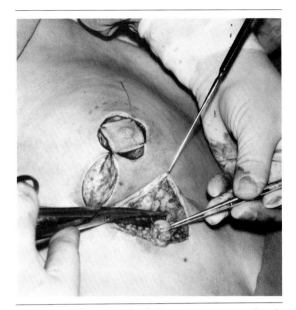

Fig. 15-57. The excess glandular tissue is removed and the dissection is carried out between the subcutaneous fat and the underlying gland, curving along the line of the new submammary fold, including the medial attachment of the gland up to the pectoral fascia. The subcutaneous layer must be preserved to make the wound margins equally thick.

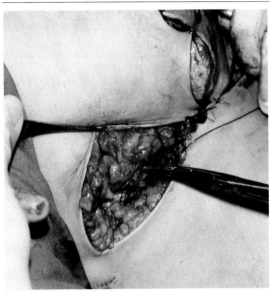

Fig. 15-59. A resorbable suture with prolonged resorption time is placed lateral of the breast meridian line in the submammary excision margin through the underlying fascia and then directed upward laterally through the subcutaneous tissue of the new submammary fold.

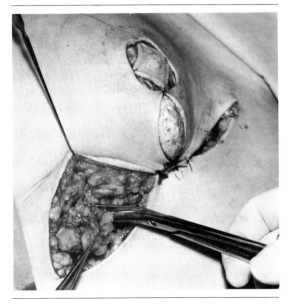

Fig. 15-58. The same procedure is carried out laterally, exposing the lateral border of the pectoralis muscle. This removal of excess tissue narrows the base of the reconstructed breast and is essential for a good aesthetic result.

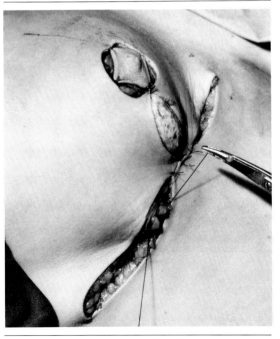

Fig. 15-60. When tightened, this suture helps to enhance the new submammary fold. A similar suture is placed medial of the breast meridian line. A more conical shape of the breast is then attained, and the breast contour is better defined.

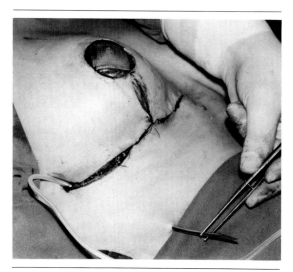

Fig. 15-61. *A drainage tube is applied to prevent formation of hematoma in the areola region, which can jeopardize the vascular supply to the areola.*

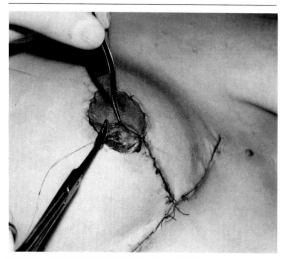

Fig. 15-62. *The areola is approximated to the surrounding skin by an intracuticular 4-0 catgut suture.*

ried out between the subcutaneous fat and the underlying gland, curving along the line of the new submammary fold, including the medial attachment of the gland up to the pectoral fascia. The subcutaneous layer must be preserved to make the wound margins equally thick (Fig. 15-57).

The same procedure is carried out laterally, exposing the lateral border of the pectoralis muscle (Fig. 15-58). This removal of excess tissue narrows the base of the reconstructed breast that is essential for a good aesthetic result.

A resorbable suture with prolonged resorption is placed lateral to the breast meridian line in the submammary excision margin through the underlying fascia and then directed upward laterally through the subcutaneous tissue of the new submammary fold (Fig. 15-59). When tightened, this suture helps to enhance the new submammary fold (Fig. 15-60). A similar suture is placed medially to the breast meridian line. A more conical shape of the breast is then obtained, and the breast contour is better defined.

Wound Closure

A drain is used to prevent hematoma in the areolar region, which can jeopardize the vascular supply to the areola (Fig. 15-61).

The areola is approximated to the surrounding skin by an intracuticular 4-0 catgut suture (Fig. 15-62).

The subcutaneous layers are closed with interrupted absorbable 3-0 sutures. The vertical wound margins are approximated very carefully by passing the suture within the dermis on the lateral side to avoid injury of subdermal vessels at the base of the nipple flap (Fig. 15-63).

The submammary incision can usually be closed without any adjustments (Fig. 15-64). A slight excess of skin is sometimes present laterally as a dogear. This can easily be eliminated (Fig. 15-65). The skin margins are approximated by an intracuticular suture of nonabsorbable material. Here we use Prolene 2-0 (Ethicon) on an atraumatic straight needle, a suture that is easy to remove (Fig. 15-66). It should be noted that the submammary incision is transverse and situated below the new submammary fold. The suture line may be more exposed in this transverse position, but scarring is less. The new submammary fold assumes a very natural configuration, and skin closure is accomplished with almost no tension.

The operation has been completed on the right

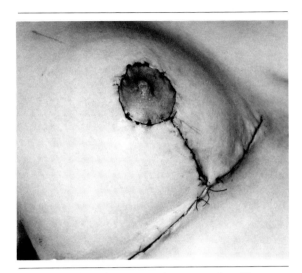

Fig. 15-63. The subcutaneous layers are closed by interrupted absorbable 3-0 sutures. The vertical wound margins are approximated very carefully, passing the needle within the dermal layer on the lateral side to avoid damage to the subdermal vessels at the base of the nipple flap.

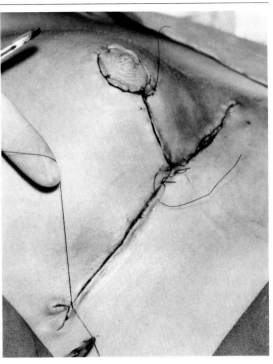

Fig. 15-65. The "dog-ear" can easily be eliminated by a small plasty.

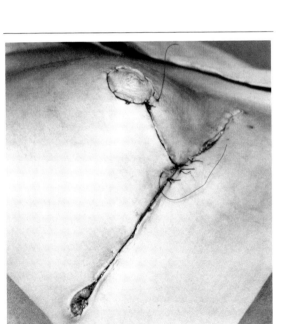

Fig. 15-64. The submammary wound can usually be closed with no adjustments. A slight skin excess is sometimes present laterally as a "dog-ear."

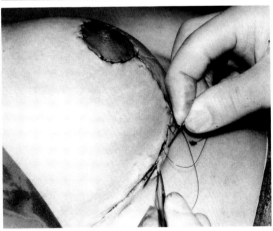

Fig. 15-66. The skin margins are approximated by an intracuticular suture of unabsorbable material. Here we use a Prolene 2/0 (Ethicon) suture on an atraumatic straight needle, a suture which is easy to remove. It should be noted that the submammary incision is transversal and situated below the new submammary fold. The suture line may be more exposed in this transverse position but scarring is less. The new submammary fold assumes a very natural configuration, and skin closure is accomplished with almost no tension.

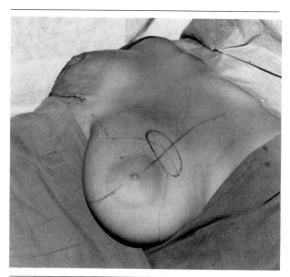

Fig. 15-67. The operation has been completed on the right side. The left breast is operated on with identical technique.

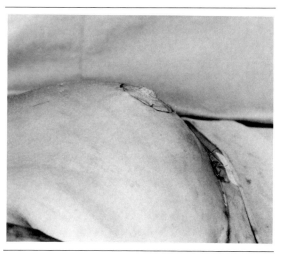

Fig. 15-69. When the nipple is raised on a cutaneous flap, skin tension is released and the lactiferous ducts are cut; this eliminates traction on the nipple. The areola then contracts in a natural way, and the nipple attains a protuberant form.

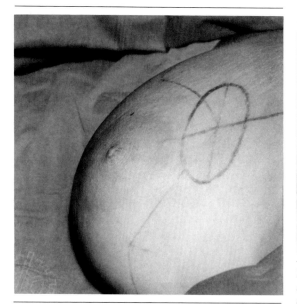

Fig. 15-68. The nipple of the hypertrophic breast to be operated on is flat and the areola distended with a smooth, even surface.

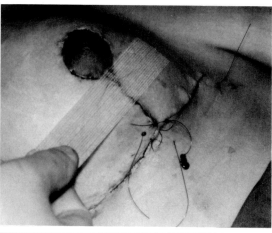

Fig. 15-70. The wounds are sealed and reinforced with sterile tape. The tapes are applied across the vertical suture line, which prevents separation of the wound edges and also helps to neutralize tension during healing.

side (Fig. 15-67). The left breast is operated on with identical technique.

The nipple of the hypertrophic breast to be operated on is flat, and the areola is distended with a smooth, even surface (Fig. 15-68).

When the nipple is raised in the cutaneous flap, skin tension is released and the lactiferous ducts are cut; this eliminates traction on the nipple. The areola then contracts in a natural way, and the nipple attains a protuberant form (Fig. 15-69).

Dressing

The incisions are reinforced with sterile tape. These are applied across the vertical suture line and help prevent separation of the wound edges and aid also in reducing tension during healing (Fig. 15-70).

Microporous tapes (Steri-Strip, 3M) are applied across the submammary suture line obliquely, medially, and laterally to the breast meridian line following the direction of the new submammary fold to support the reconstructed breast (Fig. 15-71).

Vaseline gauze is placed on the areola (Fig. 15-72), and the taped areas as well as areolas are covered with gauze pads (Fig. 15-73). For further support, a bandage of surgical tape (Microfoam, 3M) is applied (Fig. 15-74).

Slight pressure of the surgical tape is used over the areola to prevent venous congestion in the nipple flap (Fig. 15-75).

The bandage of surgical tape is left for 5 or 6 days and is then changed to a supporting bra or lighter elastic bandage for another week (Fig. 15-76).

The stitches, thus left for about 2 weeks, have been removed, and the patient is told to use a supporting bra day and night for at least 3 months (Figs. 15-77 through 15-79). After this, no bra is necessary if the patient does not wish to wear one.

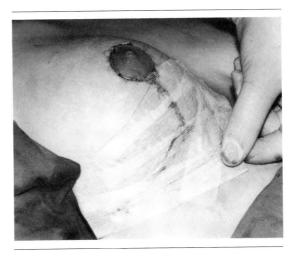

Fig. 15-71. Microporous tapes (Steri-Strip, 3M) are applied across the submammary suture line in oblique directions medial and lateral of the breast meridian line following the direction of the new submammary fold to support the reconstructed breast.

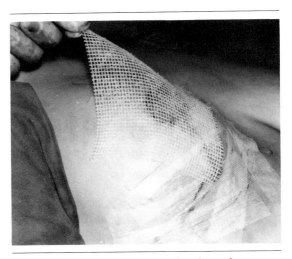

Fig. 15-72. The areolas are covered with Vaseline gauze.

Results and Comments

Skoog's technique of reduction mammaplasty with transposition of the nipple on a laterally single-based cutaneous flap has been the prevailing method at the Department of Plastic Surgery of the University Hospital in Uppsala since Skoog introduced it in 1963. His technique with a double-based cutaneous flap, however, is almost never used, as the former has been sufficient in all situations of breast reduction.

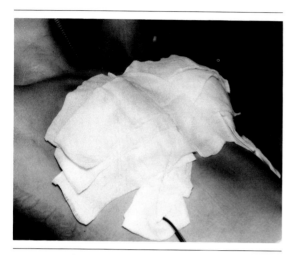

Fig. 15-73. *The taped areas and the areolas are covered with gauze pads.*

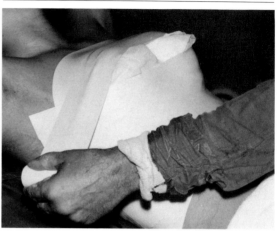

Fig. 15-75. Slight pressure of the surgical tape is applied over the areola to prevent venous congestion in the nipple flap.

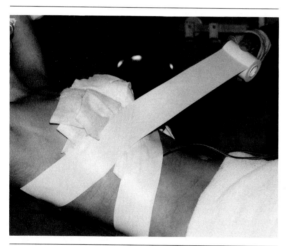

Fig. 15-74. *For further support, a bandage of surgical tape (Microfoam, 3M) is applied.*

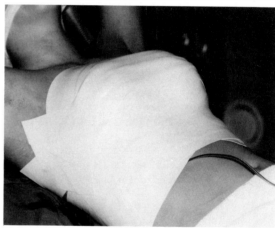

Fig. 15-76. *The bandage of surgical tape is left for 5 or 6 days and is then changed to a supporting bra or a lighter elastic bandage for another week.*

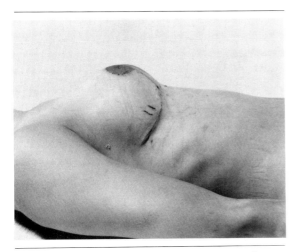

Fig. 15-77. The lighter elastic bandage is removed about 2 weeks after the operation.

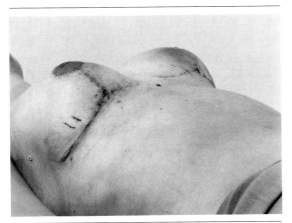

Fig. 15-78. The sutures, left for about 2 weeks, have been removed.

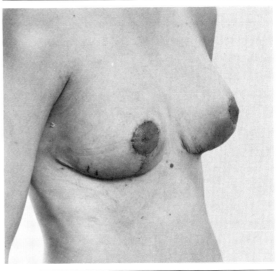

Fig. 15-79. The patient is recommended to use a supporting bra day and night for at least 3 months. After this period, no bra is necessary if the patient does not want to wear one.

Table 15-1. Symptoms of hypertrophic breasts and the effect of reduction mammaplasty according to Skoog's method

Symptoms and reasons for operation	No. of patients (%)	Mean age (years)	Cured or improved (%)
Headache	2	64	100
Neck pain	31	43	83
Shoulder-arm pain	50	42	85
Thoracic-lumbar pain	52	38	91
Indenting bra straps	41	44	98
Hygienic reasons	13	42	100
Mastodynia	6	36	80
Cosmetic reasons	41	32	98
Psychic reasons	4	37	100

Source: From I. Kinell, M. Beausang-Linder, and L. Ohlsén. The effect on preoperative symptoms and the late results of Skoog's reduction mammaplasty. A follow-up study on 149 patients. *Scand. J. Plast. Reconstr. Surg.* (in press) 1989; and L. Ohlsén, and I. Kinell. Utvärdering av den fysiska symtombilden före och efter bröstreduktionsplastik. *Svensk. Kirurgi* 42:111, 1984.

Table 15-2. Complications noted after reduction mammaplasty according to Skoog's method

Complications	Patients (no.)	(%)	Mean age (years)	Mean body weight (kg)	Mean reduced amount (gm)
Pronounced scars	7	4.4	23.3	77.3	1410
Fat necrosis	2	1.3	49.5	86.0	1525
Partial nipple necrosis	2	1.3	60.5	74.5	1730
Delayed healing	11	6.9	45.2	89.1	2312
Hematoma	4	2.5	42.0	84.5	2360
Sagging	2	1.3	37.5	70.0	1495

Source: From I. Kinell, M. Beausang-Linder, and L. Ohlsén. The effect on the preoperative symptoms and the late results of Skoog's reduction mammaplasty. A follow-up study on 149 patients. *Scand. J. Plast. Reconstr. Surg.* (in press) 1989.

Skoog chose to place the base of the flap laterally because he considered the most important blood supply of the pectoral skin to be related to the axillary vessels and the main venous return from the breast to be directed toward the axilla. The circulation of a medially based flap has, however, also proved to be adequate [19].

A retrospective study on 160 patients operated on during the period 1977 to 1979 with Skoog's technique has been carried out to evaluate the effect on preoperative symptoms and late results [10,18]. The observation time was 5 years, and the mean age of the women was 38 years (range 18 to 79 years). There was a generally occurring overweight tendency of these patients; only 25 percent had a normal or less than normal weight. The mean reduction per breast was 1100 gm, with 3800 gm as the largest total reduction. As could be expected, the amount of tissue reduction correlated positively with age and weight.

The symptoms that the patients preoperatively indicated to be caused by the hypertrophic breasts are given in Table 15-1 [10,18]. Except for headaches, of which only two women complained, pain in the neck, shoulder, and back regions was the major problem in the middle-aged women, together with indentations caused by the bra straps. It also seems natural that cosmetic and psychic reasons for operation are more common in younger women.

Of the patients, 65.1 percent were very satisfied with the result, 30.2 percent were satisfied, and 4.7 percent considered the result to be less satisfactory. The preoperative assessment of the indications for a reduction mammaplasty and the effect of the operation does not differ much from other investigations of the same type [2,11,16,28]

because the result is a subjective evaluation of the patients' expectations. This is nicely shown by the women being more happy about the outcome of the operation than was the doctor [17].

The older patients were more satisfied with the result than were the younger patients, in spite of the more often occurring complications. These also occurred more often when more than 1500 gm of tissue had been removed and when the operation had lasted more than 3.5 hours (mean operation time was 2.5 hours), which sometimes happened when an inexperienced surgeon performed the operation. The result of the reduction mammaplasty is thus also dependent on the experience of the surgeon [28].

Being overweight also entailed an increased risk for complications such as pronounced scars, infection, and nipple necrosis, as shown in Table 15-2 [10]. Women who complain of broad and pronounced scars have a very low mean age and are possibly more particular about the look of the scars. A tendency to infection was noted immediately postoperatively in four women, and fat necrosis was registered in two women. Fat necrosis is almost exclusively connected to removal of very large breasts, and special treatment is usually not necessary [17]. None of the registered fat necroses caused any postoperative difference in breast size. Partial nipple necrosis occurred as a border necrosis of the areola in two women. The necrosis was excised and then healed spontaneously. Nipple necrosis seems to be connected to a resected amount of more than 1000 gm of breast tissue [11,17]. A situation of delayed healing, including fat necrosis, nipple necrosis, and wound defects, is a complication that occurs in older women who are overweight and from whom a large amount of breast tissue was removed. The frequency of delayed healing (6.9%) is similar to that found in other studies [11].

Postoperative hematoma occurred in four women, and two of these women had to have the hematoma evacuated in a separate operation. No difference in breast size was noted afterward. Two women who complained of sagging of the breasts also showed broad and pronounced scars; inversion of the nipple was not noted in any of the women.

The postoperative inversion of the nipple and sagging of the breasts depend on the tendency of the glandular pedicles to deteriorate. The glandular mass that is pushed up to the center for reconstruction of the breast, elevating the nipple and shaping the breast cone, gradually descends owing to its weight and mobility, distending the skin below the nipple. In Skoog's technique, the breast is rebuilt with the remaining upper portion still held in place by the suspensory ligaments, reducing the possibility of sagging. When large glandular reductions are performed, these fibrous connections have a tendency to shorten, which has to be taken into account when planning the operation. Women with a juvenile breast hypertrophy should be informed that during a pregnancy, the breasts enlarge, and after delivery, a regression takes place that markedly reduces the breast volume and might have an adverse effect on the contour of the breast.

Only three women complained of reduced sensibility of the nipple. The sensibility of the nipple and the areola usually decreased postoperatively but returned slowly, and after a year, the sensibility was normal or near normal. In many cases of large hypertrophy, the women already preoperatively complained of reduced sensibility in the nipple and areola, possibly owing to nerve traction. Some women postoperatively reported increased nipple sensation, which they regarded as a positive experience. Contractility of the areola and erection of the nipple was found to be quite normal in all the women postoperatively.

In the immediate postoperative period, the sensibility and contractility of the areola may differ bilaterally despite an identical operative technique. This may be due to the preservation of an intact blood supply but a temporary insufficient nerve supply [5].

The long-term results of Skoog's technique compared to Strömbeck's technique [25,26] were reported by Hrynyschyn et al [9]. The study includes 110 patients with an observation time of 2 to 7 years. Forty-two women were operated on utilizing Skoog's technique, and in some cases, both techniques were used on the same patient for comparison. Hrynyschyn et al [9] considered the postoperative changes of the breast and nipple closely related to the histologic structure of the mammary gland. The areola was found to decrease in size about 10 to 30 percent independent of the technique. The frequency of invagination of the nipple was only 6 percent with Skoog's technique compared to 18 percent with Strömbeck's technique. They also found more often in Strömbeck's technique that the areola was pointing cranially and that there were more pronounced scars in the cranial border of the areola. Independent of technique, they found in 60 percent of patients a decrease of sensibility in the nipple.

The prolongation of the vertical scar — sagging or "herniation" of the mammary gland — did not differ between the two techniques. The sagging was found to be less in glands rich of fat tissue and more pronounced in fibrotic glands. In Skoog's technique, most of the gland is removed by the wedge excision and reconstruction is performed with the fat tissue of the lateral and medial pedicle.

Hrynyschyn et al [9] believe that the women they operated on according to Skoog's technique gave an aesthetically more attractive result with the breast more convex and better shaped. In 85 percent of cases, the women operated on utilizing Skoog's technique appraised the result as good compared to 56 percent of those operated upon utilizing Strömbeck's technique.

Other studies [2,16] regarding the result after reduction mammaplasty according to McKissock [15] and Strömbeck [25,26] and a comparative study [8] of the Biesenberger technique [3] to that of Strömbeck [25,26] show that these techniques are afflicted with some complications, which must be considered a substantial drawback. These studies show an unsatisfactory number of patients with nipple inversion (10–30%) and scar formation (8–54%). Nipple necrosis, however, shows a great variation (2–12%), and it seems that it has to be taken into account when using the McKissock technique. In these studies, reduced nipple sensibility was noted in a surprisingly high number of patients (27–60%), but a lower number (7%) has also been reported [11].

Regarding the possibility of future lactation, it is difficult to give a comparative assessment of the

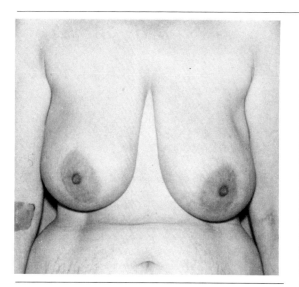

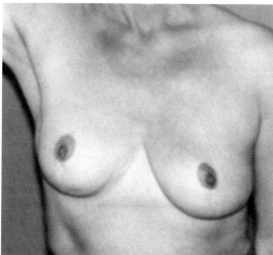

Fig. 15-80. A 44-year-old woman with ptotic and hypertrophic breasts. At operation, the nipple was placed 4 cm above the projected submammary fold and on the central meridian line of the breast. Five hundred and fifty grams of tissue was removed from the right breast, and 575 gm from the left breast. After 5 years, there is still good symmetry, no sagging, and almost invisible scars. The breasts move naturally with the position of the arms.

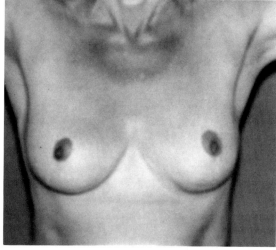

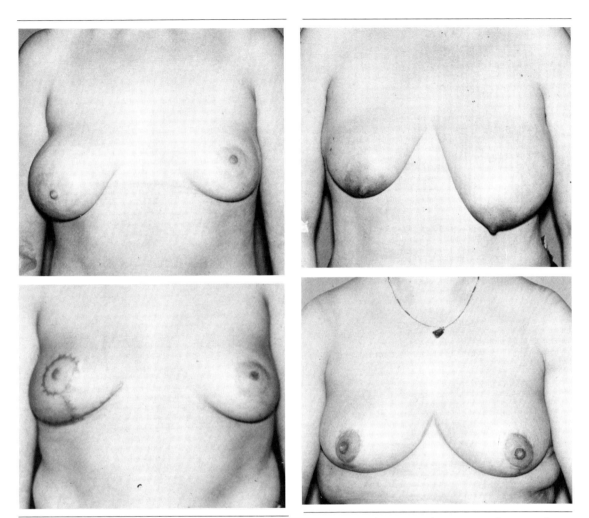

Fig. 15-81. This 18-year-old girl with asymmetric breasts was operated on with a reduction mammaplasty of the right breast. The inferior dislocation of the gland in relation to the skin was estimated to be 3 cm. Two hundred grams of tissue was resected. Six months after surgery there is good symmetry, although hyperplastic scars remain.

Fig. 15-82. With ptotic and asymmetric breasts, where the difference in breast size caused back pain, this woman, 32 years old, was operated on with a reduction mammaplasty of both breasts, in which 150 gm of tissue was removed from the right breast and 360 gm was removed from the left breast. The right nipple was placed 3 cm above the projected submammary line, and the left nipple, 2.5 cm. After 3 years, there is an excellent symmetry and, for a woman of this age, a natural shape of the breasts.

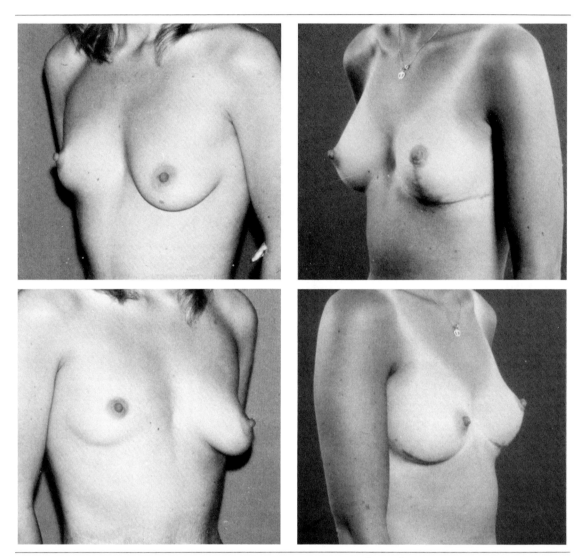

Fig. 15-83. *Suffering from asymmetry of the breasts causing both psychical and physical problems, this woman, 22 years old, was operated on with a mastopexy of the left breast, in which no breast tissue was removed but the nipple was placed 3 cm above the projected submammary line. To achieve symmetry of the breasts, the right breast was augmented with a gel-filled, round prosthesis, 160 ml (Intrashiel, McGhan), placed subpectorally. A check-up after 1 year shows good symmetry and still slightly hyperplastic scars, but no scars are visible around the areola of the left breast.*

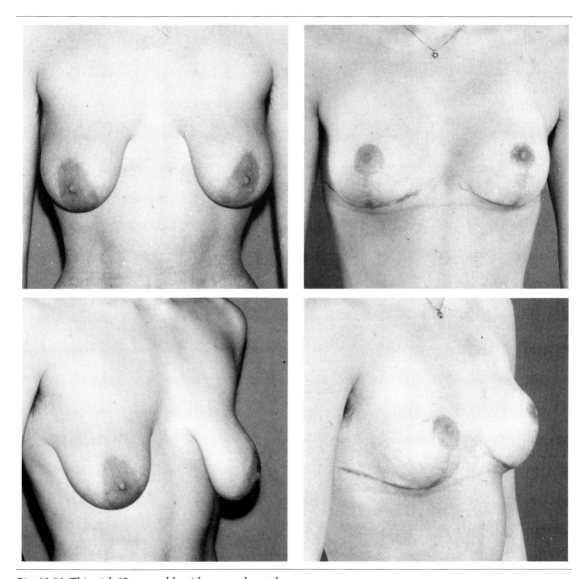

Fig. 15-84. This girl, 17 years old, with menarche at the
age of 11, developed very early tuberous breasts
causing psychical problems, including a period of
anorexia nervosa. She was operated on with a
mastopexy according to Skoog's technique, placing the
nipple 4 cm above the projected submammary line,
and removing from the right breast 160 gm of tissue
and from the left breast 140 gm. After 18 months, there
are no hyperplastic scars, but the scars in the
submammary fold are still slightly red. No scars are
visible around the areolas, there is no sagging of the
breasts, and the symmetry is good. The conical shape
of the breasts is well fitting a girl of this age.

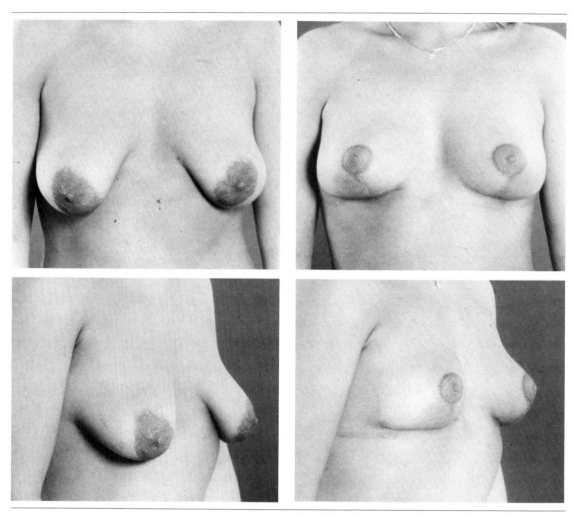

Fig. 15-85. This woman, 20 years old, had tuberous breasts and was operated on with a mastopexy, estimating the inferior dislocation of the gland in relation to the skin to be 4 cm. Only skin was excised; no breast tissue was removed. One year after the operation, there is good symmetry and shape of the breasts, no sagging, and well-healed scars.

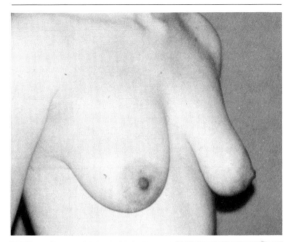

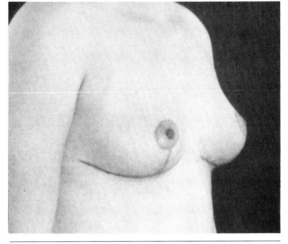

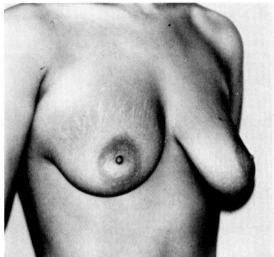

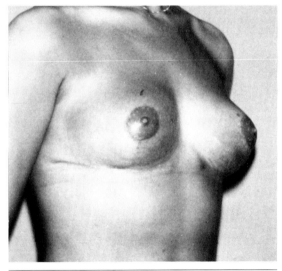

Fig. 15-86. This girl, only 15 years old, was very active in sports, including riding and volleyball. The pendulous breasts presented great difficulty in these activities. She was well built and very tall, 170 cm. She wanted a mammaplasty, which was agreed to because her body development was considered finished and the risk for recurrence owing to continuing growth of the breasts was thus reduced. The nipples were placed 4 cm above the projected submammary line. From the right breast, 170 gm of tissue was removed and from the left breast, 155 gm. No increase of breast size was noted after 1 year; there was good symmetry with a conical, natural form of the breasts, no tendency to sagging, and only slight hyperplasia of the scars. She will return for continuous check-up until she is at least 20 years old.

Fig. 15-87. This is a 28-year-old woman who has borne and nursed one child, the experience of which resulted in atrophic and ptotic breasts with visible striae. She was divorced and wanted a mammaplasty, supported by her psychiatrist, because she had very low self-esteem with aversion to exposing her body and disturbed relations to the opposite sex. With Skoog's technique, the nipples were placed 4 cm above the submammary line and a small tissue resection was performed; 95 gm of tissue was removed from the right breast and 105 gm from the left breast. Two years after surgery, a satisfactory result was noted with good symmetry and almost no scars visible. Her self-esteem had increased, and she was proud of the youthful shape of her breasts.

226

Fig. 15-88. This is a 16-year-old high-school student who was very active in athletics. The hypertrophic and ptotic breasts with the nipples 26 cm from the sternal notch caused this girl both psychical and physical problems, being a hindrance in her athletic sports and in her relations with the opposite sex. She insisted on a reduction mammaplasty and, because of her pronounced problems, the operation was performed after she had been informed about the risk for recurrence when the operation is performed on someone at this age. The nipples were placed 4 cm above the projected submammary line and on the central breast meridian line. From the right breast, 310 gm was removed, and from the left breast, 340 gm. After 2 years, she had gained a slight amount of weight, but no increase in breast volume was noted. There was a good symmetry and youthful, conical shape of the breasts and no sagging, and the scars were only slightly visible. She will return for follow-up until she is at least 20 years old.

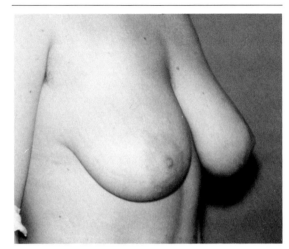

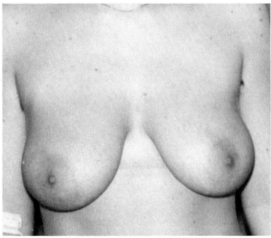

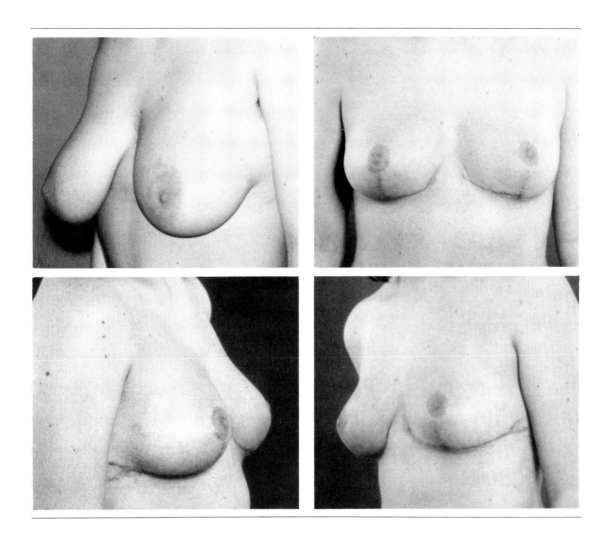

Fig. 15-89. This is a 15-year-old girl, with early menarche and breast development beginning when she was 11 years old. She was referred by her school doctor because, in addition to suffering from bronchial asthma, she also suffered both psychically and physically from her hypertrophic and ptotic breasts. The distance from the sternal notch to the right nipple was 31 cm and, to the left nipple, 29 cm. She definitely wanted a reduction mammaplasty, which was performed after she had been informed about the risk for recurrence when the operation is performed on someone this age. The right nipple was placed 3.5 cm and the left nipple 4 cm above the projected submammary line. From the right breast, 610 gm of tissue was resected, and from the left, 560 gm. At a check-up after 2 years, she had increased in weight, and she had noted an increase in size of both breasts. In spite of this, however, she was very satisfied with the size of the breasts. The symmetry and shape of the breasts were good, there was no sagging, and there was good healing of the scars, which never showed any tendency toward hyperplasia. She will be checked annually until she is at least 20 years old.

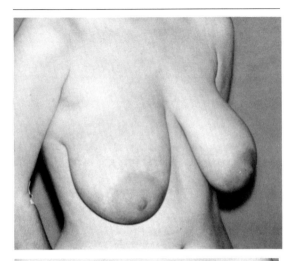

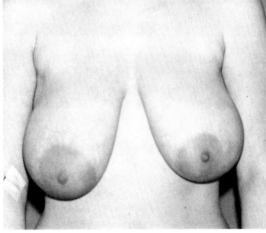

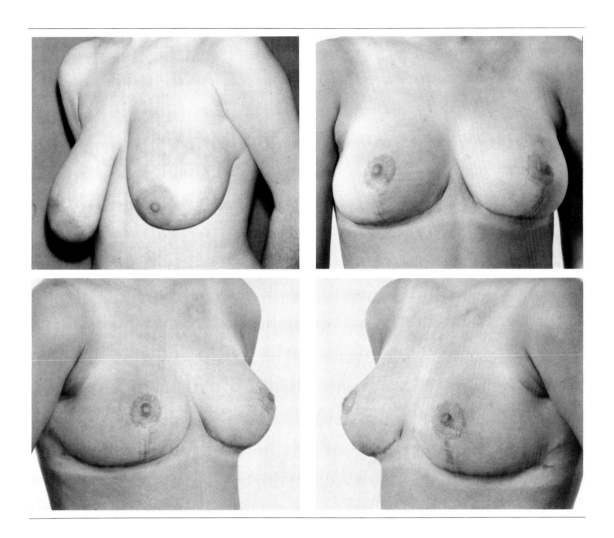

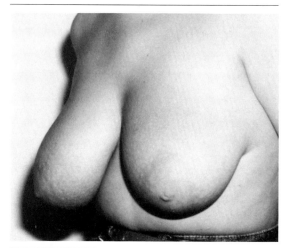

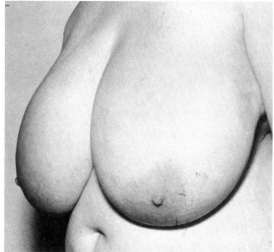

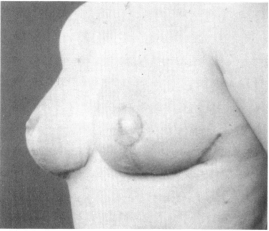

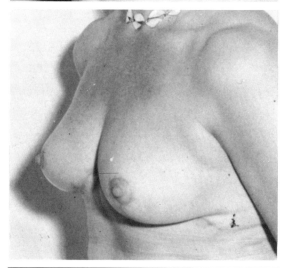

Fig. 15-90. This is a 19-year-old high-school student who was active in athletics and gymnastics. The hypertrophic breasts had given her both physical and psychical problems, being a hindrance in her sports activities and in her relations with the opposite sex. The distance from the sternal notch to each nipple was 29 cm. She was operated on with a reduction mammaplasty, removing from the right breast 440 gm of tissue, and from the left breast, 380 gm. The nipples were placed 4 cm above the projected submammary line. One year after surgery, a satisfactory healing was noted, the symmetry and shape of the breasts were good, and there was no sagging and only slight hyperplasia of the submammary scars.

Fig. 15-91. This is a multipara woman, 43 years old, who suffered from gigantic hypertrophy of the breasts causing back pain and severely indenting bra straps. She was operated on with Skoog's reduction mammaplasty, removing from the right breast 1250 gm of tissue, and from the left breast, 1075 gm. The nipples were placed 4 cm above the projected submammary line and on the central meridian line of the breast. Four years after surgery, the importance of the operation was clearly visible with a complete change of the patient's appearance. She had become very stylish and chic and had reduced her weight considerably. In spite of the reduced weight, the shape of the breasts was excellent, with good symmetry, no sagging, and only slightly visible scars.

various techniques. Many women are past the age of lactation; in others with virginal hypertrophy, it is difficult to know whether they would have lactated at all in later life. In Skoog's technique, the lactiferous ducts are cut to create the cutaneous nipple flap, and most of the gland is removed in the resection. The possibility of a reestablished lactatory system is thus very slight, although it could happen as shown in the follow-up study by Kinell et al [10], in which three women could lactate postoperatively. On the other hand, Müller [16] reported in his follow-up study of Strömbeck's technique that 10 patients became pregnant postoperatively but in none of them did any lactation occur. Women to be operated on utilizing Skoog's technique are informed that they will not be able to lactate in the future, and they accept this situation. Women who have borne and nursed one or more children often do not care for breastfeeding if they would be pregnant again after the breast reduction. Young women who have not borne any children accept not being able to lactate because of their pronounced physical and psychical problems, and their aesthetic considerations far outweigh the importance of future lactation.

From these comparative studies and follow-up reports, it can be concluded that the frequency of complications affiliated with Skoog's technique is of a satisfactory low level, which justifies the general use of this method in reduction mammaplasty. Furthermore, the technique allows for a natural convex shape and contour when rebuilding the breast. It should also be noted that the sensibility of the nipple and areola seems to be very well retained after operation with Skoog's technique. This demonstrates the accuracy in his assumption of the nerve supply to the nipple as one of the fundaments for this technique. Preserving a cutaneous bridge to the nipple leaves the nerve supply intact. Methods of reduction mammaplasty with transposition of the nipple on a broad cutaneous flap based laterally are likely to involve less damage to the lateral cutaneous nerves of the pectoral region [22], which accounts for a better preservation of the nipple sensation.

Conclusion

Skoog's technique has the advantage of permitting the surgeon to decide and individualize the size and shape of the breast and to plan and create a breast according to the patient's wish, stature, and posture.

The reduction, independent of how small or large an amount is resected, does not endanger the blood supply to the remaining tissue.

By varying the angle of the wedge resection, it gives the surgeon all possibilities for variations in the shape of the breast, from a conical and protruding to a spherical and flat breast.

The wedge resection does not disturb the superior portion of the breast, which diminishes the possibilities of future sagging. The lower portion of the breast consists of the tissue situated in the medial and lateral part of the breast joined symmetrically in the breast meridian line.

The breast tissue used for the reconstruction has a complete connection with the covering skin, as there has been no undermining and thus there will be no irregularities in the breast contour.

The base of the breast can be reduced and rounded by further slight reduction if necessary and enhanced by special sutures.

The level of the submammary fold is not changed.

The nipple is located on the central meridian line of the breast, which is not changed.

The areola and nipple are given an aesthetic protrusion because of the buttressing effect and the additional tissue under the areola with the nipple distinctly protuberant, even if it was completely flat preoperatively.

The breast moves with the position of the arm, as the suspensory apparatus of the breast tissue has not been touched.

Skoog's technique can be used in all types of asymmetric, tuberous, ptotic, atrophic, and hypertrophic breasts (Figs. 15-80 through 15-91).

References

1. Arner, O., Edholm, P., and Ödman, P. Percutaneous selective angiography of the internal mammary artery. *Acta Radiol.* 51:433, 1959.
2. Baumeister, R.G.H., Daigeler, R., Umlandt, A., and Bohmert, H. Spätergebnisse der Reduktionsplastik nach McKissock. *Langenbecks Arch. Chir.* 369:285, 1986.
3. Biesenberger, H. *Deformitäten und kosmetische Operationen der weiblichen Brust.* Wien: W. Maudrich, 1931.
4. Cooper, A.P. *On the Anatomy of the Breast.* London: Longman, Orine, Green, Brown and Longmans, 1840.
5. Craig, R.D.P., and Sykes, P.A. Nipple sensitivity following reduction mammaplasty. *Br. J. Plast. Surg.* 23:165, 1970.

6. Edholm, P., and Strömbeck, J.O. Influence of mammaplasty on the arterial supply to the hypertrophic breast. *Acta Chir. Scand.* 124:521, 1962.

7. Gillies, H., and McIndoe, A. The technique of mammaplasty in conditions of hypertrophy of the breast. *Surg. Gynecol. Obstet.* 68:658, 1939.

8. Gupta, S.C. A critical review of contemporary procedures for mammary reduction. *Br. J. Plast. Surg.* 18:328, 1965.

9. Hrynyschyn, K., Lösch, G.M., and Schrader, M. Ergebnisse vergleichender Untersuchungen bei der Mammareduktionsplastik nach Strömbeck und Skoog. *Langenbecks Arch. Chir.* 369:279, 1986.

10. Kinell, I., Beausang-Linder, M., and Ohlsén, L. The effect on preoperative symptoms and late results of Skoog's reduction mammaplasty. A follow-up study on 149 patients. *Scand. J. Plast. Reconstr. Surg.* (in press) 1989.

11. Krebs, H., and Friedl, W. Klinische und mammografische Spätergebnisse nach Mammareduktionsplastiken nach Strömbeck. *Langenbecks Arch. Chir.* 369:277, 1986.

12. Lalardrie J.-P., and Jouglard J.-P. *Plasties Mammaires pour Hypertrophie et Ptose.* Paris: Masson et Cie, 1973.

13. Maliniac, J.W. Arterial blood supply of the breast. *AMA Arch. Surg.* 47:329, 1943.

14. Marcus, G.H. Untersuchungen uber die arterielle Blutversorgung der Mamilla. *Arch. Klin. Chir.* 179:361, 1934.

15. McKissock, P.K. Reduction mammaplasty with a vertical dermal flap. *Plast. Reconstr. Surg.* 49:245, 1972.

16. Müller, F.E. Late results of Strömbeck's mammaplasty: A follow-up study of 100 patients. *Plast. Reconstr. Surg.* 54:664, 1974.

17. Müller, F.E. Spätergebnisse von 1046 Mammareduktionsplastiken. *Langenbecks Arch. Chir.* 369:273, 1986.

18. Ohlsén, L., and Kinell, I. Utvärdering av den fysiska symtombilden före och efter bröstreduktionsplastik. *Svensk. Kirurgi* 42:111, 1984.

19. Oulié, J. Utilisation d'un lambeau aréolomamelonnaire à pedicule interne au cours de plasties mammaires de reduction. *Ann. Chir. Plast.* 20:251, 1975.

20. Ragnell, A. Operative correction of hypertrophy and ptosis of the female breast. *Acta Chir. Scand.* [Suppl.] 113, 1946.

21. Salmon, M. Les artères de la glande mammaire. *Ann. Anat. Pathol.* 16:477, 1939.

22. Schwartzmann, E. Die Technik der Mammaplastik. *Chirurg* 2:932, 1930.

23. Skoog, T. A technique of breast reduction. *Acta Chir. Scand.* 126:1, 1963.

24. Skoog, T. *Plastic Surgery. New Methods and Refinements.* Stockholm: Almqvist & Wiksell, 1974.

25. Strömbeck, J.O. Mammaplasty: Report of a new procedure based on a two-pedicle procedure. *Br. J. Plast. Surg.* 13:79, 1960.

26. Strömbeck, J.O. Reduction Mammaplasty. In T. Gibson (ed.), *Modern Trends in Plastic Surgery.* London: Butterworth, 1964.

27. Strömbeck, J.O. Reduction mammoplasty: Some observations and reflections. *Aesth. Plast. Surg.* 7:249, 1983.

28. Usbeck, W., and Usbeck, B. Rechtfertigen die Ergebnisse von Reduktionsplastiken der Mamma die Indikationen zur Operation? *Langenbecks Arch. Chir.* 369:291, 1986.

29. Vesalius, A. *De Humani Corporis Fabrica.* Venetiis, F.F. Senesis & J. Criegher, 1568. P. 368. Quinti Libri figura.

16

Daniel L. Weiner

Breast Reduction: The Superior Pedicle Technique (Dermal and Composite)

In 1972, we reported our initial experience in utilizing a superiorly based dermal pedicle for nipple-areola transposition in reduction mammaplasty. The operative procedure was based on our clinical experience and supported by the work of Schwartzman, who in 1926 described the important cutaneous circulation of the nipple-areolar complex. This permitted a surgeon to design an adequate pedicle to support the nipple-areolar complex on the cutaneous circulation alone. The superior dermal pedicle seemed to be a logical next step along the path cleared by Strömbeck's work, which utilized a dermal-parenchymal bipedicle, and Skoog's experiences with a lateral cutaneous pedicle. We thought that it would be an advantage to base the pedicle superiorly, at the future site of the nipple-areolar complex.

The technique allowed for a safe, yet relatively unrestricted migration of the nipple-areolar complex and therefore could be utilized with various types of breast reduction and contouring. The folding of the superior pedicle as the nipple was migrated superiorly did not critically compromise the nipple circulation. The plastic surgery literature since that time has been filled with a number of variations of our original superior pedicle technique, confirming its safety, versatility, and acceptance.

We now utilize two modifications of the original superior based pedicle, depending on the requirements of the specific patient. One is a superior based pedicle with the nipple-areolar complex supported only by the dermis. The second is a superior based composite pedicle that includes both breast parenchyma and dermis, to support the nipple circulation and transposition (a dermal-glandular pedicle).

Our own personal series of more than 300 mammaplasties in 16 years reaffirms the original work and the adaptability of the operative procedure. There have been some improvements and modifications, but the basic operation remains the same. The superior pedicle technique can produce in almost any sized breast excellent contour and unrestricted nipple-areolar migration (up to 20 cm) free of distortion, and in most cases, maintains normal nipple sensitivity and often function. These results are shared by many, including Dr. Jorgen Gundersen's Swedish group, who have reported on a large series of patients with excellent follow-up at the referral center in Kristianstad. These women had reduction mammaplasties utilizing the superior pedicle technique. The procedure was found to be applicable in all cases and age groups, producing uniformly excellent results. Postoperative lactation was documented in their younger patients.

Method

PREOPERATIVE CONSIDERATIONS AND MARKING

All measurements and marking should be carried out with the patient in the erect position. It is important to evaluate the erect posture and to note the presence of chest wall or spinal deformities, since these findings may have an important bearing on the final result.

The midpoint of the suprasternal notch (MSP) and the midclavicular points (MCP) are marked. The inframammary crease is marked from the anterior axillary line to the sternocostal junction.

233

234

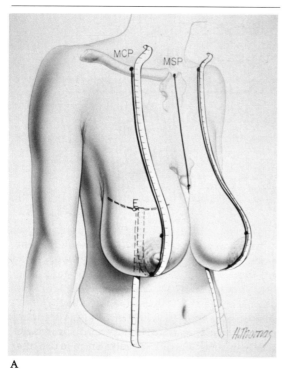

A

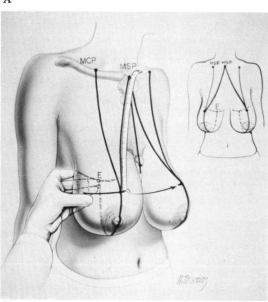

B

Fig. 16-1. A. Establishment of key reference points, breast median, and inframammary crease. B. Locating the proposed nipple site at the level of the inframammary crease.

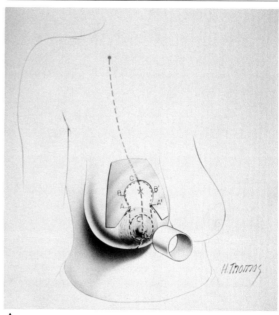

A

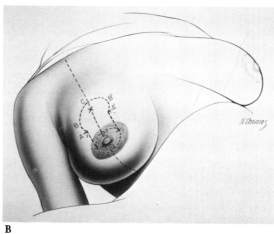

B

Fig. 16-2. A. The Wise pattern is applied 2 cm above the proposed nipple site, and a "cookie cutter" outlines the new nipple-areolar complex. B. Intraoperative marking of the pedicle and tattooing of key points.

The breast median is established by dropping a line from the MCP to the nipple. This line bisects the nipple-areolar complex and is extended to the inframammary crease, which it transects at point E. The distance from the MSP to the nipple on each side is measured and recorded, as is the distance from the nipple to the midpoint of the inframammary crease (point E) (Fig. 16-1A). The proposed nipple position should lie at the same level as the inframammary crease. Once this is established by eye and palpation, it is marked on the breast median, and a measurement is made from the MSP. A similar mark is made on the opposite breast (Fig. 16-1B). Depending on the diameter of the proposed nipple-areolar complex, a mark is then made 1.5 or 2.0 cm above the proposed nipple site at point C (Fig. 16-2A). We use Wise patterns with areola diameters varying from 37 to 45 mm as dictated by preoperative conditions such as age, parity, and the desires of the patient. This pattern is then superimposed on the breast at point C and is used only to mark the proposed areola site and the sites of the medial (A) and lateral (A′) skin closure of the inferior pole of the new areola. The rest of the pattern can also be marked preoperatively as a fail-safe check to ensure against either excessive or inadequate skin excisions. This will also facilitate a final skin closure that ensures breast symmetry.

Surgical Technique

Under general anesthesia and in the recumbent position with the arms abducted at 90 degrees, the critical marks are tattooed at points A, A′, C, C′, D, and E (Fig. 16-2B). The areola is marked with a "cookie cutter" of the same or a slightly smaller diameter than that of the Wise pattern. The breast may be put under tension by an opened lap pad wrapped around its base.

The superior dermal pedicle is deepithelialized under direct vision with meticulous care so as not to compromise the dermis. We do not use the blind technique since it can lead to "buttonholing" of the dermis, which is to be avoided. Coagulation of the dermal pedicle is neither necessary nor desirable. When completed, the dermal pedicle should have an appearance similar to the surface of a slit-thickness skin graft donor site. The dermal pedicle is then incised from B′ to D to B.

The Dermal Pedicle Verses the Dermal-Glandular Pedicle

At this point in the procedure, consideration should be given as to whether the nipple-areolar complex will be migrated superiorly to its new location on a composite pedicle of dermis and breast parenchyma, or whether the nipple's attachments to the breast will be divided and the nipple complex migrated on an isolated dermal pedicle alone (Fig. 16-3). This decision should be based on the distance of migration to the new nipple site and on the volume of breast that will need to be resected. Longer distances of movement of the nipple or larger resections of breast will usually be facilitated by use of the isolated dermal pedicle. However, it is safer and technically easier to use the composite dermal pedicle, which includes breast parenchyma; this is also the preferred choice. The composite pedicle will give better sensation and function.

If the breast reduction required is moderate and the nipple distance to be migrated is not excessive, a wedge resection with the apex of the wedge below the nipple-areolar complex and the use of a composite pedicle will suffice. However, if a larger resection is necessary and the apex of the wedge must be above the level of the nipple, or if the nipple migration will be restricted by its normal attachments to the breast, it may be necessary to isolate and move the nipple on its dermal pedicle alone. The nipple will survive on its cutaneous circulation. Then, unrestricted migration is possible as well as unrestricted breast reduction. Postoperative nipple and breast appearance will still be excellent and undistorted, although sensation may be modified. The choice of either type of superior based pedicle gives the surgeon total flexibility to meet his or her needs in any type of breast reduction operation.

The skin of the inferior hemisphere of the breast is cut longitudinally from D to E, and a plane is created between the skin and parenchyma until the inferomedial and inferolateral quadrants have been undermined. This should be accomplished at the immediate subdermal level, where bleeding will be minimal. More significant bleeding will occur both laterally and medially as the breast attachments to the chest wall are divided and the breast is mobilized. In all areas, including the breast resection, hemostasis is accomplished only

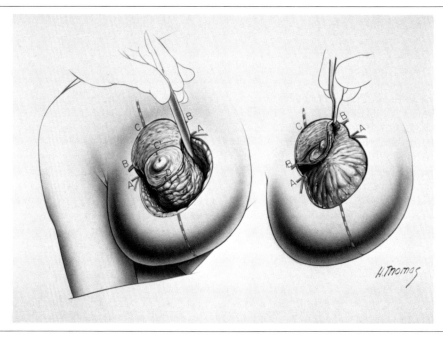

Fig. 16-3. Deepithelialization of the superior pedicle under direct vision. Creation of a dermal-parenchymal pedicle or a pure dermal pedicle.

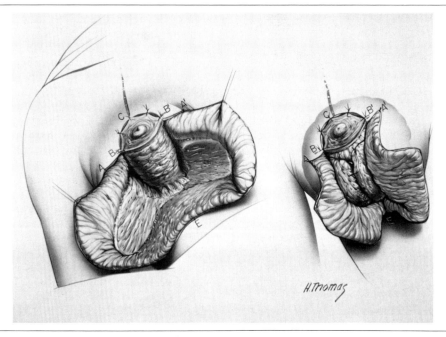

Fig. 16-4. Resection of the parenchymal wedge and reforming the breast eminence.

with the bipolar cautery. The breast has now been separated into three elements:

1. The upper hemisphere with the superiorly based dermal-parenchymal pedicle, or single dermal pedicle
2. Inferomedial and inferolateral breast skin that has been separated from the parenchyma
3. Inferior hemisphere breast parenchyma

Any single wedge or combination of wedges may be resected from the breast parenchyma. Resection may also be augmented by removal of the lateral and medial breast tails or by large transverse resections, parallel to the plane of the chest wall to reduce a breast with extreme size and forward projection. The breast should be elevated off the pectoralis fascia for a short distance so that superior transposition of the newly reconstructed and reduced breast is facilitated. The medial and lateral portions of breast parenchyma are always sutured to reconstruct and shape the new spherical breast (Fig. 16-4).

The nipple-areolar complex is now transposed superiorly by suturing C' to C and bringing A to A' to reform the areolar perimeter. The skin flaps are grasped in a series of Allis clamps. The flaps are then brought through a curved Doyen intestinal clamp until the breast has the proper three-dimensional appearance and consistency. The clamp has been marked at 6 cm, but the distance may vary from 5 to 7 cm. The flaps are marked, the clamps are opened, and the flaps are cut. The lower point of the inferomedial (E″) and inferolateral (E′) flaps are sutured to midpoint of the inframammary incision (E).

The shape and size of the new and reduced breast is determined primarily by the surgical resection and reconstruction of the breast parenchyma. The skin brassiere acts only to assist and support as the skin is redraped to conform to the new breast size and shape. Rigid adherence to predetermined marking and measurements in the skin excision phase is neither necessary nor desirable. The surgeons experience and aesthetic judgment will determine the quality of the result.

The areola to inframammary incision (D-E) is loosely closed to establish a line, usually of about 5 cm. (It may be made longer if the reconstructed breast requires it.) The medial and lateral dog-ears are resected so that the incisions lie in the inframammary crease (Fig. 16-5A). The wounds are closed after Penrose drains are brought out

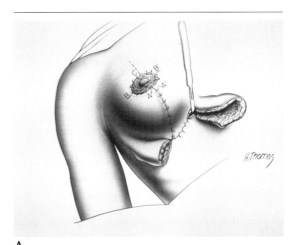

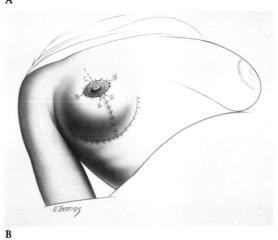

Fig. 16-5. A. Resection of medial and lateral dog-ears. B. Completed breast reduction.

through the lateral aspect of the inframammary crease (Fig. 16-5B).

Discussion

Attention to detail in the preparation of the superior dermal pedicle is, of course, critical. The deepithelialized dermal pedicle should resemble the donor site of a thick split-thickness graft. Buttonholing of the dermis is to be avoided since it may cause vascular embarrassment of the nipple-areolar complex. Despite this care in deepithelialization, the pedicle, as we now use it, is most often a dermal-parenchymal composite. This minimizes interruption of neurovascular, lymphatic, and ductal structures, which allows for greater sensibility and a more normal appearance. This is analogous to the myocutaneous concept in which skin and its underlying muscle are transposed en bloc to enhance neurovascular integrity.

Although we now prefer this composite technique, we do, at times, raise the nipple-areolar complex on a dermal pedicle as originally described if the situation necessitates it. This can be done without circulatory difficulty; however, postoperative sensibility seems to be superior when the dermal-parenchymal interface has not been violated.

Once the nipple-areolar complex has been transposed, the parenchyma is resected in one or more wedges with lateral extensions as needed. The remaining breast tissue is then reshaped and sutured into a new breast eminence. The skin is now closely redraped over this eminence and excised. This is a critical point in that we do not depend totally on a tight skin closure to determine the final breast shape. Overdependence on the skin brassiere may lead to increased tension and unaesthetic postoperative scarring and distortion. The skin assists in shaping the breast, but the parenchyma determines its primary contour.

In the last 16 years, we have found the technique adaptable to a wide spectrum of breast problems, whether they be major hypertrophy, gross asymmetry, or ptosis with involutional changes. To date, it has been used to carry out nipple-areola transpositions of up to 20 cm in major hypertrophies while still allowing for adequate resection of breast tissue for reduction.

In reviewing our cases, we find uniformly acceptable aesthetic results with none of the familiar distortions of nipple and breast contour often associated with other techniques. We have never experienced total necrosis of the nipple-areolar complex in a reduction or mastopexy. Some small partial sloughs have occurred when this technique was used in conjunction with simultaneous subcutaneous mastectomy. There have been few cases of nipple retraction, and nipple erectibility has always been present. Although specific pre- and postoperative evaluation of sensibility was not carried out, more than 80 percent of patients believed that their postoperative sensibility (after 6 months) was normal or not a problem when specifically queried.

The major postoperative complication has been with partial or full-thickness skin loss at the inverted "T" closure. This has been seen in about 15 percent of all cases and manifests itself in the second postoperative week. All resulting defects have healed by second intention and with little, if any, effect on the overall aesthetic result. Skin grafting or any other type of secondary closure has never been necessary. In one case, there was a major portion of the nipple lost secondary to a postoperative wound infection. There were no documented losses from vascular compromise.

Secondary operative procedures, involving a tightening of the skin brassiere to correct slowly progressive ptosis owing to skin relaxation or hypertrophic scar revisions, have been performed in some of these patients. The loss of original contour can occur from 5 to 7 years following the primary operation, and a simple skin and scar excision will tighten the skin brassiere and reestablish the original breast contour.

Selected Readings

Conroy, W.C. Reduction mammaplasty with superior sub-dermal pedicle. *Ann. Plast. Surg.* 2:189, 1979.

Courtiss, E., and Goldwyn, R. Breast sensation before and after plastic surgery. *Plast. Reconstr. Surg.* 58:1, 1976.

Cramer, L.M., and Chong, J.K. Unipedicle cutaneous flap areola nipple transposition on an end-bearing superiorly based flap. In N. Georgiade (ed.), *Reconstructive Breast Surgery.* St. Louis: Mosby, 1976. Pp. 143–156.

De Longis, E. Mammaplasty with L-shaped limited scar. *Aesth. Plast. Surg.* 10:171, 1986.

Dufourmentel, C., and Mouly, R. Plastique mammaire par la methode oblique. *Ann. Chir. Plast.* 6:45, 1961.

Fara, M. Reduction mammaplasty with a superior based flap. *Acta Chir. Plast.* (Prague) 16:49, 1983.

Goulian, D. Dermal mastopexy. *Plast. Reconstr. Surg.* 47:105, 1971.

Hauben, D.J. Superior based medial dermal pedicle in reduction mammaplasty. *Aesth. Plast. Surg.* 8:189, 1984.

Maliniac, J. Arterial supply of the breast. *Arch. Surg.* 47:329, 1943.

Schwarzmann, E. Die technik der mammaplastik. *Chirurg* 2:932, 1930.

Skoog, T. A technique of breast reduction-transposition of the nipple on a cutaneous vascular pedicle. *Acta Chir. Scand.* 126:453, 1963.

Strömbeck, J. Mammoplasty: Report of a new technique based on the two pedicle procedure. *Br. J. Plast. Surg.* 13:79, 1960.

Strömbeck, J.O. Reduction mammoplasty — Observations and reflections. *Aesth. Plast. Surg.* 7:249, 1983.

Weiner, D.L. Reduction mammaplasty using superior pedicle technique. *Aesth. Plast. Surg.* 6:7, 1982.

Weiner, D., Aiache, A.E., Silver, L., and Tittiranonda, T. A single dermal pedicle for nipple transposition in subcutaneous mastectomy, reduction mammoplasty or mastopexy. *Plast. Reconstr. Surg.* 51:115, 1973.

17

Daniel J. Hauben

Reduction Mammaplasty Using a Superomedial Dermal Pedicle

Evolution of the Technique

The procedures for reduction of breast tissue have undergone many changes through history. Women who have excessively large breasts have demanded reduction to "normal" size and shape because of the physical and psychological disabilities large breasts cause. In the twentieth century, more than a few dozen procedures designed to handle the problem of hypertrophic breasts have developed.

The initial stage of the operation has always been regarded as one of considerable magnitude. Surgeons have noticed untoward complications that are the result of faulty technique. Therefore, methods for achieving normal-sized and normal-shaped breasts in a short operation and with minimal complications have been sought.

Reduction mammaplasty is achieved by transposition of the areola, resection of breast tissue, and final contouring. Still many surgeons are seeking new approaches to improve and modify the available methods.

There are many variations in pedicle design for reduction mammaplasty. These can be grouped into three geometric planes: vertical, horizontal, and oblique pedicles. A vertical pedicle, either superiorly based or inferiorly based, as well as bipedicle based, has been reported and has gained much popularity [1, 10, 11, 13, 16]. The horizontal pedicle, either medially based or laterally based, or as a bipedicle, was pioneered by Strömbeck and Skoog [14, 15].

In fact, Strömbeck's procedure has become the prototype for a group of modifications, each of which was conceived to exploit more fully the pos-

sibilities of the dermal bridge and to perfect and simplify the procedure.

Strömbeck found that when there was an adequate length in the medial pedicle to allow transposition of the areola, it was safe to cut entirely the lateral end of his bipedicle. He discovered that it was better to sacrifice the lateral end rather than the medial end, which carries a better blood supply through the internal mammary artery [5]. Strömbeck's incidental modification of a medially based pedicle has been practiced for many years in the University Hospital in Rotterdam, where I learned it while serving there as a fellow with Professor Van der Meulen.

To ensure even a better viability of the pedicle, the base of the medial pedicle should be enlarged by adding more tissue thereto — that is, the superior part, as well. Thus, an oblique superomedial pedicle was created for reduction mammaplasty [4, 7, 12]. The first report of the technique was published in 1975, in a relatively small group of patients [12]. It seemed, however, to call no attention or popularity. Ten years later, I reported a larger number of patients operated on by this technique [7]. This finally brought it to the attention of others, who have just recently described their own experience with this method [4].

Objectives of the Ideal Operation

The objectives of an ideal operation have been best defined by Goldwyn as follows [6]: "To merit Michelin's four stars, it would have to be safe, simple, speedy, bloodless and relatively scarless. The results, moreover, would have to be exquisite, unchanging and normal with respect to sensation, function and palpation."

I would add more "S's": size, symmetry, suitable, sexy-shaped breasts, as well as *sine sanguis* (without blood) [8]. One now has to examine whether the results of the superomedial pedicle for reduction mammaplasty will meet these standards in the following presentation.

Indications and Symptoms

Reduction mammaplasty is performed in cases of overdevelopment of the breasts (macromastia or hypertrophy), or in cases of ptosis.

Complaints of symptoms may be regarded as an indication for reduction mammaplasty. These complaints may include physical, cosmetic, and mental complaints, as well as those relating to work and sports. The patients normally complain of too large breasts for their body shape and image. They complain of faulty posture; discomfort, including kyphosis, back pains, prominent shoulder strap markings, and submammary intertrigo; and sometimes emotional suffering and an inferiority complex about the shape of the breasts. Of no less importance are problems associated with obtaining and wearing clothing and the cosmetic improvement in the appearance of the undraped breasts. Special indications are asymmetry and ptosis of the breast.

Preoperative Assessment

A complete history must be taken, and the breasts should be carefully examined, including inquiry into a family history of breast malignancy. One must recall that in addition to appearance and function, the breast is an organ frequently involved by neoplasia.

A careful general physical examination is essential. All drug sensitivities must be known, and smoking should be stopped prior to surgery. It should be helpful to schedule the operation so that it does not coincide with menstruation, when bleeding tendency is increased. Patient weight and height are noted.

Preoperative and postoperative photographs should be obtained. The photographs should extend from the clavicles either to the rib margins or the umbilicus. Front, side, and oblique views should be taken [17].

The Markings

Guesswork in reduction mammaplasty will cause asymmetry and foster errors in size, contour, and scar location. Therefore, accurate markings are of prime importance to attain good results. Since recumbency distorts the large breast mass in all directions, the semi-sitting position (about 45 degrees) is preferable (Fig. 17-1A). In this position, the breasts are marked intraoperatively (Fig. 17-1B). The first marking is to select the new site for the nipple. It cannot be stressed strongly enough that the nipple should not be placed too high, because in that position, it is almost impossible to correct it later. The distance between nipple and intramammary fold, therefore, must be shorter than the ideal length, since there will be sagging of the breast and tension on the skin in this area. It is not unusual to notice that the areola-submammary distance has become twice as long one year later. When the areola is placed in the semi-sitting position, it is about 1 cm below the vertex of the breast compared to the usually upward position. This allows the correct compensation that the areola will achieve after the natural upward rotation of the breast, which usually begins 2 months after the operation [7].

One must bear in mind that the skin above the areola is stretched in the sitting position, so that the nipple sternal notch must be longer. The patient's arms are hanging by her sides. Care is taken to avoid brachial plexus injury and pressure on the peripheral nerves of the upper extremity.

A meridian is drawn from the midclavicular point, about 4 cm laterally from the suprasternal notch (Fig. 17-1B). However, this line should be adjusted depending on whether the nipples are judged to be more centrally placed or widely divergent. The new position of the nipple should be on the midline of the original breast.

The new location of the nipple-areola complex is usually 18 to 22 cm from the suprasternal notch depending on the height of the patient and the size and shape of the chest. The new point should coincide with the same point achieved by placing the index finger in the submammary fold and then locating the digit on the front surface of the breast.

Once again, one measures the distance from the new point to the suprasternal notch, and, according to the height of the patient, the taller the patient, the longer the distance should be; in other words, in shorter women, a shorter nipple suprasternal notch distance is recommended. Furthermore, one must be sure that the new position of

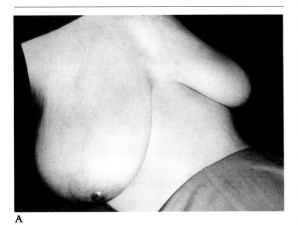

A

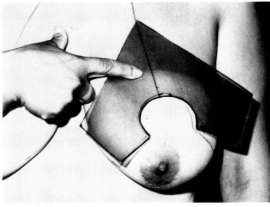

Fig. 17-2. The top of the pattern coincides with the meridian line.

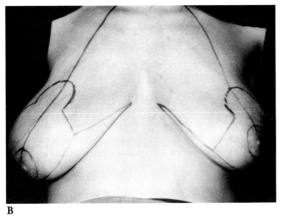

B

Fig. 17-1. The breasts are marked intraoperatively in the semi-sitting position. A. Before marking. B. After marking.

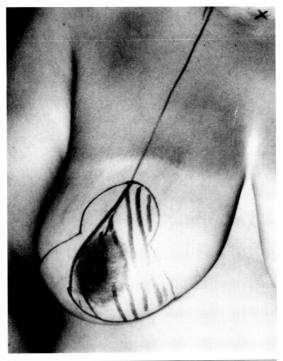

Fig. 17-3. The marking of the superomedial pedicle of the right breast within the area of the pattern surface.

both nipples is symmetric. The new point will be the upper pole of the new location of the nipple-areola complex.

A modified wise pattern is located at the point where the pole of the areola was chosen (Fig. 17-2). The midline of the pattern is placed exactly on the meridian line. The vertical limbs of the celluloid pattern are limited to 4.5 cm to avoid a high-riding nipple after the passage of time [3]. The vertical limbs are drawn obliquely outward and downward from the periphery of the areola (see Fig. 17-1B). The angle between the skin flaps is adjusted to the size of the breasts. The larger the breasts, or the more "cone" projection desired, the wider is the divergence. In large breasts, an increased divergence is allowed, but in general, one should ensure a tension-free closure beneath the areola. Then the

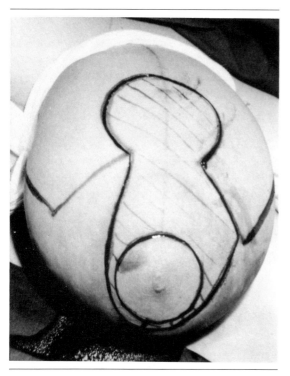

Fig. 17-4. *The breast is compressed with a tourniquet. The area to be deepithelialized is marked by incisions.*

border of the patterns are outlined on the skin with a marking pen (Fig. 17-3). The patient submammary fold is marked from its most medial point to its most lateral extension until the anterior axillary line. The inframammary crease that was marked is connected with the medial and lateral limbs by a straight line. The lateral wedge is larger than the medial wedge. The lateral and the medial end points are determined by folding the breast inward.

Operative Technique

The operation is carried out under general anesthesia with endotracheal intubation, and the patient is placed in the semireclining position, head up with her arms folded on the sides at 45 degrees, as described previously.

The patient is prepared for surgery in the standard manner and draped, exposing the chest, neck, shoulder, posterior axillary line, and upper abdomen. In this position, marking is done as described previously. The surgeon first applies a gauze tour-

niquet around the base of the breasts to distend them as much as possible (Fig. 17-4). When the breast is grasped tight with the compressed bandage, an indentation is made around the nipple by pressing a "cookie cutter" of 4 cm in diameter into the skin to determine the new areola surface. The area within the pattern designed is deepithelialized (Fig. 17-4). The incision begins along the pattern design and around the areola, continuing along the previously marked skin flap. Then, the construction of a broad, superomedial deepithelialized pedicle is performed that contains a relatively thick layer of subcutaneous breast tissue to protect the dermal blood supply and is likely to leave the superficial nerve filaments intact (Fig. 17-5A).

Preservation of the full-thickness breast tissue and dermis beneath the areola ensures a good forward projection of the nipple and augments the mediocranial volume of the breast. The full-thickness (1.5 to 2 cm) breast tissue that is left beneath the areola prevents further nipple inversion or retraction.

The pedicle is now elevated by the assistant nurse, and the inferiorly redundant transverse breast tissue and the skin are excised while undermining starts above the pectoralis fascia plane. The inferior transverse part can be resected en bloc with the lateral wedge of breast tissue. By cutting the gland down to the fascia by undermining above the plane, one aids in visualization of the perforator vessels, and a prompt hemostasis follows. If the breast tissue is found to be excessively full laterally, additional breast tissue is safely trimmed away without extending the skin incision. It should also be pointed out that it is sometimes advisable to remove glandular tissue from under the lateral skin flap to reduce excessive fullness in the lateral part of the breast.

I do not excise a core of tissue from the new nipple site, having found that the cavity alone has caused nipple retraction owing to the lack of bulk support deep to the nipple. The nipple-areola is transposed on a superomedial elevated deepithelialized pedicle. The pedicle is based on the full extent of the medial skin flap, part of the superior part, and the entire new nipple site except for a small lateral portion. The lateral portion of the new nipple-areola site must be incised to obtain easy mobility in transposing the nipple.

The superomedial pedicle is now easily rotated upward and laterally to its newer position. The superior aspect of the areola is advanced to the top

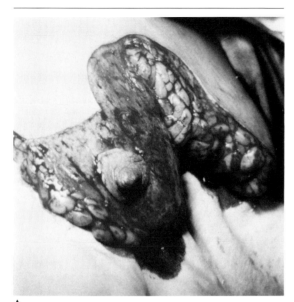

A

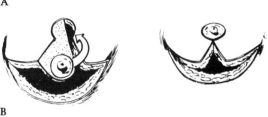

B

Fig. 17-5. A. A superomedial pedicle has been separated from the adjacent breast parenchyma. The glandular tissue can now freely be resected. B. The superomedial pedicle of the left breast is prepared for transposition into the new areola location.

of the "keyhole" to sit on the deepithelialized bulky dermal platform and is tacked in position (Fig. 17-5B). No back cut of the pedicle is required to facilitate mobilization. Additional sculpturing of the medial and lateral flaps can be done as necessary. If good repositioning of the nipple has been achieved, the skin envelope can be closed but not before careful hemostasis is achieved. To assess volume and shape, staples or temporary sutures of 3-0 nylon are used. It is easier to operate on the second breast before completing closure on the first one so that an accurate comparison can be made and symmetry achieved. Weighing the specimen from the first side may be helpful to determine the amount of tissue to be resected from each side. The closure begins with a staple joining the

lower corners of the skin flaps, and the areola is repositioned. The relocation of the nipples must be in a manner such that they face slightly outward and downward to look natural. One can now judge the shape of the breast. If there is still excessive breast, it is preferable to resect laterally than medially.

Sutures should commence laterally and medially, working any excess skin toward the meridian rather than beginning at the T junction. This also achieves appropriate compensatory or adjusting sutures for inequities in incision length. Furthermore, when the laterally excessive skin is pushed medially, it also allows relief of tension at the tripod point. This maneuver has several advantages: It prevents dog-ear formation at the lateral ends, and it permits a tension-free closure of the inferior aspects of the flaps. The incisions are closed in layers.

Finally, I prefer placement of hemo-vac drains across the full width of the breast, out of the extreme lateral end of the submammary wound.

Reinforcement of sutures is done with sterile adhesive Steri-Strips. Further support can be applied with padding and a compressing bandage with Tenso-plast or elastic binder as a sort of external brassiere. The bandage is applied for 1 day; then the patient is allowed to wear an elastic brassiere. The patient is kept in bed for 24 hours, but as soon as the drains are removed (normally after 24 hours), the patient may ambulate. Sutures are removed between the first and second week postsurgery. No antibiotics are used.

In cases of ptosis or macromastia of a lesser degree, the operative procedure in these cases is the same as described previously and is continued as follows: Only the skin in the area of resection is excised down to the subcutaneous fat. It was found that this pedicle is equally applicable to dermal mastopexy operation with similar results. Then, skin closure follows. In cases of mastopexy, one should not use an angle of 110 degrees of the pattern but, rather, a small angle adjusted to the breast.

Postoperative Care

Drains are usually removed after 24 hours, and the patient is discharged with instructions on minimizing home activities. The patient wears a continuously soft brassiere for the next 6 weeks, day and night. Follow-up examination is at 1 week. The dressings are removed, and the breasts are fur-

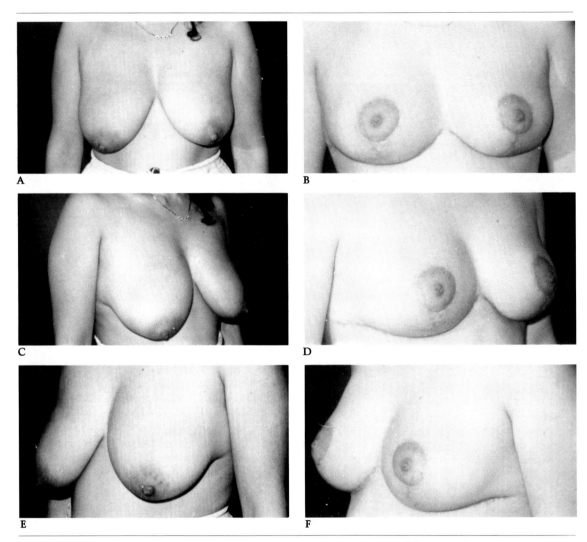

Fig. 17-6. Patient with hypertrophic and ptotic breasts. A. Frontal view before surgery. B. After surgery. C. Oblique view before surgery. D. After surgery. E. Oblique view of the other side before surgery. F. After surgery. G. Right lateral breast before surgery. H. After surgery. I. Left lateral view before operation. J. After surgery.

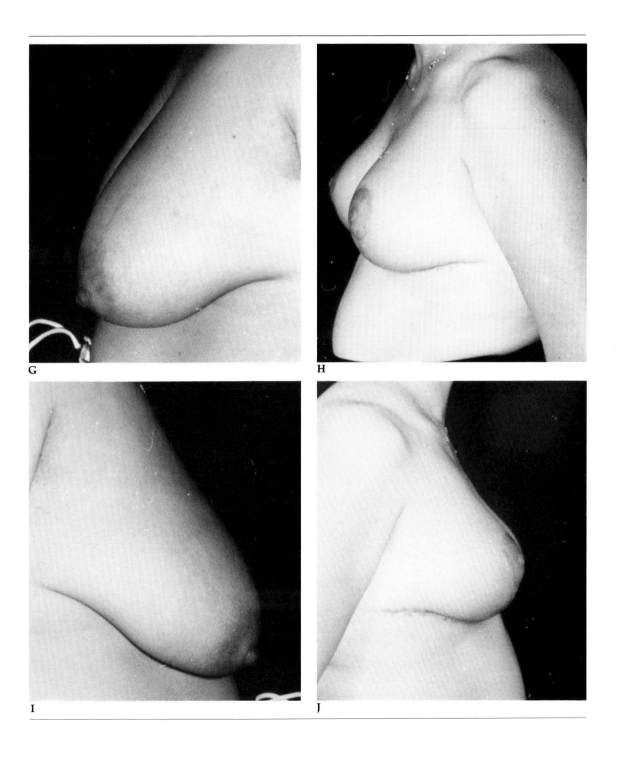

G

H

I

J

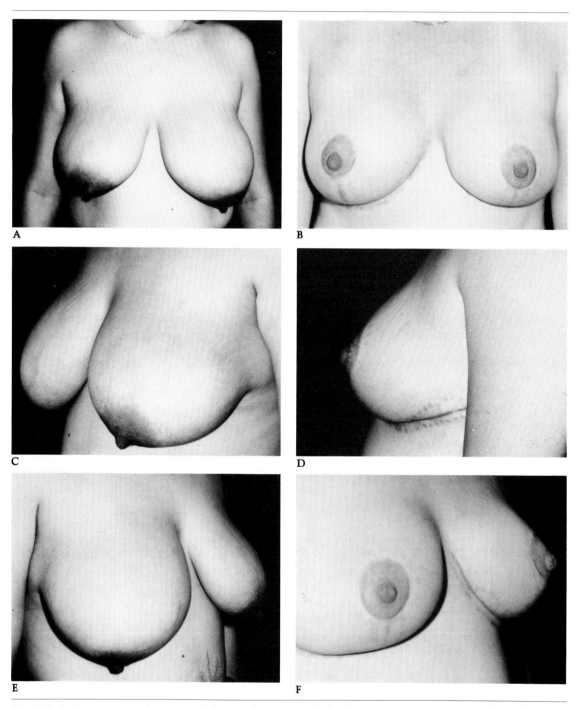

Fig. 17-7. A. Large ptotic and asymmetric breasts. B. After surgery. Closure was done with staples. C. Same patient in the oblique view before surgery. D. Lateral view post surgery. Staple markings are conspicuous. A good nipple position and projection is observed. E. Oblique view before surgery. F. Postsurgery, after removal of 700 gm from each breast.

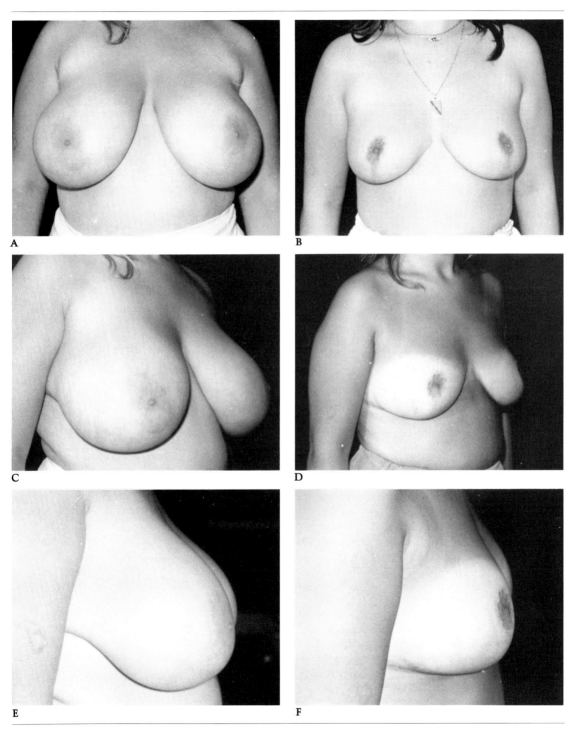

Fig. 17-8. A. Large hypertrophic breasts. B. Postsurgery, after removal of 1000 gm from the right breast and 800 gm from the left breast. C. Oblique view of the same patient before surgery. D. After surgery. E. Lateral view before surgery. F. After surgery, closure was performed with cutaneous running sutures.

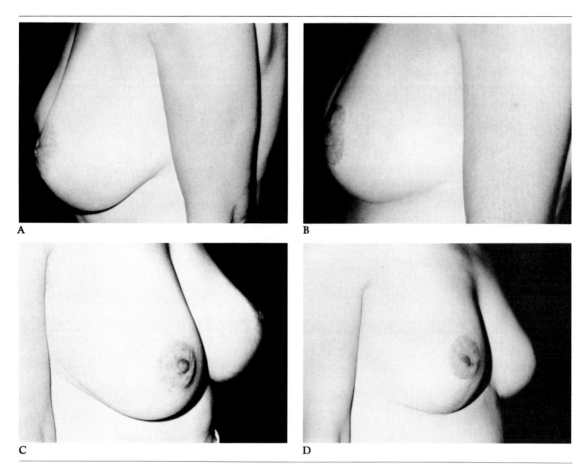

A

B

C

D

ther cleaned. Activities are moderately increased after 6 weeks. Follow-up examinations are at 3 months, 6 months, and 1 year.

Representative cases of varying sizes and shapes of breast hypertrophy and ptosis are presented in (Figures 17-6 through 17-11).

Results

The result of a comprehensive evaluation must include all factors extending from immediate postoperative complications to the final attitude of the patient. During the past 4 years, 212 patients were operated on using the superomedial pedicle technique. The ages of the patients ranged from 13 to 66 years, with an average age of 26 years. The height of the pedicle varied from 4 to 26 cm, with a median of 12 cm. This technique was applied to reductions ranging from 320 to 1800 gm per breast.

None of the patients required blood transfusion.

Fig. 17-9. A. A 50-year-old woman with ptotic breasts —lateral view. B. After mastopexy with the superomedial technique. C. Oblique view before surgery. D. After surgery.

As with many other techniques, healing has been the normal expectation, except for a few complications that will be discussed later. There were no major complications, and postoperative wound infection was surprisingly rare.

The operation produced consistently well-shaped normal-appearing breasts without lateral fullness, with round, nondistorted nipples, which have retained moderate or normal sensation in the majority of the cases.

Complications
HEMATOMA
Postoperative hematoma may occur. Usually, postoperative bleeding is limited, causing only discoloration of the skin. The incidence of hema-

toma in 212 patients was 2.26 percent, all cases of which resolved spontaneously without the need for surgical evacuation. Hematoma usually lengthens the convalescence but does not worsen the end result.

SKIN COMPLICATIONS
Minimal wound dehiscence was observed, especially in the vertical scar. Occasionally, there is a mild loss of tissue at the lower corners of the skin flaps. Significant dehiscence of sutures was observed in one patient, probably the result of their premature removal.

NECROSIS
Of 212 cases of hypertrophy and ptosis, a single case had a complete areola loss. (Unfortunately, it was the first patient in whom this method was performed.) Another patient had in one breast a mild partial areola loss that healed spontaneously and did not require surgical revision. This patient had a pedicle of more than 26 cm and was a heavy smoker.

No fat necrosis was observed. Necrosis of parenchyma alone or loss of overlying skin did not occur.

Scars
Almost all possible closure techniques were used, including intradermal sutures (see Fig. 17-11), running sutures (see Fig. 17-8), and staples closure (see Fig. 17-7). The latter allowed for speedier surgical technique and shorter operative time. However, all have resulted in scars that, at the early postoperative period, were red but have later faded over a period of more than 2 years. Scars are always present. The horizontal scar in the submammary crease is long and extends close to the midline. The medial portion of the scar is most likely to thicken and become prominent. Some of the scars were discouraging, painful, and itchy, but relief came later, when skin tension decreased with time. One patient required scar revision a year after the operation for the medial portion of the scar.

It would seem that the only way to ameliorate scar formation is to try to decrease the scar length as much as possible. Significantly shorter scars can be achieved in cases of mammary ptosis. In these cases, the technique is such that long scars are totally unnecessary.

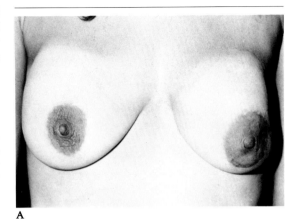

A

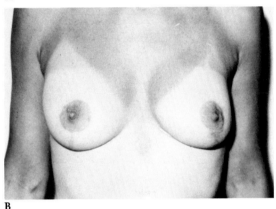

B

Fig. 17-10. A. A 30-year-old patient after retromammary augmentation. Note the capsular deformity of the left breast. Both breasts are ptotic as well. B. Replacement of new prosthesis of 220 ml in each side behind the pectoralis muscle and mastopexy with a superomedial pedicle.

Sensation
The majority of the patients studied had not had a preoperative evaluation of nipple sensation. However, postoperative examination by pinprick and light touch demonstrated diminished sensation then determined by careful patient questioning.

The principal cutaneous nerves are preserved with this method, especially when one does not use undermining of the lateral and medial cutaneous flaps. It was of interest that nipple sensation gradually improved in the majority of the patients (83.3%) over a period of 3 to 8 months postoperatively. Perhaps of greatest interest was the fact that more than 85 percent of patients who experienced altered sensation stated that this was of no concern to them.

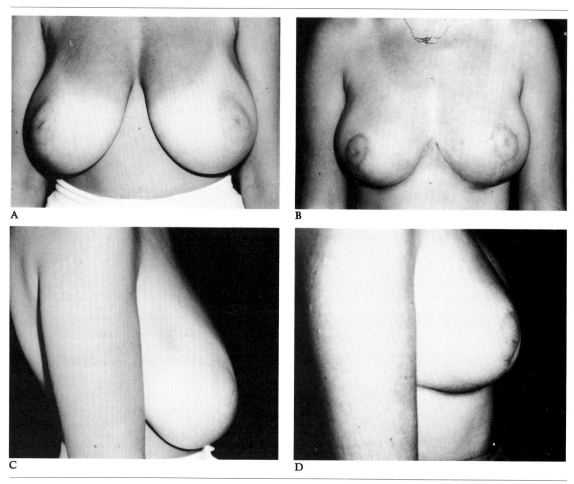

A

B

C

D

Fig. 17-11. A. Hypertrophic breasts. Note the bifid nipple. This kind of nipple will have the tendency to invert and retract after the operation. B. After surgery. Intradermal closure was carried out. C. The same patient before surgery in the lateral view. D. After surgery.

Preservation of sensation in the majority of the cases is most likely a result of the fact that the medial aspect of the dermal pedicle carries fibers from the anterior cutaneous branches of the fourth and fifth intercostal nerves [2].

Inverted and Retracted Nipples

When one removes an exceedingly large amount of breast parenchyma, especially below the central part of the breast, nipple retraction and inversion will occur. The tissue around the nipple will retract and will pull the breast into the area where breast tissue is least well preserved. Furthermore, one must examine the nipples before operation. Some will have a tendency to retract and to invert after surgery, especially those that already show a mild degree of central retraction, or those that appeared slightly bifid (see Fig. 17-11).

Care must be taken to preserve a relatively thick pedicle to support the areola-nipple complex. Nipple inversion occurred in about 2 percent of our patients and was corrected by the author's technique [9].

Discussion and Final Thoughts

A gradual evolution has taken place in the management of the large breast. The superomedial pedicle technique of reduction mammaplasty has a few advantages: it is safe, simple, speedy, suitable, and bloodless. Safety is achieved with a larger pedicle, which is based superiorly and medially. After the elevation of the pedicle, the remaining exposed breast tissue is easily resected, making the operation rather simple. It allows en bloc excision of the breast tissue and, hence, results in speed and spare operative time. The medially based pedicle carries cutaneous branches of the fourth and fifth intercostal nerves, which result in better preservation of sensation. The thick superomedial pedicle will further augment the mediocranial volume of the breast. An excessive resection of the lateral breast with a well-maintained medial volume of the breast will shape the breast in a suitable, symmetric size and in an aesthetically "sexy" fashion. However, the limiting factor with this technique might be the length of the pedicle that can comfortably be enclosed by the cutaneous breast envelope. The skin envelope design therefore should include geometric and artistic considerations as well as the anticipation of tissue behavior. Thus,

besides inherent drawbacks such as scarring and decreased lactability, this method is limited to moderately hypertrophic breasts and to rather significantly large breasts. In severe gigantomastia with pedicle length reaching up to 30 cm, it is not advocated because of the risk of vascular compromise of the relative narrow and long pedicle. Preservation of nerve and blood supply to the nipple must be weighed against removal of a greater bulk of tissue. The superomedial pedicle for reduction mammaplasty, like any other technique, requires practice. But, because of its ease, versatility, and dependability, it can be readily recommended, since it gives consistently satisfactory results. Actually, it is technically easy and quite capable of producing a longer lasting aesthetic effect.

The areola-nipple complex usually lies in the vertex of the breast cone. Thus, there is almost no tendency for mammary ptosis, and with time, the nipple continues to be in its normal position and the medial breast pole remains particularly full, creating an aesthetically pleasing appearance.

Breast reduction does not necessarily result in a well-contoured breast. Proper contour is the result of careful design, depending on thoughtful analysis of factors that influence the desired effect. It is designed to avoid late loss of projection while allowing easy transposition of the nipple-areola complex.

As with other procedures, it was found that an inferior wedge resection allows reconstruction of a spherical breast. The superomedial pedicle, with the nipple freely movable, grants the surgeons more freedom to resect breast tissue. Wedge resection can be of any magnitude and if necessary can be safely carried laterally where there almost always is an excessive fullness of breast parenchyma. Once an adequate wedge of tissue has been removed, conical reconstruction is ensured by closure without objectionable lateral fullness.

It seems, therefore, that the combination of a superomedial pedicle also avoids the kinking that can occur with the superior pedicle alone, particularly in larger reductions. Furthermore, it seems that with the superomedial pedicle, a better nipple sensation is retained.

The technical details presented here make reduction mammaplasty and the migration of the nipple-areola complex simpler, safer, suitable, and speedy, with relatively little blood loss. It has resulted in a pleasing appearance of the breasts, which maintain, in the majority of cases, their sensory and palpatory qualities.

Beauty may lie in the eye of the beholder, but diligent attention to proper surgical technical detail and careful aesthetic evaluation and planning are responsible for the shape of things to come.

References

1. Courtiss, E.M., and Goldwyn, R.M. Reduction mammaplasty by the inferior pedicle technique. *Plast. Reconstr. Surg.* 59:500, 1977.
2. Craig, R.D.P., and Sykes, P.A. Nipple sensitivity following reduction mammaplasty. Br. J. Plast. Surg. 23:165, 1980.
3. Dinner, M.I., and Chait, L.A. Preventing the high riding nipple after McKissock breast reduction. *Plast. Reconstr. Surg.* 59:330, 1977.
4. Finger, R.E., Vasquez, G., Drew, G.S., and Given, K.S. Superior medial pedicle technique for reduction mammaplasty. *Plast. Reconstr. Surg.* 83:471, 1989.
5. Goldwyn, R.M. *Plastic and Reconstructive Surgery of the Breast.* Boston: Little, Brown, 1976. Pp. 195–209.
6. Goldwyn, R.M. *Plastic and Reconstructive Surgery of the Breast.* Boston: Little, Brown, 1976. P. 147.
7. Hauben, D.J. Experience and refinements with the supero-medial dermal pedicle for nipple areola transposition in reduction mammaplasty. *Aesth. Plast. Surg.* 8:189, 1985.
8. Hauben, D.J. Discussion on superior medial pedicle technique of reduction mammaplasty. *Plast. Reconstr. Surg.* 83:479, 1989.
9. Hauben, D.J., and Mahler D. A simple method for the correction of inverted nipple. *Plast. Reconstr. Surg.* 71:556, 1983.
10. Labandter, H.P., Dowden, R.V., and Dinner, M.L. The inferior segment technique for breast reduction. *Ann. Plast. Surg.* 6:493, 1982.
11. McKissock, P.K. Reduction mammaplasty with a vertical dermal flap. *Plast. Reconstr. Surg.* 49:245, 1972.
12. Orlando, J.C., and Guthrie, R.H. The superomedial pedicle for nipple transposition. Br. J. Plast. Surg. 28:42, 1975.
13. Robbins, T.H. A reduction mammaplasty with the areola nipple based on an inferior dermal pedicle. *Plast. Reconstr. Surg.* 59:64, 1977.
14. Skoog, T. A technique of breast reduction. *Acta Chir. Scand.* 126:1, 1963.
15. Strömbeck, J.O. Mammaplasty: Report of a new technique based on the two pedicle procedure. Br. J. Plast. Surg. 13:79, 1960.
16. Weiner, D.L., Ariache, A.E., Silver, R., and Tittis T. A single dermal pedicle for nipple transposition in subcutaneous mastectomy, reduction mammaplasty or mastopexy. *Plast. Reconstr. Surg.* 51:115, 1973.
17. Zarem, H.A. Standards of photography. *Plast. Reconstr. Surg.* 74:137, 1984.

COMMENTS ON CHAPTERS 15, 16, AND 17

Robert M. Goldwyn

The preceding three chapters are a logical grouping since each of them describes a method of breast reduction utilizing a superior dermal flap. In the method of Tord Skoog, described by Ohlsén and Valdemar Skoog, the superior dermal flap is laterally based; in Weiner's method, the pedicle is centrally based, and in Hauben's procedure, it is medially based. In all these techniques, the nipple-areola survives because of its cutaneous vessels.

In their introduction to the description of the Skoog method, Ohlsén and Skoog summarize Tord Skoog's reasoning for the design and success of his method. These concepts about blood supply to the nipple-areola are extremely important not only in regard to performing his technique and other superior dermal procedures but also in understanding all methods of breast reduction. The rationale for breast reduction by a superior dermal flap containing the nipple and areola is that the breast is ectodermal in origin and therefore the nipple and areola are essentially components of the pectoral skin. These points and their ramifications are discussed in greater detail in my comments following Chapter 2.

In discussing his method of breast reduction, Tord Skoog wrote [7]: "The presence of a well-developed superficial vascular system related to the nipple and areola is clearly demonstrated in the described operative procedure, whose subcutaneous vessels by themselves proved sufficient to supply the nipple and areola."

The other important consideration is that the pectoral skin contributes not only arteries and veins to the nipple and areola but nerves as well. How good is that cutaneous nerve supply in the superior dermal techniques compared to that in other methods, such as the inferior pedicle or the McKissock procedure? The authors of these three chapters present evidence that their patients did have adequate sensation if followed from more than 6 months after operation.

However, Lalardrie and Jouglard [4] believe that "the anatomical disposition of the mammary nerves accounts for the fact that at large glandular resections, particularly behind the areola and nipple, there is a temporary and sometimes permanent reduction in nipple sensitivity." Hrynyschyn et al [3], however, found that 60 percent of patients having had the Skoog method of reduction as well as the Strömbeck procedure had decreased sensibility (no significant difference between both methods). The fact is that in the chapters by Ohlsén and Skoog, Weiner, and Hauben, no systemic objective determination of sensibility was done preoperatively. Nevertheless, postoperative sensation seemed to be satisfactory to the majority of patients. Hauben reasons that the medial aspect of his kind of superior dermal pedicle contains the anterior cutaneous branches from the fourth and fifth intercostal nerves.

Weiner has stressed the importance of not buttonholing the dermis and removing the epidermis and superficial dermis. He has also stated that, in many instances, he uses a composite flap of parenchyma and dermis. He has been able to transpose the nipple and areola, on dermis alone, 20 cm, and in no case in his series did he have total necrosis of the nipple and areola. A common difficulty with his operation as with many other kinds of reduction is the skin necrosis, usually not significant, at the point of the inverted T closure. His incidence rate of that complication, 15 percent, could be reduced if closure was under less tension either by leaving more skin or by approximating from medial to lateral. However, the type of tension he puts on his closure may give a better shape to the breast. Not surprisingly because of the elasticity of skin, Weiner has observed and reported honestly that over a period of 5 to 7 years, some patients experience a loss of contour.

In reporting his method of reduction by the superomedial dermal flap, Hauben has stated that patients seem to bleed more during their menses, and he tries to avoid operating at that time. I have never seen a study to document this impression, but I believe that it is correct. In most hospitals in the United States, few of us have the luxury of postponing a procedure because of the occurrence of menstruation. Bed availability and scheduling are too difficult.

Hauben advises not excising tissue from the keyhole to avoid subsequent nipple-areola retraction. Incidentally, he begins his closure laterally in order, I suppose, to reduce the dog-ear laterally and the necrosis medially. In thinking about the superomedial dermal pedicle, credit should also be given to Oulié, who, in 1973, reported at a meeting and later published his successful experience with this method [5, 6]. Van der Meulen in Rotterdam, however, as mentioned by Hauben and stated by himself [8], has used this technique since the 1960s.

Regarding the upper limit of the pedicle length, Hauben feels that 30 cm would not be advisable, as in cases of gigantomastia. His method, he feels, is best for patients with moderate and large hypertrophy. After having followed his patients, he concludes that the nipple stays in its position and the breast remains full medially without sagging. A point he reiterated in discussing [2] an article by Finger et al [1], who had described using the superomedial technique for "resections as large as 4100 gm per breast with nipple-areola transposition up to 30 cm . . . with reliable nipple-areola survival, including preservation of sensation."

Ohlsén and Skoog have given a complete, step-by-step description of their procedure, which involves, as mentioned, a laterally based supero dermal pedicle. Tord Skoog thought that the more important blood supply was lateral. As the authors have noted, their incidence of complications is no greater than that with other methods. Furthermore, those patients have been very thoroughly and objectively followed. Of 160 patients operated on between the years 1977 and 1979, 65 percent were very satisfied with their result; 30 percent were satisfied, and 5 percent were dissatisfied. In his series, older patients were happier than younger patients, despite a higher incidence of complications. As in most studies, obesity was associated with more complications in terms of infection, nipple and fat necrosis, and poor scarring. Whether or not patients were smokers is not known because, in those years, that factor in relation to vascular supply and necrosis was poorly appreciated.

Regarding lactation, Ohlsén and Skoog point out that in their technique, the lactiferous ducts are cut to fashion the cutaneous nipple-areola flap, and most of the glandular tissue is removed. Lacta-

tion, although possible, is uncommon, and they inform their patients that they will likely not lactate.

In summary, these three methods of using a supero dermal pedicle have been well described in the preceding chapters. Each of the methods gives the surgeon full access to the breast. That these techniques are versatile and safe and produce predictably good results are their great advantages. Having used each of these techniques, I can attest to the fact that they are excellent methods for doing reduction mammaplasty. I must admit, however, that I feel more secure in having a blood supply to the nipple and areola that comes from more than a cutaneous source. This feeling is admittedly unscientific but nevertheless shared by many surgeons who are always looking for that additional safety factor with regard to nipple and areola viability. Furthermore, I think that a more objective assessment of sensation should be done before and after using the various supero dermal techniques for breast reduction.

REFERENCES

1. Finger, R.E., Vasquez, B., Drew, G.S., and Given, K.S. Superomedial pedicle technique of reduction mammaplasty. *Plast. Reconstr. Surg.* 83:471, 1989.
2. Hauben, D.J. Discussion of above paper. *Plast. Reconstr. Surg.* 83:479, 1989.
3. Hrynyschyn, K., Losch, G.M., and Schrader, M. Ergebnisse vergleichender Untersuchungen bei der mammareduktionsplastik nach Strombeck und Skoog. *Angenbecks Arch. Chir.* 369:279, 1986.
4. Lalardrie, J.-P., and Jouglard, J.-P. *Plasties Mammaires pour Hypertrophie et Ptose.* Paris: Masson et Cie, 1973. P. 26.
5. Oulié, J. Utilisation d'un lambeau areolo-mamelonnaire a pédicule interne au cours de des plasties mammaires de reduction. Presented at the 19th annual meeting of *Société Francaise de Chirurgie Plastique et Reconstructiv.* Marseilles, October 20, 1973.
6. Oulié, J. Utilisation d'un lambeau areolo-mamelonnaire à pédicule interne au cours de des plasties mammaires de reduction. *Ann. Chir. Plast.* 20:251, 1975.
7. Skoog, T. *Plastic Surgery, New Methods and Refinements.* Stockholm: Almqvist & Wiksell International, 1974. P. 338.
8. Van der Meulen, J.C.H. Superomedial technique for reduction mammaplasty (letter). *Plast. Reconstr. Surg.* (in press).

18

Reduction Mammaplasty by the Inferior Pedicle (Pyramidal) Technique

Inferior Pedicle Technique

Robert M. Goldwyn and
Eugene H. Courtiss

Within 2 years of each other but without knowledge of the others' work, Ribeiro [22], Robbins [23, 25] and Courtiss and Goldwyn [6], published their descriptions of the inferior pedicle technique for breast reduction. In retrospect, Joseph had utilized the same principle a half century before — another example of Jacques Joseph's extraordinary ingenuity, still pertinent to what we plastic surgeons do today (Figs. 18-1 and 18-2).

In the United States and elsewhere, the inferior pedicle technique and its variants currently are a popular, if not the most popular, method of reduction mammaplasty [1–4, 7–9, 13, 17–20, 27–29]. Its advantages are that it has a rich, axial pattern blood supply [21, 30] to the nipple, areola, and remaining breast tissue from the internal mammary artery and intercostals, the fifth particularly, and from the external branches from the lateral thoracic artery; it allows the surgeon latitude to resect breast tissue wherever required; it preserves normal or almost normal sensation to the nipple and areola because it spares the important cutaneous branches of the third, especially the fourth, and the fifth intercostal nerves; it can be used for breasts that are mildly or moderately large or those that are gigantic, without recourse to nipple and areola grafting; the aesthetic results are generally excellent; and the operation is relatively easy to learn.

The pedicle in the "inferior pedicle" technique can be of dermis, with glandular tissue at its base under the nipple and areola, as we have described and prefer [10], or it can be a glandular pedicle without dermis. That the nipple-areola survives on any single quadrant of breast tissue was shown

many years ago by Kaplan [12] and later by Climo and Alexander [5].

Technique
MARKING

A major advantage of the inferior pedicle technique is that it can be used to predetermine the site of the new nipple-areola, thereby eliminating guesswork during operation.

With the patient standing or sitting, a line is drawn from the middle of the clavicle through the nipple. A finger is placed behind the breast in the inframammary fold, and with the breast *partially supported*, the level of the fold is marked across the first line drawn (Fig. 18-3). This becomes the future upper level of the areola. Thus, the nipple is 22.5 to 25.0 cm from the sternal notch on the midclavicular line, depending on the habitus of the patient and her inframammary fold. *When in doubt, locate the nipple lower.*

A keyhole wire pattern (McKissock Keyhole Pattern, Padgett Instruments, Kansas City, Missouri) is placed on the breast with its top at the upper level of the areola so that the medial limb goes directly inferiorly and the lateral limb goes somewhat outward. By this method, the horizontal length of the medial and lateral flaps will be equal (Fig. 18-4). The limbs should not diverge excessively or closure will be too tight. If the areola is very large, it may not be possible to eliminate all the redundancy; the patient should be informed about this possibility preoperatively.

To prevent the final location of the nipple from being too high, the medial limb should not be more

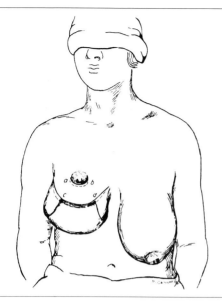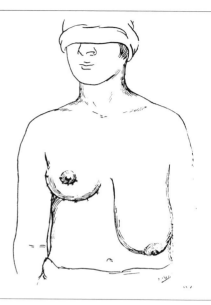

Fig. 18-1. Joseph's markings to show the extent of nipple-areola transposition (left) and outline of the inferior pedicle flap (right). This was the first stage of his two-stage reduction mammaplasty described in 1925. (From J. Joseph. Nasenplastika und Sonstige

Gesichtsplastik nebst einem anhang uber Mammaplastik und einige weitere operationen aus dem gebiete der gebiete der ausseren Korperplastika. Ein Atlas und Lehrbuch. *Leipzig: Curt Kabitzsch, 1931.* P. 735.)

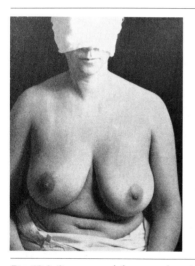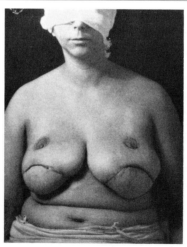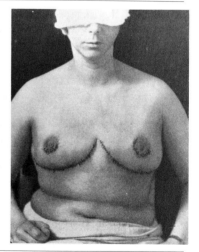

Fig. 18-2. Sequence of the procedure in a patient: preoperatively (left) and after the first stage (middle). Note the inferior pedicle with its nipple-areola having been pulled through the skin ridge and sutured to its new higher location. Completion of final stage (right). (From J. Joseph. Nasenplastika und Sonstige

Gesichtsplastik nebst einem anhang uber Mammaplastik und einege weitere operationen aus dem gebiete der gebiete der ausseren Korperplastika. Ein Atlas und Lehrbuch. *Leipzig: Curt Kabitzsch, 1931.* P. 768.)

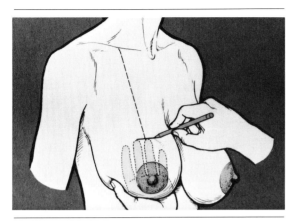

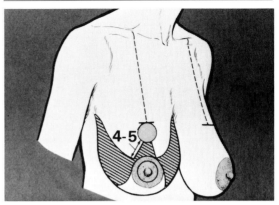

Fig. 18-3. With the breast partially supported, the proposed upper margin of the new areola site is marked where the level of the inframammary crease transsects the mid clavicular line. The nipple is usually 24 to 25 cm from the sternal notch toward the mid clavicular line, but this measurement will differ with the shape and size of the breasts and the habitus of the patient. (This figure and Figs. 18-4 through 18-8 are from R.M. Goldwyn and E.H. Courtiss. Inferior Pedicle Technique. In P. Regnault and R.K. Daniel (eds.), Aesthetic Plastic Surgery. Boston: Little, Brown, 1984. Pp. 522–523.)

Fig. 18-4. The keyhole and the future medial and lateral skin flaps are marked with limbs about 4.5 cm.

than 5 cm long. The inferior borders of the lateral and medial skin flaps are drawn relatively straight without lazy-S extensions, which will cause closure to be tight and the ultimate scar to be hypertrophic. The combined length of the medial and lateral flaps should be 1 to 2 cm longer than those of the inframammary fold to which they are sutured.

As mentioned in Chap. 8, the patient should be fully awake and not medicated so she may cooperate in the marking. Again, the surgeon should ask her what size she wants to be, but no guarantees should be given.

OPERATIVE TECHNIQUE

When the patient is anesthetized, the markings can be reinforced with a No. 25 needle dipped in methylene blue so that prepping will not wash them away.

The circumference of the nipple-areola can be outlined with a "cookie cutter" or with washers or various diameters easily purchased at a hardware store or with methylene blue traced on a round medicine glass, whose diameter happens to be 4.5 cm. It is important not to have the areola either

too large or too small; the critical factor in this determination is how much pressure is applied to the breast and how much stretch is placed on the areola-nipple during marking. The circumference of the areola also depends on the breast size that the patient desires. An areola of 4.5 cm in diameter may be ideal for a breast that will be a B or C cup but may be slightly large for a size A cup.

The base of the inferior dermal pedicle is marked with a line running 1 cm above the inframammary fold so that the final scar is not irritated by the brassiere (Fig. 18-5). Its width is usually 8 to 10 cm but should be slightly greater in patients with gigantomastia.

A split-thickness graft is taken from the inferior pedicle by sharp dissection. It is important to keep a generous rim of pedicle above the outlined nipple-areola to ensure its blood supply to it (Schwarzmann procedure).

How one removes the epidermis and superficial dermis depends on the surgeon's preference. The breast can be held upward with a Velcro band or a Penrose drain tightening its base; multiple vertical incisions into the dermis facilitate this process. It has been shown that the blood supply to the nipple-areola is preserved whether the skin removed from the inferior pedicle is full thickness or split thickness [5]. Bleeding, however, is less with taking just split-thickness skin. In addition, handling the pedicle is easier when the dermis is left.

The upper border of the dermal pedicle is then incised to the subcutaneous fat. A cutting electric current is used to dissect the breast pedicle, which is held forward away from the chest. If the vertical

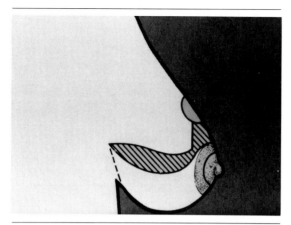

Fig. 18-5. In the operating room, the inferior pedicle is outlined with its inferior margin 1 cm above the entire length of the inframammary fold. Alternatively, for very large reductions and greater transpositions, more of the inframammary fold may be used as the inferior margin. A split thickness skin graft is removed from the surface of the inferior pedicle. Note the rim of dermis left superior to the areola.

length of the inferior pedicle is less than 15 cm, the inferiorly based flap can and should remain attached to the pectoralis muscle at the base, retaining a thickness of 8 to 10 cm (Fig. 18-6). The dermal pedicle should be kept about 3 cm thick beneath the nipple-areola. Maintaining this thickness helps to avoid inversion as well as ischemia. Preserving bulk at the base ensures not only good contour but also adequate vascularity and sensation because the crucial vessels and nerves remain uninjured. The attachments to the pectoral muscle provide support for the flap and added blood supply through perforating vessels.

It is important not to damage the vessels and the pedicle that go to the nipple and areola as one dissects the dermal flap. Therefore, it is best to dissect slightly outward and laterally from the pedicle and to preserve, as mentioned, the rim of dermis.

Redundant breast tissue is resected laterally and medially as well as superiorly. Contouring laterally by suction can minimize the length of the scar in that location. A better projection of the breast will be obtained if no tissue is removed from under the breast superior to the keyhole. Occasionally, however, this area has to be thinned slightly, but it should never be gouged; otherwise, the result will be unpleasant hollowness and nipple-areola inversion. Taking too much medially will also cause a problem: a displeasing concavity.

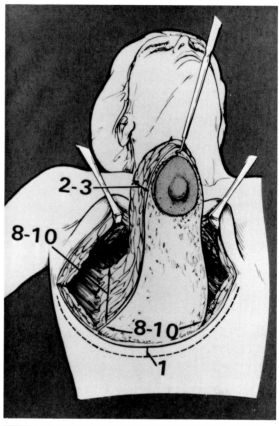

Fig. 18-6. The inferior pedicle is dissected through the breast to the pectoral muscle. Care is taken to maintain a 3-cm thickness beneath the nipple-areola complex and 8 to 10 cm at the base of the pedicle. It is better to leave more tissue on the pedicle initially and trim it later in the operation if required.

The patient should be placed in a semiupright position as final contouring is done.

Hemostasis should be meticulous. This is a basic principle in all surgery and should not be ignored during reduction mammaplasty. The careful use of the cautery aids hemostasis. Blood transfusion is not necessary, and neither is the local infiltration of epinephrine, although one of us (Courtiss) has found it useful.

Employing a stapler for temporary closure saves time and allows comparison with the other breast after it is finished.

The surgeon should remember the patient's preoperative appearance, which should have been noted at the time of the initial consultation as well as immediately prior to operation during marking. Photographs in the operating room are a useful reminder of any asymmetry that was present preoperatively and that should now be corrected.

At the time of closure, if more projection of the nipple-areola is desired, the rim of dermis can be sutured backward to the tissue behind the areola or, alternatively, onto the deepithelialized dermal platform if preserved in the keyhole. Although advocated as a means of increasing projection and decreasing inversion [26], the dermal platform is useful also as a convenient substrate. However, Robbins [24] and others, such as ourselves, have found that too often the resultant areola-nipple after the inferior pedicle technique is too prominent and puffy; putting it on this dermal platform is liable to increase this outpouching. If one observes that the nipple-areola is too bulky, it is wiser to revise it later than to attempt to do so now with the likelihood of causing ischemia.

Closure proceeds in the usual fashion. Some surgeons, however, prefer a Y-type skin approximation at either end of the inframammary incision to shorten the eventual scar medially and laterally. Another alternative is to close from laterally toward the midline in order to bring extra tissue centrally. By this means, the lateral extension of the incision will be shortened; the disadvantage, however, is that unless one is careful, the nipple and areola will rise with the addition of the extra skin brought in from the lateral end of the wound.

Although the nipple-areola site has been predetermined, the surgeon must check its position for symmetry and to be certain that the distance from the nipple to the inframammary line does not exceed 6.5 cm. One of us (Courtiss) predetermines the location of the nipple-areola complex but does not cut the keyhole until after the medial and lateral flaps and inframammary incisions are temporarily sutured. This places tension on the flaps and allows an additional opportunity to assess the final location of the nipple-areola. Establishing tension makes creating a round areola easier than cutting and closing the keyhole beforehand.

Final closure should not be done until the patient has been placed almost at 90 degrees (Fig. 18-7), with the surgeon viewing her from the foot of the table. It is also useful to palpate both breasts to get an idea of the quantity and location of the remaining tissue.

A multilayered closure is performed (Fig. 18-8) with buried 3-0 Vicryl and with an intradermal pullout of 4.0 Prolene. If drainage is desired, a

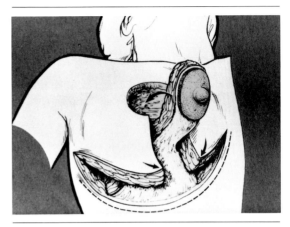

Fig. 18-7. The nipple and areola on an inferior pedicle are raised and attached to the circular part of the keyhole. The medial and lateral skin flaps are approximated beneath the areola.

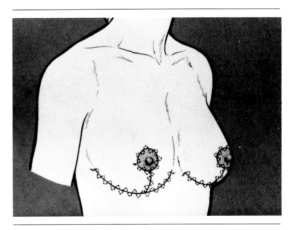

Fig. 18-8. Closure. Drains may be used, depending on the surgeon's preference, and they should be of the vacuum type inserted through a separate stab wound.

Jackson-Pratt suction can be brought out separately below the inframammary incision but not at its extreme lateral end; otherwise, the resulting scar will be visible and may be hypertrophic.

Nipple-areola vascularity should be assessed by observation and by testing its capillary filling.

Throughout the operation, the surgeon, when resecting tissue, should be mindful of the ultimate contour to be achieved. No operation, and certainly not this one, should be performed by rote. The surgeon should not simply cut on a dotted line but must take into account the specific problems of each patient as well as the three-dimensional nature of the body. To achieve an optimal result, small adjustments are usually necessary throughout the operation.

AXILLARY BREAST

If axillary breast tissue is prominent, it should be removed. We prefer using liposuction only or in combination with dissection through a separate incision in the axilla. In an older patient whose axillary tissue may be principally fat, liposuction alone will accomplish the task via a small incision.

UNILATERAL REDUCTION

The inferior pedicle technique is useful to reduce one breast to match the other. The situation commonly arises in patients who have had breast reconstruction for a mastectomy or who have asymmetry, whether it be congenital, developmental, or acquired.

Because the inferior pedicle technique allows easy access to all parts of the breast, it is versatile. Yet because this method has a generous inframammary incision that will scar, it is best reserved for a large breast. In reducing a small breast, particularly in a young patient who is prone to hypertrophic scarring, the surgeon should consider other techniques that involve volume reduction (see Chap. 29) and shorter scars (see Chaps. 21, 23, 25, and 28).

CAVEATS

To achieve the desired result with the inferior pedicle technique, the surgeon should not commit the following errors:

1. Placing the nipple-areola too high. This point cannot be stressed sufficiently. As mentioned, when in doubt, site the nipple-areola lower.
2. Dissection at the base of the pedicle should not compromise its width nor injure the vessels and nerves emerging through the fascia. It is far better to leave a small amount of tissue superficial to the muscle layer than going too deeply with the possibility of subsequent nipple necrosis or numbness. A very common mistake in performing inferior pedicle operation is cutting the flap at its base too medially and encroaching on the nutrient vessels to the nipple.
3. Excessive thinning of the tips will cause them to necrose.
4. Before final closure, the surgeon must look at

the patient in an upright position and think about symmetry as well as location of the nipple-areola complex. Having someone else assess the appearance of the breast at this stage is helpful.
5. The surgeon should not forget to observe the vascularity of the nipple-areola before dressings are applied in order to assess possible ischemia and congestion.

TECHNICAL VARIATIONS TO IMPROVE RESULTS

Preventing the Teardrop or Inverted Areola

Hallock and Altobelli [11] have suggested a useful maneuver that prevents the displeasing appearance of a comma-shaped or inverted teardrop areola, commonly noted with the inferior pedicle method. If one splits the dermis and dissects the pedicle away from the areola, the areola immediately assumes a circular shape as closure proceeds and as healing occurs. The excellent vascularity of the inferior pedicle technique will not be jeopardized by this maneuver.

Another way of minimizing inversion of the nipple-areola, as mentioned earlier, is to suture it backward. This should be done with minimal tension and with an absorbable stitch.

We have already mentioned suturing the flaps before cutting the keyhole as another and perhaps better way of ensuring a round areola. It should be noted, however, that not all women who have normal-sized breasts have round areolae.

We agree with McKissock [15, 16], who has stated that the final diameter of the areola (and even the shape) cannot always be predicted because it is the product of several factors, including (1) the diameter of the new nipple-areola window as it is being cut, which varies with the amount of stretching that the assistant applies and is also affected by the temperature of the room; and (2) the tension of the closure, which depends on the relationship between the area of the skin envelope and the mass of the gland it contains.

Avoiding a Conspicuous Medial Incision

To avoid a scar that will be visible on the sternum, the surgeon, while the patient is asleep but in a semisitting position, should carefully trace the proposed incision so that at its end medially it will be hidden by the breast.

Achieving or Preserving a Cone-Shaped Breast

Ribeiro's original description of his technique (see Chap. 24) emphasized folding the pedicle into a cone. Although this maneuver will give a better shape to the breast, it might also compromise the blood supply to the nipple-areola. In our experience, folding the pedicle on itself has not been necessary if one leaves a generous amount of tissue at the base of the pedicle and if one remembers the ultimate contour desired when resecting tissue.

Reus and Mathes [21], in 22 patients followed for an average of 4.7 years, noted a gradual increase in the distance from the inframammary fold to the areola. Since the midclavicle to nipple distance did not lengthen, their conclusion was that the breast parenchyma had descended along with the displacement of the nipple-areola superiorly. In our opinion, this problem can be lessened and perhaps avoided by not placing the nipple-areola site too high and by resecting enough tissue. These considerations are more important than suturing the pedicle to the chest wall. If one does the operation carefully, one can preserve the fascial attachments of the pedicle to the chest. One is also more likely to preserve sensation to the nipple-areola and the breast skin.

In an attempt to avoid what they call "flat breast" in reduction mammaplasty, Mathes, Nahai, and Hester [14] have used a combination of the superior pedicle that retains the nipple-areola complex folded over an inferior pedicle. We have not found this necessary and agree with McKissock, [15] who questions the need to remove and then replace central breast bulk when it is already present.

The surgeon as well as the patient must keep in mind that no matter how well the inferior pedicle technique has been performed, the breast changes with time, aging, loss of elasticity, weight fluctuation, pregnancy, and systemic diseases.

WOUND SEPARATION AND NECROSIS

The inferior pedicle technique has, like many other procedures for reduction mammaplasty, the disadvantage of an inverted T closure. With excessive tension on perhaps partially devascularized tips on the skin flaps, the tissue at the junction of the T may not heal primarily because of necrosis. Infection may result; one should distinguish between secondary and primary infection. In most instances, the drainage that we see at the junction

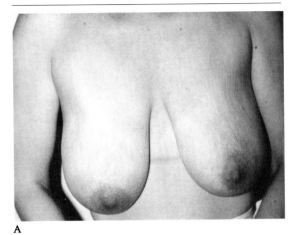

A

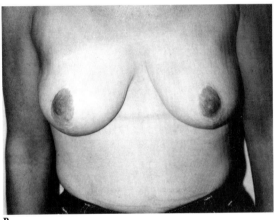

B

Fig. 18-9. A. Preoperative, 30-year-old woman. B. Postoperative, 1 year after removal of 390 gm of tissue from the right breast, and 420 gm from left.

of the inverted T is the result of necrosis. Ways of reducing ischemia in that area are to close laterally to medially, decreasing the tension centrally but also, as previously mentioned, perhaps causing the nipple and areola to rise slightly because of the additional skin brought toward the center of the breast. Another means of reducing the incidence of necrosis is to put fewer stitches in the area of the tips of the flaps. The best way of preventing this problem is to leave the flaps long in the beginning of the operation and to trim them later as needed.

The careful use of the cautery aids hemostasis and decreases bleeding. We have not needed to transfuse blood or to inject epinephrine locally prior to operation.

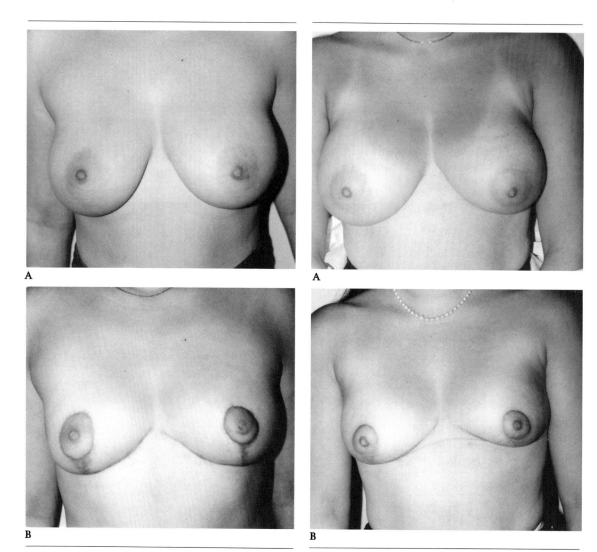

Fig. 18-10. A. Preoperative, 26-year-old woman. B. Postoperative, 11 months after removal of 320 gm of tissue from the right breast and 330 gm from the left breast. The left breast is still slightly larger.

Fig. 18-11. A. Preoperative, 21-year-old woman. B. Postoperative, 11 months after removal of 320 gm of tissue from the right breast and 365 gm from the left breast.

DISADVANTAGES

The chief disadvantage of the inferior pedicle technique is the length of the scar in the inframammary fold. Although the scar can be lessened by varying the closure as just discussed, it is still a longer scar than in other techniques described elsewhere in this book. However, in general, most surgeons have found that shorter scar procedures are more easily applied to patients in whom resection of breast tissue per side will be less than 550 gm. The inferior pedicle technique, despite the drawback of a relatively long inframammary scar, has the versatility of reducing breasts whose size ranges from comparatively small to spectacularly large (gigantomastia) (Figs. 18-9 through 18-17). Many authors have documented the safety, simplicity, versatility, and teachability of the inferior pedicle method of breast reduction as well as its excellent results and high patient satisfaction.

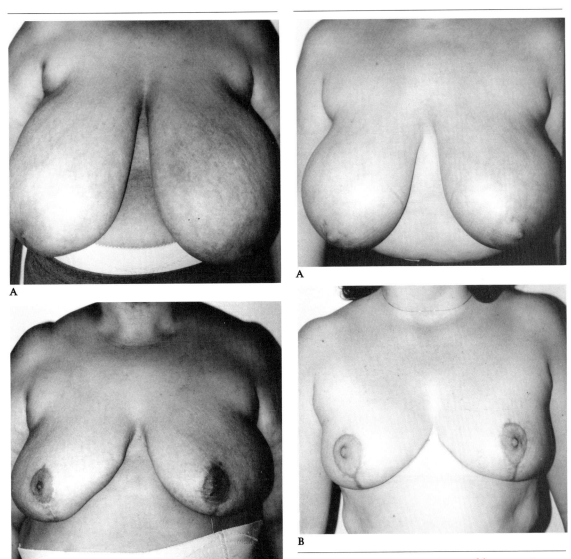

Fig. 18-12. A. Preoperative, 64-year-old woman. B. Postoperative, 18 months after removal of 2,100 gm of tissue from the right breast and 2,200 gm from the left breast. Although more could have been excised, this older patient feared becoming too small, a reaction she nevertheless initially experienced.

Fig. 18-13. A. Preoperative, 22-year-old woman. B. Postoperative, 6 months after removal of 775 gm of tissue from the right breast and 785 gm from the left breast. This early result shows slight areola distortion, which can be avoided by steps described in the text.

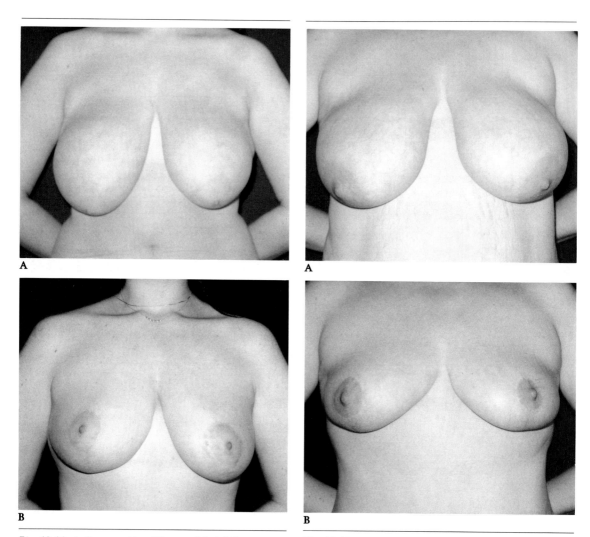

Fig. 18-14. A. Preoperative, 18-year-old girl. B. Postoperative, four years after removal of 637 gm of tissue from the right breast and 580 gm from the left breast.

Fig. 18-15. A. Preoperative, 37-year-old woman. B. Postoperative, 5½ years after removal of 550 gm of tissue from the right breast and 535 gm from the left breast.

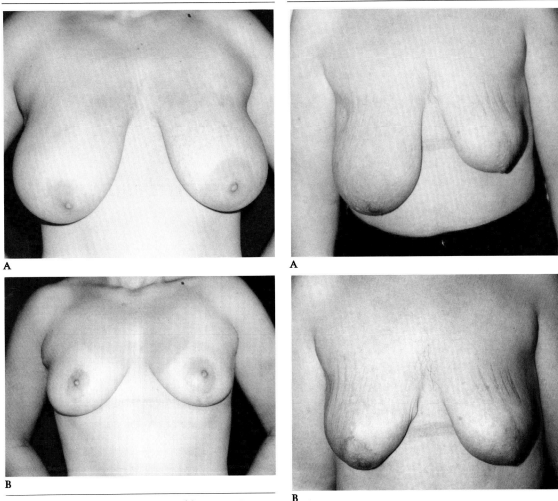

Fig. 18-16. A. Preoperative, 28-year-old woman. B. Postoperative, 8 years after removal of 587 gm of tissue from the right breast and 542 gm from the left breast.

Fig. 18-17. A. Preoperative, 22-year-old woman with asymmetry who wanted only the right breast reduced. B. Postoperative, 15 months after removal 320 gm of tissue. Note the small dog-ears; the patient, however, refused revision. (From R.M. Goldwyn and E.H. Courtiss. Inferior Pedicle Technique. In P. Regnault and R.K. Daniel (eds.), Aesthetic Plastic Surgery. Boston: Little, Brown, 1984. Pp. 522–523.)

References

1. Amar, R., and Bosch DelMarco, G. Plastie mammaire de reduction utilisant un lameau dermo-glandulaire a pedicule inferieur. *Ann. Chir. Plast.* 26:243, 1981.
2. Ariyan, S. Reduction mammaplasty with a nipple-areola carried on a single, narrow inferior pedicle. *Ann. Plast. Surg.* 5:167, 1980.
3. Bolger, W.E., Seyfer, A.E., and Jackson, S.M. Reduction mammaplasty using the inferior glandular "pyramid" pedicle: Experiences with 300 patients. *Plast. Reconstr. Surg.* 80:75, 1987.
4. Bruschi, S., Muti, E., and Bocchiotti, G. Mastoplastica reduttiva con lembo inferiore. *Riv. Ital. Chir. Plast.* 17:69, 1985.
5. Climo, M.S., and Alexander, J.E. Intercostothelial circulation: Nipple survival and reduction mammaplasty in the absence of a dermal pedicle. *Ann. Plast. Surg.* 4:128, 1980.
6. Courtiss, E.H., and Goldwyn, R.M. Reduction mammaplasty by the inferior pedicle technique. An alternative to free nipple and areola grafting for severe macromastia or extreme ptosis. *Plast. Reconstr. Surg.* 59:500, 1977.
7. Crepau, R., and Klein, H.W. Reduction mammaplasty with inferiorly based glandular pedicle flap. *Ann. Plast. Surg.* 9:463, 1982.
8. DiGiuseppe, A., Cobbett, J., Cochrane, T., et al. La mastoplastica riduttiva secondo Robbins, McKissock E. Pitanguy modificata: tre diverse filosofie interpretative della riduzione del volume mammario riviste alla luce di un'esperienza casistica quadriennale. *Riv. Ital. Chir. Plast.* 18:51, 1986.
9. Georgiade, M.G., Serafin, T., Morris, R., and Georgiade, G. Reduction mammaplasty utilizing the inferior pedicle nipple-areola flap. *Ann. Plast. Surg.* 3:211, 1979.
10. Goldwyn, R.M., and Courtiss, E.H. Inferior Pedicle Technique. In P. Regnault and R.K. Daniel (eds.), *Aesthetic Plastic Surgery*. Boston: Little, Brown, 1986. Pp. 522, 526.
11. Hallock, G.G., and Altobelli, J.A. Prevention of the teardrop areola following the inferior pedicle technique of breast reduction. *Plast. Reconstr. Surg.* 80:531, 1988.
12. Kaplan, I. Reduction mammaplasty: Nipple-areola survival on a single breast quadrant. *Plast. Reconstr. Surg.* 61:27, 1978.
13. Labandter, H.P., Dowden, R.V., and Dinner, N.I. The inferior segment technique for breast reduction. *Ann. Plast. Surg.* 8:493, 1982.
14. Mathes, S.J., Nahai, F., and Hester, T.R. Avoiding the flat breast in reduction mammaplasty. *Plast. Reconstr. Surg.* 66:63, 1980.
15. McKissock, P.K. Discussion of avoiding the flat breast in reduction mammaplasty by S.J. Mathes, F. Nahai, N.T. Hester. *Plast. Reconstr. Surg.* 66:63, 1980.
16. McKissock, P.K. Discussion of J.M. Ramselaar's precision in breast reduction. *Plast. Reconstr. Surg.* 82:642, 1988.
17. Moufarrege, R., Beauregard, G., Bosse, J.P., et al. Reduction mammoplasty by the total dermoglandular pedicle. *Aesth. Plast. Surg.* 9:227, 1985.
18. Moufarrege, R., Muller, G., Beauregard, G., et al. Plastie mammarie a pedicule dermo-glandulaire inferieur. *Ann. Chir. Plast.* 27:249, 1982.
19. Ramsellar, J.M. Precision in breast reduction. *Plast. Reconstr. Surg.* 82:631, 1988.
20. Reich, J. Mammaplasty with the retention of a lower central breast. *Br. J. Plast. Surg.* 36:196, 1983.
21. Reus, W.F., and Mathes, S.J. Preservations of projection after reduction mammaplasty: Long-term follow-up of the inferior pedicle technique. *Plast. Reconstr. Surg.* 82:644, 1988.
22. Ribeiro, L. A new technique for reduction mammaplasty. *Plast. Reconstr. Surg.* 55:330, 1975.
23. Robbins, T.H. A reduction mammaplasty with the areola-nipple based on an inferior pedicle. *Plast. Reconstr. Surg.* 59:64, 1977.
24. Robbins, T.H. A platform for nipple projection. Letter to editor. *Plast. Reconstr. Surg.* 69:906, 1982.
25. Robbins, T.H. Reduction mammaplasty by the Robbins technique. Letter to editor. *Plast. Reconstr. Surg.* 79:308, 1987.
26. Schulz, R.C., and Markus, M.J. Platform for nipple projection modification of the inferior pedicle technique for breast reduction. *Plast. Reconstr. Surg.* 68:208, 1981.
27. Silversmith, P.E., and Crepau, R. Reduction mammaplasty. *Ann. Plast. Surg.* 11:266, 1983.
28. Smith, G.A., and Schmidt, G.H. Experience with the Ribeiro reduction mammaplasty technique. *Ann. Plast. Surg.* 3:260, 1979.
29. Versaci, A.D. Reduction mammaplasty for moderate macromastia. *Ann. Plast. Surg.* 6:253, 1981.
30. Zelnick, J.N., Pearl, R.M., and Johnson, D. Use of an axial flap for reduction mammaplasty. *Ann. Plast. Surg.* 7:204, 1981.

COMMENTS ON THE INFERIOR PEDICLE TECHNIQUE

Thomas H. Robbins

The idea of the inferior pedicle technique of reduction mammaplasty seems to have evolved independently and about the same time in several widely separated parts of the globe. It also seems to have been accepted quickly and widely. This would suggest that it represents a natural development from previous techniques.

When a procedure is widely and frequently performed, differences in details of technique must occur. It is the principles of the techniques, which are here clearly illustrated by Goldwyn and Courtiss, rather than the details, that characterize the technique.

The procedure does have the advantages of simplicity, safety, and versatility. This does not mean that the operation is always easy. Other advantages are retained sensitivity of the nipples and, in many cases, retention of the ability to breastfeed.

The freedom of the retained breast segment from the encumbrance of attachments to other parts of the breast except at the chest wall promotes the simplicity, safety, and versatility of the procedure. The retention of substantial breast tissue on the undersurface of the dermal pedicle (in my case the full thickness of the breast down to the chest wall) promotes the safety of the procedure as well as the retention of some mammary ducts. The fact that the T junction overlies the dermal pedicle also promotes the safety of the procedure. In my experience, breakdown of this junction does not occur often, but when it does, it usually heals because of the reepithelialization of the dermal pedicle where it is exposed. (I find it interesting that this pedicle reepithelializes where it is exposed up to the edges of the area exposed but epithelium does not regenerate in the buried part of the pedicle.) The exposed deepithelialized area of the inferior pedicle, if large owing to gross error in marking, is the "perfect" bed for regrafting with some of the discarded breast skin. This occurred once in my experience when a nurse secretly replaced the markings after they had been washed away.

Some of the advantages of the inferior pedicle technique have been well-illustrated in this chapter. I agree with the authors that the retained deepithelialized dermis of the pedicle is probably not essential for the viability of the pedicle and the nipple, but I have always retained it because I do suspect that the subdermal plexus is very important, and retention of the dermis ensures the safety of this plexus.

In summary, the procedure does offer the sophistication of simplicity as clearly demonstrated by Goldwyn and Courtiss.

Inferior Pyramidal Technique

Gregory S. Georgiade,
Ronald E. Riefkohl, and
Nicholas G. Georgiade

The state of the art in the design and execution of satisfactory breast reduction has improved significantly over the past 20 years. A properly contoured, balanced, and predictable aesthetic result is one that the patient in this era has come to expect.

The development of the technique to be described is a compilation of many surgeons' ideas, which we have incorporated and modified for a safe, easy, and predictable result. In 1973, Ribeiro and Bacher [11] reported on their technique of enhancing the projection of the breast in the reduction mammaplasty technique. At that time, they were using a technique that was modified after the technique of Arié [1] and Pitanguy [8]. Their modification utilized dermal breast pedicle placed behind a superiorly based nipple-areolar pedicle for optimum projection of the nipple-areola. Later, in 1975, Ribeiro [10] described his technique with an inferiorly based dermal pedicle. This was followed with reports of the nipple-areola based on an inferior dermal flap by others [3, 12] in the reduction mammaplasty technique. In 1979, Georgiade et al [6, 7] described the use of a pyramidal breast tissue flap in combination with a dermal pedicle. Reich [9], in the same year, described his preferred technique utilizing a combination of dermal pedicle with breast parenchyma. The importance of a suitable base of breast parenchyma attached to the pectoralis muscle for assurance of adequate blood supply and innervation to the nipple-areola area was stressed by Georgiade et al [5, 6] in 1979, and later by Ariyan in 1980 [2]. From these initial observations and techniques described more than 10 years ago has evolved the improved technique for breast reduction we now use. More than 1,000 breast reductions have been carried out with these concepts in mind.

Technical Aspects
PREOPERATIVE EVALUATION AND MARKINGS
The routine now used involves the marking of the breast with the patient in an upright position. In patients with larger breast hypertrophies, a dermal flap and inferior mammary lines can be marked more easily if the patient is in a supine position.

The initial markings are made with a methylene blue skin marker at the point of the sternal notch. The midsternal location is then marked in a vertical manner. The inferior mammary crease is then palpated, and a mark is made on the superior skin surface slightly higher than the inframammary crease line and at the midclavicular point or slightly more medial in the larger breasts, as the nipple-areola complex is usually lateral to the midclavicular line (Fig. 18-18). The circumference of the new areola is then determined and marked with a stainless steel loop (Duke design), which has been used for approximately 15 years [4]. These loops are made in two diameters — 4.0 and 4.5 cm — with the larger diameter used in the older patients with larger areolae (Fig. 18-19). At this point, it is necessary to determine the amount of breast tissue to be excised. This determination is made by estimating the distance between the new breast flaps, by approximating the flaps with the thumb and forefinger of each hand. The degree of tension will now determine the distance to be marked between each arm of the wire loop marker. The distance between the arms of the wire loop will vary from 8 cm in a breast reduction of approximately 400 gm to a distance of 10 to 12 cm in a 700-gm breast reduction. A distance of 14 or more cm is necessary for a breast reduction of approximately 2,000 gm (Fig. 18-19). Once this distance has been established and marked, a distance from each areolar marking to the midsternal line is adjusted as necessary to equalize each eventual nipple-areola distance from the midline. The patient is then placed in a supine position, and the inferior dermal pedicle flap is marked with a base of 7 cm for a resultant small breast (A cup). The base of the dermal pedicle is increased up to 9 cm for the larger (C cup). A margin of 1.5 cm of dermis is maintained around the superior areola, not only to protect the areola but also to expedite the closure. The inferior mammary markings are made slightly above the inframammary crease line, and a slight triangular projection is marked in

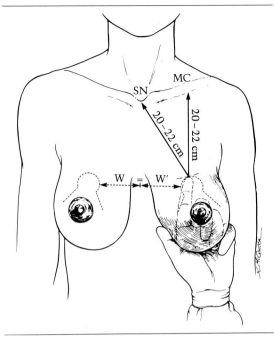

Fig. 18-18. *The distance to the superior portion of the new areolar position from the sternal notch is shown. Note that this position is slightly more medial than the unoperated position of the areola. The distance to the midline must be the same from each areolar marking.*

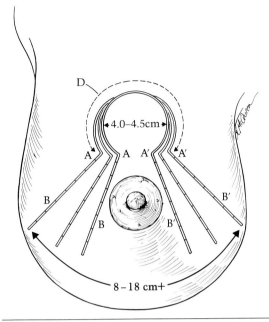

Fig. 18-19. *The flexible steel wire is shown in various positions of expansion, simplifying the marking of a breast for reduction. The serrations on the wire are at centimeter distances, allowing the simple marking of the areola to the inframammary crease line.*

the middermal pedicle area. The lateral and medial markings are maintained in the inframammary crease, care being taken not to extend the marking past the anterior axillary area laterally and medially. The marking is maintained in the breast shadow but never extending to the midline. The length of the areolar inframammary is marked at 5 cm. A horizontal slightly S-shaped line is extended laterally to meet the inframammary line. All the markings are then reinforced with a brilliant green dye so that they will not be removed during routine skin preparation at the time of surgery.

OPERATIVE PROCEDURE

Following suitable skin preparation, the base of each breast is infiltrated with approximately 40 ml of 1:300,000 epinephrine solution (1 ml of 1:000 epinephrine mixed with 300 ml of saline). This technique yields excellent vasoconstriction and results in minimal blood loss so that even an individual breast reduction of 700 gm or more will

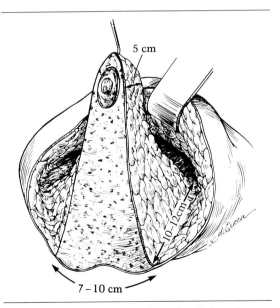

Fig. 18-20. *The basic inferior dermal pedicle and pyramid of breast tissue is shown. Note the sloping sides away from pyramid.*

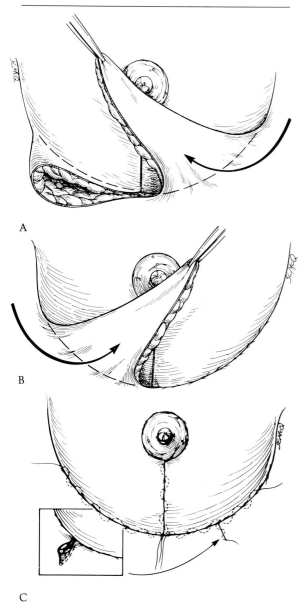

A

B

C

Fig. 18-21. A. The excision of the redundant tissue is carried out with tension exerted medially as shown. This technique will minimize the extension of the scar medially. B. The same technique is carried out laterally, incising the flap initially medially and gradually extending the incision, supported by 4-0 Dexon dermal sutures. C. The final closure is carried out by subcuticular running sutures. Note that occasionally a small excision of inferior redundant skin will improve the aesthetic appearance and limit the medial and lateral extension of the scars.

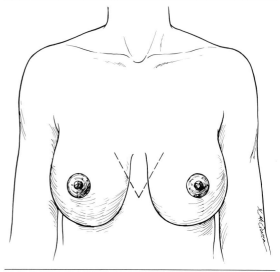

Fig. 18-22. The inverted midline triangle represents the area that must be resected without extension of the scar.

usually not necessitate blood replacement. The initial phase of the surgery involves the deepithelialization of the previously marked dermal pedicle. Following this, the other markings are incised with the exception of the lateral "lazy S" markings, which are excised only at the time of the final tailoring of the breast flaps. The pyramidal breast mound is developed by incising in a tangential fashion from the dermal flap laterally, medially, and superiorly, with an increasingly wide base attached to the pectoralis musculature. Following the development of a widely based flap attached to the inferiorly based dermal pedicle, the excess breast tissue is excised in a semicircular manner, maintaining a uniform thickness of 1.5 cm of the skin flaps (Fig. 18-20). Any residual tissue in the corners of the medial and lateral breast areas are excised to minimize an ovoid appearance of the completed breast when redundant tissue is allowed to remain in these areas. The medial and lateral flaps are approximated with 4-0 Dexon or Vicryl sutures, and the nipple-areola is brought under these flaps to the new keyhole position and maintained in position with multiple 5-0 dermal sutures. The dermal pedicle is incised lightly at its base to allow the buried sutures coverage at the time of the flap approximation. Once the two flaps of each breast have been approximated, any disparity in size between the breasts is adjusted. The

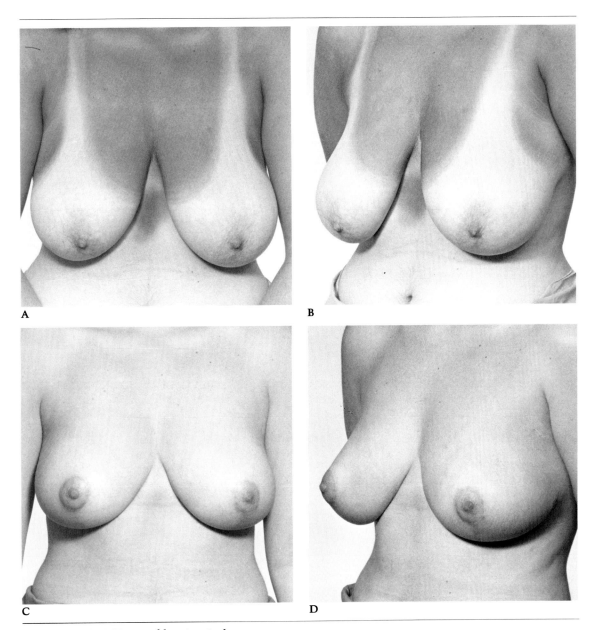

Fig. 18-23. A, B. A 25-year-old patient is shown
preoperatively with moderately hypertrophied breasts
with a significant degree of ptosis. C, D. One and one
half years post–reduction mammaplasty of 500 gm of
tissue from each breast.

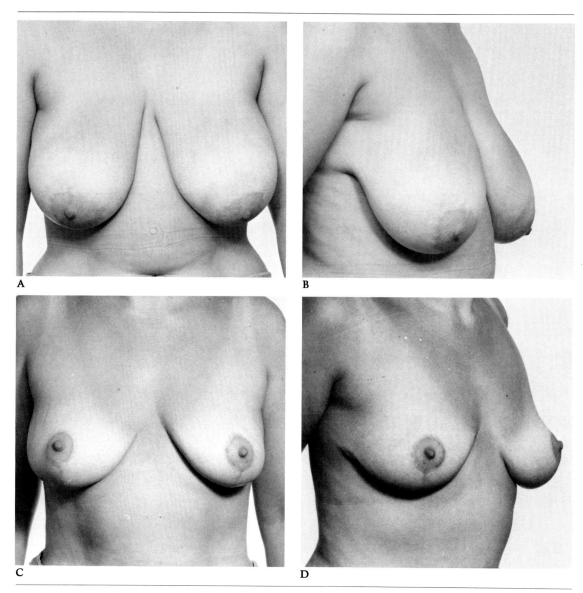

Fig. 18-24. A, B. A 25-year-old patient is shown with a greater degree of hypertrophy and ptosis prior to breast reduction. C, D. Three years post–reduction mammaplasty of 700 gm of tissue from the right breast and 800 gm from the left breast.

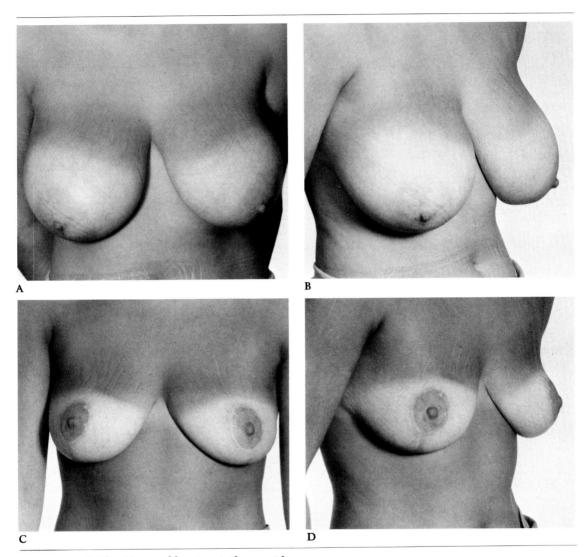

Fig. 18-25. A, B. This 18-year-old patient is shown with large hypertrophied and asymmetric breasts with associated ptosis. C, D. Two years post–reduction mammaplasty of 1225 gm of tissue from each breast. Note the well-concealed inframammary scars both medially and laterally.

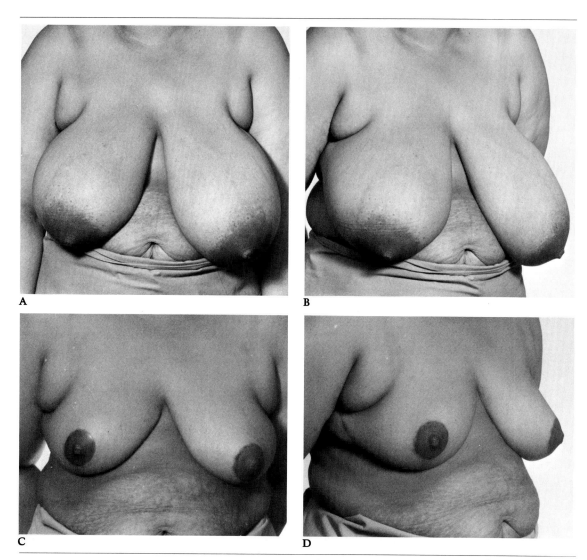

A   B

C   D

final tailoring of the breast is carried out on the medial portion of the breast flap, with slight lateral pressure being maintained on the breast to keep it in a midposition so that the breasts' contour can be evenly maintained and following the breast curvature. A few 4-0 dermal sutures are used to approximate the flaps along the inframammary crease line. The final tailoring of the redundant tissue is accomplished by utilizing traction toward the midportion of the breast, minimizing the extension of the scars medially (Fig. 18-21A, B). The same maneuver is carried out on the lateral aspect of the new breast mound, carefully following the breast contour. Bringing the excess mam-

Fig. 18-26. A, B. A 19-year-old patient is shown with massive breast hypertrophy and associated ptosis, with associated breast asymmetry and ptosis. C, D. Fifteen months post–reduction mammaplasty with excision of 1900 gm of tissue from the right breast and 2250 gm from the left breast.

mary tissue into the midportion of the inframammary area will cause some redundancy to be present, especially in the inframammary areas when a larger reduction has been carried out. A moderate degree of this redundant tissue will gradually redrape over a period of months; however, it is occasionally necessary to excise a small wedge of redundant inframammary tissue on the medial or lateral, or both, areas, which is nicely concealed in the inframammary areas (Figs. 18-21C and 18-22). A suction drain is inserted at the time of closure at the lateral position of the breast. Dermal running sutures are used to approximate the skin edges, and sterile paper tape strips are placed across the lines of incisions for adequate support. The dressing consists of bulky mechanic's waste shaped around the breast cone and maintained in position with a figure-of-eight bias cut stockinette dressing. The dressing is changed the following day, and the wound is examined for any signs of hematoma or undue pressure. The suction drains are usually kept in place for 24 to 48 hours. The sutures are removed on the tenth postoperative day, and the wound is reinforced with sterile tapes for an additional 10 days. The patient wears a comfortable brassier for the next 3 to 4 weeks continuously (Figs. 18-23 through 18-26).

UNTOWARD RESULTS

There is always the possibility of less than desirable results occurring, although this is uncommon. In our experience, we have had the following problems occur with decreasing frequency as our technical abilities have improved: (1) The most common undesirable result has been an inadequate excision of the hypertrophied breast tissue, particularly in the lateral position, but also in the medial aspect of the contoured breast. The problem has been largely corrected by placing the patient in a sitting position prior to finishing the closure and comparing both breasts. Any adjustments as to volume and shape are carried out at that time. (2) Nipple inversion has occurred when insufficient breast tissue was present beneath the nipple-areola (see Fig. 18-21). A thickness of at least 5 cm must be present to prevent this problem. (3) Superficial loss of the areola occurred in three patients in this series, but no permanent full-thickness loss occurred. It was postulated that the pyramidal base was not developed in a sufficient tangential manner, increasing the base along the superior aspect of the pyramid. (4) Occasional loss of approximately 1.5 cm of medial and lateral

flaps at the inverted T position has occurred, particularly in older patients with less dermis (6%). The use of a triangular projection of the inframammary skin in the inferior midportion of the dermal pedicle minimizes the frequency of this occurrence (see Fig. 18-20).

Discussion

The utilization of a dermal pedicle inferiorly based with an accompanying large pyramid of breast parenchymal appears to offer the safest technique for breast reduction. Although the incorporation of dermis is probably not essential for viability, the dermis does offer stability of the pedicle with greater support to the medial and lateral flaps.

References

1. Arie, G. Una Nieva Tecnica de mammaplastica. *Rev. Lib. Anovica* 12:23, 1958.
2. Ariyan, S. Reduction mammoplasty with the nipple-areola carried on a single, narrow inferior pedicle. *Ann. Plast. Surg.* 5:167, 1980.
3. Courtiss, E.H., and Goldwyn, R.M. Reduction mammaplasty by the inferior pedicle technique. *Plast. Reconstr. Surg.* 50:500, 1977.
4. Georgiade, N.G. *Breast Reconstruction Following Mastectomy.* St. Louis: Mosby, 1979. P. 101.
5. Georgiade, N.G., and Georgiade, G.S. Reduction Mammoplasty Utilizing the Inferior Pyramidal Dermal Pedicle. In N.G. Georgiade (ed.), *Aesthetic Breast Surgery.* Baltimore: Williams & Wilkins, 1983. Pp. 291–299.
6. Georgiade, N.G., Serafin, D., Morris, R., and Georgiade, G.S. Reduction mammaplasty utilizing an inferior pedicle nipple areola flap. *Ann. Plast. Surg.* 3:211, 1979.
7. Georgiade, N.G., Serafin, D., Riefkohl, R., and Georgiade, G.S. Is there a reduction mammoplasty for all seasons? *Plast. Reconstr. Surg.* 63:765, 1979.
8. Pitanguy, I. Surgical treatment of breast hypertrophy. *Br. J. Plast. Surg.* 20:78, 1967.
9. Reich, J. The advantages of a lower central breast segment in reduction mammaplasty. *Aesth. Plast. Surg.* 3:47, 1979.
10. Ribeiro, L. A new technique for reduction mammaplasty. *Plast. Reconstr. Surg.* 55:330, 1975.
11. Ribeiro, L., and Bacher, E. Mastoplasia con pediculo de seguridad. *Rev. Esp. Cirurg. Plast.* 6:223, 1973.
12. Robbins, T. A reduction mammaplasty with the areola-nipple based on an inferior dermal pedicle. *Plast. Reconstr. Surg.* 59:64, 1977.

COMMENTS ON INFERIOR PYRAMIDAL TECHNIQUE

Robert M. Goldwyn

The authors have documented once again their satisfaction with the inferior pedicle technique (the "inferior pyramidal technique" in their terms) for breast reduction. They consider it a reduction mammaplasty "for all seasons" [1]. Indeed, it is difficult to controvert their experience and results.

The senior author's concept of a pyramidal breast tissue flap in combination with a dermal pedicle does give the reduced breast a pleasing shape. If one adheres to the suggested dimensions of this flap, sufficient tissue at the base and behind the areola, one avoids a flat breast, an inverted nipple-areola, or, worse, an ischemic one. Being careful not to dissect too deeply below the pectoralis fascia will ensure adequate sensation. Being cautious not to resect too much tissue from under the superior flap at the keyhole will prevent an unsightly concavity.

The authors' injunction to cut the flap tangentially, especially toward the base, is important advice to avoid encroaching on the critical blood supply — a very common and serious error that should not occur if the surgeon continually keeps in mind not only where he or she is incising but what he or she is leaving behind. It is easy to place incorrect traction on the pedicle at its base, thereby misleading one to overestimate the amount of tissue remaining at the base.

The suggestion of making the areola larger in an older patient is logical since those women usually have very large, slack breasts and will have a resultant breast that is seldom small, a size that the patient may have requested ("make me as small as you can") but one that she would not have liked since it would not have been appropriate to her habitus. Making an excessively large nipple for a small breast is also unsightly. Therefore, the surgeon must vary the size of the areola in relation to the size of the breast.

In deciding how much breast tissue to resect in any patient, the authors offer helpful guidelines, including measuring the distance between the ends of the arms of the wire loop marker. I would emphasize that it is better to leave more skin for resection later, if necessary, than to struggle during closure — an unpleasant experience that most of us have had at least once, but that is enough. The balance between leaving sufficient skin and breast tissue for proper closure and shape and leaving too much is easier to achieve the greater the surgeon's experience. However, simply sitting the patient up prior to closure, as the authors instruct, and being critical about the appearance and symmetry of the breasts is not only helpful but necessary to get the best result.

To reduce the length of the horizontal scar as well as to improve the shape of the breast and to forestall or prevent later bottoming out, the authors close with traction medially, as do most of us, but they have added the clever suggestion of resecting any extra tissue in the inframammary fold with small vertical excisions.

Their use of a triangular projection of skin from the inframammary fold in the midline is one that I have also found useful in decreasing the incidence of necrosis at the junction of the inverted T. Obviously, if the height of this tissue is excessive, the nipple will be too high.

The patient shown in Figure 18-26A and B would have benefited by removal of her axillary tissue, which characteristically becomes more noticeable after the breasts have been made smaller.

REFERENCES

1. Georgiade, N.G., Serafin, D., Riefkohl, R., and Georgiade, G.S. Is there a reduction mammoplasty for all seasons? *Plast. Reconstr. Surg.* 63:765, 1979.

19

Paule C. Regnault and
Rollin K. Daniel

Breast Reduction:
B Technique

The B technique of reduction mammaplasty and correction of ptosis has been used by the senior author for more than 20 years with excellent results. This technique has been published several times in plastic surgery journals and in some books and has been used by many surgeons around the world. Each publication has brought a few variations in the concept of the technique owing to the author's desire to improve and clarify certain details. This chapter also follows that desire. There is no end to improvement. Since perfection does not exist, improvements are constantly occurring; the most recent ones are presented in this chapter. We have said and written that the general concept of the B technique was mainly a vertical reduction with a lateral prolongation. Unfortunately, some drawing may have given the wrong impression that the technique is more oblique than vertical. In this chapter, we hope to clarify this important point.

The B technique combines the advantages of several previous classical techniques as well as attempting to reduce the submammary scar. The procedure combines reduction of the Strömbeck mammaplasty with no skin undermining, the verticality of the Arié technique with no horizontal scar, and the obliquity of the Marc-Dufourmentel technique with no medial scar.

Pinching the tissues at the lower pole of a large breast in a vertical way leaves an inferior lateral wedge that can be located easily above the submammary crease so that the overall excess of breast tissue forms a thick crescent open laterally. This maneuver demonstrates excision of the lower quadrants. The idea of taking the measurements of the new periareolar limits instead of the classical measurement of the new nipple site location has been imagined as a safe protection against the dangers of locating the nipple too high or too medially. It is a fundamental basic principle of the B reduction mammaplasty technique.

Indications

This technique is indicated in all cases of breast reduction and mastopexy, except in cases in which excision of a maximum of 1500 ml is required. In these cases, nipple grafting is safer. The absence of a medial submammary scar makes this technique especially advantageous in patients subject to hypertrophic scarring.

As with all reduction techniques, the B reduction technique is easier in smaller reductions and mastopexies. The surgeon should master the technique in these cases, becoming familiar with the markings, resection, and suturing. Because of its limited dissection and short scars, it is recommended for patients who prefer local anesthesia and has often been used in smaller reductions and mastopexies.

Examination

The patient is examined nude from the umbilicus to the neck so that the proportions between the breast and the body are well visualized and can be measured accurately. It is obvious that the hip-breast proportion is very important to establish the desired breast size. The breast perimeter at the nipple level should be about the same as the hip perimeter, or a little less. Thus, breast size is measured at the nipple level with the brassiere on, and thorax size is measured at the submammary fold or above the breast at the axillae level. The difference between the measurements of the breast and the thorax give the cup size. One-inch difference is an A cup; two inches is a B cup; and so on. One discovers that patients do not always wear the correct size brassiere. According to the classical beauty standards, an average-sized woman should have a 34 B breast. Whatever the torso perimeter, it is advisable to reduce the breast to a B cup. Breast symmetric volume is verified and measured, if useful, by measuring each half perimeter (spine-sternum) at the nipple level. The breast skin is examined to verify the elasticity, texture, and looseness. Skin tumors and visible veins are noted and pointed out to the patient. Areolae and nipples are examined: The pigmentation, the size, and the symmetry are studied so that some modifications might be planned in agreement with the patient. Nipple invagination correction may also be planned, as well as nipple hypertrophy correction.

The breast parenchyma quality is evaluated by careful palpation. Mainly glandular and firm in young patients, it becomes soft, adipose, and flabby in postmenopausal women. In a large percentage of patients, some small cysts may be found. These should be noted and explained to the patient. They are not a contraindication to the reduction unless they constitute the only motivation for surgery; then, a more radical excision may be indicated. The presence of a distinct tumor must be ruled out. Based on the authors' experience, a breast cancer will be discovered in one case of every thousand cases.

Discussion with the Patient

Although the surgeon should give his or her opinion, he or she should never impose his or her views about breast size. It is better to let the patient be involved in this decision, because many patients have a predetermined concept. Showing photographs to the patient helps her to get a better understanding about breast size as well as nipple and areola modifications. It is equally important to explain the location of the scars on postoperative pictures and, if necessary, to draw the location of the scars on the patient's skin.

Complications should be explained in depth. The quality of the scars vary with each patient, and scar revision is necessary in about 10 percent of cases. Diminution or loss of sensation around the nipple-areola complex is usually temporary and rarely permanent. Uneven size or uneven shape of the breasts is transitory and rarely permanent. Secondary correction should be discussed. Although lactation is possible with the B technique, it is not recommended since volume variations are always followed by ptosis.

It should be pointed out that the upper breast quadrants will remain the way they are, not more rounded, unless an implant is used. In contrast to hypotrophy and ptosis cases, an implant should be inserted only secondarily when the operative result of the reduction is final, usually 1 year postoperatively.

Preparation for Surgery

The routine preparation is used, including vitamins C and K for 1 week before surgery. Forbidding aspirin for 2 weeks before and after surgery is recommended. In large reductions, it is advised to avoid operating in the premenstrual period. Blood transfusions are rarely necessary. Since local infiltration is always used in conjunction with general anesthesia, significant bleeding is extremely rare. However, in very large breast reductions, it may be useful to have one or two units of autologous blood available.

Aesthetic Anatomy

As previously discussed, currently, the optimum breast size is one that can fill a B cup brassiere. The distance from the sternal notch to the nipple varies from 18 to 24 cm according to the patient's build. The areola size is an average of 4 cm in diameter. The distance from the inframammary crease to the nipple is about 7 cm. The location of the inframammary crease should be at the level of the fifth intercostal space in young women. It migrates down to the sixth rib or even lower with weight and aging.

Objectives of the B Reduction

The main objective of the B reduction technique is the removal of glandular and fatty tissue in order to leave the desired size of the breast. Although the size may be judged at the time of surgery, it is quite difficult with the patient in the horizontal position and with the skin incised. It is better to calculate the excess volume at the time of the examination by following the table of the brassiere size. The predicted size of reduction may, of course, be somewhat modified at the time of surgery. For example, according to Table 19-1, a patient having a preoperative breast size of 36 D has a volume of about 1,000 ml and should be reduced by about 400 ml to obtain a size 36 B.

Attaining an aesthetic shape is a question of leaving the tissues equally distributed, with a well-projected nipple at the apex of a hemispheric mound. To get this result when using the B tech-

Table 19-1. Approximate volume of breasts according to well-fitted brassieres

	100	200	300	400	500				
32	A	B	C	D					
34		A	B	C	D				
			400	600	800	1000	1200		
36			A	B	C	D			
38				A	B	C	D		
					1100	1400	1700	2000	2300
40					A	B	C	D	
42						A	B	C	D

nique, care is taken to remove more tissue medially than laterally since the tissues are stretched laterally while they are gathered medially. If the removal was symmetric, the breast would appear flat in the lateral portions and bulgy in the medial quadrants.

Small well-located scars are normally achieved since the inframammary incision is located in a newly elevated submammary fold and located centrally and laterally with no medial component. In the cases of extremely flabby tissue, it may be useful to resect a small triangle of skin at the lower medial curve of the B. The periareolar skin is much longer than the areola, so that in very large reductions, it is better to keep the areola at its natural size.

It is a relatively simple procedure once the planning is done. There is very little undermining (only at the lower medial quadrant owing to thickness reduction), so that bleeding is minimal and operative time very short compared with that of other techniques. For the same reasons, it is a very safe procedure.

Sensation is rarely impaired since the entire periareola dermis is left intact except at the lower quadrants, where the full thickness of tissues is removed, leaving only a 1-cm margin below the areola. Sensation may be reduced temporarily but rarely permanently.

Lactation is possible, the nipple remaining at its natural glandular basis. There has never been any problem regarding this function.

The result may be considered *permanent*. Breast changes are natural, with no tendency for upward migration of the nipples. It is only in cases of body changes that a secondary revision may be useful.

Altogether, the special characteristics and principles of the B technique are:

1. Nipple transposition on a wide dermaglandular pedicle, from upper, lateral, and medial parts of the breast.
2. Preservation of a wide periareolar area of dermis.
3. Glandular resection done mainly from the lower quadrants.
4. Closure in a Z-plasty manner, with stretching of the lateral flap downward and medially, while the medial flap is gathered and brought laterally and horizontally.

Marking

All the markings are done preoperatively with a heavy felt pen. Only one mark is done with the patient in the sitting position (Fig. 19-1). It is the new upper limit of the periareolar skin (not the new nipple site, as is done in the classical techniques). This upper limit (point V on the figures) is obtained by measuring a distance corresponding to the patient's thorax and taken from the sternal notch on the line sternal-notch-to-nipple, symmetrically on both breasts. According to the patient's size, it may vary from to 15 to 22 cm. This measurement may be verified by placing the fingers under the breast, at the submammary fold. It should be about 3 cm above the fingers. Once the upper areolar limit has been found, the patient is asked to lie down and may, at this moment, be anesthetized.

The second important mark is the new medial limit of the areola, which is found by measuring its

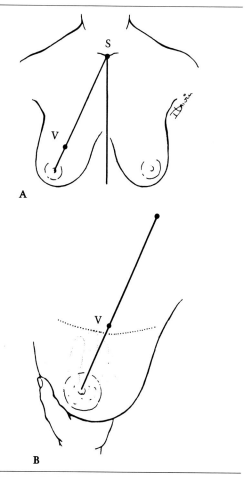

A

B

Fig. 19-1. A. The distance (SV) from the sternal notch to the new upper limit of the areola is measured. B. It is verified by placing the fingers in the submammary fold. (From P. Regnault and R. K. Daniel (eds). Aesthetic Plastic Surgery. Boston: Little, Brown, 1984.)

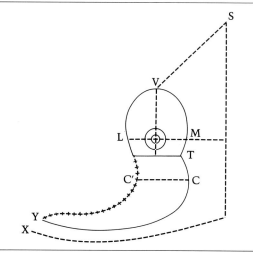

Fig. 19-2. Drawing of the incision is completed on the patient supine: V is a new upper limit of the areola; M is the new medial limit; L is the lateral limit, symmetric to M. Point C is at the vertical from M. T is an angle of about 1 cm lateral to the vertical MC. From the apex of this angle is traced the medial lower curve of the excision, down to the new submammary fold. Line X is the previous submammary fold. Line V is the new submammary fold.

distance from the midsternal vertical line, on a horizontal line at the new nipple level. The new periareolar limit at this level varies from 9 to 12 cm, according to the patient's thorax. This point is point M on the figures (Fig. 19-2).

Symmetric to point M, in relation to a vertical line traced from point V (first mark) downward, is marked the lateral limit of the periareolar skin on a *horizontal line* from point M. This mark has, unfortunately, not been well marked in some previous publications, somewhat changing the orientation of the whole operation, causing it to resemble an oblique technique. This point is L on

the drawings. In case of abnormal location of the nipple-areola complex, point L should be placed to establish symmetry.

These three points (V-M-L) define an oval, more or less elongated figure, according to each case. It should be clear that these points are only landmarks for drawing and excision but *not for suturing*, since there will be a rotation of the periareolar tissues before closing.

The areolar circle is marked using a diameter of 3.5 to 5.0 cm. The vertical and horizontal axes of the areola are marked to ensure equal tension at the time of closure.

The new submammary fold is marked parallel to the existing fold, which is also marked, and about 1.0 to 4.0 cm above, according to age, looseness of tissues, and importance of the reduction. In young firm breasts, this new fold is sometimes left at the same level as the previous one, whereas in older or very flabby tissues, it may be elevated 4.0 cm; this is easily determined by palpation of the breasts in the horizontal position. If one does not elevate the fold, as with most techniques, a mistake is made

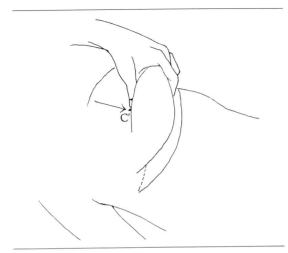

Fig. 19-3. Pinching the lower quadrants gives the measurement C-C'.

that creates old-looking breasts located too low on the thorax.

A vertical line M-C is drawn from point M downward.

A horizontal line is drawn 1 cm below the areola indicating the lower limit of the periareolar deepidermization, which is also the upper limit of the glandular resection. On this line, 1 cm lateral from the vertical MC is marked point T.

Joining points M-T-C defines an angle of about 90 or 100 degrees, separating the upper and lower curves. This angle is one of the most important characteristics of the B drawing.

The lower curve is completed downwards to join the new submammary fold. It is the medial limit of the glandular resection.

By pinching the breast lower poles, at this lower curve, one can define point C', which gives an approximate idea of the lateral limit of the full gland-skin resection (Fig. 19-3). From point L to C' down to the submammary fold, an S curve is drawn in a dotted line, the approximate limit of the lateral section. It may be changed after the glandular flap has been dissected from its upper medial and deep attachments.

The completed drawing resembles the letter B on the right breast. A symmetric drawing is then done on the opposite side or according to any difference that might exist. Although the whole drawing may seem complicated at first, it is learned quite fast, utilizing the preceding instructions.

Surgical Technique

The use of local infiltration at a low percentage (0.25% lidocaine with 1:400,000 dilution of epinephrine) has been routine with the senior author. When the patient is not under general anesthesia, the intercostal blocks of the third, fourth, fifth, and sixth nerves are always added. The large breast reductions are always done under general anesthesia with local infiltration, whereas the smaller reductions (less than 300 ml) and mastopexies are done under local anesthesia and sedation.

The operation is done in four steps: (1) deepithelialization, (2) breast tissue section and dissection, (3) resection, and (4) closure.

Following the preoperative markings, the whole upper portion of the B is deepithelialized, leaving a large dermal area around the areola, taking care to preserve the 1-cm margin of dermis below the areola, which is a warranty against partial areolar necrosis.

Complete division of breast tissue is then done following the horizontal infra-areolar deepithelialized margin across from the lateral end and continued in the medial lower curve of the B, where the scalpel is used slightly oblique to remove more deep than superficial tissue medially and between the new and previous submammary folds. The incision is continued laterally to the end of the marking.

The preceding incisions have created a flap of breast tissue attached laterally (Fig. 19-4). This flap is now detached from its base on the pectoralis, leaving some areolar tissue over the muscle and pulled medially with moderate tension over the medial edge of the incision so that one can estimate the optimum resection to be performed to get satisfactory breast size and an easy closure. By pulling medially and downward on the lateral flap, the periareolar tissue, following the same pulling, is reduced and one can estimate how the upper part of the breast will be sutured. In case of excessive tension, it is advisable to remove more breast tissue. Once the flap has been removed and size adjustment has been done, the excised tissues are measured volumetrically since the density may be somewhat different on the other side.

In case of firm breasts or smaller excision cases, it is necessary to incise the periphery of the dermis to close the areola area with no tension or distortion. In large breasts or very flabby ones, incising the dermis is unnecessary (Fig. 19-5).

Complete hemostasis is done very carefully,

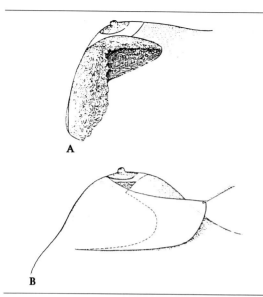

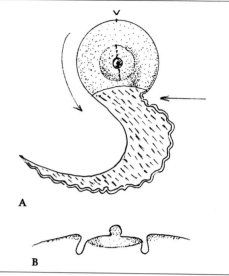

Fig. 19-4. A. The full-thickness skin-gland flap has been dissected with excess tissue and remains attached laterally. B. Pulling on the flap indicates where the optimum resection will be (dotted line). (From P. Regnault. Breast reduction: B technique. Plast. Reconstr. Surg. 65:840, 1980.)

Fig. 19-6. A. The lateral flap is pulled downward and medially, while the medial angular flap is pulled laterally. The medial skin edge is longer than the lateral; some folding appears. B. The periareolar dermis is folded by approximation of the periareolar skin to the areola. (From P. Regnault. Breast reduction: B technique. Plast. Reconstr. Surg. 65:840, 1980.)

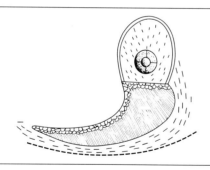

Fig. 19-5. After resection of the flap, it may be useful to defat more between the previous and the new submammary folds and at the medial area.

after all adjustments of tissues are completed. The medial lower quadrant often needs some deep tissue removed at the very end of the lateral submammary incision.

The only preoperative landmark used in the suturing is point V, which is sutured to the upper end of the areola vertical axis. Closure is then started at the lower quadrants, bringing the lateral flap maximum convexity into the medial maximum concavity by pulling the lateral flap downward and medially in the same manner as was done to esti-

mate the resection. The triangular medial flap T is pulled laterally straight across, so that the closure is somewhat like a Z-plasty. These two flaps are attached by two key sutures on the parenchyma, using an 00 heavy absorbable material (Fig. 19-6).

The upper periareolar closure is facilitated by suturing first the four ends of the vertical and horizontal axis of the areola to the periareolar skin with equal tension and equal gathering of the periareolar skin.

At this stage, skin modifications may be easily done. A split silicone drain tube is left at the lateral part of the submammary incision. Closure is completed by a subcutaneous running suture along all the incisions (usually 0000 Vicryl). The edges of the skin are unequal, mainly around the areola and at the lower curve, creating a moderate folding. The folds will disappear in a few weeks. However, in case the folds are exaggerated at the lower part of the inferior curve (in very flabby large reductions), a small triangle of skin may be resected or the possibility of a secondary scar revision may be planned. In case of excessive tension or unaesthetic shape, additional breast tissue may be removed.

To avoid tension on the suture lines, adhesive

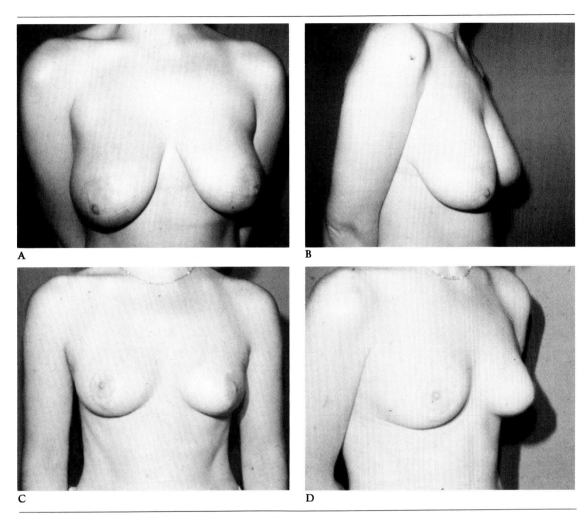

A   B

C   D

Fig. 19-7. A, B. A 28-year-old patient with asymmetric
breasts with small hypertrophy. C, D. Four years after
B reduction; 320 ml were removed from the right
breast and 200 ml from the left breast.

paper tape is always used. Nonadhesive gauze is
used on the areola, then padding is used to obtain a
moderate pressure. Elastic tapes are then used
with moderate tension, and the whole dressing is
changed after 48 hours. A well-fitted brassiere is
recommended for several weeks.

Results and Advantages

In average cases, results of the B breast reduction
are excellent, giving a natural-looking breast with
no tendency to secondary deformity (flatness of

the upper quadrants and upward migration of the
nipple-areola complex). This superior result is because the lateral lower flap is holding down the
nipple-areola complex, which is also maintained
strongly downward by the triangular medial flap.
Because no breast tissue is being removed from the
upper pole, this area remains like it was before
surgery and will follow the same evolution as nonoperated on tissues (Figs. 19-7 through 19-10).

Like all breast reduction techniques, it is easier
in small reductions and mastopexies. It should be
used in these cases at first, progressively increasing the reduction size as one becomes more familiar with the technique. Although it has been used
in very large breasts by the senior author, it is not
advisable above 1500-ml removal by inexperienced surgeons.

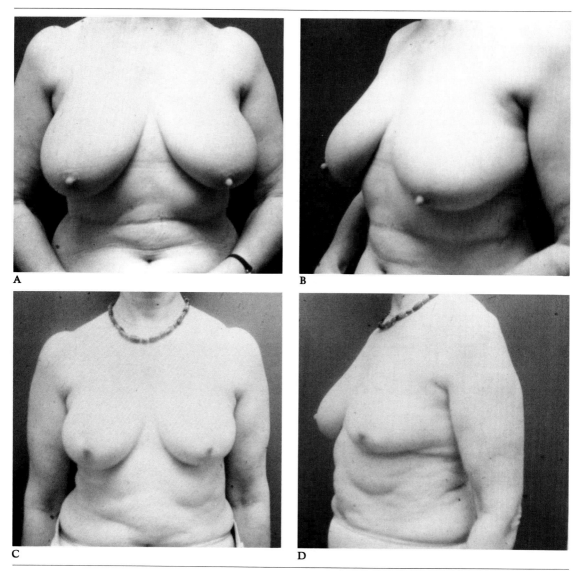

Fig. 19-8. A, B. A 54-year-old patient with moderate hypertrophy. C, D. Three years after B reduction; 550 ml were removed from the right breast and 500 ml from the left breast.

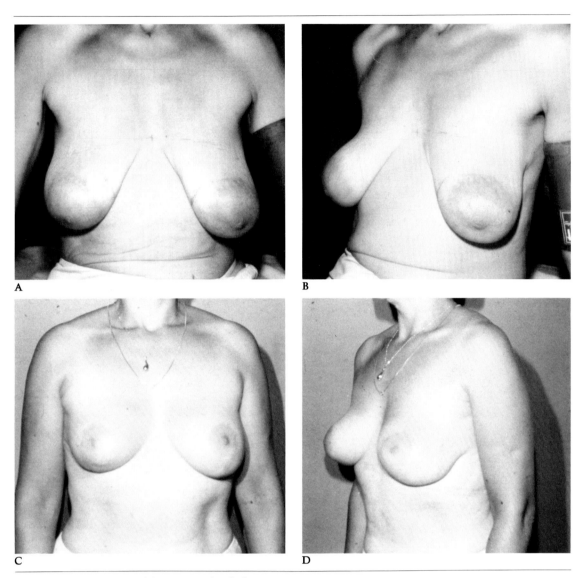

A   B
C   D

Fig. 19-9. A, B. A 38-year-old patient with tubular
breasts with small hypertrophy. C, D. Nine years after
B reduction; 175 ml were removed from the right
breast and 200 ml from the left breast.

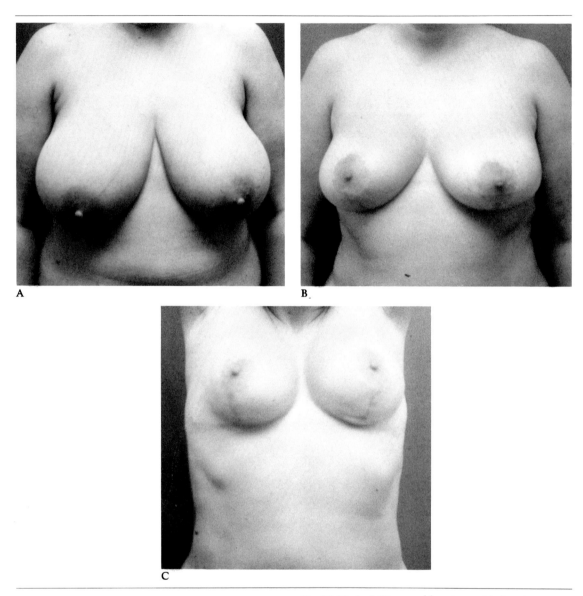

A

B

C

Fig. 19-10. A. A 32-year-old patient with firm large hypertrophy. B, C. One year after 650 ml were removed with B reduction on each side.

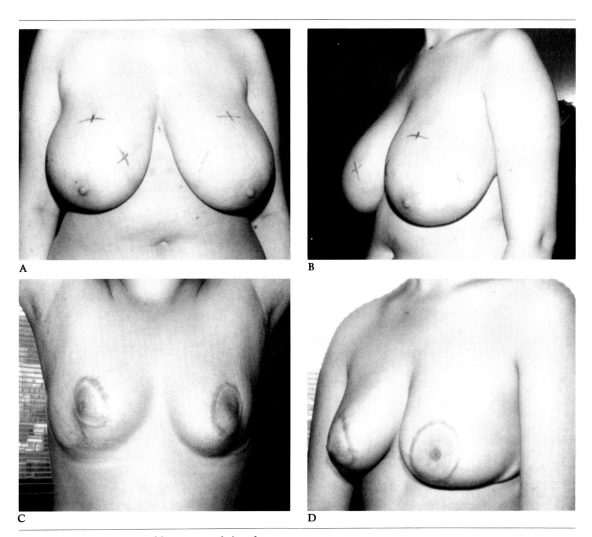

Fig. 19-11. A, B. A 24-year-old patient with firm large
hypertrophy. C, D. One year after 900 ml were
removed with B reduction on each side. There are
hypertrophic scars and some deformity at the lower
quadrants.

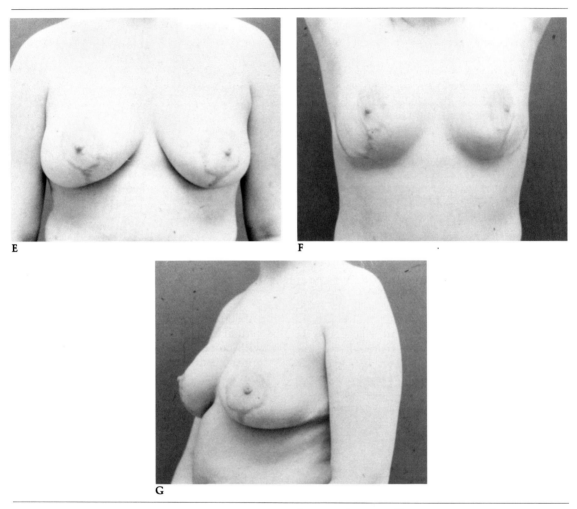

E

F

G

Fig. 19-11 (continued). E–G. One year after correction.

Complications and Disadvantages

Complications are about the same as with any breast reduction technique of proven value, although on a minimal scale. Complete nipple loss has not occurred in more than three thousand cases. Partial areolar necrosis occurred in three cases of very large reductions. Scar revision is required in about 10 percent of the cases, mainly periareolar, in young firm breasts. Usually scars are hypertrophic, in these cases for a few months, followed by resolution. It is advisable to wait at least 1 year for revision of scars (Fig. 19-11).

Shape revision has been done in 5 percent of cases and consisted mainly of correction of bulginess of the medial quadrants or flatness of the lateral lower quadrant. These deformities are often temporary, and one should not attempt to correct them before 1 or 2 years. Bulging of the medial quadrants is corrected by removing some excess deep tissues and excess skin at the lower vertical scar and sometimes, in the medial periareolar area. Removing a small triangle of skin medially to the lower curve is sometimes useful. Flatness of the lower lateral quadrant is due to removal of too much deep tissue in this location. It may be corrected by a complete revision of the whole operation, excising all scars and dissecting the deep tissues to be able to move a deep flap from the medial and central part of the breast to the lateral part of the B. In case the flatness may be extreme, it may be necessary to insert an implant.

In addition to the complications just mentioned, other disadvantages include:

1. The necessity for defined measurement and marking, especially the upper and medial limits of the areola, which are final and determine the location of the nipple-areola complex.
2. The suturing of unequal edges may seem uneasy to be handled satisfactorily. The foldings that appear may look unpleasant in the early postoperative period. Although they disappear in a few weeks, it is better to warn the patients about the evolution before surgery.

B technique advantages are numerous:

1. It is a very safe technique because it preserves a large area of periareolar dermis with vascularization and innervation to the nipple-areola complex. The absence of skin undermining and the absence of suprapectoral undermining of the upper quadrants also preserve vascularization and innervation to the gland.
2. The operating time is short once the markings and local infiltration are done. In the authors' hands, it takes about 1 hour for a moderate reduction to be completed on both sides.
3. The use of local anesthesia alone is possible owing to simplicity of the dissection of tissues.
4. This technique is universal for all kinds of breast reductions up to about 1500 ml as well as for mastopexies and asymmetries. It is the ideal technique for the correction of asymmetry requiring a unilateral reduction, since all the landmarks are taken exactly from the normal breast. The volume difference may be estimated easily once the lower flap has partially been separated from the medial, upper, and lower areas.
5. Postoperative pain has been minimal most of the time, rarely requiring sedatives, probably because of the very limited amount of undermining.
6. Durability of the results is excellent, and the natural look of the breast remains with aging, with no tendency to secondary flatness of the upper quadrants or secondary upward migration of the nipple-areola complex.

Selected Readings

Aufricht, G. Mammaplasty for pendulous breasts: Empiric and geometric planning. *Plast. Reconstr. Surg.* 4:13, 1949.

Dufourmentel, C., and Mouly, R. *Chirurgie Plastique* Paris: Flammarion, 1959. Pp. 325–359.

Dufourmentel, C., and Mouly, R. Dévelopements Récents de la plastie mammaire par la méthode oblique latérale. *Ann Chir. Plast.* 10:227, 1965.

Dufourmentel, C., and Mouly R. Modification of "periwinkle shell operation" for small ptotic breast. *Plast. Reconstr. Surg.* 41:523, 1968.

Letterman, G., and Schutter, M. Facilitation of the upward advancement of the nipple areola complex in reduction mammaplasty by Kiel resection. *Plast. Reconstr. Surg.* 67:793, 1981.

Marc, H. La plastique mammaire par la méthode oblique, L'imprimerie centrale commerciale. Paris: J. London Imp., 1952.

Marchac, D., and De Olarto, G. Reduction mammaplasty and correction of ptosis with a short inframammary scar. *Plast. Reconstr. Surg.* 69:45, 1982.

Meyer R., and Kesselring, U. Reduction mammaplasty with an L-shaped suture line. *Plast. Reconstr. Surg.* 55:139, 1975.

Peixoto, G. Reduction mammaplasty: A personal technique. *Plast. Reconstr. Surg.* 65:217, 1980.

Pitanguy, I. Surgical treatment of breast hypertrophy. *Br. J. Plast. Surg.* 20:78, 1967.

Pitanguy, I. Breast hypertrophy transactions, 5th International Congress of Plastic Reconstruction Surgery. Melbourne: Butterworths, 1971. Pp. 1180–1187.

Regnault, P. Breast Reduction. In J.Q. Owsley and R. Peterson (eds.), *Symposium on Aesthetic Surgery of the Breast.* St Louis: Mosby, 1968.

Regnault, P. Reduction mammaplasty by the B technique. *Plast. Reconstr. Surg.* 53:19, 1974.

Regnault, P. Reduction Mammaplasty by the B Technique. In R.M. Goldwyn (ed.), *Plastic and Reconstructive Surgery of the Breast.* Boston: Little, Brown, 1976. Pp. 269–285.

Regnault, P. Gigantomastia by the B technique. *Aesth. Plast. Surg.* I:115, 1977.

Regnault, P. Breast reduction B technique update. *Plast.*

Reconstr. Surg. 65:840, 1980.

Schatten, W., and Hartley J. Jr. Reduction mammaplasty by the Dufourmentel-Mouly method. *Plast. Reconstr. Surg.* 48:306, 1971.

Strömbeck, J.O. Mammaplasty: Report of a new technique based on a two pedicle procedure. *Br. J. Plast. Surg.* 13:79, 1960.

Strömbeck, J.O. Late Results after Reduction Mammaplasty. In R.M. Goldwyn (ed.), *Long-Term Results in Plastic Surgery.* Boston: Little, Brown, 1980. P. 722.

Strömbeck, J.O., and Rosato, F.E. *Reduction Mammaplasty in Surgery of the Breast.* New York: Thieme, 1986. Pp. 277–311.

COMMENTS ON CHAPTER 19   *Jean-M. Parenteau*

When I began doing breast reductions and mastopexies at the start of my practice in 1968, I looked for a technique that could be used safely in large reductions and give a pleasant aesthetic result in skin lifting–type mastopexy, with and without the need for a prosthesis. The Biesenberger technique gave excellent cosmetic results but seemed to be accompanied by a high ratio of complications; others, such as the Strömbeck method, gave, in my hands, less-than-hoped-for cosmetic results. Before 1968, most reductions were of the anchor or inverted T-shape incisions, giving me a median scar too obvious even when the patient was wearing a bra.

While questioning these facts and watching with critical eyes the immediate and longer term results of surgeons around me, Paule Regnault exposed me to her way of doing the reductions with the B technique. Working at the same surgical clinic, I observed her surgery and was convinced to at least try her way in breast reductions. The immediate results were obviously pleasant with minimal scars (a must for aesthetic surgeons) and the surgery was efficiently performed (as Regnault does) — blood loss and length of time being minimal.

Graciously, Regnault came over for the markings in my first cases and assisted me a couple of times. Without this help, I doubt that I would have persisted in doing this technique because some difficulty existed in understanding the measurements and then executing the surgery.

I believe that what makes this technique so interesting in performing is also what makes it difficult — that is, its ability to adapt itself to various cases and circumstances. The experience and personal judgment of the individual surgeon play a most important factor. To me, the technique's main qualities are versatility, maneuverability, and adaptability, with minimal permanent scarring.

I now use it exclusively for all my cases of breast reductions (the largest has been resection of 1300 gm of tissue in one breast) and mastopexies, with and without reductions and supplemented, if necessary, in the latter cases, by breast augmentation with a prosthesis placed immediately under the pectoral muscle. Since 1968, I have done more than 1000 breast reductions of all sizes, shapes, asymmetries, age group, and so on.

This most excellent review of the B technique by Regnault and Daniel leaves little to add. The paragraphs on markings and surgical technique make clear what can be difficult to understand. A strong point is made when they insist on taking the measurements of the new upper limit of the periareolar skin instead of the new nipple-site location. Of course there are slight differences between their way and mine, if not in the essence of the text, then in technical details. Personally I like the nipple diameter larger than 4 cm, so my measurements of the nipple will vary from 4.5 cm to even larger than 6.5 cm. I find it difficult to reduce a nipple from more than 12 cm in diameter (which happens) to a radical sizing down. Also, a longer perimeter of the areola helps in the closure.

My measurement of point M, that is, the median periareolar marking, is never less than 10 cm, knowing that it is so much easier to correct a nipple that appears too laterally than too medially placed.

The marking of my new submammary fold might not be as high as 4 cm. Very little is to be added in the description of the surgical technique except for minor preferences (i.e., use of subcuticular sutures with Prolene instead of absorbable sutures and the immediate use of a soft bra as a dressing).

My patients are warned about the danger of smoking, which results in more frequent skin necrosis, and are advised strongly to quit smoking previous to surgery.

I would not pretend that the B technique for breast reductions is the ultimate and exclusive way, but I believe that its advantages outweigh its inconveniences once one understands the measurements and the principle of the rotating flaps. It has given me satisfaction both in ease of execution and cosmetic results.

SELECTED READING
Parenteau, J.M., and Regnault, P. The Regnault "B" technique in mastopexy and breast reduction: A 12-year review. *Aesth. Plast. Surg.* 13:75, 1989.

20

Jean-Pierre Lalardrie

The Dermal Vault Technique

In every reduction mammaplasty, the operative techniques involve the three structural components of the breast: (1) the mammary gland or mass—the "content"—consisting of glandular or fatty tissue; (2) the skin—the "container"; and (3) the nipple-areola complex—the "keystone" of the mammary vault.

The Mammary Gland

In regard to the mammary gland, two conditions must be fulfilled: correction of the residual mammary volume and total vascular security.

CORRECT RESIDUAL MAMMARY VOLUME

The golden rule here is "what is left is more important than what is removed." Without a correct residual volume, a good result can never be achieved. It has always been a matter of some surprise to me that this is so seldom emphasized in the literature. What is required is a technique in which no limit is placed on resection by the vascularization of the tissues. This technique now exists; it combines quasitotal subcutaneous mammectomy with cutaneous remodeling.

TOTAL VASCULAR SECURITY

Ensuring vascular security is now an easy matter, provided that the subdermal cutaneous vascularization, which alone is constant and fully effective, is respected; vascularization may be cranial or caudal in origin.

Anatomically, it has been demonstrated that the retromammillary glandular vessels over a thickness of 1 cm are instrumental in safeguarding the nipple-areola complex, since the fatty plane is not present at this level—hence, the importance of ensuring cutaneous continuity with the areola and of leaving a glandular thickness of at least 1 cm behind it.

A nipple vascularized solely by a dermal flap would simply not be viable, since the vascularization is subdermal; a "dermal flap" would be disastrous technically, and it is hoped that those who use this term are simply using incorrect terminology.

Controversial Aspects of Reduction Mammaplasty

Aside from these two imperatives, there are four other practices whose merits are still being discussed and debated: intercutaneoglandular undermining, choice of a glandular resection, glandular suspension, and glandular remodeling.

INTERCUTANEOGLANDULAR UNDERMINING

Intercutaneoglandular undermining was a common operational practice from the 1930s to the 1960s but is seldom desirable. Not only does it destroy the embryologic and anatomic cutaneoglandular unity, it also severs Cooper's ligaments, which are essential to glandular suspension.

CHOICE OF GLANDULAR RESECTION

Whether the resection should be external, upper, lower, and so on, is still hotly debated. My preference is for a homogeneous resection over the entire surface, leaving, in the case of major hypertrophies, a central glandular stump with a volume of about 100 ml and a thickness of 2 cm; this is normally sufficient to give a harmonious residual volume.

GLANDULAR SUSPENSION

It is my view that the only effective suspension is that provided by the skin.

Glandular Remodeling

Attempts to remodel the gland by means of "tucks" and "periwinkle shell devices" have all, in the long run, proved disappointing, since the gland, particularly in the younger woman, is inherently plastic and the most ingenious constructions tend ultimately to collapse.

The Skin

In regard to the skin, there are the following two imperatives:

1. The need for a perfect match between skin and gland. The prime aim of any mammaplasty is to reduce the breast to an appropriate volume and to tailor the cutaneous surface to fit. Preoperative markings will be of scant use in determining the cutaneous resection, since the glandular resection has not yet been made. It would be putting the cart before the horse! No one would deny the value of preoperative markings as a precautionary measure, particularly for the inexperienced practitioner.
2. The need to keep scar length to a minimum and to ensure that scars are discreetly placed. I am constantly amazed that the literature so seldom makes mention of this obvious requirement. One way of minimizing scar length is to adjust the cutaneous resection around the areola, although this solution is admittedly not ideal. It is important that the scars be sited discreetly so that they are concealed by the scantiest brassiere; this rules out "anchor" scars or scars that project too far out to the side. My own preference is for an inverted T scar, with an extremely short internal branch.

Although the lateral approach has its merits in reducing scar length, I tend to favor the lower vertical approach.

Dermopexy depends on the quality of the dermodermal adhesions. These serve to reinforce the glandular suspension through the skin and glandular connections. It has been demonstrated that dermodermal adhesions are more effective than dermofatty or dermomuscular adhesions.

The Nipple-Areola Complex

The imperative for the nipple-areola complex is to place it properly at the end of the operation to avoid unfortunate dysmorphies. It is important to reduce the distance between the areola and the submammary fold since the areola should point slightly downward at the end of the operation.

Most techniques tend to construct the breasts by first determining the site of the areola. In my technique, I place it only at the end of the operation.

Nipple sensitivity can be a problem whatever the technique used, and no one can guarantee that it will not be affected. Some claim that the transglandular nerve can be conserved by a technique involving the lower pedicle, but I believe this to be unrealistic.

Historical Review

Before discussing my own technique — the dermal vault — which evolved from the technique of subtotal mastectomy with simultaneous prosthetic inclusion and skin modeling described in 1970, I will briefly discuss the three phases in the fascinating history of reduction mammaplasty.

Prior to 1930, surgeons were groping forward empirically. Among the famous pioneers are such great names as Morestin, De Quervain, and Aubert.

In the ensuing years, mammary surgery made a major leap forward, thanks to the work of Biesenberger. Schwarzmann was the first to realize the vascular potential of periareolar deepithelialization, but this path ultimately proved to be a dead end, since cutaneoglandular undermining implied the separation of content from container. It was misconceived from the embryologic standpoint (the breast is, after all, a cutaneous gland) and from the vascular standpoint (vascularization of the breast and nipple is essentially cutaneous) as well as pathogenically. (Its exclusive reliance on glandular remodeling often resulted in failure since the cutaneoglandular connections necessary for mammary stability were always severed.)

It was only in 1960, with Pitanguy and Strömbeck, that the unity between skin and gland came to be respected. But the type of glandular resection proposed and the fact that their techniques did not allow unlimited periareolar deepithelialization set a limit to the volume that could be resected, and breast stability could not always be guaranteed.

The techniques of Skoog and the subsequent development of subcutaneous mammectomies that presented no risk to the areola and nipple laid the groundwork for reduction mammaplasty as it is practiced today.

The 1970s saw the emergence of a variety of techniques, all of which rely on subdermal cutaneous vascularization. Some of the most recent techniques conserve a lower pedicle and appear to hold great promise. My only caveat is the inherent difficulty of achieving sufficiently short scars.

The Technique

Eighteen years have now elapsed since I first presented the dermal vault technique, and I have now performed it on about 2,500 patients with hypertrophic or ptotic breasts and on about 200 patients who required remodeling of the contralateral breast in cases of reconstruction after amputation. I can safely claim that the technique is suitable for all cases of mammary hypertrophy and ptosis.

In cases of hypertrophy, glandular resection can be unlimited and the reduction can be tailored to the patient's morphology. The only contraindication might be a rigid gland where there is a risk of subsequent concavity of the nipple-areola complex. This problem could be obviated by reducing the thickness of the glandular flap bearing the nipple-areola complex, since a thinner flap is more supple.

The technique is eminently suited to cases of ptosis, since the nipple-areola complex may be raised by as much as 15 cm through extensive deepithelialization.

DESCRIPTION

No preoperative markings as such are made. The patient is placed in a three-quarters sitting position and the surgeon traces:

1. The breast meridian (which will not pass through the nipple if this is off-center) (Fig. 20-1).
2. An areolar circle (radius 2 to 2.2 cm).
3. A circle indicating the extent of deepithelialization (radius 5 to 7 cm); its radius is determined in the same way as the vertical excision in Biesenberger's technique.

In cases of substantial ptosis, the upper part of the outer circle is extended into an ellipse, bringing the upper pole to a point 14 to 16 cm from the midclavicle (see Fig. 20-1). The skin between the two circles is then deepithelialized. The breast is raised by a retracting suture or skin hook placed above the areola (Fig. 20-2). The skin is cut on the breast meridian between the lower pole of the outer circle and the inframammary fold. On either side of the incision, the skin is separated from the gland sufficiently to free the lower part of the

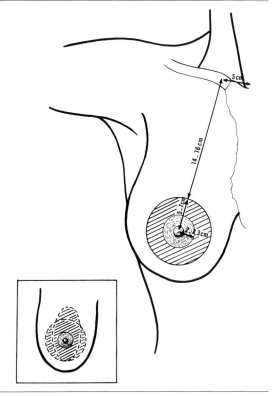

Fig. 20-1. Preoperative markings showing the extent of deepithelialization. The circle of deepithelialization is made oval in cases of serious ptosis.

gland (see Fig. 20-2). The cut is extended along the semicircumference of the outer circle.

The gland is now cut horizontally 1 cm below the lower pole of the areola, over the whole width of the area freed. When the depth of the incision reaches 1 to 1.5 cm, the upper lip is raised by a suture. The surgeon holds this lip between the index and forefinger of one hand while placing the other two fingers on the surface of the breast; he then turns his hand so that the palm is toward him. The surgeon now places the scalpel in the existing incision and cuts the gland parallel to its surface. This gives a slice whose thickness may be controlled by the surgeon's opposite hand, and the gland to be resected falls progressively (Fig. 20-3).

The remaining cutaneoglandular thickness must be homogenous but thicker at the center than at the periphery. The scalpel is brought toward the surface of the gland, first laterally then at the level of the upper pole, but once the surgeon

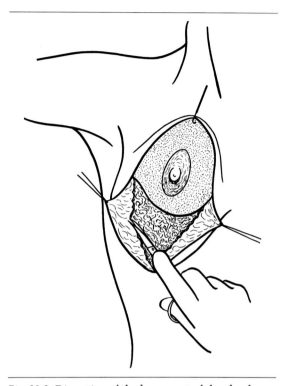

Fig. 20-2. Dissection of the lower part of the gland.

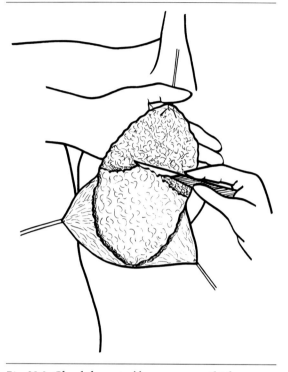

Fig. 20-3. Glandular cut of homogeneous thickness, leaving a glandular disk of controlled thickness.

reaches the fatty tissue, he must be careful not to come too near the skin. With practice, the surgeon can use his left hand to gauge both the thickness of the cut and its homogeneity. This is important in that it can ensure equal resection of the two breasts. If the breasts are not identical, a symmetric result may be achieved without having to weigh the resected gland or having to operate simultaneously on both breasts.

This resection is, in a sense, a subtotal mastectomy. The new breast is formed from a dermal and fatty thickness and a glandular stump. When hypertrophy is considerable, the latter is confined to the central area, and there is no gland at the periphery; the volume of the glandular stump determines the residual mammary volume. When hypertrophy is moderate, however, some gland must be left over the whole surface of the cut, especially at the upper pole; there is also a need for complete undermining between the gland and the pectoral muscle. In major hypertrophies, this is done automatically in the course of glandular resection.

The glandular stump and nipple remain vascularized by the subdermal blood supply from the cutaneous vessels of the external mammary, acromiothoracic, and internal mammary arteries. The technique respects subdermal vascularization and is, hence, totally safe.

In remodeling the skin, the upper edge of the areola is brought to the top of the deepithelialized area (Fig. 20-4). Two points situated 6 to 8 cm from this point on the edges of this area are brought together by a temporary suture at point B. Any invagination of the skin edges immediately below point B may be corrected by deepithelialization. The lower skin flaps are then brought forward and pulled toward the front and sides (Fig. 20-5). A curved clamp, similar to that used in McIndoe's operation, is now applied (Fig. 20-6). The skin of the two flaps is cut along the line of the clamp. In cutting the skin, the dermis should be preserved, since this makes for a better suture through dermodermal adhesion; a glandular suture is out of the question, since no gland is left at the lower pole.

The horizontal skin resection is performed in the usual way, but the central part of the lower

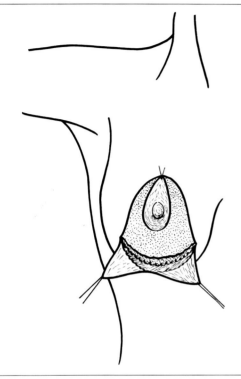

Fig. 20-4. Elevation of the nipple. Folding of the upper zone of deepithelialization.

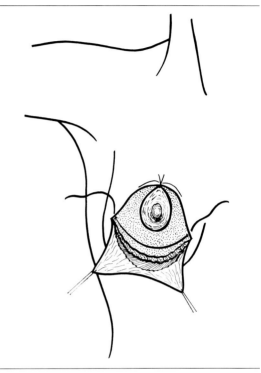

Fig. 20-5. The edges of the circle of deepithelialization are brought together at a point determined by the surgeon.

edge must be accurately placed in the submammary fold. The skin excision should be horizontal and not curved upward; in this way, it will be invisible and there will be no keloid scarring at the extremities. Any internal skin resection should be reduced to a minimum.

The final step involves a further area of deepithelialization to bring down the lower edge of the areola to a point 4 to 5 cm from the inframammary fold (Fig. 20-7). This has the advantage of bringing skin tension to bear on the areola—enhancing breast stability—but can cause puckering around the areola suture in the case of major reductions. Although the puckering usually disappears after a few weeks, it can lead to scars that tend to widen.

The suture is now cut, and a dermoglandular cylinder comes forward (Fig. 20-8); the greater the ptosis, the longer the cylinder. This cylinder constitutes the whole volume of the remaining breast, and its invagination creates the "dermal vault", (Fig. 20-9) which has given its name to this technique, even though it is by no means the unique feature of the operation. The vault is formed by

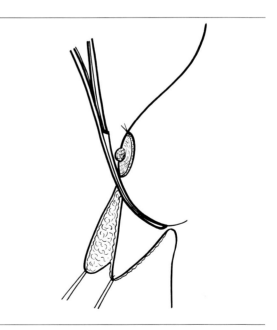

Fig. 20-6. A curved clamp is applied. Vertical cutaneous resection.

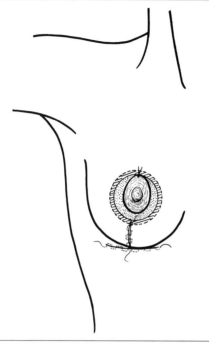

Fig. 20-7. Secondary deepithelialization for final positioning of the "key" of areolar vault. Horizontal cutaneous suture with external lift of the lower edge.

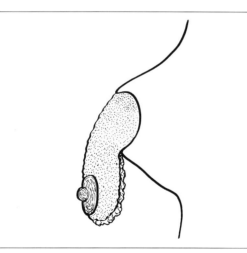

Fig. 20-8. Exteriorization of the dermoglandular cylinder.

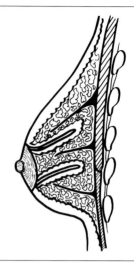

Fig. 20-9. Cross-section. The dermal glandular cylinder constituting the dermal vault is re-invaginated.

dermodermal adhesion and serves to create the breast mound. Drainage is normal practice in the operation and may be left in place for 48 hours.

Elastic adhesive bandages or steri-drapes are used as a dressing and are changed a week later. Two to 3 weeks after the operation, the intradermal sutures are removed.

Discussion

It is perhaps appropriate here to call attention to some of the merits of the technique as well as to some minor drawbacks.

Its main merit is the absolute vascular security that it provides, since the subcutaneous vascularization is respected with the preservation of a large superior pedicle. It also ensures excellent vascularization of the glandular stump and the nipple-areola complex. I have so far operated on 5,200 breasts and have experienced only one case of partial areolar necrosis following a resection of 2.3 kg. Anatomic studies carried out since 1970 have confirmed the existence and consistency of subdermal vascularization from the acromiothoracic artery as well as the internal and external mammary arteries.

A further advantage is the unlimited glandular resection that the technique affords. Many techniques do not permit sufficient reduction in the case of large breasts, and although some surgeons

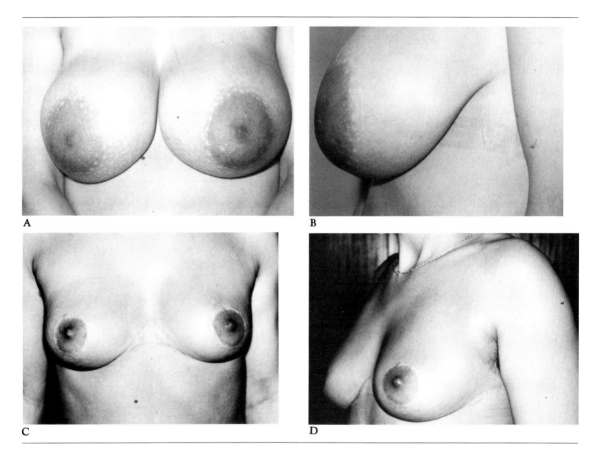

Fig. 20-10. A, B. A patient with mammary hypertrophy. C, D. Ten years postoperative; 1300 gm of tissue was removed from the right breast and 1450 from the left breast.

exculpate themselves on the grounds that they are simply respecting the patient's preference, this, for me, is a poor excuse. The breast should be adapted to the patient's build, and if she is overweight, she should be encouraged to slim down.

The technique provides a pleasing form, evoking more an apple than a pear (Figs. 20-10 and 20-11). Use of the curved clamp will help achieve an ideal match between the skin (the container) and the glandular stump (the content). The technique is hence eminently suitable for correcting mammary asymmetry. Another feature is the remarkable stability of the new breast. If the breast is to remain stable, the forward projection should never be greater than one third of the diameter of the mammary base. If this is so, a brassiere is nor-

mally unnecessary (provided that the breast does not undergo variations in volume as a result of pregnancy, slimming, and so on).

The dermal vault technique is inherently "plastic" and flexible, leaving the surgeon's hands free to the end of the operation. The absence of preoperative markings has already been noted, and the initial marking — indicating the first area of deepithelialization — is no more than a guideline; adjustments are possible at the stage of periareolar deepithelialization. This said, a step-by-step approach is imperative to avoid any resection, whether glandular or cutaneous, that would irrevocably compromise the outcome.

One last advantage that deserves mention is that scars are quite short and discreetly placed. All too often in other techniques, the submammary scar is too long, extending too high into the mammary cleft and into the axillary area. My technique creates a true inverted T scar, with the internal branch as short as possible.

300

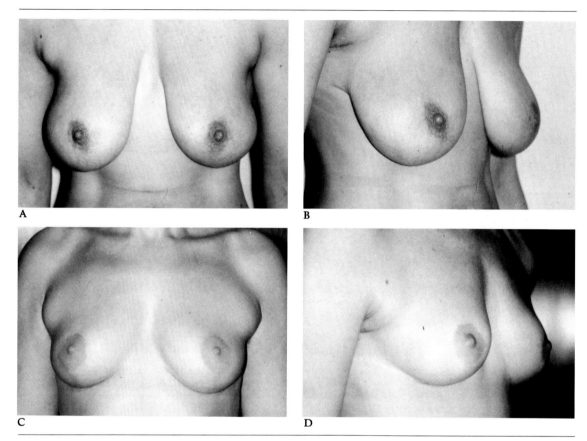

Fig. 20-11. A, B. Patient with mammary ptosis. C, D. Eight years postoperative; 345 gm of tissue was removed from the right breast and 320 gm from the left breast.

I would never claim that the technique is totally problem-free. Its very simplicity can make it difficult to execute, especially by a novice. Only after having seen many such operations and having performed a number oneself can one hope to achieve a perfect result. But cannot the same be said of all techniques?

The scars, particularly the periareolar scar, may be of poor quality. In the early days, my prime concern was to reduce the length of the submammary scar by means of extensive secondary deepithelialization. One unfortunate result was a wide periareolar scar. This problem has been remedied by diminishing the area of secondary deepithelialization, although the submammary scar is necessarily longer. When ptosis is particularly marked, the two scars may in fact meet in a single horizontal scar. Many may disagree, but I prefer this to scars that rise into the mammary cleft. Returning to the question of scar quality, it should be noted that the ingestion of estrogens, especially oral con-

traceptives, can produce a hypertrophic reaction. I always ask patients to refrain from taking estrogens 2 months before the operation and not to resume them until 6 to 12 months after surgery.

One last problem is the risk of nipple hypesthesia or anesthesia as a result of the operation. Although lactation has never presented any problem (it is well known that a smaller breast lactates better than a hypertrophic breast), in about 5 percent of cases, there has been a temporary or permanent loss of specific nipple sensation. In most cases of anesthesia, the phenomenon affected one breast only and I am at a loss to explain why.

To conclude this discussion of the dermal vault technique and to help the novice avoid a number of pitfalls, I will point out some of the specific problems that may be encountered in its performance:

1. In tracing the preoperative markings, the line of the outer circle will depend on the degree of hypertrophy and ptosis; it is important not to remove too much skin at the outset. The outer circle serves to reposition the nipple-areola complex when this is too medial.
2. Especially when there is initial asymmetry, it may be difficult to determine the volume of gland to be resected from the second breast. Weighing resected tissue is not going to solve the problem! If the volume of the second breast is insufficient at the end of the operation, extra volume can be provided by using a dermofatty flap from the mammary and thoracic skin as proposed by Longacre.
3. The technique cannot correct a supermammary preaxillary adipose cushion, but if present, this may be removed by excision leaving a scar in the natural preaxillary skin fold. The scar is normally invisible.
4. Perhaps the most difficult aspect of the operation for the inexperienced surgeon is the placing of the curved clamp. I would not be so bold as to lay down hard-and-fast rules for all cases but simply offer a few words of advice:

   a. Avoid excessive tension on skin edges since this impairs the quality of the vertical scar.
   b. Do not take up too much skin in the clamp since the end of the clamp determines the position of the future submammary sulcus, which, in turn, determines that of the nipple-areola complex.
   c. Avoid placing the curved clamp too horizontally (with the risk of too great a reduction of the mammary base and secondary ptosis) or too vertically (risk of too extensive a mammary base and too great a distance between the inframammary sulcus and areola).

5. Care must be taken to secure the superior edge of the submammary sulcus to the underlying muscle to avoid glandular laxation in the postoperative phase.
6. The complementary areolar deepithelialization

must not be too extensive, since this could create excessive skin tension and, hence, a poor-quality periareolar scar.

Conclusion

Although it is not without its problems for the inexperienced surgeon, the dermal vault technique is inherently simple in its conception, affording absolute vascular security and allowing unlimited glandular resection. In its respect for the unity of skin and gland achieved through a subdermal superior vascular pedicle, it represents a synthesis of modern techniques.

Selected Readings

Georgiade, N.G. Aesthetic Breast Surgery. Baltimore: Williams & Wilkins, 1983. P. 408.

Georgiade, N.G., Serafin, D., Morris, R., et al. Reduction mammaplasty utilising an inferior pedicle nipple-areolar flap. Ann. Plast. Surg. 3:211, 1979.

Georgiade, N.G., Serafin, D., Riefkhol, R., et al. Is there a reduction mammaplasty for "all seasons"? Plast. Reconst. Surg. 63:765, 1979.

Lalardrie, J.P. The "dermal vault" technique. Reduction mammaplasty for hypertrophy with ptosis. Transacta der III Tagung der Vereinigung der Deutschen plastichen. Köln: Chirurgen, 1972. Pp. 105–108.

Lalardrie, J.P. Reduction mammaplasty by "dermal vault" technique after 425 cases. Transactions of the Sixth International Congress of IPRS. Paris: Masson, 1976. Pp. 519–523.

Lalardrie, J.P., and Jouglard, J.P. In D. Marchac and J.T. Hueston (eds.), Chirurgie Plastique du Sein. Paris: Masson, 1974. P. 290, Fig. 142.

Lalardrie, J.P., and Morel-Fatio, D. Mammectomie totale souscutanée suivie de reconstruction immédiate ou secondaire. Mém. Acad. Chir. 96:651, 1970.

McKissock, P.K. Reduction mammaplasty with a vertical dermal flap. Plast. Reconstr. Surg. 49:245, 1972.

Pitanguy, I. Breast hypertrophy. Transactions of the second International Congress of Plastic and Reconstructive Surgery, London. Edinburgh: Livingstone, 1960. Pp. 509–522.

Skoog, T. A technique of breast reduction. Acta Chir. Scand. 126:453, 1963.

Strömbeck, J.O. Mammaplasty: Report of a new technique based on the two pedicle procedure. Br. J. Plast. Surg. 13:79, 1960.

COMMENTS ON CHAPTER 20   *Robert M. Goldwyn*

Lalardrie's description of his "dermal vault" procedure for reduction mammaplasty reveals the considerable thought he has given to his conception and execution. This quality of thinking is one that is not an attribute possessed by all surgeons, unfortunately. The book that Lalardrie authored with his confrere Jouglard [4] should be read by every surgeon performing reduction mammaplasty because their analysis and classification of various techniques provides a much needed perspective.

Lalardrie's dermal vault method utilizes the principles of subcutaneous mastectomy and applies them to breast reduction. The nipple-areola survives because of its subdermal vascularization. Lalardrie makes the important distinction, which most of us who are less precise usually do not, between "dermal" and "subdermal." Most pedicles that we call dermal, as in the superior dermal technique for breast reduction, have the more important subdermal arteries and veins in addition to the strictly intradermal extensions of those vessels, which are much less important and by themselves would unlikely nurture the nipple-areola.

The advantages that Lalardrie [3] claims for his technique are that it permits unlimited resection (as for breasts with significant hypertrophy and ptosis); it provides vascular safety for the nipple-areola; it avoids intercutaneous-glandular undermining; it minimizes the length of the horizontal scar because it involves skin resection around the areola; it allows dermis-to-dermis healing, which maintains breast shape; it permits unchanged or adequate sensation in 95 percent of patients; and it frees the surgeon from predetermined markings so that he or she can have the latitude to obtain an optimal result as dictated by interoperative events.

To many surgeons, the last advantage of giving freedom carries also the disadvantage of not furnishing security, especially for the inexperienced surgeon, who, Lalardrie admits, is liable to find the dermal vault difficult at first, even though it is "inherently simple in its conception."

In commenting on their experience with this procedure, Maillard, Montandon, and Goin [5] wrote:

The technique has no advantage over the others in cases of moderate hypertrophy and ptoses — it is more complex and time consuming. . . The shape is often difficult to form: the deepithelialized cylinder is fragile and the use of the clamp is traumatic, especially when placed several times. When we first began using this technique, inadequate glandular resection was frequent. Periareolar scar widening is possible and often needs revision.

The obvious paradox is that the beginner needs experience before being able to perform the procedure well without anxiety or error. This is true, obviously, with learning every new operation.

One of the advantages of Lalardrie's technique is the short inverted T, placed "discretely." In the patient shown in Figure 20-10, who had a large reduction, however, the medial and lateral extensions are visible. This perhaps picayune point aside, the more important question is, practically speaking, how much effort should be expended to minimize or eliminate the horizontal scar, when other methods with which the surgeon is familiar give comparable results except for the submammary scar? Each surgeon must answer that for himself or herself. This query becomes even more compelling if, in reducing the length or, ideally, the presence of the submammary scar, we produce worse scarring around the areola, as seems to be the drawback in this method, a point Lalardrie also honestly makes. Even with the most imaginative intradermal suturing, one cannot usually prevent the spreading and possible hypertrophy of the periareolar scar if there had been significant tension at the time of closure.

In reporting their experience with the dermal vault procedure in 100 patients selected randomly from 250 patients done between 1969 and 1979, Forli et al [2] found that the average distance between the medial end of the horizontal scar of one breast and that of the other was 10.6 cm, with 55 percent of patients in the range of 10 to 20 cm. Almost all patients were able to wear décolleté clothes. The length of the horizontal scar both laterally and medially, however, varies with the amount of tissue removed, which is usually related to the degree of hypertrophy. In general, larger breasts require larger excision and the result of horizontal scar will be longer. The article by Forli and co-authors unfortunately failed to give data of weight removed, but it is interesting that the authors thought that they have left too much tissue in one of every three patients.

Regarding nipple-areola sensitivity, Forli et al [2] found it unchanged in 50 percent of patients; therefore, it must have been altered in the other 50 percent. None of these 100 patients had nipple necrosis; only one developed partial necrosis of areola, none requiring revision or reconstruction. This confirms one of the virtues of this technique: vascular security for the nipple and areola.

Regarding scars, Forli et al [2] concluded that in 40 percent of patients, the scar around the areola and the scar that was vertical were of "poor quality." To get better scarring in those areas, the authors proposed better subcutaneous and intradermal closure as well as adhesive tape support for 2 months postoperatively.

In another study, Dreant et al [1] reported their results with the dermal vault procedure, but they varied it by citing the nipple-areola with fixed markings preoperatively. However, they modified Lalardrie's procedure in other ways, so that their results cannot be considered a true evaluation of the procedure as described in this chapter by its innovator. One point, however, in that article is relevant: If one tries to eliminate the medial extension of the horizontal incision in an effort to get a better scar, postoperatively the patient may have ptosis medially — namely, a bulge.

In summary, the dermal vault technique as described and performed by Lalardrie gives consistently good results, but other surgeons may have trouble with the technique until they gain sufficient experience. Knowing where to apply the clamp is difficult to learn at first, but even more important, in patients with significant hypertrophy, ending with a truly short horizontal incision without producing prominent periareolar or vertical scarring remains a challenge, at least for surgeons who lack Lalardrie's experience.

REFERENCES

1. Dreant, J., Magalon, G., Latil, F., and Bureau, H. Un procédéde correction de l'hypertrophie mammaire par la voûte dermique avec dessin pré-établi. A propos 180 cas. *Ann. Chir. Plast.* 24:231, 1979.
2. Forli, V., Carlin, G., Echinard, Ch., and Jougliard, J.-P. Étude critique de 100 mammoplasties de reduction par la méthode de la voûte dermique. *Ann. Chir. Plast.* 25:241, 1980.
3. Lalardrie, J.-P. Reduction Mammoplasty: The "Dermal Vault" Technique. In N.G. Georgiade, (ed.), *Aesthetic Breast Surgery.* Baltimore: Williams & Wilkins, 1983. Pp. 166–174.
4. Lalardrie, J.-P., and Jouglard, J.-P. *Chirurgie Plastique du Sein.* Paris: Masson et cie, 1974. Pp. 115–121.
5. Maillard, G.F., Montandon, D., and Goin, J.-L. *Plastic Reconstructive Breast Surgery.* Paris: Masson, 1983. P. 106.

21

*Ulrich Kesselring and
Rodolphe Meyer*

Reduction Mammaplasty with L-Shaped Suture Line

Today, reduction mammaplasty must be not only an operation to give relief from an overweight breast but must also produce an aesthetically pleasing result. For this reason, plastic surgeons in the early years already tried to minimize scarring and to obtain an ideal cone in the reduced and newly shaped breast [1]. The history of the evolution of reduction mammaplasty has been related comprehensively elsewhere [2] (see Chap. 1); we need not dwell on those facts.

Principles

Our technique features three important basic principles: (1) minimization of scar length, (2) volume reduction in en bloc across the whole base of the breast, and (3) diminution of the breast at its base, with elevation of the inframammary crease in many cases. Geometric patterns quite often give false security, because the parameters for a good result are just as much the skin resilience as the exact application of three-dimensional geometry. It is useful, however, to remember some elementary principles, which are discussed below.

AREOLA CIRCUMFERENCE

The circumference of a circle doubles with its diameter — that is, if one draws a concentric circle with double diameter around the areola, the half-circumference of the outer circle equals the circumference of the areola. Owing to skin resilience, we may, however, add up to about 35 degree sectors on either side and distribute this additional length over the whole arch. This maneuver helps eliminate some of the vertical skin redundancy (Fig. 21-1). By removing volume and thus diminishing vertical projection, the skin margins converge toward the areola (Fig. 21-2).

SCAR LENGTH

Because the vertical scar is a fairly standard 5 to 8 cm from the inferior areolar border to the inframammary fold, the horizontal scar length is determined by the laxity of the skin and therefore by the amount of ptosis. Volume and width of the breast influence to a much lesser degree the length of this scar (Fig. 21-3). This also means that the greater the amount of skin overhang that can be taken up toward the areola, the shorter the compensating horizontal inframammary scar will be. This principle is used by all techniques that feature a vertical scar only or a very small horizontal scar.

BREAST SHAPE

There is an antagonism between good breast shape and short scars; it may not be very important in the hypertrophic and moderately ptotic breast but can be quite frustrating in the slack long breast. This is one of the reasons why the authors of all the fascinating new modifications of old techniques rarely show this type of mammaplasty in their representative series. It has been demonstrated by Peixoto [8] and others that a breast that appears to be somewhat formless at the end of the operation can shrink down to a breast cone with a natural appearance. Here again, it is skin resilience that does the trick, and the experienced surgeon knows just how much skin redundancy he or she can leave to be taken care of by this phenomenon.

Technique

The key point for the topography of the remodeled breast is the new nipple site. Once this is determined (Fig. 21-3), everything else is planned

305

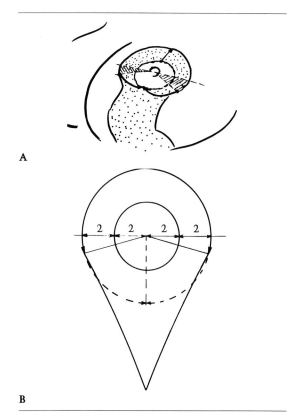

A

B

Fig. 21-1. A. The circumference of a circle doubles with its diameter. B. Skin resilience allows, however, for distribution of additional length along the areola margin, thus eliminating some vertical skin redundancy.

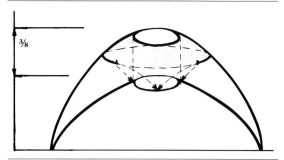

Fig. 21-2. Theoretically, such a skin resection combined with the appropriate volume reduction reduces projection by three eighths.

however, to stay away from the midsternal line by at least 7 cm.

Prior to the resection of the adipoglandular tissue, the whole periareolar and vertical areas are deepithelialized (Fig. 21-5). On the pectoro-fascial level, the gland is then bluntly undermined and mobilized along its whole width. As we pull the surface of the breast taut, the basal portion of the redundant breast tissue is resected in a parallel plane to the thorax (Fig. 21-6). Lateral wedge resections facilitate the plication of the flap and the areolapexy. To avoid undue pull on the areola, the dermal flap can cautiously be severed laterally, taking care to spare the radial vessels, which can be identified at the 10 and 2 o'clock positions (Fig. 21-7).

With a key suture at the 12 o'clock position, we pull the areola into its new site and then approximate the lateral skin borders and the areola at the 6 o'clock position with a subcutaneous resorbable suture (Fig. 21-8). At this time, the remaining adipoglandular tissue can be modeled. For this purpose, its lower portion has to be well mobilized, especially toward the sternum (Fig. 21-9). The distal portion of the nipple carrier flap is rolled beneath the nipple-areola complex and attached with a strong resorbable suture to the pectoral fascia (Fig. 21-10). If a prolonged breast-supporting function of these sutures cannot be proved, they are still very helpful to keep the newly shaped breast cone in place while the skin is being draped around it (Fig. 21-11). The skin is closed (Fig. 21-12) and the dressings are applied (Fig. 21-13).

Discussion

For almost 20 years, we have used and refined a breast reduction technique that produces short

around this center. What we have shown as a concentric circle around the areola might become an eccentric circle if the nipple was originally situated too far laterally. The principle remains the same. The vertical skin resection should be wide enough to maintain equal tension between the top and the bottom suture of this line. The horizontal resection area with its inevitably too long lower skin border needs a strongly curved upper skin border to make up partially for this difference in length (Fig. 21-4). This suture line can be placed anywhere in the inframammary fold from the sternum to the axilla. We chose to add it like the horizontal L line to the vertical suture line. If a great amount of redundant skin has to be taken up, the L gets a short medial "heel"; otherwise, the horizontal scar will reach too far laterally. We take care,

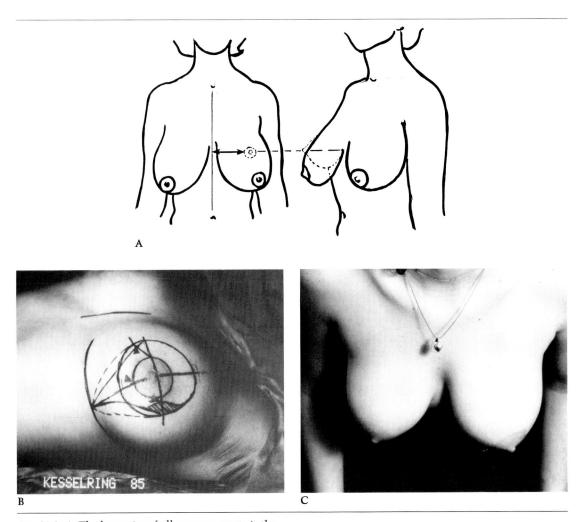

A

B

C

Fig. 21-3. A. The key point of all measurements is the
new nipple site, which is determined when the patient
is standing and usually is situated on the height of the
inframammary fold. B. The cautious beginner will not
perform the probable skin resection immediately but
will leave a security margin. C. Besides the
measurements, weight control of the resected tissue
helps to achieve a symmetrical result. For this
purpose, volume difference of the breasts has to be
assessed preoperatively; this is best done when the
patient is leaning forward.

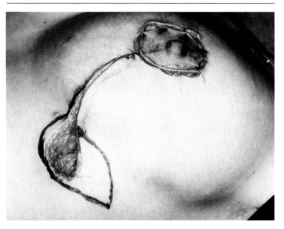

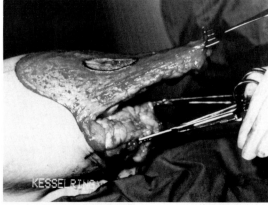

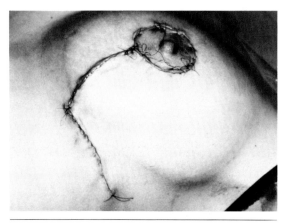

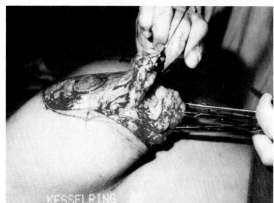

Fig. 21-4. In the L-shaped suture line, we are faced
with a lower skin border that exceeds in length its
upper counterpart. To partially make up for this
discrepancy, we perform a curved upper skin reduction.

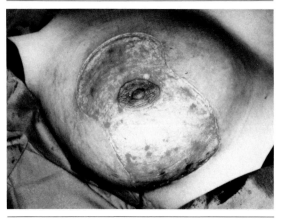

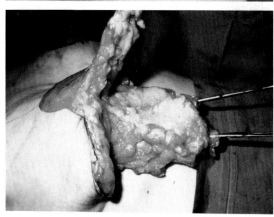

Fig. 21-6. While the nipple carrier flap is held taut, the
resection is performed in a plane parallel to the
thoracic wall—the adipoglandular tissue having been
previously mobilized from the pectoral fascia.

Fig. 21-5. Prior to the reduction of the adipoglandular
tissue, the whole periareolar and vertical area is
deepithelialized.

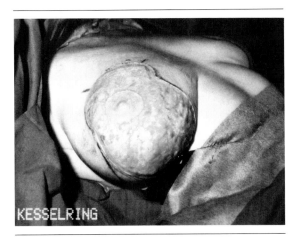

Fig. 21-7. The dermal pedicle can be severed along its margins up to about the 10 and 2 o'clock positions.

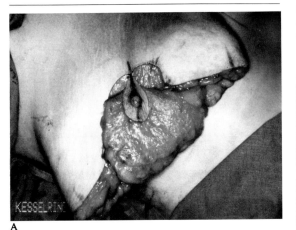

A

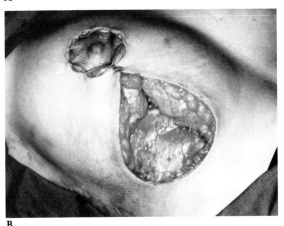

B

Fig. 21-8. The areolapexy is performed first at the 12 o'clock position (A), followed by an approximation of the lateral skin borders at the 6 o'clock position (B).

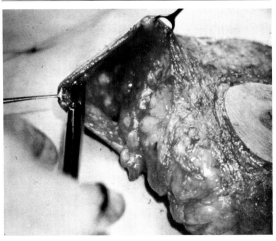

Fig. 21-9. To permit optimal shaping of the new breast cone, the remaining tissue has to be well mobilized, especially toward the sternum, where additional defatting is often beneficial.

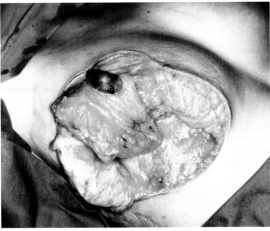

Fig. 21-10. The nipple carrier flap is rolled beneath the nipple areola complex and attached to the pectoral fascia with a strong resorbable suture (shown here prior to complete areolapexy for better view).

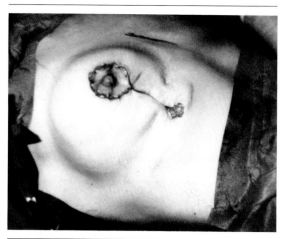

Fig. 21-11. *Once the cone is modeled, the skin can be draped around it.*

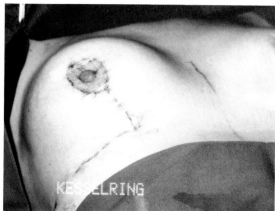

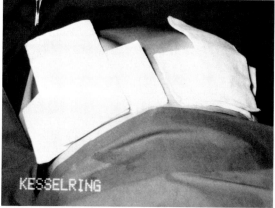

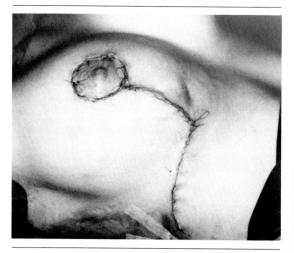

Fig. 21-12. *Closure along the planned lines is achieved in three layers: for the deep and subcutaneous layers, resorbable sutures are used; the skin is closed with intradermal running nonresorbable sutures. Single interrupted key stitches ensure a perfect approximation. In the areola, they are half buried with the knot on the areolar side.*

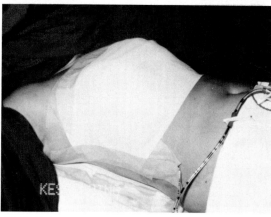

Fig. 21-13. *The dressing consists of Steri-Strip, gauze, and Sparelast bandages, which remain untouched for 10 to 14 days. The suction drainage is removed after 48 hours.*

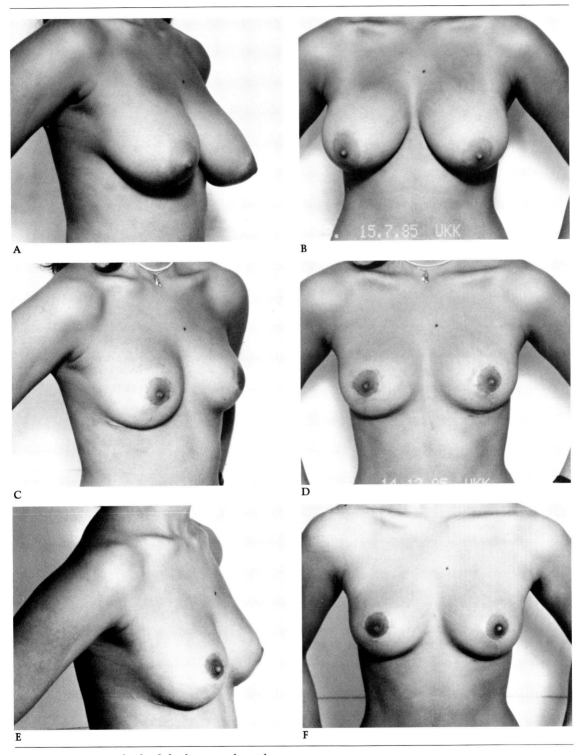

Fig. 21-14. A,B. Juvenile glandular hypertrophy and
ptosis. C,D. Postoperative result after 5 months. E,F.
Postoperative result after 2½ years.

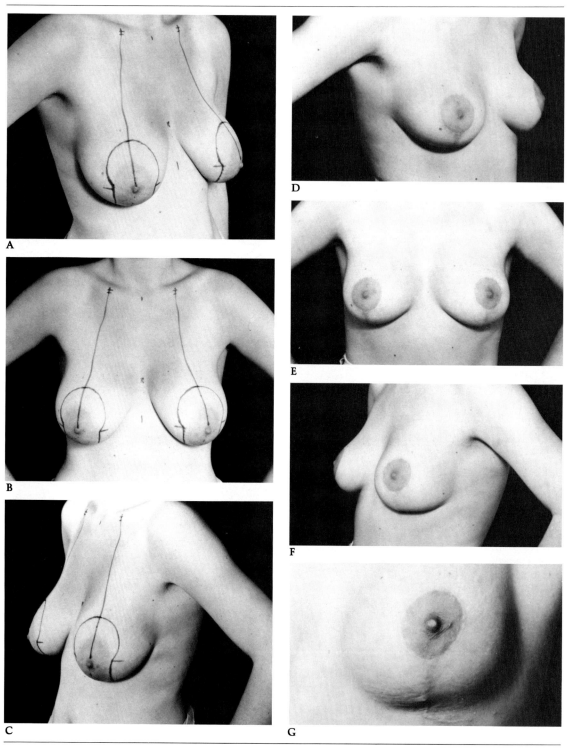

Fig. 21-15. A–C. Adipose hypertrophy and ptosis. D–F.
Result 11 months postoperative. G. The L-shaped scar
11 months postoperative.

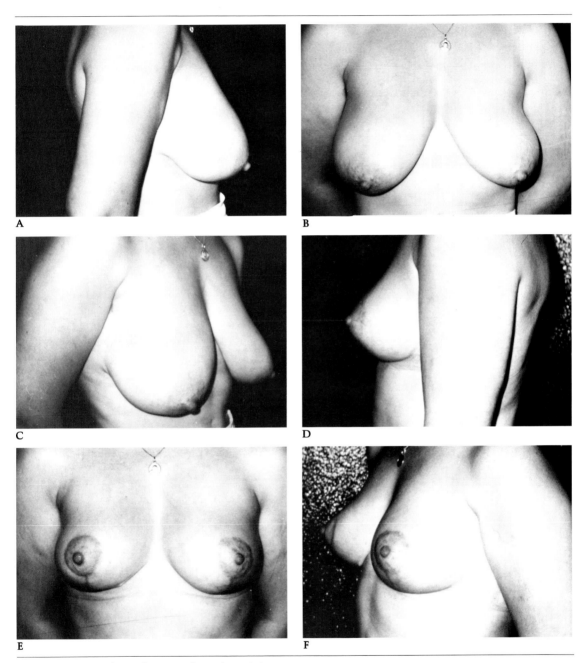

Fig. 21-16. A–C. Adipose hypertrophy and ptosis in a
middle-aged patient. D–F. Result 3 months
postoperative.

and well-concealed scars [4–7]. It is encouraging to observe that worldwide many of the more recent publications [3, 8] use the same basic principles, that is, basal volume resection, reduction of the breast base, and, of course, scar minimization. We do not believe that a single vertical scar line can give satisfactory results in any breast with more than a mild hypertrophy and ptosis. In large ptotic breasts, the amount of redundant skin will require an undue prolongation of the scar, and attempts to condense the scar will cause bad scarring. Our method is technically not easy and requires proper assessment of the breast preoperatively, precise planning, and meticulous execution. The experienced surgeon will be rewarded with a happy patient who appreciates an aesthetically pleasing breast of attractive contour and minimal scarring (Figs. 21-14 through 21-16).

References

1. Holländer E. Die Operation der Mammahypertrophie und der Hängebrust. *Dtsch. Med. Wochenschr.* 50:1400, 1924.
2. Lettermann, G., and Schurter, M. History of reduction mammaplasty. In J.Q. Owsley and R.A. Peterson (eds.), *Symposium on Aesthetic Surgery of the Breast.* St. Louis: Mosby, 1978.
3. Marchac, D., and De Olarte, G. Reduction mammaplasty and correction of ptosis with a short inframammary scar. *Plast. Reconstr. Surg.* 69:45, 1982.
4. Meyer, R., and Kesselring, U.K. Reduction Mammaplasty. In N.G. Georgiade (ed.), *Aesthetic Breast Surgery.* Baltimore: Williams & Wilkins, 1983.
5. Meyer, R., and Kesselring, U.K. Reduction Mammaplasty with L-shaped suture line. *Plast. Reconstr. Surg.* 55:139, 1975.
6. Meyer, R., and Kesselring, U.K. Various dermal flaps with L-shaped suture line in reduction mammaplasty. *Aesth. Plast. Surg.* 3:41, 1979.
7. Meyer, R., and Martinoni, G. Mastoplastica di Riduzione. Atti XXI Congr. Nazionale della Società Italiana di Chirurgia Plastica, 1971.
8. Peixoto, G. The infraareolar longitudinal incision in reduction mammaplasty. *Aesth. Plast. Surg.* 9:1, 1985.

COMMENTS ON CHAPTER 21   *Robert M. Goldwyn*

The authors of this chapter have noted here and elsewhere that the lateral method of reduction mammaplasty is not original with them — a fact that should be evident to those who have read other chapters in this book (e.g., by Bricout and Mouly, Schatten, Regnault and Daniel).

As Kesselring and Meyer have stated, Holländer is generally considered the originator of the oblique approach to breast reduction. Later, Glasmer and Amersbach together (1928) and then singly described resecting a lateral wedge of gland and skin and rotating the nipple 90 degrees upward [1]. A quarter century afterward, Marc wrote about *la méthode oblique* and her satisfaction with it. A few years later, in the 1960s, Dufourmentel and Mouly popularized the oblique technique (see Chap. 13). Kesselring and Meyer have stated that they modified the Lotsch (1928)-Gohbandt operation by conceiving of an "L-shaped suture line which avoided the lateral flattening of the breast, a feature inherent in the more lateral approaches. The curved horizontal branch of the L also avoids the backcut used by Hollender [sic] which makes a U out of L. In the last years modified lateral approaches have been reported and they are gaining acceptance (Elbaz and Regnault)" [3].

This L-shaped suture line thereby results in a shorter scar than the traditional horizontal scar of the inverted T also because of the reduction in breast volume at its base and the elevation of the inframammary fold "in many cases," as Kesselring and Meyer state. This principle of raising the inframammary crease is a keystone in other techniques that attempt to avoid a long horizontal scar, for example, that of Marchac and Sagher [2]. By having the breast higher on the chest wall, some of the length of the horizontal scar is now converted into the length of the vertical scar. In every technique of breast reduction, the surgeon must contend with the problem of eliminating excess skin. In the L-shaped suture line technique of Kesselring and Meyer, the redundancy is removed from around the areola. The more skin that can be excised there, the less needs to be eliminated in the sulcus and, therefore, the shorter the horizontal scar.

Kesselring and Meyer make the important point — one that should be obvious but is not always so to surgeons doing reductions — that the more skin one has to eliminate to achieve a firm, well-shaped breast, the more difficult the operation if one of the prime objectives is to end with a short horizontal scar or even without one. Not all redundant skin has to be cut away; some will shrink with time and that, of course, is the basis of the volume reduction method of Cloutier (see Chap. 29). The procedure of Kesselring and Meyer and of others, including Peixoto, is also important but obviously not so crucial as in the Cloutier procedure.

In extremely large breasts with a great amount of skin excess and laxity, the authors acknowledge that a horizontal medial "heel" to the L scar may be necessary. They have correctly concluded that the amount of skin and its slackness are more important factors in determining the length of the horizontal scar than are the volume and width of the breast.

In any technique that raises the inframammary fold, one may see in the interval between the new and the former fold an unwanted bulge or wrinkling of the skin. This problem can be avoided by meticulous skin excision (see Figs. 21-11 and 21-12).

The authors' final caveat should be heeded: "In large ptotic breasts the amount of redundant skin will require an undue prolongation of the scar [and] attempts to condense the scar will cause bad scarring." As they have written, their method is technically not easy and requires accurate evaluation of the breast along with precise planning and careful performance.

We plastic surgeons are continually trying either to get more skin, by using flaps or expansion, or eliminating skin by excision. Perhaps some day we shall have a method that allows us to shrink skin immediately during the operation in order for us to minimize our incisions and the scars our patients have to bear.

REFERENCES

1. Letterman, G., and Schurter, M. History of reduction mammaplasty. In J.Q. Owsley and R.A. Peterson (eds.), *Symposium of Aesthetic Surgery of the Breast.* St. Louis: Mosby, 1978. Pp. 3–29.
2. Marchac, D., and Sagher, U. Mammaplasty with a short horizontal scar. Evaluation and results after 9 years. *Clin. Plast. Surg.* 15:627, 1988.
3. Meyer, R., Kesselring, U.K. Various dermal flaps with L-shaped suture line in reduction mammaplasty. *Aesth. Plast. Surg.* 3:41, 1979.

22

Daniel Marchac

Reduction Mammaplasty with a Short Horizontal Scar

When a surgeon is faced with a patient requesting a reduction of breast hypertrophy or ptosis correction, or both, the ideal would be to obtain the desired contour correction without leaving visible sequelae, as we do for breast augmentation or rhinoplasty.

The only area where a scar on the breast could be hidden would be the periphery of the areola, but, to my knowledge, no techniques have been able to correct hypertrophy or ptosis through the single preareolar incision with a satisfactory residual scar. It must remain our aim, and we must someday be able to achieve the desired breast correction without leaving visible scars. The periareolar scar should also be improved; even if it is a fine hardly visible line, it is too perfect a circle, and we should be able someday to copy the slightly irregular areolar limit. I must say that I have tried it with many incisions, without much success, but someday a surgeon will find the trick. And, in the satisfactory long-term result I have observed with my technique, this too perfect periareolar circle was practically the only visible sequela of the surgery at normal eye distance examination. The inverted T scar has become practically invisible in these long-term favorable cases. We know through experience that to obtain this result, several factors are required:

1. Limited tension on the skin sutures.
2. Short incisions not going vertically below the inframammary line, or showing medially or laterally on a standing patient.
3. Favorable healing with no undue hypertrophic reaction.

I have been utilizing (since 1977) the technique I will describe later. It has been inspired by previous techniques I first utilized.

During my plastic surgery training, I was first taught by Claude Dufourmentel and Roger Mouly their lateral approach, with an ellipse excision going from the areola to the axilla. Through this skin approach, initially a Biesenberger type of correction was performed, the breast being nourished by an inner thoracic pedicle.

A simpler and safer approach was developed later by Dufourmentel and Mouly [3], with a wedge resection of glandular tissue corresponding to the skin excision. In case of pure ptosis, the gland was overlapped or infolded. Some results were excellent, but I was not satisfied because of (1) the unpredictability of the results, with a tendency of the nipples to look inward, and (2) the long lateral scar with a tendency of spreading at its end.

Having helped Ivo Pitanguy demonstrate a case in Miami while I was Ralph Millard's fellow in 1968, I adopted his technique. The results were satisfactory, but I was not happy with the length of the horizontal scar. I was finally able to shorten this horizontal scar through an approach that is a blend of three procedures: (1) the vertical resection of Arié [2], narrowing the breast transversally instead of the usual horizontal movement, (2) the ellipse excision of skin and breast tissue of Dufourmentel and Mouly performed vertically instead of laterally, and (3) the breast tissue resection advocated by Pitanguy [7] under the nipple-areola complex and, as much as necessary, from the deep aspect of the gland.

My only contribution was the idea of stopping the vertical excision well above the inframammary line and to let some extra skin of the lower portion of the breast retract and be converted into abdominal skin, below the new inframammary line.

Since the publication of the technique in 1982 [5], some modifications and simplifications have been introduced, but the basic technique has not been changed.

Technique

PRINCIPLE

A vertical resection is performed mainly below the areola, including skin and breast tissue, followed by a careful glandular suturing to create a conical shape. A suspension stitch to the pectoralis fascia lifts the breast tissue while the lower part of the suture is adjusted, a new inframammary fold being created about 2 cm above the previous one. The empty horizontal skin pocket located between the new and the old inframammary fold retracts and flattens out rapidly with the help of a brassiere with a wide lower strap.

DETAILED DESCRIPTION

The technique is described here in a case of moderate hypertrophia with marked ptosis.

The *preoperative examination* includes a clinical assessment with palpation of the breasts and axilla as well as echography and x-rays to detect a possible malignancy. Size, shape, and symmetry of the breasts will be evaluated. The degree of ptosis will be measured from under the inframammary fold. The quality of the breast tissue, supple or rigid, glandular or fatty, will be evaluated. The skin must also be examined in regard to thickness and the presence of striae.

At this time, expectations of the patient in terms of volume and future location of the breast must be understood. One should discuss with the patient the principle of the operation, the location of scars specific to the technique, and the following points:

1. The necessity of wearing a special brassiere with a wide lower strap, which the patient is requested to buy and bring with her to the hospital.
2. The fact that the breast will be initially high, with an areola looking often slightly downward. It is explained to the patient that the breast weight and skin distention will give the breasts a more natural appearance after a few months, with a stable result thereafter.
3. The possibility of minor imperfections, especially at the end of the horizontal incision, eventually requiring correction at about 6 months after the surgery.

The markings are performed in the operating room, the patient being put in a semisitting position after intubation. The legs are slightly flexed, the arms remaining vertical, slightly aside from the thorax, with a careful posterior padding. It is important that the head be maintained in a normal position with a posterior cushion and a frontal strap to avoid cervical distortion. The drapes are placed in the usual way, and we have long avoided stitches in the shoulder and clavicle areas; we use adhesive tapes because of the risk of keloids. The markings will include the following (Fig. 22-1):

1. The midline, from umbilicus to sternal notch.
2. The vertical axis of the breasts. By that, we mean the line on which we wish to see the nipple on the standing patient. In cases of ptosis, the breasts tend to drop laterally, even in the semisitting position. One should lift up the breast with the left hand to put the nipple-areola complex in the final desired position and draw a vertical line below the inframammary line, with the nipple as reference. This vertical line is usually 8 to 10 cm from the midline, depending on the width of the thorax. It will be our reference line to determine the width of the skin excision and should indicate the location of the future vertical branch of the inverted T.
3. The vertical side of the excision. The left hand will push the breast first laterally, and a vertical line will be drawn on the medial part of the breast in continuity with the previously determined axis of the breast. The same maneuver will be repeated for the lateral vertical line, the breast being pushed medially. One should avoid pushing too much, keeping a fullness corresponding to the desired residual breast tissue volume. This is how we determine the width of the vertical ellipse to be resected. It is checked; it can also be determined by pinching the skin or lightly applying Allis clamps. If in doubt, it is better to make this resection a little too wide and to recut it later than to have it too narrow with subsequent skin tension. The width of the excision varies usually between 5 and 12 cm.
4. The horizontal bottom line d-e usually is drawn 5 cm above the inframammary fold (Fig. 22-2). One checks by pinching that the bringing together of points d and e determines a new inframammary fold of proper location for the proposed size and shape of the new breast. The tension between d and e should not be exces-

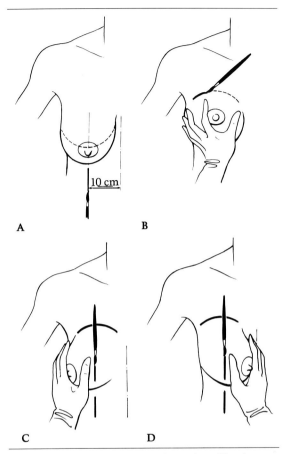

A   B

C   D

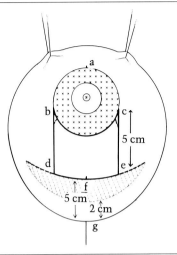

Fig. 22-2. The horizontal inferior line d-e is usually located 5 cm above the inframammary fold. The hatched area located below represents the skin that will be resected at the final adjustment. There is, therefore, only about 2 cm of skin not resected above the inframammary fold. Point a is located at the summit of a curve joining b to c slightly above the areola. Note an indent of 0.6 to 0.8 cm made at the level of b and c to diminish the tension of the suture below the areola.

Fig. 22-1. The markings are made on the table, the patient being in a semisitting position. A. The axis of the breast corresponds to the vertical of the desired nipple position and is located 8 to 10 cm from the midline. B. The upper limit of the breast is self-evident when the breast is lifted up. C. The inner side of the vertical resection is determined by pushing the breast laterally, keeping some fullness medially, and drawing a line in continuity with the axis of the breast. D. The same maneuver is done laterally.

sive; these two points should come together easily.

5. From the point d and e, a distance of 5 cm is marked upward on the vertical sides of the drawing. This represents the future vertical suture. An indent of about 0.8 cm is made at this point to diminish the tension at the upper limit of this vertical suture, where it joins with the areola. We then have points b and c, and we will join them by a curved line passing above the areola. Sometimes the areola is not in the middle of the vertical lines b-d and c-f. It is because

of the differences of skin excess between the lateral and medial sides of the breast. The important point is that the vertical lines when pinched together correspond to the vertical axis of the breast carefully determined at the beginning of the procedure.

6. The curved upper line joining b and c should then be drawn as a portion of a circle as if the areola would be in the center of the marking, the higher portion a of this curved line being on the vertical axis of the breast and at an equivalent distance between b and c. It should be only slightly higher than the areola, about 4 cm above the nipple level. In moderate ptosis, when the width of the vertical excision is a moderate 7 to 8 cm, the curved line between b and c will represent four fifths of a circle and the final drawing looks like an Islamic window. When the ptosis is severe, on a large breast, the distance between b and c can reach 10 to 14 cm, and the line above the areola will be moderately curved.

7. To avoid asymmetry of the vertical level of the future areola, a measurement is made from the

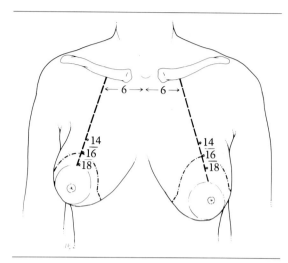

Fig. 22-3. *The distance between the midclavicular point and the areola is measured, and a scale is tattooed every 2 cm above the areola. This is to ensure that one ends up at the same level at the completion of the operation.*

midclavicular point (6 cm from the sternal notch) to the nipple. From point a upward, a tattooed mark will be made every 2 cm (Fig. 22-3). One can also check the symmetry or asymmetry of the breasts.

8. The symmetry of the markings in regard to the midline umbilicus sternum is now checked.
9. The upper limit of the breast, corresponding to the upper limit of our retroglandular undermining. This limit will be determined by pushing the breast upward: a fold marks the upper limit of the glandular tissue, often quite high, not far from the clavicle (see Fig. 22-1B).

Tattooing of the key points a, b, c, d, e, f of the vertical axis and the inframammary fold is performed with a needle whose tip is immersed in surgical ink.

Infiltration of the operative area is performed with lidocaine and epinephrine. This infiltration is made in the dermis around the areola to facilitate deepithelialization; it is done along the skin incision lines, under the skin down to the inframammary fold and behind the breast, in front of the pectoralis major.

The mammostat described by Michel Costagliola is then placed around the base of the breast. It provides an even breast pressure that facilitates the preareolar undermining. The periareolar circle is marked first with a circular device. We prefer to draw a rather larger circle to diminish the final periareolar tension, and we utilize a 4.5-cm circle in small breasts and 5.5-cm circle in larger breasts.

Deepithelialization around the areola is then performed as a circle, up to the limit of the drawing, to a, b, c superiorly, and about 2 cm below the areola inferiorly.

In making the skin incision, in the lower part, the vertical sides b-d and c-e are incised, as well as the horizontal line d-e, through the full thickness of the skin, but without removing the area of skin then delimited. It will go away with the glandular tissue and will be utilized for traction in the meantime.

The mammostat is removed, and the lower undermining from d-e to the lower pole of the gland will be performed next. To facilitate this maneuver, a traction stitch will be passed at a and pulled up by the assistant. This lower undermining should be done close to the breast tissue rather than subcutaneously. One should find the lower pole of the breast and the thoracic wall, and start the dissection between the gland and the pectoralis fascia upward. The skin undermining is not performed on the vertical sides b-d and c-e, but just 1 or 1.5 cm above d and e, to help free the lower pole of the breast on all its length, medially and laterally. This good freeing of the lateral and medial lower part of the gland from the posterior and lower adherences is important to permit the conical reconstruction of the gland. The posterior undermining should be extensive laterally, medially, and superiorly. The superior undermining must reach the upper limit of the breast drawn previously.

Breast tissue resection is performed in two stages:

1. *The lower full thickness resection.* The left hand being placed behind the breast, incisions are made laterally in continuity with the skin lines b-d and c-f, as if cutting a full-thickness slice of an orange. Superiorly, a horizontal incision 1.5-cm deep is made 2 cm below the areola (Fig. 22-4).
2. *The retroareolar resection.* At this stage, the level of the nipple-areola complex should be carefully controlled to perform the resection under it with safety. The traction suture pulling at point a and the skin hook placed at the lower part of the deepithelialized area will be utilized to lift the nipple-areola complex horizontally.

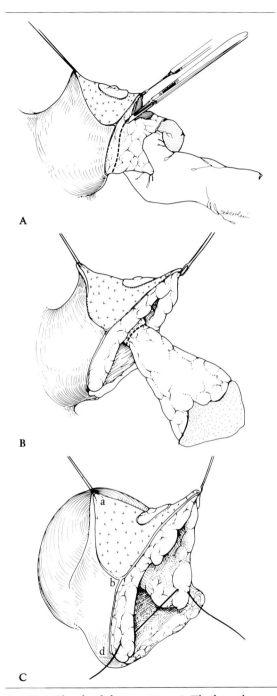

A

B

C

The central resection will then be performed cutting one side and then the other. This resection made at the deep part of the breast is continued until a satisfactory residual volume is obtained, taking off as much breast tissue as necessary.

The following three points must be considered during this resection:

1. The two lower lateral glandular pillars corresponding to b-d and c-e must be carefully preserved even if thinning is necessary at their deep aspect.
2. The area of breast tissue resection must be carefully adjusted to each particular case. When the breast implantation is very wide, it may be advisable to thin the breast tissue from the deep aspect at the periphery, whereas in the case of a concentrated breast, more will be resected at the center. One should always keep enough tissue in the center to allow sufficient projection of the nipple-areola complex.
3. Symmetry of the resection must be checked carefully.

Suspension of the breast tissue to the pectoralis fascia is the next step, after a careful hemostasis (Fig. 22-5). One central stitch seems to be sufficient. It should be placed superiorly at the upper limit of the posterior undermining, in line with the axis of the breast, and taking a strong bit of fascia and muscle. The lower stitch is inserted in the posterior aspect of the residual breast tissue, slightly above the areola and also carefully on the line of the axis. While the knot is tied, one should obtain a bulging at the superior part of the breast. The areola should not be attracted inward. If these two objectives are not reached, one should replace the knot. We utilize an absorbable stitch for this maneuver, this suspension being considered as a temporary help for the remodeling of the breast in the early postoperative period. If the breast tissue

---

Fig. 22-4. The glandular resection. A. The lateral section is performed perpendicularly to the skin. At the upper level, a horizontal cut starts below the areola. The nipple-areola complex must be carefully elevated and maintained horizontally by the assistant to ensure maintenance of an even thickness. B. The resection continues at the deep aspect of the gland, *superiorly and laterally, as much as necessary—the blood supply coming from the surface. C. After completion of the glandular resection, one is left with a sort of grotto, with two lateral glandular pillars at the entrance. These pillars will be carefully brought together after the suspension has been performed.*

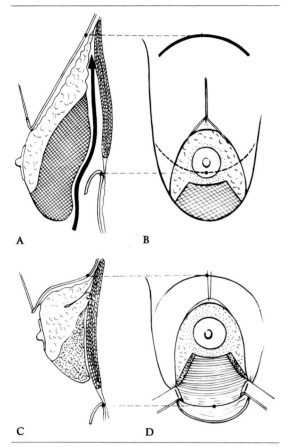

A　　　　　**B**

C　　　　　**D**

Fig. 22-5. Suspension of the breast tissue to the
pectoralis major fascia allows an elevation of all the
breast and produces a superior convexity. A. The
hatched area represents the glandular resection in the
central part of the breast, and the arrow goes to the
point of placement of the suspension stitch. B. The
breast hanging below the inframammary fold before
the suspension. C. The plication of the upper part of
the gland owing to the suspension. D. This illustrates
how the suspension elevates the gland, bringing it
tangential to the upper limit of the breast, and raising
the glandular lower pillars above the original
inframammary line.

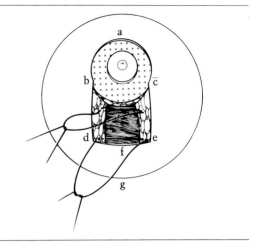

Fig. 22-6. Glandular remodeling is an essential part of
the procedure. The glandular pillars are sutured
together in several layers, taking care to be symmetrical.

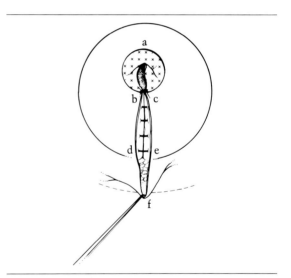

Fig. 22-7. Vertical line suturing. After the glandular
pillars have been sutured, lower pulling on point f (on
the axis of the breast) helps to suture the vertical line,
with suturing of point b-c and d-e together.

is too rigid to fold on itself for this suspension, attracting the nipple, we will cut off this suspension stitch, usually after the glandular remodeling.

The glandular remodeling is performed by suturing together the two glandular pillars corresponding to b-d and c-e (Fig. 22-6). The tattooed points are clearly visible and will help to suture the glandular tissue symmetrically. Usually we put a stitch at b-c and one at d-e, each time taking a large bit of glandular tissue with a 3-0 absorbable Maxon stitch and then a few intermediate stitches. This suturing will give a conical shape to the breast and, for this purpose,

1. The lower part of the remaining breast tissue must be well freed from its position and lower adherences.
2. The glandular suture must be meticulous, including all the thickness of the gland at b-d and c-e levels, and also going down enough, with an especially good suturing at the d-e level, the future junction point of the inverted T scar.

Since there was no undermining, the skin will follow the glandular tissue and will come in contact on the vertical line b-c – d-e. A few dermal stitches are additionally placed on this vertical line b-c – d-e (Fig. 22-7).

The horizontal skin incision is then performed. The new inframammary line is usually obvious at the level of d-e when the width of the resection has been well calculated. It corresponds to the base of the reconstructed mammary cone and is even more visible with up and down mobilization of the breast. If the new inframammary line does not show itself clearly, this may be due to several reasons, including (1) the glandular pillars have not been brought together correctly, especially at the lower part, and have not been freed sufficiently laterally and medially; (2) there is glandular tissue hanging below the d-e line; and (3) the skin resection is not wide enough. With a well-reconstructed cone, the new inframammary line shows itself, and the incision is made at the d-e key stitch level. It is horizontal, the inner branch being shorter than the lateral one. The average length is 2 to 3 cm medially and 3 to 5 cm laterally, depending on the size and width of the breast. Once this incision is performed, the remaining lower skin presents itself like a quadrangular flap (Fig. 22-8).

The lower guadrangular skin flap is excised (Fig. 22-9). The two angles of the flap are lifted up, and

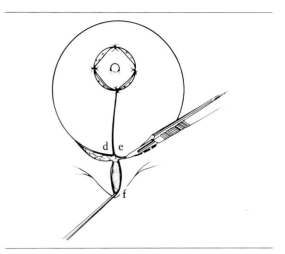

Fig. 22-8. The horizontal incision. The new inframammary line is usually obvious. The incision is usually 2 to 3 cm long medially and 3 to 5 cm laterally.

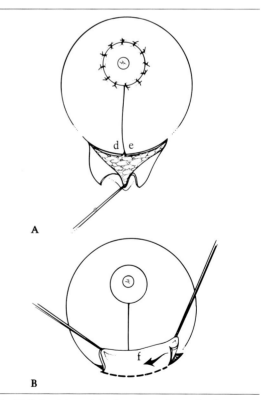

Fig. 22-9. Excision of the lower quadrangular flap. A. After horizontal incisions at the d-e level, the lower skin excess is unfolded. B. It is lifted up, and a line as short as possible is drawn and incised across the base of this quadrangular flap.

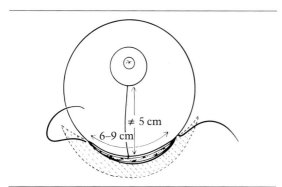

≠ 5 cm

6–9 cm

Fig. 22-10. The new inframammary line is located approximately 2 cm above the previous one. The hatched area represents the excess skin of the lower part of the breast, which is transformed into thoracic skin. It also represents the area to defat carefully and to flatten out with the dressing and the lower strap of the brassiere. An intradermal running suture is used after closure of the deep dermofatty layer.

one pulls the flap up gently. A line is drawn across the flap horizontally, joining, by the shortest possible line, the two ends of the horizontal incision of the new inframammary fold. The cut across the lower quadrangular flap is done under tension, one skin hook at the end of the horizontal incision, being careful to incise perpendicularly to the skin. One obtains a horizontal ellipse whose lower edge is slightly longer than the upper one.

The new inframammary fold must be sculpted out. Medially and laterally, one should usually remove some fat under the new inframammary line to improve its contour. This can be done with scissors or by liposuction. One should also check that the breast tissue is not going below the inframammary line, and, if so, it is excised. Some fullness must always be kept at the lower part of the vertical glandular suture, where the junction of the T will be. Eventually, a lower excess of breast tissue can be rotated and sutured at this level instead of being excised, if one believes that there is not enough fullness at the lower part of the vertical glandular suture, where the junction of the T will be.

The horizontal ellipse is then sutured after a retroglandular suction drainage has been installed (Fig. 22-10). Because of the slight discrepancy between the edges, the suture is begun at the ends by buried inverted sutures at the dermis level. We now use 4-0 Maxon, an absorbable suture presenting itself like nylon.

The areola is then adjusted. The location of the areola is determined by its position above the vertical line. In this technique, instead of starting the procedure by locating the desired position of the areola and then adjusting the breast below, we proceed the other way. We start by locating the new inframammary line. Then we usually measure 5 cm on the vertical suture and locate the new areola above it. Five centimeters is the average length of the vertical suture in a medium-sized breast. It usually corresponds to the length of the third and second phalanx of the index fingers, as taught to me by Dr. Morel-Fatio. In large and wide breasts, this distance can be increased to 6 cm, and reduced to 4.0 to 4.5 cm in smaller breasts; however, 5 cm is used in the majority of cases. It corresponds to points b-c tattooed during the markings, with a 1-cm indent to diminish transversal tension. The areola will therefore be located above. Our aim is to resect the extra skin around the areola but to avoid excessive tension. The suture together of points b-c has converted the arched line, joining them initially through point a in a circular line. Sometimes it is sufficient to suture the areola to this circular line, with minor adjustments at the lower part.

In many cases, one may think that there is still some extra skin to be resected beyond the deepithelialized line, especially at the upper level. A stitch can then be run at the limit of the deepithelialized area, passing through point a and the sutured points b-c, and then pulled on gently like closing a purse (Fig. 22-11). It is tied at the desired tension, the areola remaining buried underneath. No undue tension must be applied, and we often tie it at an intermediate position, leaving open a hole of 1 to 2 cm of diameter. A circle of 3.5 cm is then drawn with a circular marker, its inferior limit being tangential to b-c. The level of the upper limit will be carefully compared to the previously tattooed scale of distances between the clavicle and nipple (see Fig. 22-3). It is essential to finish with the same end up at the same level on the opposite side. The running stitch is then removed, and the deepithelialization is extended to the new periareolar drawing (Fig. 22-11D).

If there is some resistance of the areola to being elevated to the desired position, a cut through the dermis is performed from points b-c upward, medially and laterally, for 2 to 3 cm (Fig. 22-12). This will allow an easy adjustment of the areola without compromising the blood supply. Sometimes, especially in firm breasts, one feels that the areola

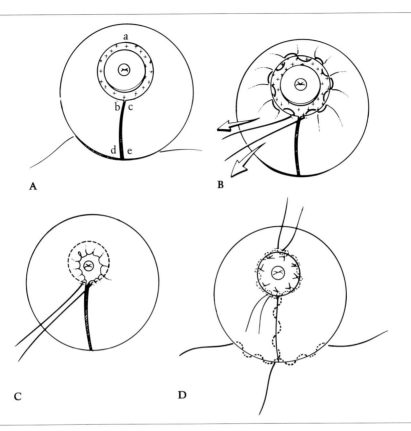

Fig. 22-11. Adjustment of the areola. A. Sometimes the areola adjusts itself with the desired tension to the edges of the deepidermized area below point a. B. In many cases, one feels that some extra tension would be preferable. A stitch is then run around the edges of the deepithelialized area. C. The stitch is pulled until the desired tension is obtained, like closing a purse. A circular marking is made, the knot is untied, and the supplementary deepithelialization is performed. D. The areola is sutured with intradermal running stitches.

is retracted inward by the suspension stitch. If a pull on the nipple does not allow the areola to come outward, one can cut out the suspension stitch at this stage. One should then be even more careful to obliterate the lower inframammary pocket, because there is an increased risk of sliding down of the breast. If this suspension stitch is left, with a slight inward attraction of the areola, this will correct itself spontaneously in a few weeks.

The minimization of scars depends on two main factors: (1) minimal tension on the sutures, and (2) precise epidermal approximation with prolonged

dermal support. As explained previously, with transversal tension on the vertical line being applied on the glandular pillars and minimal tension being exerted at the horizontal and periareolar levels, the skin suture can easily be done without tension. We perform sutures in two layers. On the vertical and horizontal lines, we utilize interrupted inverted 4-0 Maxon in the dermal layer and an intradermal running 3-0 Prolene suture superficially. Around the areola, we had microabscesses with all deep sutures; we use now eight U-stitches of 5-0 Prolene tied on the areola and an intradermal running 4-0 Prolene. Generous taping is performed with wide straps of Steri-Strips.

The dressing is important for only one area: the inferior skin pocket located between the new and old inframammary fold. This must be flattened down by a pressure dressing. One can use compresses and Elastoplast or, even better, a brassiere with a wide lower strap.

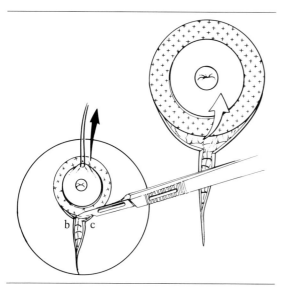

Fig. 22-12. Releasing of the areola. A dermal incision is made at the junction of the deepithelialized area, and skin is often useful to help in elevating the areola to the desired position.

Cases of Pure Ptosis

The drawing of the skin incision is performed in the same way. In most cases, the breast is small and all the existing volume must be preserved. We then deepithelialize all the area included in the drawing to keep the volume of the dermis.

After incision through the dermis, along b-d, d-e, and e-c, dissection of the lower pole of the gland and its posterior aspect is performed like that described previously for reduction and ptosis.

Once the superior suspension is completed, a splitting of the lower part of the breast is performed, going vertically up to the areola (Fig. 22-13).

Two hanging flaps of breast tissue are obtained, and they will be overlapped. Usually we start by suturing the end of the lateral flap to the deep aspect of the medial flap, and then the end of the medial flap is pulled laterally above the lateral flap.

A wide dissection of the lower part of the breast is important to allow a good mobilization and reconstruction of a conical shape.

In small breasts, any breast tissue or fat hanging below the planned inframammary line will be lifted up and fixed under or above the lower part of the reconstructed breast.

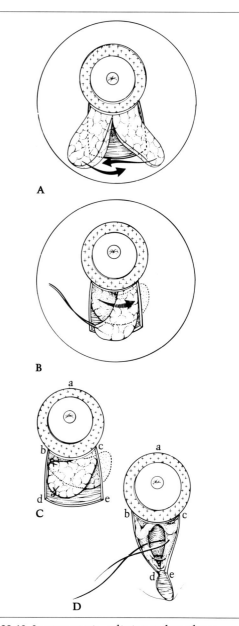

Fig. 22-13. In pure ptosis, splitting and overlapping. A. After freeing of the gland and its suspension, a vertical incision along the axis of the breast is performed. B. The lateral lower flap is sutured under the medial flap. C. The medial flap is sutured over the base of the lateral flap. D. A plication of the breast tissue is made to reinforce the lower support and to bring in contact the skin edges b-d and c-e.

The suturing of the vertical line and adjustment of the horizontal line and areola will be done as in other cases. In small breasts, the vertical distance may have to be reduced to 4 cm to keep the areola at the summit of the reconstructed mammary cone.

When the mammary tissue is insufficient in volume, it is possible to combine this correction of ptosis with the placement of a prosthesis.

The width of the vertical resection must be calculated accordingly, and it may be wise to plan a rather narrow skin resection. One will then be able to adjust precisely the skin tension at the end of the procedure.

Very Large Breasts

The technique can be used for reduction up to 800 gm on each side. Two technical points must be mentioned:

1. Nearly all the breast tissue can be removed from the deep aspect of the gland, the areola being vascularized superficially by the subdermal tissue. Nevertheless, one should preserve the two glandular pillars corresponding to the vertical line and also keep enough tissue beneath the areola to obtain a sufficient forward projection.
2. It is fundamental to free sufficiently the remaining inferior breast medially and especially laterally to be able to bring inward the lateral axillary prolongation and to reconstruct a conical shape.

POSSIBLE PROBLEMS AND THEIR SOLUTIONS

Retraction of Areola

1. It can be due to a lower dermal attachment and can easily be released by cutting through the dermis a few centimeters on each side, starting from points b and c (see Fig. 22-12).
2. The suspension stitch may be wrongly placed, too low behind the areola and retracting it. It must be replaced higher.
3. Sometimes in some very rigid breasts, the plication of the breast tissue above the areola is difficult, creating a retraction, and one has to release the suspension stitch at the end of the procedure, before suturing the areola (Fig. 22-14).
4. Enough breast tissue must be kept behind the areola, especially in large and wide breasts, to avoid areola retraction.

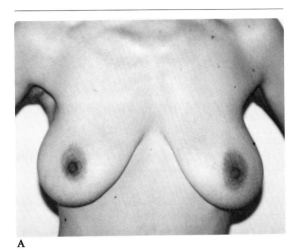

A

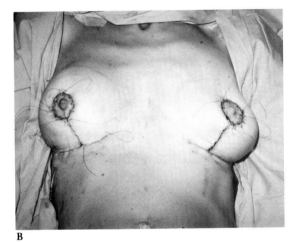

B

Fig. 22-14. The effect of the suspension. A. Hypertrophy and ptosis in a 35-year-old woman. B. The suspension stitch has been released on the left side. One sees the difference in shape and how the superior convexity has disappeared.

Sliding of the Gland

Sliding of the gland beneath the inframammary fold can be due to three causes:

1. Insufficient conical reformation of the breast. When the glandular pillars are well brought together, down to the lower part of the vertical, the gland stands by itself and does not tend to slide down.
2. Insufficient removal of the breast tissue, which may be "hanging" below the new inframammary line.

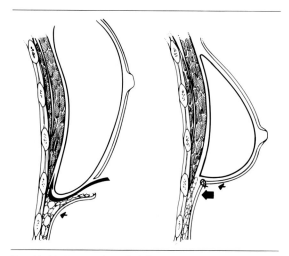

Fig. 22-15. To avoid medial depression, one should leave some fat tissue under the skin while dissecting down to the inframammary line from line d-e.

3. Defective dressing. The lower pocket between the new and old inframammary line must be obliterated by a pressure dressing and, as soon as possible, by a brassiere with a wide lower strap. This will be worn continuously for 2 weeks and during the day for another 6 weeks.

Medial Depression

When the patient raises her arms, a depression appears at the level of the junction of the T. This can be due to two mistakes:

1. Excessive removal of fat under the skin located below the horizontal line d-e when dissecting down the lower part of the breast. One should remain close to the glandular tissue and leave some subcutaneous fat under the skin (Fig. 22-15).
2. Insufficient approximation of the glandular pillars at the lower part of the vertical suture. If there is a glandular gap at the lower part of the vertical suture, a depression will appear.

Asymmetry

It is usually an asymmetry of the superior level of the areolas. To avoid it, we now mark a tattooed scale from the clavicle to the areola on both sides to be sure to end up at the same level.

Table 22-1. Evaluation of aesthetic results on 176 patients

Operations	Excellent	Good	Mediocre	Bad
Ptosis	44	20	4	—
Moderate hypertrophy	50	20	6	—
Hypertrophy greater than 50 gm	19	11	2	—

Evaluation of Results (with U. Sagher, M.D.)

We have tried to evaluate the results of our technique after 10 years and have been able to review 176 patients. Among them are 51 with more than 4 years follow-up.

The questions raised refer to the quality of shape, location, stability, length, and quality of scars and sensitivity.

Evaluation of the aesthetic quality of the operated on breast is the most difficult to perform. As for all our aesthetic evaluations, we use a four-grade scale: excellent, good, mediocre, and bad.

Excellent is when shape, location, and quality of scars are good and correspond to what was expected. Good corresponds to an acceptable result but with some minor imperfections that could eventually require a minor revision. A mediocre rating is given when both the patient and the examiner are dissatisfied with an obvious shortcoming requiring partial revision. Bad represents a defective result that may justify complete reoperation.

This appreciation is, of course, subjective. It is best performed by the patient and an examiner who is not the surgeon — the surgeon always being influenced by the previous condition and the improvement. We are not rating an "improvement," but a result as such.

AESTHETIC RESULT (SHAPE AND LOCATION) (TABLE 22-1)

The satisfactory results (excellent and good) have been the vast majority, especially as can be expected in moderate reductions and pure ptosis (Figs. 22-16 through 22-19).

STABILITY OF RESULTS (TABLE 22-2)

Stability of results has been remarkable. Our previous experience with other techniques and examination of patients having been operated on elsewhere have shown, in addition to stable results, a

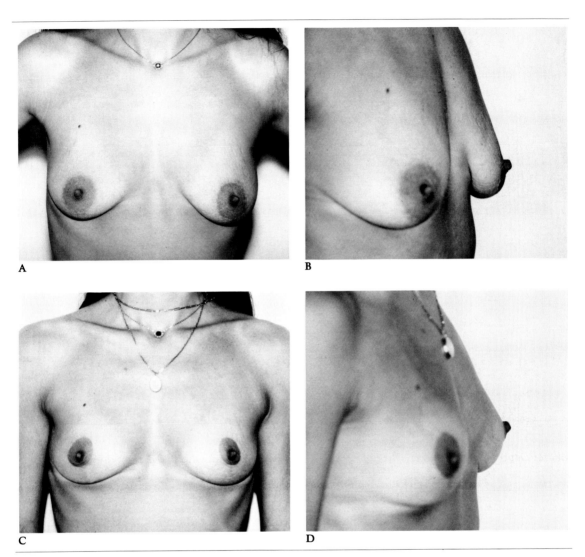

Fig. 22-16. A, B. A 28-year-old patient presenting with ptosis after pregnancies. C, D. Eighteen months after correction by the described technique with splitting of the gland.

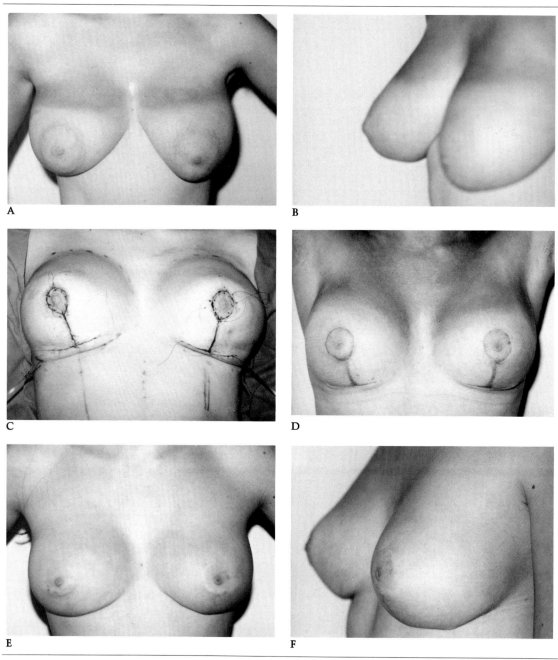

Fig. 22-17. A, B. A 17-year-old girl presenting with asymmetry, moderate hypertrophy, and ptosis. C. The subcutaneous pocket located between the new and the primary inframammary fold is clearly visible at completion of operation. Owing to asymmetry, the right breast is more pronounced. D. One month after the operation, the inframammary pockets have flattened out. The continuous pressure of a brassiere with a wide lower strap is fundamental. E, F. Eighteen months after surgery, the shape, location, and symmetry are satisfactory.

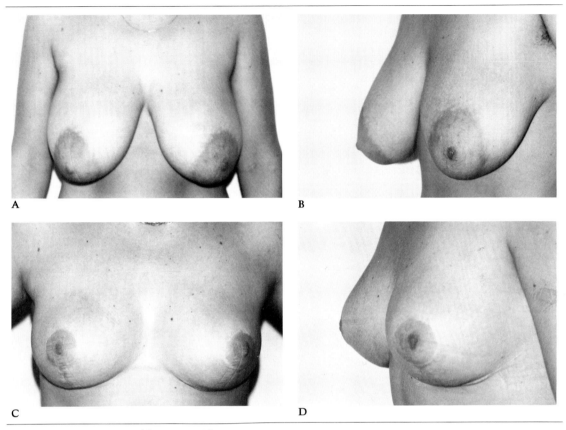

Fig. 22-18. *A, B. A 20-year-old woman with hypertrophia and severe ptosis. C–D. One year after a 600-gm reduction and ptosis correction.*

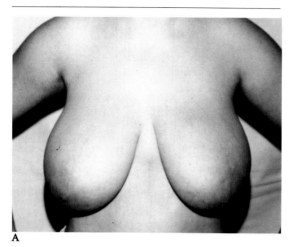

A

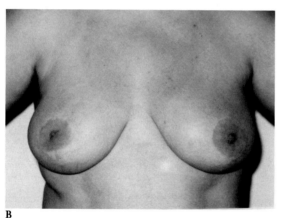

B

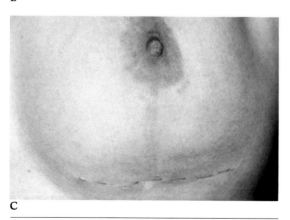

C

Fig. 22-19. A. A 19-year-old woman with heavy pendulous breasts. B. Six years after an 800-gm reduction. She has gained and lost 20 kg in the meantime. C. The short horizontal scar had to be marked to make it more visible. Note how it is well hidden under the breast.

Table 22-2. Average scar length on 176 patients

Condition	Average scar length (cm)
Ptosis	7.1
Moderate hypertrophy	9.3
Hypertrophy above 500 gm	11.1

significant deterioration with time in many patients. Especially frequent is the sliding down of the breasts, migrating below the inframammary fold, with time. It was therefore especially pleasing to observe that a good result obtained during the first year postoperatively will remain as such. We think that this is due to the glandular remodeling, which is producing a strong lower vertical buttress. (Figs. 22-20 and 22-21).

LENGTH OF SCARS (TABLE 22-3)
The length of scars is of course bigger in larger breasts. Our main goal is to keep the scar hidden beneath the breast when the patient is standing. In a small breast, a scar longer than 8 cm will show medially and laterally, whereas in a large breast, a 11-cm scar will remain well hidden.

SENSITIVITY (TABLE 22-4)
This has been appreciated by tactile examination with paper and feather. The number of patients with permanent hyposensitivity is rather low. It has to be noted that sensitivity is often low preoperatively in large and ptotic breasts. Sensation to the areola is provided through two main sources: (1) the intercostal nerves, and (2) the subcutaneous network. The intercostal nerves are obviously cut, as when putting a retroglandular prosthesis, but the dermal network is sufficient to provide good sensation in most cases.

Indications
This technique is mostly indicated to correct ptosis. The lower midline skin resection and the reformation of a conical gland with a superior suspension and a strong lower buttress aim to maintain the gland in higher position.

The best indication is therefore represented by pure ptosis, or ptosis with moderate hypertrophy, up to 500 gm.

When there is no ptosis, especially in young girls, a glandular reduction according to Peixoto

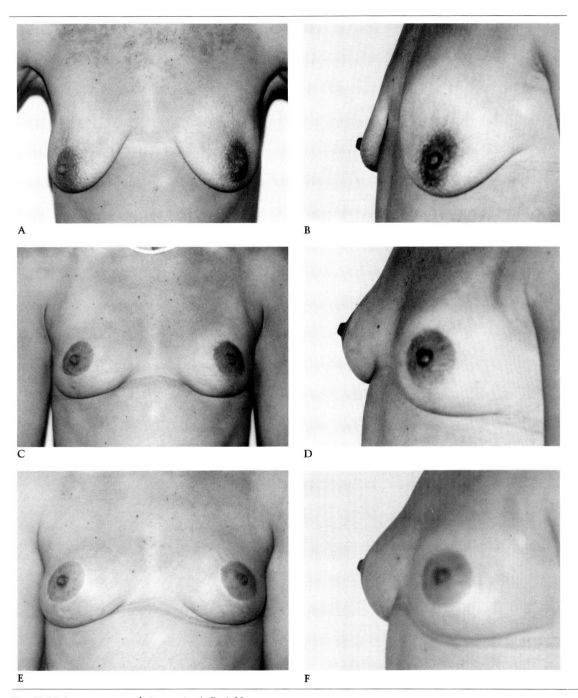

Fig. 22-20. Long-term result in ptosis. A, B. A 38-year-old woman presenting with severe ptosis. C, D. One year after surgery. E, F. Five years after surgery, there is no deterioration.

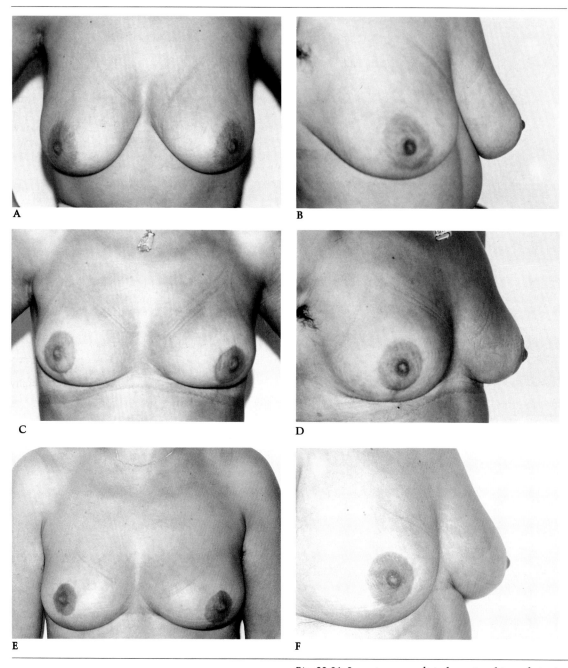

Fig. 22-21. Long-term result in hypertrophia and ptosis. A, B. A 45-year-old woman presenting with mild hypertrophia and ptosis. C, D. Ten months after a 300-gm resection on both sides. E, F. Six years after surgery, the result is stable, with a good convexity in the superior part of the breasts.

Table 22-3. Stability (evaluated after 4 years
on 51 patients)

Operation	Excel-lent	Good	Medi-ocre	Bad
Ptosis (23)	15	6	2	—
Moderate hypertrophy (19)	12	5	2	—
Hypertrophy greater than 500 gm (9)	3	4	2	—

Table 22-4. Sensitivity of areola

Sensation	Percentage
Remained normal	51
Transitory diminution	24
Moderate permanent diminution	18
Significant diminution	7

[6], through a vertical or horizontal lower approach, is sufficient.

In very large breasts, the technique described can be utilized with success, as demonstrated by d'Angierri Basile, [1], but is more difficult to execute, especially with soft breasts, and requires experience.

Reproducibility and easiness to teach is, of course, important for a technique of mammaplasty.

At the beginning of our experience, it was a cut-as-you-go approach, but with time, we have better determined what has to be done and we have simplified the technique in comparison with our initial description [5]:

1. *Predetermined design.* We now rarely recut our vertical lines, and often keep the upper curve b-a-c.
2. *Limited undermining.* Contrary to our initial description, we no longer undermine, except at the lower portion.
3. *One central suspension* is sufficient instead of three.

These simplifications allow an easier operation and teaching, and we were very happy to know that Madeleine Lejour's [4] residents are easily learning how to perform this type of mammaplasty.

Many more techniques will be described, and perhaps some day it will be possible to perform a satisfactory mammaplasty with only a periareolar scar as sequelae, but, in the meantime, we believe that our short scar technique is a footstep in the general effort for correcting deformities with minimal sequelae.

References

1. D'Angierri-Basile R. Mammaplasty: Large reduction with inframammary scars. *Plast. Reconstr. Surg.* 76:130, 1985.
2. Arié, G. A new technique of mammaplasty. *Rev. Latinoam.* 3:28, 1957.
3. Dufourmentel, C., and Mouly, R. Plastie mammaire par méthode oblique. *Ann. Chir. Plast.* 6:45, 1961.
4. Lejour, M. Personal communication, 1986.
5. Marchac, D., and De Olarte, G. Reduction mammaplasty and correction of ptosis with a short inframammary scar. *Plast. Reconstr. Surg.* 69:45, 1982.
6. Peixoto, G. Reduction mammaplasty: A personal technique. *Plast. Reconstr. Surg.* 65:217, 1980.
7. Pitanguy, I. Surgical treatment of breast hypertrophy. *Br. J. Plast. Surg.* 20:78, 1967.

Selected Readings

Georgiade, N.G., Serafin, D., Riefkohl, R., and Georgiade, G.S. Is there a reduction mammaplasty for "all seasons"? *Plast. Reconstr. Surg.* 63:765, 1979.
Lalardrie, J.P., and Jouglard, J.P. *Chirurgie Plastique du Sein.* Vol. 1. Paris: Masson, 1974. P. 156.
Maliniac, J.W. Arterial blood supply of the breast: Revised anatomic data relating to reconstructive surgery. *Arch. Surg.* 47:329, 1943.
Maillard, G, Montandon, D, and Goin, J.L. *Plastic Reconstructive Breast Surgery.* Volume A. Geneva: Medecine & Hygiène, 1983. P. 112.
Mitz, V., and Lassau, J.P. Vascularisation du sein: Etude des rapports entre les vascularisations artérielles, glandulaires et cutanées du sein. *Arch. Anat. Cytol. Pathol.* 21:365, 1973.
Salmon, M. Les artères de la glande mammaire. *Ann. Anat. Cytol. Pathol.* 16:477, 1939.
Wise, R.J. A preliminary report on a method of planning the mammaplasty. *Plast. Reconstr. Surg.* 17:367, 1956.

COMMENTS ON CHAPTER 22 *Robert M. Goldwyn*

In my comments following Chap. 21, I remarked on Marchac's technique, whose evolution has just been described. One of the ideas of this book was to have authors relate how they arrived at their current preferred method for reduction mammaplasty. Usually, as in Marchac's instance, a new technique does not spring de novo.

I would second Marchac's observation that reduction via only a periareolar incision, theoretically ideal, is followed too often by periareolar scars that are too wide and hypertrophic and breasts that remain too large. As Marchac further notes, the bigger the breast, the larger the horizontal scar. Therefore, a shorter scar will likely result if the breast is already small or can be made smaller prior to making the horizontal incision. In his technique, Marchac diminishes the breast volume by resecting it vertically to narrow it, by resecting the breast also transversely to reduce its volume, and by stopping the vertical incision above the inframammary line, allowing more extra skin of the lower portion of the breast to retract or become abdominal skin. By these maneuvers, one can reduce satisfactorily breasts whose amount of tissue resection does not exceed 800 gm per side.

I have found Marchac's method useful and easy for small and moderately hypertrophic breasts and for correcting pure ptosis. I did have a problem with bunching of the skin and the interval between the new and old inframammary folds. His suggestion of having the patient wear a bra with a wide lower strap may obviate this problem and I shall try it.

Another key factor in producing a short horizontal scar is to elevate the breast on the chest wall. This can be done internally, as he does, or only externally, as is often done in ptosis operations by excising skin and pulling it together with tension, thereby creating a skin brassiere elevating effect. As most of us who have treated patients with ptosis find, the results are far better initially, and are better later if the breast is actually raised on the chest wall and fixed there [1]. However, as Marchac has stated, all this has to be done with symmetry. For this purpose, he alludes to a marking scale. I use a long suture with its fixed point in the sternal notch so that it can be swung in pendulum fashion to site the new location of the nipples in order to get symmetry.

In performing Marchac's procedure correctly, an excellent conical breast will result if one adheres to his directions. However, the cone is much more difficult to achieve in very large breasts, whose skin has lost much of its elasticity. To make the breast conical, Marchac has emphasized the important point of freeing "sufficiently the remaining inferior breast medially and especially laterally to bring inwards the lateral axillary prolongation."

In the first part of his chapter, Marchac has remarked that the areola shape and periareolar scar after reduction almost always looks artificial — "too perfect a circle." Knowing his ingenuity, I would predict that he will be the person who will fulfill his own prophecy: "Some day a surgeon will find the trick."

REFERENCE
1. Marchac, D., and Sagher, U. Mammaplasty with a short horizontal scar. Evaluation and results after 9 years. *Clin. Plast. Surg.* 15:627, 1988.

23

Gerardo Peixoto

Reduction Mammaplasty: A Personal View

The majority of breast reduction techniques currently in use are more than 25 years old [3, 16, 21]. These procedures continue to be used, maintaining their original characteristics or, what is more frequent, being subjected to innumerable modifications [1, 4]. Sometimes, these modifications are also improvised during the execution of the surgery, in an effort to adapt them to the type of breast being operated upon.

Many of the most used techniques do not permit great modifications due to their inherent limitations. The results obtained are extremely varied: sometimes good, sometimes poor. To us, this seems to occur due to the absence of a necessary elasticity of procedures, in view of the great variations that the breasts present from patient to patient. In our view, these techniques fail due to a lack of flexibility, an indispensable factor necessary for the adaptation to the peculiarities of each case.

After the appearance of the techniques of Strömbeck [21], Pitanguy [16, 17], Dufourmentel and Mouly [3], and MacKissock [10], which are today universally used, always with innumerable modifications, and in spite of the brilliant contributions by plastic surgeons of various countries that followed [2, 7, 15, 18, 19], little has evolved in this quarter-century in terms of reduction mammaplasty. It is true that variations of those procedures have been improved and perpetuated [5, 9].

The fact is that no plastic surgeon is completely satisfied with the present state of reduction mammaplasty. Lalardrie and Jouglard's book *Chirurgie Plastique du Sein*, published in 1974 [6], lists more than 80 different techniques and procedures. One wonders if there were a similar number for the execution of a face lifting or a rhinoplasty.

The conclusion that is reached is that much has to be changed in the way the current surgeon-patient binomial is viewed, with respect to what can be considered a good reduction mammaplasty result. There is an unconsciously established consensus that the breast has to have the same specific shape and appearance in all cases. It is demanded that the neobreast present an imaginary ideal of perfection that escapes the natural aspect of the organ. The desire is to obey a single sculptural beauty standard, as if all individuals have structures that are absolutely alike.

The role of the surgeon is not to make a new organ but to seek to return to the breast its own intrinsic normality of form and size, endeavoring to preserve its specific characteristics, correcting, in addition to its size, only those distortions that can be remedied, as, for example, the reduction in the diameter of the areola or the size of the nipple. Each individual has her own area of breast implantation on the thorax. To attempt to change this location is an effort to change the anatomy. When the Galtier meridian is followed and a divergence is observed between the areolomammillary complex, no effort should be made to modify this fact. With the elimination of the ptosis, the divergence will continue but to a lesser extent, maintaining this additional anatomical characteristic of the patient.

In reduction mammaplasty, as in aesthetic rhinoplasty, we repeat: What must be done is not create a new organ, but improve the existing one, respecting the anatomical characteristics of each of these. Otherwise, it will be the eternal "torture of Tantalus," which haunts all plastic surgeons in this field. It is to desire the impossible instead of perfecting the possible.

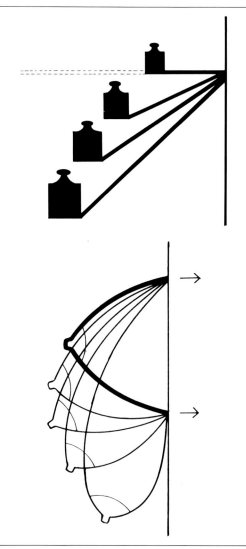

Fig. 23-1. *The normal placement of the breast in relation to the thorax depends on the stable equilibrium between the content-continent (glandular adipose tissue and skin). When this equilibrium is broken, whether it be due to the increase of the mammary volume or to the reduction of the strength of the skin, a progressive ptosis takes over in direct proportion to the importance of these factors. The law of gravity plays a part in this action.*

An important factor that is not always taken into consideration is that the normal position of the organ on the thoracic wall depends, fundamentally, on the equilibrium of the content-continent (glandular adipose tissue and skin) (Fig. 23-1). When the mammary tissue grows and increases in

weight, it encounters the natural resistance of the skin, which, in spite of expanding, is able to maintain the balance, still holding the breast in its proper position. Once the resistance of the skin is overcome by the weight of the content, added to the force of gravity, the elastic fibers of the cutaneous tissue are broken (the development of striae) and the skin yields, which breaks the existing equilibrium and gives rise to an irreversible ptotic process.

This appraisal, which has been developed over 25 years of constant interest in this field, has led us to a concept [11–14] we believe can be useful in this effort: to obtain better results in this area of aesthetic surgery, which is so inspiring, and yet so contradictory.

Principles of Our Method

Since its first presentation in Paris in 1975, during the Sixth International Congress of Plastic and Reconstructive Surgery, and through subsequent publications, our method has undergone innumerable improvements, both in design and execution. These improvements make the method more effective, contribute to the ease of operation, and give more desirable results.

Our concept encompasses the breast as a whole, taking into full account its specific components. We emphasize the following items as fundamental points of the concept:

1. The normal position of the breast in relation to the thorax depends on the stable equilibrium between its content and the continent (see Fig. 23-1).
2. The design of the skin excision varies according to the characteristics of each case. In our experience, the quantity of skin to be removed can be a considerable quantity, or there may be no need to remove any skin tissue at all (Figs. 23-2 through 23-9).
3. It is of the greatest importance to take the distance between the base of the nipple and the inframammary fold into consideration. It normally varies between 5 and 14 cm (Fig. 23-10).
4. We systematically sever the entire base of the mammary gland, leaving it totally free from the deep planes (Figs. 23-11 and 23-12).
5. We proceed, as a means of reduction, to the amputation of the base of the mammary cone, leaving, therefore, a cone of smaller size (Fig. 23-13).

6. The resection line at the base of the breast should be inclined toward its lateral external part. This is necessary to keep more mammary tissue in the external quadrants, so as to obtain a better accommodation to the rib cage (Figs. 23-14 and 23-15; see Figs. 23-11 and 23-12).

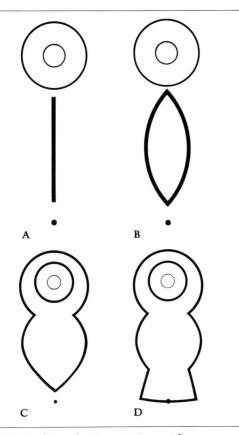

Fig. 23-2. Markings that I use. A. In turgid hypertrophies with intact skin, without striations, in young (15 to 25 years old) nullipara patients, when through bidigital pinching, we do not encounter any skin to be removed, both in the superior and inferior poles. B. When there is some skin to be removed in the inferior pole, an ellipse rises at the border of the areola and goes to 1 cm above the inframammary fold. C. Design used in 90 percent of cases in small, medium, and large hypertrophies, when the distance between the base of the nipple and the inframammary fold measures from 10 to 12 cm, and when there is no skin to be removed on line B (see Fig. 23-5A), the conclusion that is reached after bidigital pinching at this level. D. In giant hypertrophies, when this distance is greater than 12 cm and skin must be removed, I use this design.

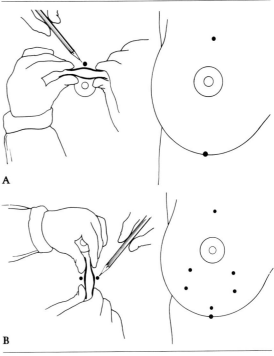

Fig. 23-3. A. Bidigital pinching to calculate the excess of skin in the superior pole. B. Similar procedure with respect to the skin in the inferior pole.

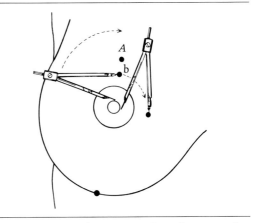

Fig. 23-4. Distance A-b represents the reduction in the amount of skin that remains between the fingers during digital pinching. This distance, in poor-quality skins with striae, is approximately 1 cm. In good-quality skins, principally in young patients, owing to the vigor of the specific function of the elastic fibers, the same distance A-b should be 2 cm to avoid the widening of the scar. Point b is transferred to the cardinal and collateral points, which, when joined, will originate the cupula of the design.

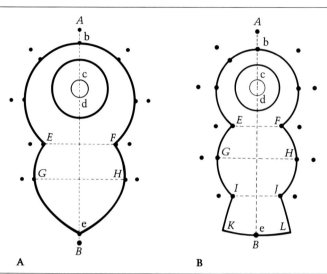

A   B

Fig. 23-5. A. Discount of the skin A-b that remains between the fingers during bidigital pinching. Distance b-c to be transferred to the cardinal and collateral points. Distance d-e, from the base of the nipple to a point, which, when the breast is in repose, with the patient supine, is approximately 1 cm distant from the inframammary fold. At the level of e-B, it can be observed, through bidigital pinching, that in the predominant majority of cases, there is no skin to be removed. Thus, the end of the longitudinal scar is above the inframammary fold line. B. When the distance d-B is greater than 10 or 12 cm, and this happens most in large or giant hypertrophies, the design is modified in its inferior part. With bidigital pinching, we encounter line I-J, which has the same length as line E-F. The distances K-B, B-L, I-K, and J-L measure 3 cm each, which calls for a complementary horizontal incision of 6 cm (distance K-L). This line can measure a little more — 1 or 2 cm — when the distance from the base of the nipple to the inframammary fold is bigger than 12 cm. Lines E-F and I-J represent the narrowed points of the mammary contour, by virtue of a slight "ovoid tendency," when the patient is in the orthostatic position. This ovoid tendency has an appearance similar to an American football with one fourth of one extremity amputated (see Fig. 23-6). In both designs, line G-H represents the greatest diameter of the breast in its inferior pole.

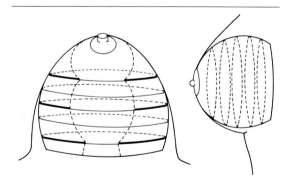

Fig. 23-6. The dark lines indicate the points of narrowing of the breast contour, which must be considered at the time of marking. The lack of observance of these points could result in localized stress, with deformation of the shape of the neobreast, with tissue tension and widening of the scar at these points. Observe (on the right) the ovoid form of the breast design, severed at the attachment base.

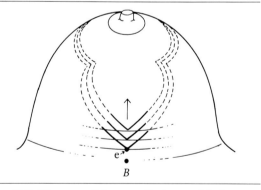

Fig. 23-7. Distance e-B is generally 1 cm, with the breast in repose and the patient supine. Normally there is not any skin to be removed at this level. Through bidigital pinching, it can be noted that point e can rise, with line e-B reaching as much as 3 cm.

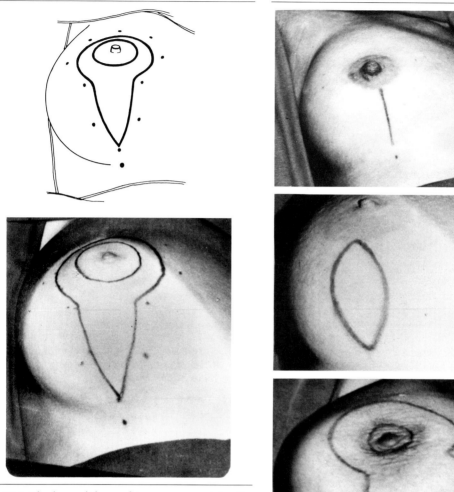

Fig. 23-8. The form of the marking may vary, giving the method greater flexibility. Here, the amount of skin to be removed from the inferior pole is less than usual, this fact being determined by digital pinching.

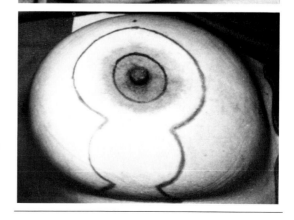

Fig. 23-9. Preoperative aspects of various designs. (The top figure is from G. Peixoto. The infra-areolar longitudinal incision in reduction mammoplasty. Aesth. Plast. Surg. 9:1, 1985.)

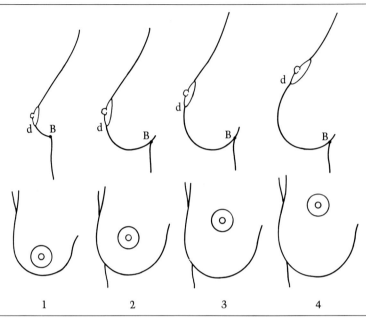

Fig. 23-10. The distance between the base of the nipple and the inframammary fold varies between 6 and 14 cm. In small hypertrophies, this value is in the range of 6 to 7 cm; 7 to 8 cm for medium hypertrophies; 10 to 12 cm for large hypertrophies; and reaching 14 cm in giant hypertrophies. With distances in the range of 6 to 8 cm, all techniques that require a transverse resection of the skin should be avoided, because this sometimes produces a reduction of as much as 3 cm, which results in the downward traction of the areolomammillary complex.

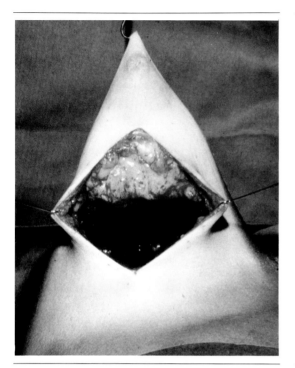

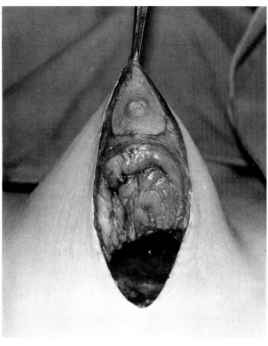

Fig. 23-11. Separation of the gland from the thoracic wall and the resection of the base of the mammary cone in a case in which the infra-areolar longitudinal incision was used (see Fig. 23-2B). Note the existence of an excellent surgical field, which favors the removal of the excess content and at the same time permits good hemostasis. The areolar diameter, which in this case is large, will become reduced spontaneously in proportion to the skin retraction. Observe the use of the jaw-hook above the areola.

Fig. 23-12. Breast separated from the deep planes, and the cone base amputated. The height of the remaining glandular adipose tissue, measured from the base of the nipple downward to the line of resection, should vary between 5 and 7 cm in accordance with the wish of a smaller or larger neobreast. At times, a central wedge is removed to narrow the organ in those cases in which it is extremely wide.

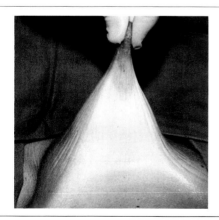

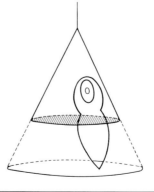

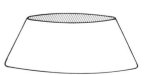

Fig. 23-13. The conical shape of the breast leads us to amputate its base to obtain the desired reduction of the organ. It is, I believe, the best manner in which to reduce it, maintaining its original form.

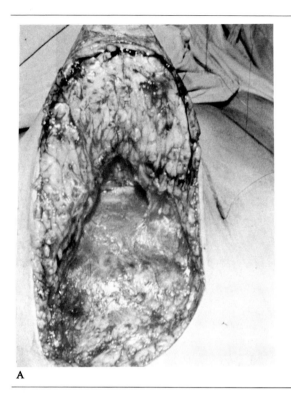

A

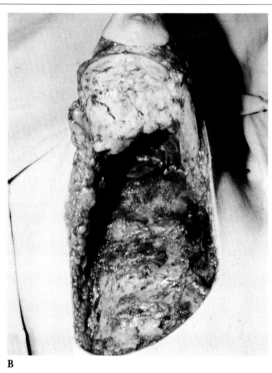

B

Fig. 23-14. A. In a longitudinal cut of the organ made to accompany the horizontal line, we observe the predominance of glandular adipose tissue in the external quadrants. B. In the reduction treatment of the organ, this disposition should be maintained to avoid future deformation of the neobreast.

7. It is our belief that all good and lasting results in a mammaplasty depend on the "feeling" of the surgeon in the evaluation, with relative precision, of the exact point at which the equilibrium of the content-continent is established, after an adequate resection of a gland from its envelope.

8. We take into consideration the ability of the skin to stretch and to contract, which permits its retraction over the remaining content. This capacity is impaired by the presence of striae as a result of the rupture of the elastic fibers or owing to the premature or natural senility of the cutaneous tissue (Figs. 23-16 through 23-18).

9. We consider the necessity of complete maintenance of organ function, avoiding separations and incisions, which may place its anatomical and physiological integrity in jeopardy (Fig. 23-19).

10. We give major importance to the size of the scar: the smaller, the better. A small scar is a factor of undeniable importance in the final results of a reduction mammaplasty. We have exhaustively shown that the reduction in the scar size does not produce any impairment

with relation to the shape of the breast. To the contrary, an excellent aesthetic aspect is obtained as a result of the natural form imparted (Figs. 23-20 and 23-21).

Analyses of Some Items

1. It is not possible to use a single design for all breasts. The design will have to vary, obeying the specific demands of each case. In our method we use four designs (see Fig. 23-2).

2. The severing of the breast from the deep planes does not affect the arterial and venal circulations but does permit a good visualization for the resection of the glandular adipose excess, eases hemostasis, and, above all, permits the location of the new base on its normal site (see Fig. 23-19).

3. The reduction of the glandular adipose excess takes into consideration the fact that the breast

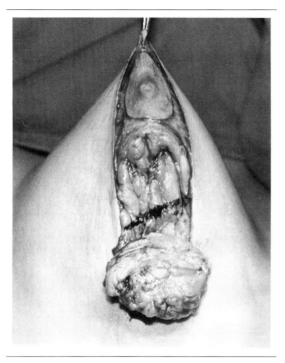

Fig. 23-15. Amputation of the inferior pole, which was necessary in this case due to the predominance of glandular tissue. The marking of the future resection line of the mammary cone base can be noted.

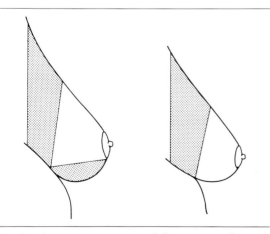

Fig. 23-16. Transverse section of the resection showing the amputation of the base and the inferior pole. The amputation of the base is executed in all cases. The amputation of the inferior pole is executed only in turgid breasts with a predominance of glandular tissue. In the case of flaccid breasts, we utilize the remaining inferior pole as fill to increase the consistency of the organ.

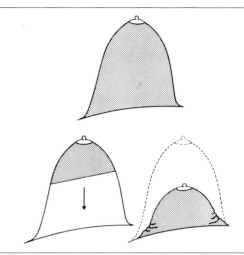

Fig. 23-17. Under normal conditions, intact skin has the ability for total retraction after a subcutaneous mastectomy on a breast of medium proportions, the normal skin stretching itself over the thorax as though the gland had not existed. The degree of contractibility varies, however, with the quality of the skin. The greater the number of striae, the greater the degree of skin senility—thus, the smaller the degree of contractibility. This capacity, however, never disappears completely. Thus, when the skin is intact, we resect it a little or none at all. When the skin tissue is anatomically and physiologically impaired, the amount of resection is directly proportional to the intensity of the impairment. This illustration shows the process of accommodation after the amputation of the base of the cone until its adjustment onto the thorax.

resembles the geometric form of a cone (see Fig. 23-13). Thus, the best way to reduce the size of this cone is to amputate its base, in this manner obtaining a smaller cone.

4. The stretching and retracting ability of the skin is consciously or unconsciously taken into consideration in any plastic surgery. What would be the result in rhinoplasty if the skin did not retract over the remaining content? Could good results be obtained if these properties did not exist? We do not affirm that the skin retracts equally in all cases. There are cases in which this capacity has been impaired (e.g., the presence of striae, cutaneous senility), which obliges us to remove larger quantities of skin. There are other cases in which the skin maintains the fullness of its anatomical and physiological functions of specific elasticity and contractibility.

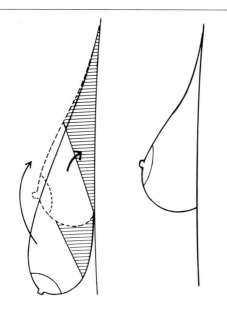

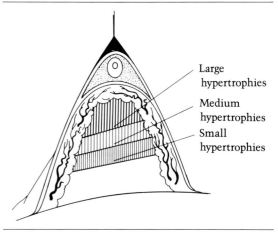

Fig. 23-19. Resection of the glandular adipose tissue in small, medium, and large hypertrophies. Observe the retention of an adequate thickness of the subcutaneous cellular tissue, which is necessary for the protection of the principal vascular network of the organ. The observance of the Schwartzmann maneuver is essential for the vascularization and innervation of the areolomammillary complex.

Large hypertrophies

Medium hypertrophies

Small hypertrophies

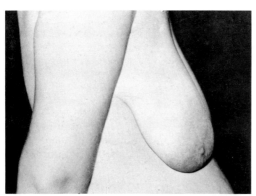

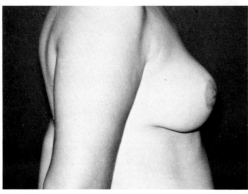

Fig. 23-18. Repositioning of the neobreast on the thorax, forced by the retraction of the skin and by the reestablishment of the equilibrium between the weight of the gland and the resistance of the skin after the removal of the adequate excess of each.

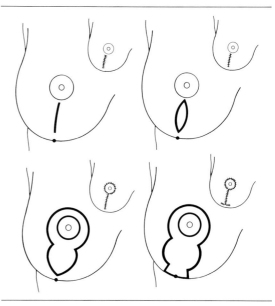

Fig. 23-20. Grouping of the four markings we utilize, showing the form of the corresponding scars.

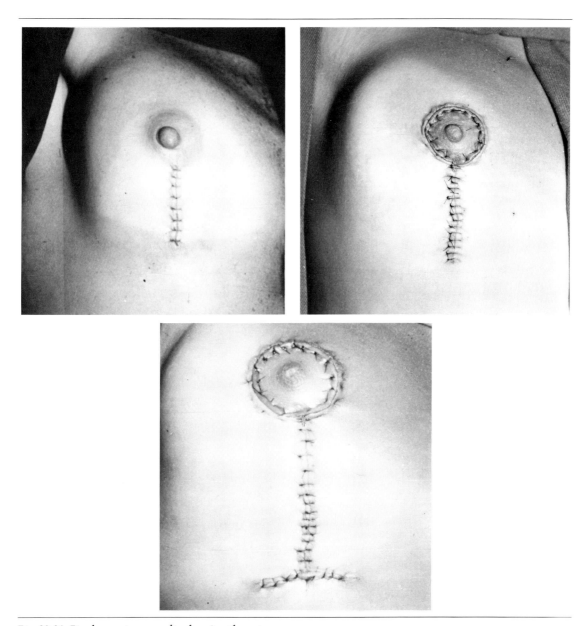

Fig. 23-21. Final operatory results showing the sutures
that will give rise to the future scars.

These cases are more common in young or nullipara patients, and the amount of skin that will have to be removed will be less or nil.

5. We believe that any practices that involve the dissociation of the skin-gland should be avoided, as well as those that involve the use of flaps of any type.

6. It is important to consider the decisive role that the careful preservation of the blood supply has in maintaining the integrity of the neobreast. Salmon's [20] and Maliniac's [8] studies about the blood circulation of the breast brought a decisive contribution to its understanding and made possible great progress in the evolution of reduction mammaplasty. The breast has a rich blood supply, with its origin from the internal mammary artery and branches from the subclavicular, lateral thoracic artery via the axillary artery along with intercostal branches. It is clear that all principal blood supplies run parallel to the skin, inside the connective tissue, which forms Cooper's ligaments. The perforating arteries reach the breast in its medial part when the breast is in its normal position. When ptosis occurs, its progression subjects these arteries and veins to constant stretching and subsequent atrophy, making them almost disappear, thereby making them less important to the vascularization of the breast. This fact causes a true "mute zone" centrally. The same phenomenon happens with innervation so that there is atrophy of the central ramification of the nerves. The absence of surrounding structures, in relation to the veins and nerves inside the subcutaneous cellular tissue close to the skin, leaves them without protection, covered only by loose connective tissue, becoming scarcer with increasing ptosis. This being so, it is possible to displace the gland completely from the muscular surface and to amputate the base without damage to its vascularization and innervation.

7. Every time the scar remains within the area of the breast proper, its quality is indisputably better. In our experience, we have observed the obvious aesthetic advantage of a longitudinal scar over a horizontal one. One way of improving the quality of a horizontal scar is to reduce its size and reduce the tension at its edges. In cases of giant hypertrophies, when the distance between the base of the nipple and the inframammary fold is greater than 12 cm, the design in Figure 23-2D should be used.

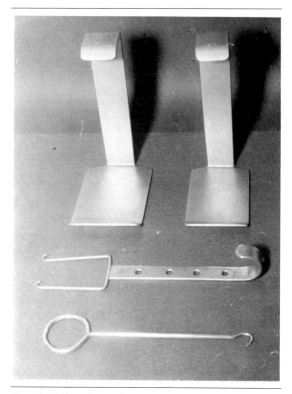

Fig. 23-22. Set of complementary instruments for mammaplasty surgery. The two spreaders, of our own design, each have a height of 11 cm at their handles. The blade of the smaller one is 7 × 4 cm and of the larger one 8 × 5 cm. The double hook (d'Assumpção) is the jaw-hook previously described.

Surgical Technique

The operation is performed with the patient in the supine position, with her back slightly elevated. Her arms are abducted at right angles with her trunk. Normally, general anesthesia is used.

SKIN MARKING

Skin varies according to the patient. We use four propositions that follow definite criteria but give more flexibility to the technique.

Two important factors should be taken into consideration for selecting the type of design:

1. The previous evaluation of the quantity of skin that will have to be removed, as demonstrated by a bidigital pinch, using both hands (see Fig. 23-3A and B).
2. The distance between the base of the nipple and the inframammary fold.

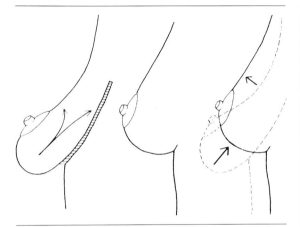

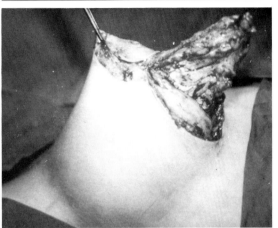

Fig. 23-23. In intact skin that is highly elastic, ptosis tends to occur. The intervention consists exclusively of skin resection in the amount necessary, and all the content of the organ is used to fill it, eliminating the ptosis while increasing the consistency of the breast.

In the case of mammary hypertrophy in young patients (15 to 25 years old), with intact skin of good quality, and where little or no skin needs to be excised, the design chosen will be either that shown in Figure 23-2A or B, according to the case.

We use the design shown in Figure 23-2C in approximately 90 percent of cases. It is indicated for breasts with flaccid and striated skin, with small, medium, or large hypertrophy, accompanied by ptosis, and when the distance between the base of the nipple and the inframammary fold is between 7 and 10 cm, approximately.

In giant hypertrophy, this distance is normally greater than 12 cm, reaching as much as 14 cm. In these cases, we use the design shown in Figure 23-2D, in order to reduce the height of the breast.

In these last two categories, the Schwarzmann maneuver is used routinely.

All skin markings are done with the patient supine and already anesthetized, and with the breast in repose.

SOME NECESSARY INSTRUMENTS

To facilitate the removal of the glandular-adipose tissue, we use a set of spreaders (Fig. 23-22), a jaw-hook, and a double hook (d'Assumpção hook). The jaw-hook and the double hook are used only on breasts with a single infraareolar longitudinal incision. The simple hook is placed right above the areola to lift the breast. The double hook is used on

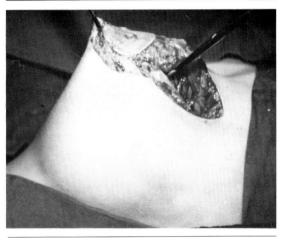

Fig. 23-24. Intraoperative aspect of the case formulated in the drawing in Figure 23-23. The skin incision follows the marking in Figure 23-2C. The entire mammary gland is separated from the thoracic wall; then we bury the inferior pole within the lateral columns, which forms a type of pedicle for the superior base. We never fix the gland directly onto the thoracic wall.

350

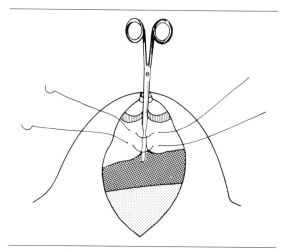

Fig. 23-25. Closure of the glandular adipose tissue. We unite the columns to each other, with absorbable thread, and without fixation to the thoracic wall.

the inferior end of the incision. The two spreaders are of the greatest importance with any type of design. They help to view the inside of the breast, facilitating hemostasis, and making it possible to accurately model the remaining content. A head light is equally indispensable for the best possible exposure of the breast.

REMOVAL TECHNIQUE

After resecting the skin in accordance with the selected design, and following the Schwartzmann maneuver, we pull the breast upward with a strong Kocher clamp placed at the superior pole, near the areola, exactly on the median line of the breast, in the deepithelialized area. We then dissect the entire glandular-adipose tissue from the deep planes. We calculate the height of resection of the glandular-adipose tissue to be kept. This height is measured from the base of the nipple downward. The height may vary between 5 and 7 cm. Naturally, the physical build of the patient must be taken into account, as well as wishes expressed by the patient, and the surgical practicability of the resection, considering the equilibrium of the content-continent. We never make this height less than 5 cm, nor more than 7 cm. Sometimes, in ptosis without hypertrophy, we do not resect any content, but only skin is removed (Figs. 23-23 and 23-24).

With the height marked, making the line slightly oblique outwardly, in order to follow the

anatomy of the breast, which has a greater amount of tissue in the external quadrants (see Fig. 23-14), we proceed to the amputation of the base of the breast, using a scalpel, following the oblique line, while preserving the subcutaneous cellular tissue (approximately 2 cm), on the lateral and upper walls of the organ, in order to protect the principal blood supply through the internal mammary and thoracic lateral arteries. This resection should be carried out so that a perfect cone is left, with an even base. Once hemostasis is accomplished, we proceed with the closing of the glandular-adipose tissue, approximating the columns and burying the inferior pole (Fig. 23-25). When the breast is flaccid, the superior pole is used to fill the breast, increasing its consistency. In the case of turgid breasts, with predominance of glandular tissue, we do not carry out the internal approximation and nearly always amputate the inferior pole. Absorbable sutures are used for internal closure. The skin is approximated with 5-0 nylon.

RESECTION OF GIANT HYPERTROPHY CONTENTS

The surgical treatment of giant hypertrophies is always a problem for every plastic surgeon. In addition to the immense size of the organ, the skin is striated and has lost a great deal of its anatomical and physiological integrity. We classify as true giant hypertrophy those breasts from which we expect to remove 1,000 gm per side.

We have obtained excellent results with our method in these cases — results that we consider significantly better than we would have achieved with other techniques. These good results are more frequent in young patients with better quality skin. With elderly patients and those whose skin that has lost much of its elasticity, there is great difficulty in reestablishing a balance between skin envelope and content: residual ptosis is usually observed 6 months postoperatively. Thus, in giant hypertrophy we consider it advisable to inform the patient of the possibility of a later revision, which can be accomplished with local anesthesia. This touch-up will consist exclusively of the removal of excess skin remaining, or even some glandular-adipose tissue to reduce the breast still more. We reaffirm the fact that the quality of the skin has a great influence on the result. If the skin has good texture, even in the presence of a giant hypertrophy, good results can be obtained without the need of a later touch-up.

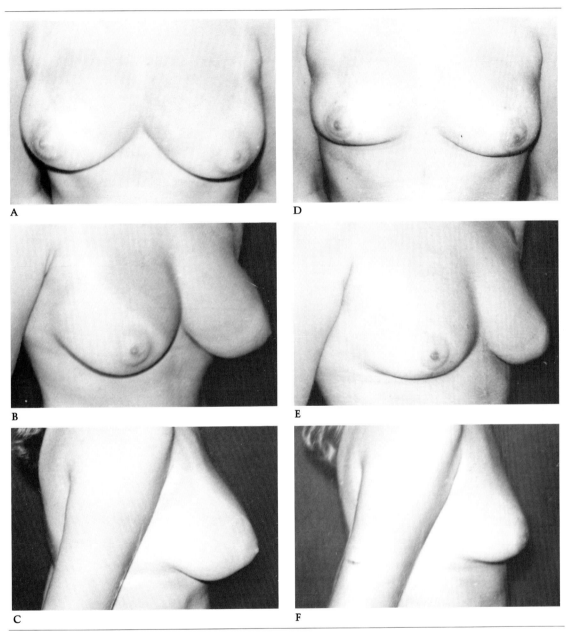

Fig. 23-26. A–C. A 22-year-old patient with moderate
hypertrophy. D–F. Postoperative result after 2 years.
For marking used, see Figure 23-2B. (From G. Peixoto.
The infra-areolar longitudinal incision in reduction
mammoplasty. Aesth. Plast. Surg. 9:1, 1985.)

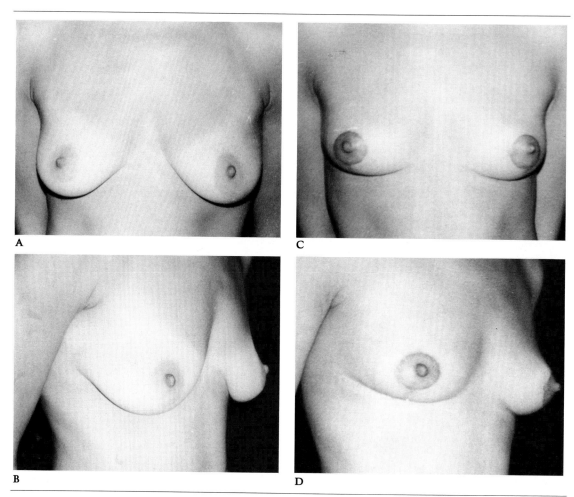

Fig. 23-27. *A,B. A 31-year-old patient with ptosis and asymmetry. C,D. Small resection of the right breast was performed. Internal treatment followed what is explained in Figure 23-24. For marking used see Figure 23-2C.*

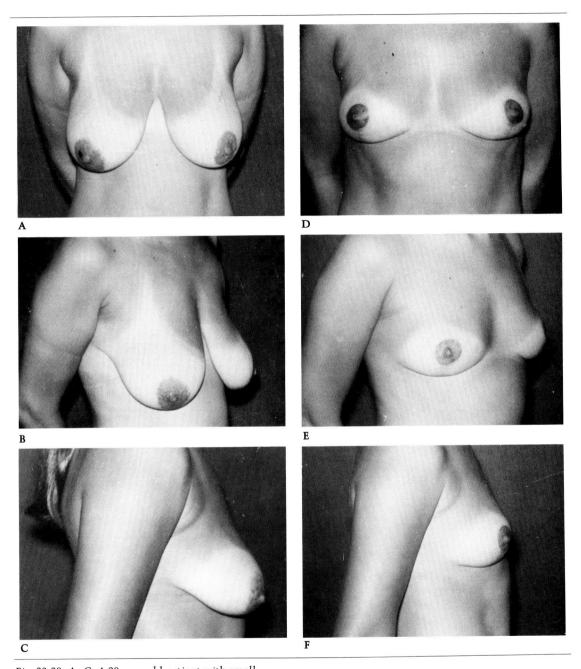

Fig. 23-28. A–C. A 28-year-old patient with small
hypertrophy and ptosis. D–F. Postoperative results
after 2 years. For marking used, see Figure 23-2C.

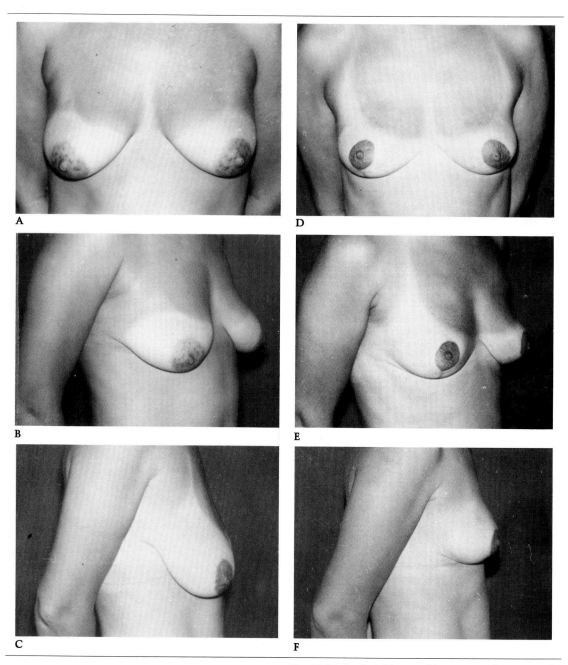

Fig. 23-29. A–C. A 36-year-old patient with ptosis and medium hypertrophy. D–F. Postoperative results after 11 months.

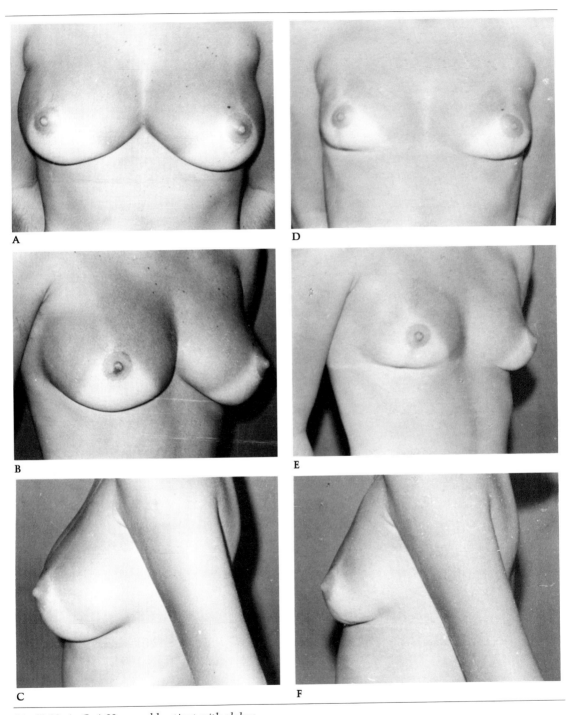

Fig. 23-30. A–C. A 22-year-old patient with globus
breasts. Medium hypertrophy. D–F. Postoperative
results after 2 years. For marking used, see Figure 23-2C.

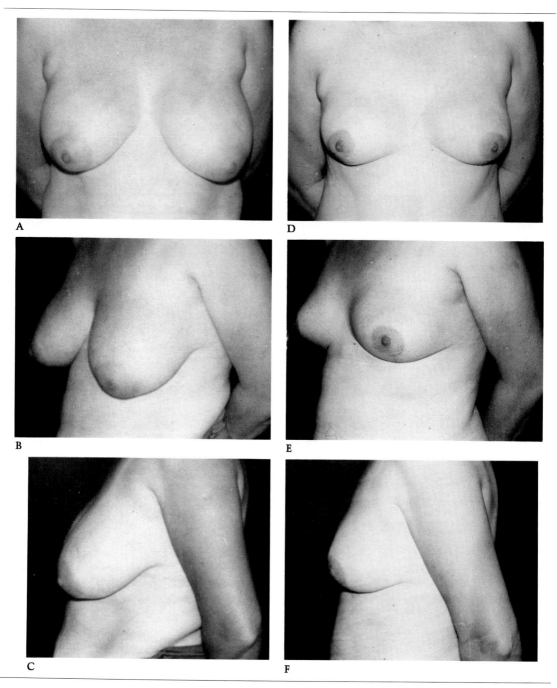

Fig. 23-31. A–C. A 40-year-old patient with medium hypertrophy and ptosis. D–F. Postoperative results after 5 years. For marking used, see Figure 23-2C.

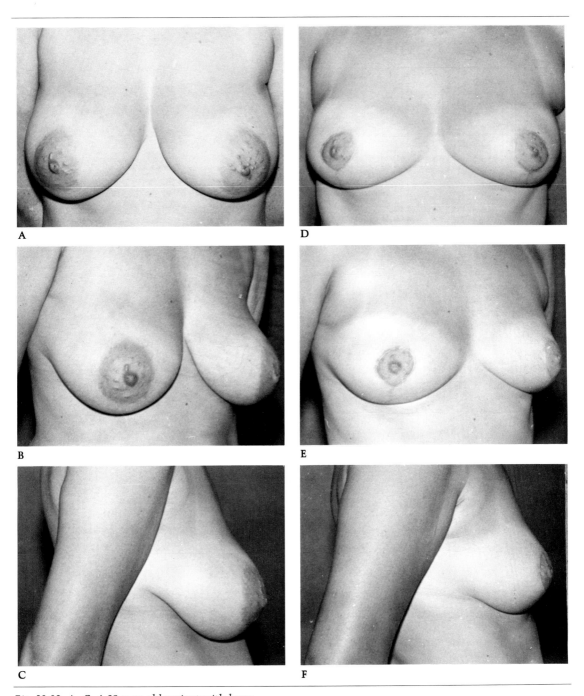

Fig. 23-32. A–C. A 39-year-old patient with large hypertrophy and ptosis. D–F. Postoperative results after 3 years. For marking used, see Figure 23-2C.

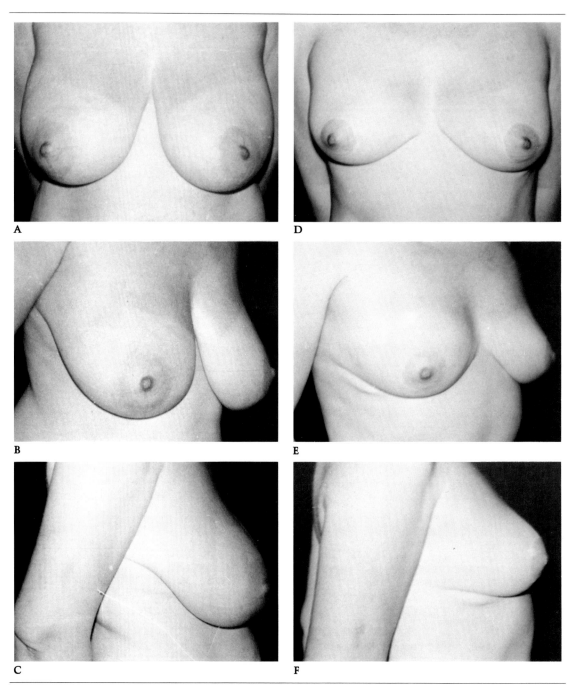

Fig. 23-33. A–C. A 39-year-old patient with giant hypertrophy and ptosis. D–F. Postoperative results after 1 year and 8 months. For marking used, see Figure 23-2C.

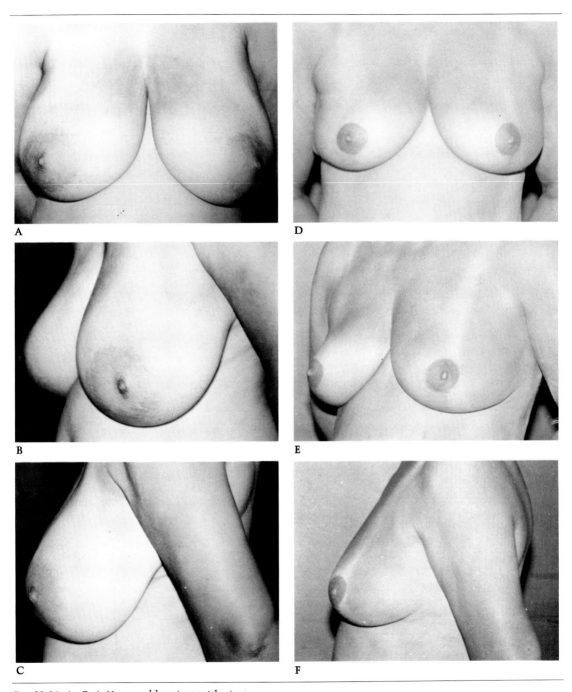

Fig. 23-34. A–C. A 41-year-old patient with giant
hypertrophy. D–F. Postoperative results after 4 years.
For marking used, see Figure 23-2D.

Be that as it may, immoderate hypertrophy will continue being a challenge to the plastic surgeon. In those cases in which it is not possible to foresee a good final aesthetic result, we think it wise to do the procedure in two steps. In the second step, which can be performed 6 months after the first, the surgeon will be working with only moderate residual hypertrophy, with every expectation of success.

Complications

From the beginning to its present stage, the method has undergone modifications and improvements with the objective of correcting some inconveniences, which are described in the following paragraphs.

During the first years of its evolution, we observed widening of the scar and areola, residual ptosis, minimal necrosis of the areolar periphery, insufficient removal or excessive removal of content, and concavities. These cases were not evaluated on a percentage basis because they were scarce, the total number was very small, and, most of all, they were not common to the same patient. It became easy to control such problems after we had discovered their causes. In this way, the widened scar and the exaggerated expansion of the areolas were corrected with techniques such as that shown in Fig. 23-11 and by carefully calculating the amount of excess skin to be removed (see Fig. 23-3). Residual ptosis was corrected with a better evaluation of how to get an equilibrium between the volume and the container (see Fig. 23-1). The insufficient or exaggerated removal of the volume was avoided with a greater attention when using the Schwartzmann maneuver. The depressions were avoided with a more careful modeling of the remaining glandular adipose tissue. These difficulties were gradually corrected on a scale in proportion to the experience of the surgeon using the method. If, in the present stage of the method we are faced with some of these cases once in a while, however minimized, this is certainly due to the specific characteristics of the case, as it occurs in all branches of surgery, in any area of the human body.

The problems previously mentioned were consequences of the surgeon's lesser experience with the technique when he or she first started using it. When an experienced surgeon follows the rules of the method, complications usually are avoidable.

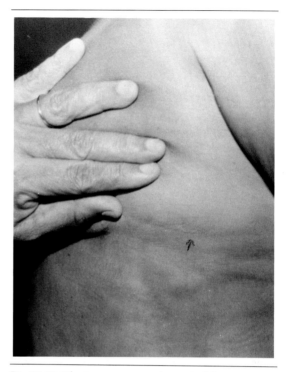

Fig. 23-35. The transverse scar (arrow) of the patient in Figure 23-34, where the design B was used (see Fig. 23-5), measures 7 cm because the distance between the base of the nipple and the inframammary fold was 14 cm. Being so, in the inverted T, the longitudinal scar had 7 cm, and the transverse scar had 7 cm on each side (b-c or K-B). They add 14 cm (K-L). This case of such a big distance is not common, even in giant-sized breasts. The median distance between the base of the nipple and the fold is about 12 cm. In giant-sized breasts and enormous hypertrophy, it is usually 8 cm for the longitudinal line and 4 cm for the transverse line. The shorter the distance between the base of the nipple and the fold, the smaller the transverse line.

It is possible that my experience overcoming difficulties will help others using this method to obtain the same results my patients and I have enjoyed and with which I am completely satisfied (Figs. 23-26 through 23-35).

Final Considerations

We do not pretend to affirm that we have found the philosopher's stone to the problem. There is still a long way to go. The relative simplicity of this method, the natural look of the resultant breast, the small size of the scar, and the logic of the concept, and the method give us the feeling that this contribution might be a new road to follow. As with all methods, and this happened with us, improvement of results occurs with increased experience. We believe that the creativity and experience of each practitioner will permit him or her to have ample leeway for exploring this method, which can lead to the attainment of still better results than those we have achieved.

References

1. Arufe, H., and Juri, J. Modification of the Strömbeck technique. *Plast. Reconstr. Surg.* 46:604, 1970.
2. Basile, R.D. Mammaplasty: Large reduction with short inframammary scar. *Plast. Reconstr. Surg.* 76:130, 1975.
3. Dufourmentel, C., and Mouly, R. Plastie mammaire par la mèthode Oblique. *Ann. Chir. Plast.* 6:45, 1961.
4. Hirshowitz, B., and Moscona, R. Technical variations of the MacKissock operation for reduction mammaplasty. *Aesth. Plast. Surg.* 3:149, 1983.
5. Hollander, E. Die operation der mammahipertrophie und derHangerbrust. *Dtsch. Med. Wochenschr.* 50:1400, 1924 (Apub Robert M. Goldwyn, Cirurgia de la Reconstruction de la Mama. Barcelona: Salvat, 1981).
6. Lalardrie, J.P., and Jougland, J.-P. *Chirurgie Plastique du Sein.* Paris: Masson, 1974.
7. Maillard, G.F. A Z-mammaplasty with minimal scarring. *Plast. Reconstr. Surg.* 77:66, 1986.
8. Maliniac, J.W. Arterial blood supply of the breast. *Arch. Surg.* 47:329, 1943.
9. Morestin, H., and Guinard, A. Hypertrophie mammaire traitée par la resection discoide. *Bull. Mem. Soc. de Chir.* Paris 33:649, 1907.
10. MacKissock, P.K. Reduction mammaplasty with a vertical dermal flap. *Plast. Reconstr. Surg.* 49:245, 1972.
11. Peixoto, G. Reduction mammaplasty. A personal method. Translation of Seventh International Congress of Plastic and Reconstructive Surgery. Rio de Janeiro, 1979.
12. Peixoto, G. Reduction mammaplasty. A personal technique. *Plast. Reconstr. Surg.* 65:217, 1980.
13. Peixoto, G. Reduction mammaplasty. *Aesth. Plast. Surg.* 8:231, 1984.
14. Peixoto, G. The infra-areolar longitudinal incision in reduction mammaplasty. *Aesth. Plast. Surg.* 9:1, 1985.
15. Piotti, F. Experience with vertical technique in mammaplasty. *Aesth. Plast. Surg.* 4:349, 1981.
16. Pitanguy, I. Mamaplastias. Estudo de 245 casos consecutivos e apresentação de técnica pessoal. *Rev. Bras. Cir.* 42:201, 1961.
17. Pitanguy, I. Surgical treatment of breast hypertrophy. *Br. J. Plast. Surg.* 20:78, 1967.
18. Pontes, R. A technique of reduction mammaplasty. *Br. J. Plast. Surg.* 26:365, 1973.
19. Regnault, P. Reduction mammaplasty by the "B" technique. *Plast. Reconstr. Surg.* 53:19, 1974.
20. Salmon, M. Les artères de la glande mammaire. *Ann. Anat. Pathol.* 16:477, 1939.
21. Strömbeck, J.O. Mammaplasty: Report of a new technique based on the two pedicle procedure. *Br. J. Plast. Surg.* 79:90, 1960.

COMMENTS ON CHAPTER 23   *Robert M. Goldwyn*

Peixoto has emphasized several important points concerning his technique:

1. A major objective is to inflict as small a scar as possible on the patient. The scar should be vertical, as vertical scars heal better than horizontal scars.
2. Although four basic designs are used, depending on the size, shape, and elasticity of the breast, one is used predominantly (see Fig. 23-2C).
3. The skin is not dissected free from the breast tissue itself, thereby helping to ensure an adequate blood supply to the nipple and areola.
4. The mammary gland is completely separated from its deep attachments.
5. The base of the mammary cone is amputated, thus creating a smaller cone. By inclining the line of resection obliquely, more breast tissue is left in the outer quadrants, which gives the breast a better shape.
6. The final contour of the breast depends on the ability of the skin to retract; the more the elasticity, the greater the capacity of the skin to shrink. Women who are young, without excessive hypertrophy, without ptosis, and without striae are the best candidates.
7. Although the surgeon uses preexisting markings, he or she cannot simply cut along the dotted lines and expect to get the desired result. The direction and extent of the glandular resection vary with the patient, as does the closure, to some degree. The new nipple site is not premarked or predetermined.

Although Peixoto states that he has used the procedure in giant hypertrophy (more than 1,000 gm resected per breast), he admits that it is more difficult, especially in elderly patients, in whom he advises a two-stage effort. The last stage can be done under local anesthesia and would generally involve resecting more skin or more breast tissue or both. If we accept Peixoto's word that he uses a specific design (see Fig. 23-2C) in 90 percent of patients, the remaining patients would necessarily have had to be done using one of the three remaining designs. This means that those with extremely large breasts constitute only a relatively small proportion of Peixoto's series. In my experience, his technique is much more difficult in patients in whom one expects to remove a great amount of tissue. In fact, unless one has previously used the technique in patients with less dramatic hypertrophy, performing it on a very large-breasted woman would take an unnecessarily long time and would be very difficult to do. Indeed, this is what Cumberscure and Lamarche [1] reported in their series of 165 patients, in whom 94 breasts had reduction by a modified Peixoto method and were able to be followed beyond 6 months. They noted that the horizontal scar widened more than in other techniques, but because it was shorter and in a favorable position, it was not prominent with the patient either sitting or standing.

In discussing Peixoto's technique [2], Pitanguy made the point that although "many authors have been concerned about reducing the submammary scar . . . [p]ersonally I think that the aphorism, 'the smaller, the better' should not always be applied in plastic surgery. Sometimes a longer scar, if well hidden in a natural skin fold, will look better than a shorter one, harder to conceal" [3]. Pitanguy was referring specifically to the horizontal limb of the Peixoto design, which is slightly above the submammary fold.

My own experience with the Peixoto technique is not extensive. The first patient in whom I utilized it had partial areola necrosis bilaterally because I removed too much breast tissue below the bridge of the gland in order to get the nipple and areola moved to its new location because I was having trouble in doing so. Subsequently, in patients with smaller breasts, when the need to transpose the nipple-areola has been no more than 6 cm, this is less of a problem. In all those patients, however, sensation has not been normal. If one is removing the breast from all its attachments at its base, it would seem reasonable that the sensory nerves would be interrupted. Admittedly, I do not have Peixoto's experience and have to rely on his observations and those of other authors.

For patients with extremely large breasts, the Peixoto method may be more difficult to apply for most surgeons. In my experience, those women do not mind a longer scar, particularly if one does the operation speedily, easily, and safely, with particular regard to the viability of the nipple-areola. Figure 23-34F shows a patient who had large breasts but who also seemed to require a scar going laterally, as one would normally have in the McKissock or the inferior pedicle methods.

Peixoto correctly talked about the "torture of Tantalus." His story is worth recalling. Once the favorite of the gods, this wealthy king, presumably a son of Zeus and Pluto, was allowed to participate in the deliberations of the gods and to share their meals. His good fortune made him overbearing, and he insulted them and had to suffer the consequences. One version has him in the world below with unappeased hunger and thirst, being at the same time immersed in water to the chin, while the finest fruits were hanging before him.

Whenever he opened his mouth to enjoy them, the water dried up and the fruits vanished. Another version, no less pleasant, has him suspended in air, while above his head hangs a huge rock, threatening to fall and crush him. In these times, and in my country, the rock would obviously be the threat of malpractice.

REFERENCES

1. Cumberscure, C., and Lamarche, J.P. Notre technique de Peixoto modifiée pour la correction des hypertrophies mammaires. Indications et resultats. *Ann. Chir. Plast. Esthet.* 32 : 30, 1987.
2. Peixoto, G. Reduction mammaplasty: A personal technique. *Plast. Reconstr. Surg.* 65 : 217, 1980.
3. Pitanguy, I. Discussion of Peixoto, G. Reduction mammaplasty: A personal technique. *Plast. Reconstr. Surg.* 65 : 217, 1980.

24

Liacyr Ribeiro

The Lozenge Technique

Throughout the last decade, all authors, particularly Ariyan [2], Lassus [14], and Peixoto [18–20], writing on reduction mammaplasty and recording their experiences, preferences, or techniques have reported good cosmetic results in terms of the shape of the breasts [10]. The work of Biesenberger [4] and Burian [7] was important in that regard. However, technical difficulties in achieving the desired size and shape along with minimal scarring have remained in certain patients. Proponents of various methods have argued the advantages of their respective methods. Most did not believe or still do not believe that a pleasing shape of the breast is possible with reduced scars. At first we did not believe it either, since we considered that the horizontal scar was essentially irreducible. Later, however, based on Peixoto's philosophy and concepts, we became convinced that scars could be shortened at no detriment to the end result.

So that these concepts could include all patients desiring reduction mammaplasty, we conceived the "lozenge" technique, which was derived from other methods in addition to our own experience over the past 20 years [21–23].

In addition to the scar around the areola, the technique produces a single vertical scar that never extends beyond the submammary fold. This feature distinguishes the procedure from that of Lotsch [16], Joseph [11], Arié [1], and Juri et al [12]. With those procedures, scars always extended further than the submammary fold and prevented patients from wearing bathing suits or bikinis.

The lozenge technique can be described briefly as a combination of Arié's method of marking, Peixoto's concept of the subsequent contraction of the skin and gland after reduction, Bozola et al's [5, 6] technique of inverted sutures, and our inferiorly based pedicle method (pedicle 1) similar to those described by Arufe [3], Courtiss and Goldwyn [8], Georgiade et al [9], Robbins [24], Labandter et al [13], Longacre et al [15], and Maliniac [17].

Peixoto pioneered a method whereby the end result depended on tissue retraction after resection. However, despite all his experience and mastery, we found his technique useful only for specific kinds of patients.

The introduction of the inferiorly based pedicle by ourselves in 1973 has given good cosmetic results early and even better later after the tissues have shrunk completely. Despite our satisfaction with the lozenge technique, we are certain that there will be subsequent improvements. We offer our technique as a contribution to reduction mammaplasty today and possibly a bridge to better procedures in the future.

Indications

The lozenge technique cannot be used for every patient. Best results are attained in young women with juvenile hypertrophy, with good skin elasticity, where the amount of tissue to be excised will not be greater than 500 gm per breast. The technique is also useful in simple cases of ptosis, with small or medium hypertrophy, and as an adjunct when a prosthesis is used along with correction of ptosis. If a patient fits any of the categories just mentioned but has loose skin with striae, the surgeon should be sure that she understands that a good result will occur only in the long-term.

Operative Technique

The patient should preferably be operated on under general anesthesia in a semiseated position.

Marking begins at the areola, whose diameter should be between 3.5 and 4 cm (Figs. 24-1A and 24-2).

A line is drawn from the midclavicular point to the upper border of the areola (Fig. 24-3). Next, we designate point a, which is a projection of the mammary fold on the upper pole of the breast (see

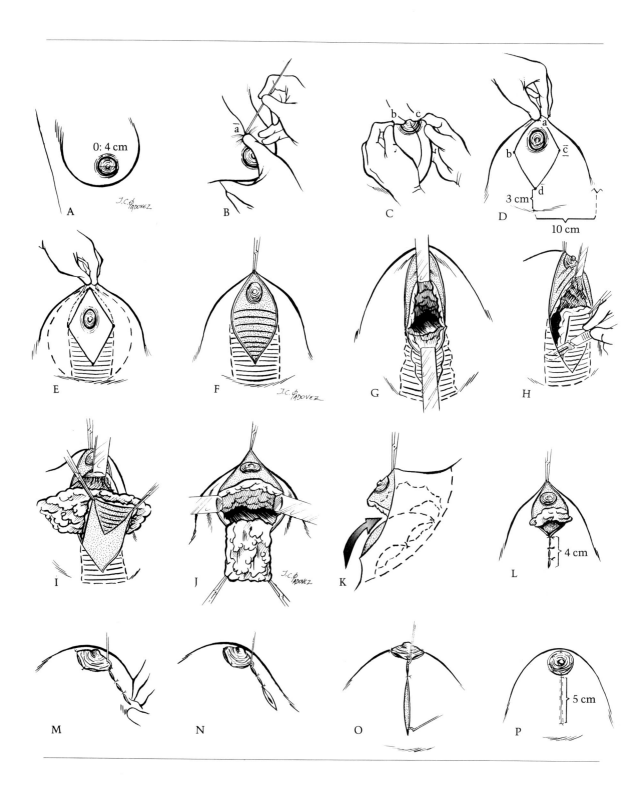

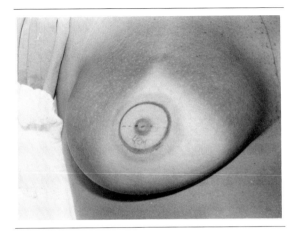

Fig. 24-2. The new areola is outlined, with about a 4-cm diameter.

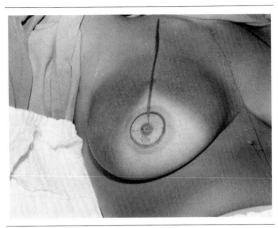

Fig. 24-3. The marking is done from the midclavicular line to the new areola border.

Fig. 24-1B). This is accomplished through the widely used bidigital maneuver (Fig. 24-4).

By sight and by moving the breast, we align two imaginary points that will cross diametrically (Figs. 24-5 through 24-8; see Fig. 24-1C).

Point d is marked at 2.5 or 3.0 cm superior to the submammary fold, corresponding to the inferior pole of the breast (Fig. 24-9; see Fig. 24-1D).

By joining all our points in a straight or curved line, we achieve a lozenge-shaped outline (Fig. 24-10; see Fig. 24-1D). With the breast now pulled upward at point a, the area to be resected is determined (Fig. 24-11; see Fig. 24-1E).

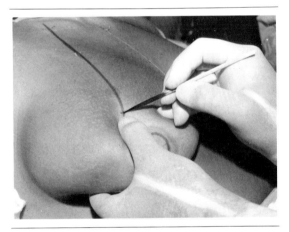

Fig. 24-4. By means of a bidigital maneuver, point a is marked to correspond to the submammary projection of the line formerly drawn.

Fig. 24-1. A. The new areola is outlined with about a 4-cm diameter. B. Point a is marked. C. Points b and c are marked. D. Point d is determined 3 cm up from the submammary fold and 10 cm from the xiphoid appendix. E. The inferiorly based pedicle is outlined. F. The area corresponding to the lozenge outline is deepithelialized. G. Horizontal incision below the areola is carried to the muscular plain. H. Medial lateral undermining of the inferior pole of the breast is done. I. Both the inferior pole and the marked area are undermined to allow formation of the pedicle. J. The pedicle is formed by lateral and medial incisions and resection toward the inferior pole. K. Fixation of the pedicle on the muscular wall. L. The vertical suture is carried 4 or 5 cm from the new fold. M. The dog-ear to be excised is marked. N. Area of skin to be resected for correction of the dog-ears. O. Skin and intradermal sutures are placed. P. Vertical suturing begins 4 or 5 cm from the new fold. The areola anchoring suture should be checked.

The transposition of points a, b, and c to the second breast is accomplished by stitching two sutures at the sternal notch and at the xiphoid appendix, bringing them together with a hemostat, and moving them to the opposite side (Figs. 24-12 and 24-13).

Point D is transposed and located 10 cm (measured with a ruler) laterally to the xiphoid appendix (Figs. 24-14 and 24-15).

The next step is to outline the inferiorly based pedicle (see Fig. 24-1E).

The lozenge area is deepithelialized (Fig. 24-16), followed by forming the pedicle (Fig. 24-17; see Fig. 24-1F).

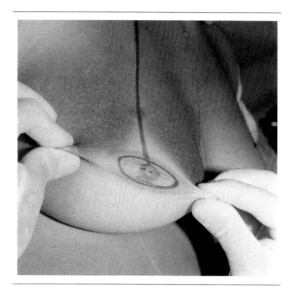

Fig. 24-5. With a bidigital maneuver, an imaginary line crosses the nipple. This is a significant part of the procedure, since it depends on one's ability to visualize the extent of skin to be removed.

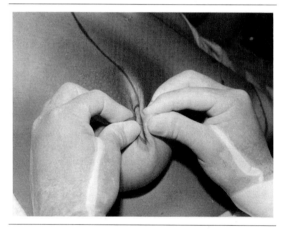

Fig. 24-6. Joining two points, with projection of point a.

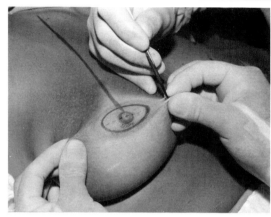

Fig. 24-7. Points b and c are marked.

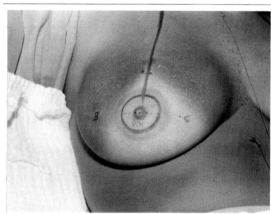

Fig. 24-8. Points a, b, and c are marked.

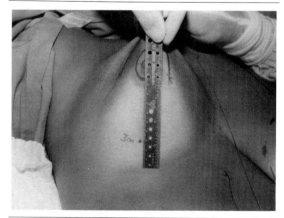

Fig. 24-9. Point d is marked 3 cm above the submammary fold beginning the line and future incision that will extend to the nipple.

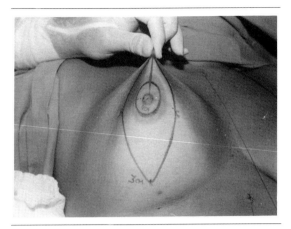

Fig. 24-10. Points a, b, and c are joined in a straight or curved line, producing a lozenge-shaped outline; hence, the designation "lozenge technique."

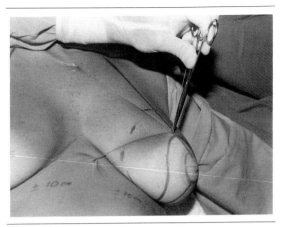

Fig. 24-13. Point a is transposed to the opposite breast as are points B and C.

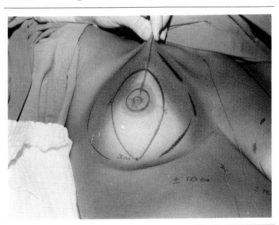

Fig. 24-11. Marking along the mammary area, staying close to the chest wall, outlines the area for resection that corresponds to the base of the mammary cone.

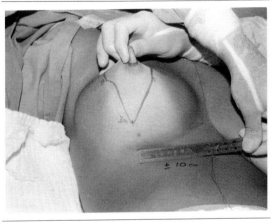

Fig. 24-14. Point d is also transposed. By using a ruler, we determine 10 cm from the xiphoid appendix.

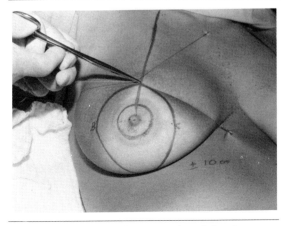

Fig. 24-12. Points a and b are transferred, by aligning two sutures stitched at the sternal notch and at the xiphoid appendix. Observe the transposition of point a.

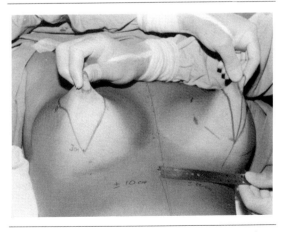

Fig. 24-15. Transposition of point d from side to side.

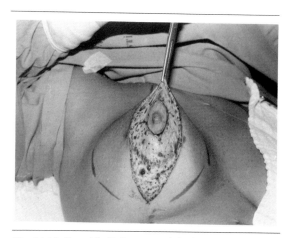

Fig. 24-16. Deepithelialization of the lozenge area.

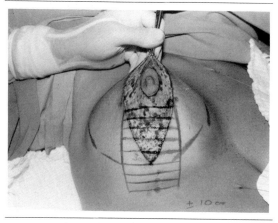

Fig. 24-17. The inferiorly based pedicle is drawn, whose outline corresponds to that part of the flap behind the skin.

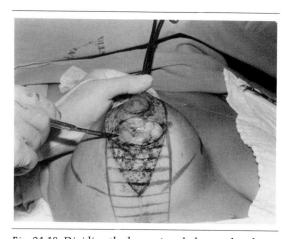

Fig. 24-18. Dividing the breast into halves and making the pedicle take place simultaneously.

A horizontal incision immediately below the areola is carried down to the muscular layer as if to divide the breast in half (Figs. 24-18 and 24-19; see Fig. 24-1G).

The lateral and medial margins of the flap are now in size (see Fig. 24-1H), with care taken to preserve the thickness of the dermal skin flap (approximately 2 cm).

Following mediolateral undermining (Fig. 24-20; see Fig. 24-1I), the inferior border close to the skin should be freed very carefully in order not to injure the fourth and the fifth intercostal perforating vessels, which account for the pedicle's viability (Fig. 24-21).

The pedicle is now complete (Fig. 24-22) and should be transposed to the upper pole of the ptotic and hypertrophic breast. In the instance of hypertrophy, the pedicle is transposed after excess tissue has been excised.

One can now judge the vascularity of the flap, which should also be noted throughout the operation.

Constructing the second pedicle is now begun. As soon as that has been accomplished, one must verify the viability of the first pedicle. In the event that ischemia is noted, because of a technical failure, one should change the procedure or choose another kind of marking, utilizing a part of the breast not touched surgically (see Fig. 24-22). If no vascular complications have occurred, one can begin resecting the upper pole (Fig. 24-23; see Fig. 24-1J). Mammary tissue is resected from the base of the mammary cone, corresponding to the supramuscular portion of the breast (Fig. 24-24).

The breast should be reconstituted now, with the patient placed in a horizontal position.

Fixing the pedicle is done first. This will vary with the patient, not only with regard to the number of stitches but also to its position. The pedicle should droop naturally. Lateral and medial stitches are required only if the pedicle has a tendency to slide sideways (Fig. 24-25; see Fig. 24-1K).

While the vertical incision is being closed, beginning at its lower end, the entire mammary complex is pulled upward. Suturing is begun four or five cm superior to the new fold, thereby causing the new breast to retract (Fig. 24-26; see Fig. 24-1L).

Note: The stitching should not begin in the original fold.

Once the pedicle has been secured and the vertical stitching begun, the areola-nipple complex

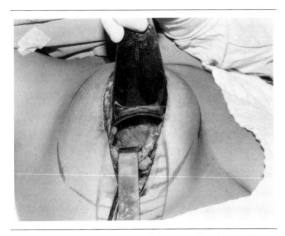

Fig. 24-19. An incision is made perpendicular to the level of the muscle, as can be observed posteriorly.

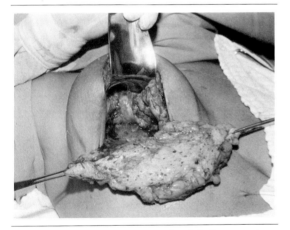

Fig. 24-20. The whole inferior pole of the breast is free, as are its lateral and medial segments.

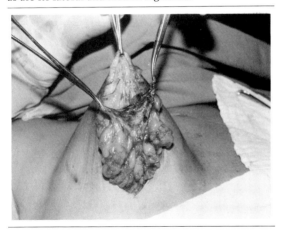

Fig. 24-21. The inferior portion is also freed, with caution taken as the incision goes close to the skin, down to the original fold.

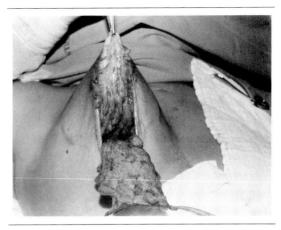

Fig. 24-22. The inferiorly based pedicle is formed with resection of the medial and lateral segments. The pedicle should be 3 cm at its base so that its viability is not compromised by division of the perforating intercostal vessels.

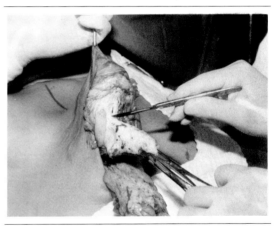

Fig. 24-23. Excess mammary tissue is resected beginning with the central area of the superior pole.

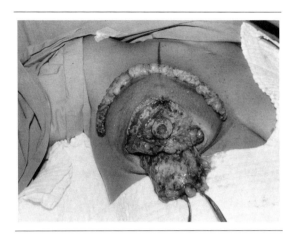

Fig. 24-24. Mammary tissue is resected from the base of the mammary cone, corresponding to the supramuscular portion. After resection, tissue is placed over the skin, exposing the area of resection.

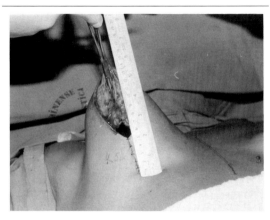

Fig. 24-26. Starting from the new fold (breast retraction is already beginning), the position of the new areola is determined. The diameter should be 4 to 5 cm.

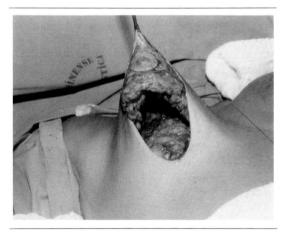

Fig. 24-25. After resection, the pedicle is fixed to its new position and should remain there spontaneously, without tension. Subsequently, it will be fixed to the muscle wall, with one or two nonabsorbable stitches.

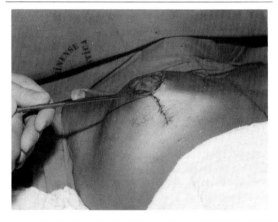

Fig. 24-27. The main stitches are placed on the new areola, where no skin resection will be required. The areola-nipple complex should droop naturally into its new position.

should be fixed in its new position. No skin resection will be required. The periareolar incision is closed by stitching in such a way as to compensate for the excess of skin surrounding the areola (Fig. 24-27).

As the stitching on the areola and the vertical incision are being completed, a hook should be placed at the areola incision junction to pull the breast upward (Fig. 24-28).

In most instances, a dog-ear has developed (Fig. 24-29; see Fig. 24-1M) and must be excised (Figs. 24-30 and 24-31; see Fig. 24-1N), with no adverse effect on the end result (see Fig. 24-1O). Afterward, the vertical incision, which is usually 5 or 6 cm, will not extend beyond the submammary fold (Figs. 24-32 and 24-33; see Fig. 24-1P).

The breast must be immobilized upward (Fig. 24-34); this is done by applying adhesive microporous tape. This is the same method used to immobilize the nasal skin after rhinoplasty. With regard to the breast, the technique is also based on skin retraction (Fig. 24-35). The tape should remain for 10 days; the patient should then be placed in a brassiere.

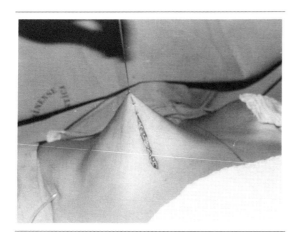

Fig. 24-28. Suturing is done in two ways. The illustration shows the intradermal stitch with nonabsorbable material and inverted knots.

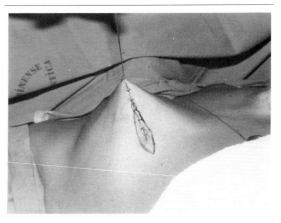

Fig. 24-30. The dog-ear is present and outlined. Care should be taken not to extend the line of resection beyond the submammary fold.

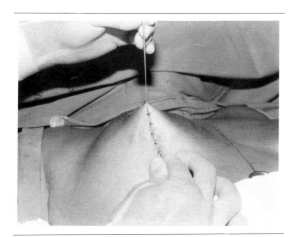

Fig. 24-29. After suturing and by means of a bidigital maneuver, we note that excess skin is present at the distal end of the incision. This maneuver helps in determining whether or not a dog-ear remains in this location.

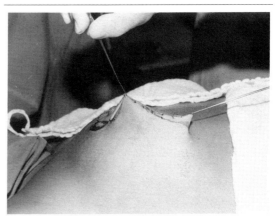

Fig. 24-31. Side view of the dog-ear remaining at the distal end of the incision. The skin resection outlined does not extend beyond the fold.

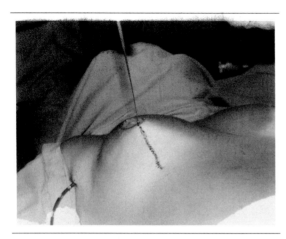

Fig. 24-32. End result. Areola and vertical suturing is completed.

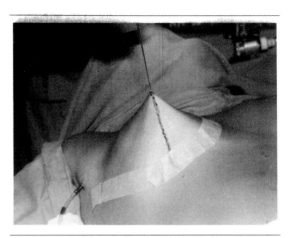

Fig. 24-34. Immobilization is done with microporous adhesive tape with upward tension on the breast to give an optimal cone shape. Adhesive tape is applied in the vertical direction, from the lower to the upper end.

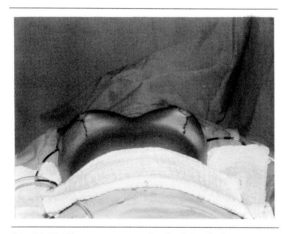

Fig. 24-33. The operation is finished. With the patient lying on the table, we observe symmetry and the ends of the incision, which do not extend beyond the fold.

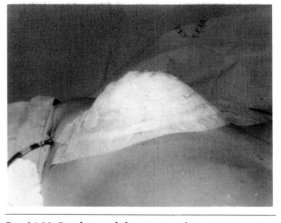

Fig. 24-35. Final immobilization, with microporous adhesive tape, which should remain until the tenth day.

Drainage is accomplished through suction. The drain should emerge from the axillary area, *never* from the incision (Fig. 24-36).

Complications

Since we have been using this technique, we have had no instances of total or partial necrosis of the nipple-areola complex, no fat necrosis or skin necrosis, no atrophy of the pedicle, and no infection.

However, the most frequent unfavorable results have been enlargement of the areola and vertical scars in 5 percent of the patients we have done; improper positioning of the nipple-areola in 6 per-cent; and excess skin remaining inferiorly in 10 percent.

With regard to the problem of postoperative scarring, we believe this to be a technical matter — either because of improper closure or inadequate compensation for the excess skin around the areola. The solution is simple: revision, with new anchoring of the skin and immobilization. If scar hypertrophy or a frank keloid occurs, betatherapy is advisable.

To correct an anomalous position of the areola, a secondary procedure is required. Point a is put in its normal position, and a wedge of skin is resected in the vertical direction, from the upper area. We

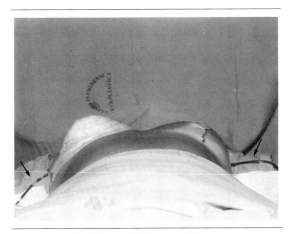

Fig. 24-36. The efficacy of the immobilization is verified by comparing the immobilized breast, with more projection and a better cone shape, with the other one, not immobilized. We also note that drainage is done through suction via the axilla; the drains are removed after 24 hours.

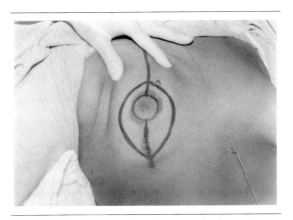

Fig. 24-37. Revision mammaplasty in which a wedge is resected to correct an anomalous positioning of the areola-nipple complex.

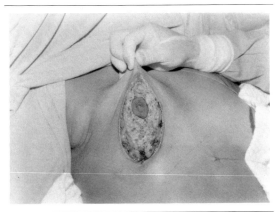

Fig. 24-38. Deepithelialization of the outlined area.

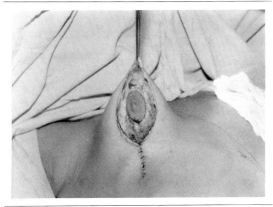

Fig. 24-39. Suturing is begun from the lower to the upper end to raise the areola.

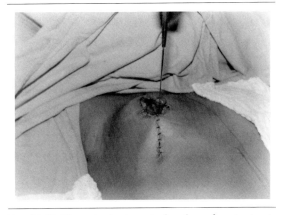

Fig. 24-40. The principal vertical and areola suturing is shown, not extending beyond the submammary fold.

anchor our dermal stitches with inverted knots, and we find that, as after the original procedure, immobilization is indispensable after a revision (Figs. 24-37 through 24-40).

The most frequent complication, as mentioned, is excess skin on the inferior pole of the breast. Two factors cause this: (1) a too high positioning of the pedicle, producing dead space in the area of excess skin; and (2) an insufficient excision of skin from the inferior end of the vertical incision. It is absolutely essential at operation to observe very

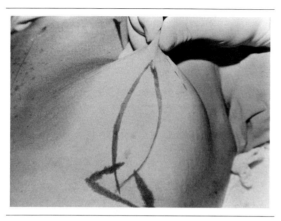

Fig. 24-41. The area of the skin for resection is marked in the form of a wedge or some other outline, which will result in an inverted T-shaped scar. The resection should not extend beyond the submammary fold.

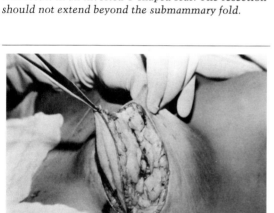

Fig. 24-42. Excision of skin and glandular and fat tissue. Both lateral and medial incisions should be extended to produce an inverted T that will not go beyond the fold.

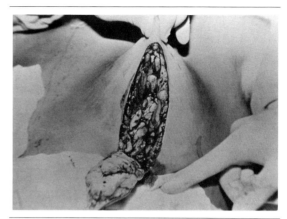

Fig. 24-43. Resection is almost complete.

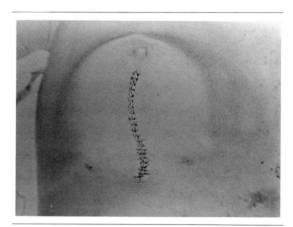

Fig. 24-44. End result without going beyond the submammary fold. In this instance, the edges of the scar remain untouched and a small inverted T was avoided.

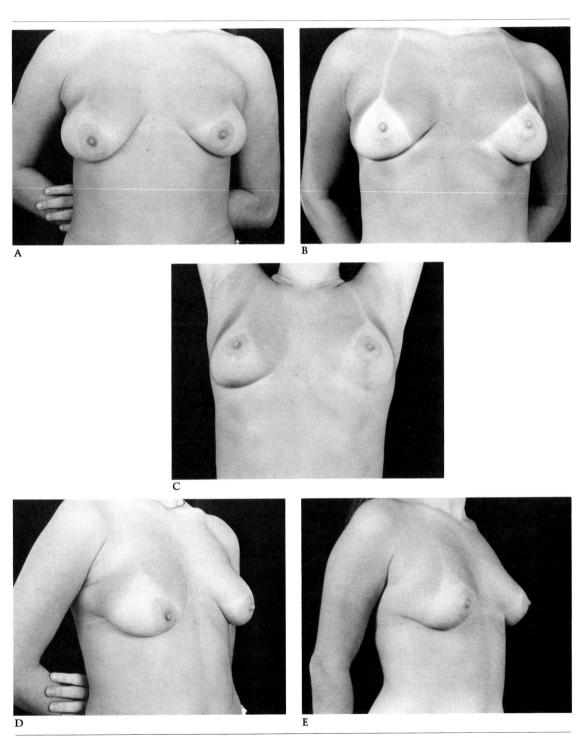

*Fig. 24-45. A. Preoperative view of a ptotic breast
with asymmetrical areolar position and size.
B. Postoperative view 2 years later. The right breast is
still slightly larger. C. Arms are elevated to allow
visualization of the vertical scar, which does not
extend beyond the submammary fold. D, E.
Preoperative and postoperative side views.*

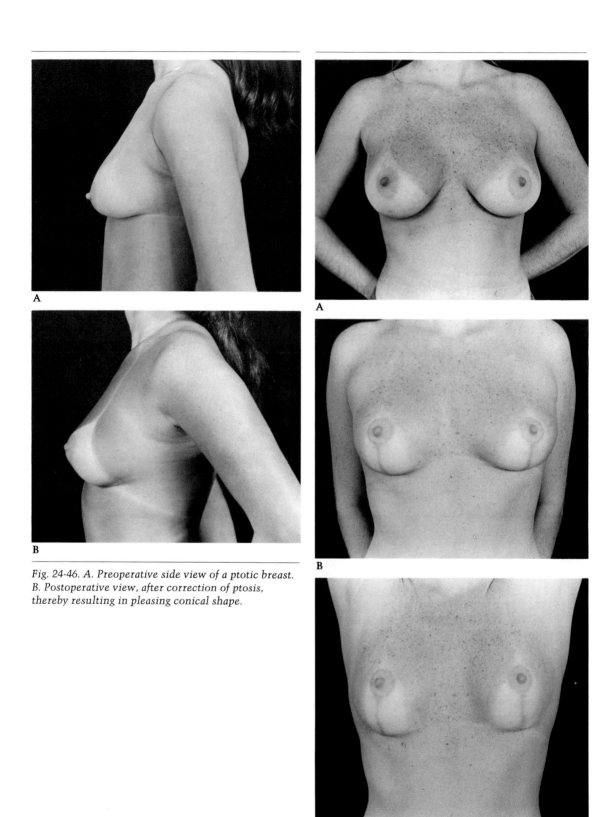

Fig. 24-46. A. Preoperative side view of a ptotic breast. B. Postoperative view, after correction of ptosis, thereby resulting in pleasing conical shape.

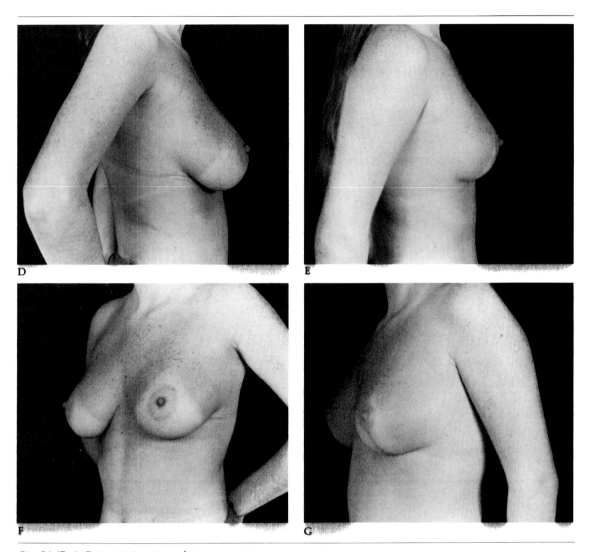

Fig. 24-47. A. Preoperative view of a young patient
with hypertrophy and ptosis (juvenile hypertrophy).
B. Postoperative view, 20 months later. C. Arms
elevated to show vertical scars. D. Side view of same
patient for better visualization of the ptosis and degree
of hypertrophy. E. Postoperative view, 20 months later,
with pleasing shape and fullness of the superior pole.
F. Postoperative oblique view, opposite side.
G. Postoperative, same view, with clear view of the
retracted breast, with a good superior pole and an
excellent conical shape attained.

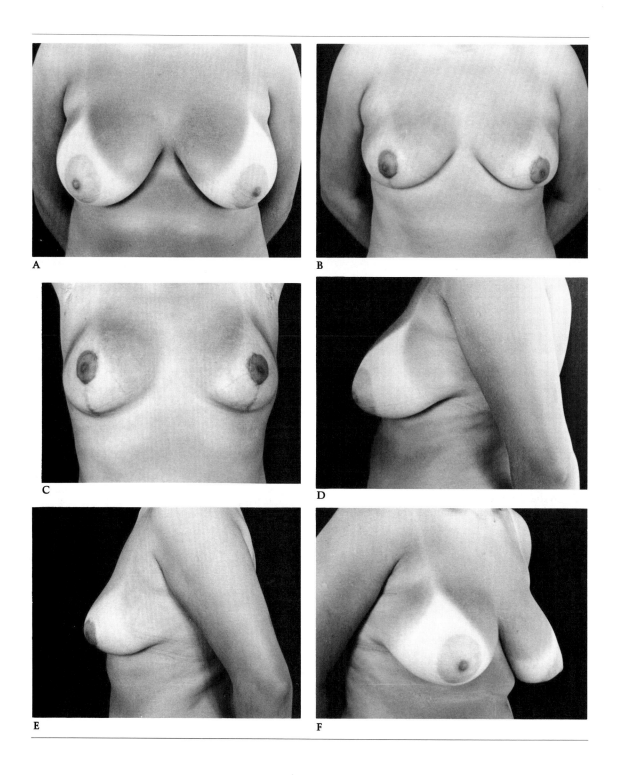

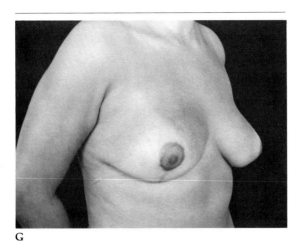

G

Fig. 24-48. A. Preoperative view of a patient with large hypertrophy and ptosis. B. Postoperative view, 10 months later, after a resection of 500 gm from each side. C. Postoperative view, with arms elevated, to show vertical and areolar scars. D. Preoperative view of the patient. E. Postoperative, same view to show the amount of reduction achieved. F. Preoperative oblique view of globular breast on the opposite side. G. Postoperative oblique view in which a good reduction and conical shape were attained.

carefully for the presence of a dog-ear at this point (see Fig. 24-1M, N, and O).

Revision is accomplished through a vertical excision that should not extend beyond the submammary fold. If such a maneuver cannot be performed, a T-shaped outline is made to permit the excision of the excess tissue without adversely risking a change in the shape of the breast or the cosmetic result (Figs. 24-41 through 24-44).

No revision should be done until at least 6 months have elapsed after the original operation because, by that time, skin retraction might still eliminate the excess skin and the need for revision. Prior to operation, patients must understand that a revision is possible and that the end result takes many months. The single vertical scar is an advantage and can be achieved only if patience is the key word for both the patient and the surgeon (Figs. 24-45 through 24-48).

References

1. Arié, G. Nueva técnica en mammaplastia. *Rev. Latam. Cir. Plast.* 3:28, 1957.
2. Ariyan, S. Reduction mammaplasty with the nipple areola carried on a single, narrow inferior pedicle. *Ann. Plast. Surg.* 5:167, 1980.
3. Arufe, H. Mammaplasty with a single vertical superior based pedicle to support the nipple areola. *Plast. Reconstr. Surg.* 60:221, 1977.
4. Biesenberger, H. *Deformitäten und Kosmetische Operationen der Weiblichen Brust.* Wien: Maurich, 1931.
5. Bozola, A.R. Sistematização tática da mamoplastia em L. *Anais da 1a. Jornada Sul. Bras. Cir. Plast.* 365:374, 1984.
6. Bozola, A.R., Oliveira, H.C., Sanchez, W.H., et al. *Mamoplastia em L: contribuição pessoal. A.M.R.I.G.S.* 26:207, 1982.
7. Burian, F. *The Plastic Surgery Atlas.* New York: Macmillan, 1986.
8. Courtiss, E.H., and Goldwyn, R.M. A reduction mammaplasty by the inferior pedicle technique. An alternative to free nipple and areola grafting for severe macromastia and extreme ptosis. *Plast. Reconstr. Surg.* 59:500, 1977.
9. Georgiade, G., Serafin, D., Reifkohl, R., and Georgiade, D. Reduction mammaplasty utilizing an inferior pedicle nipple-areolar flap. *Ann. Plast. Surg.* 3:211, 1979.
10. Goldwyn, R.M. *Plastic and Reconstructive Surgery of the Breast.* Boston: Little, Brown, 1976.
11. Joseph, J. In Biesenberger, H. (ed.), *Deformitäten und kosmetische Operationen der weiblichen Brust.* Wien: Maudrich, 1931.
12. Juri, J., Jari, C., Cutini, J., and Colagno, A. Vertical mammaplasty. *Ann. Plast. Surg.* 9:298, 1982.
13. Labandter, H.P., Dowden, R.V., and Dinner, M.I. The inferior segment technique for breast reduction. *Ann. Plast. Surg.* 8:493, 1982.
14. Lassus, C. New refinements in vertical mammaplasty. *Aesth. Plast. Surg.* 10:9, 1986.
15. Longacre, J.J., Stefano, G.A., and Holmstrand, K. Breast reconstruction with local dermal and fat pedicle flaps. *Plast. Reconstr. Surg.* 24:563, 1959.
16. Lotsch, G.M. Über Hängelbrustplastik. *Zentralblatt fur Chir.* 50:1241, 1923.
17. Maliniac, J. The use of pedicle dermo-fat in mammaplasty. *Plast. Reconstr. Surg.* 12:110, 1953.
18. Peixoto, G. Reduction mammaplasty: A personal technique. *Plast. Reconstr. Surg.* 65:217, 1980.
19. Peixoto, G. Reduction mammaplasty: Conceptual evolution. Transactions of the VIII International Congress of Plastic Surgery. Montreal, 1983.
20. Peixoto, G. Reduction mammaplasty. *Aesth. Plast. Surg.* 8:231, 1984.
21. Ribeiro, L. Pedicles in mammaplasty. In Transactions of the International Congress of Plastic and Reconstructive Surgery. Montreal, 1983.
22. Ribeiro, L., and Backer, E. Mastoplastia con pedículo de seguridad. *Rev. Esp. Cir. Plast.* 16:223, 1973.
23. Ribeiro, L., and Backer, E. Inferiorly Based Pedicles in Mammaplasties. In N.G. Georgiade (ed.), *Aesthetic Breast Surgery.* Baltimore: Williams & Wilkins, 1983. Pp. 260–270.
24. Robbins, T.H. A reduction mammaplasty with the areola-nipple based on an inferior dermal pedicle. *Plast. Reconstr. Surg.* 59:64, 1977.

COMMENTS ON CHAPTER 24   *Robert M. Goldwyn*

In an attempt to reduce and, if possible, eliminate, the horizontal scar that usually accompanies reduction mammaplasty, Ribeiro evolved a technique that, as he acknowledges, is based partly on Peixoto's method (just described) and its concept of tissue retraction-shrinkage and consolidation of the breast and its integument following reduction mammaplasty. A major component of Ribeiro's operation is the imaginative use of an inferiorly based pedicle, which he pioneered. This pedicle provides bulk and natural fullness inferiorly so that the breast will not look pinched after the tissues contract and the wounds have healed.

Ribeiro's technique is safe with respect to nipple and areola viability, since he reports no necrosis, even partial. However, he honestly concedes that the operation is not for every patient, especially elderly women with loose, nonelastic skin and massive hypertrophy. He admonishes us to use his method only in patients who will not require more than a 500-gm removal of tissue per side. Otherwise, there will be a struggle to avoid a moderately long horizontal scar — the objective of the Ribeiro procedure.

Another point to remember about Ribeiro's technique is that marking is not done before operation but during it. This fact undoubtedly accounts for the 6 percent incidence rate he reports of malpositioning the nipple and areola — a problem that commonly requires revision. The fact that this complication occurs with that frequency in the hands of the originator of the technique suggests that the operation is not easy to perform and that others less knowledgeable about the method would undoubtedly have more difficulty with correctly situating the nipple-areola.

As in every technique whose objective is to lessen or eliminate the inframammary scar, the ultimate periareolar scar is usually wider than that in the McKissock or inferior pedicle techniques. The reason is the need to resect much of the excess skin around the areola that other methods would have removed in the submammary fold, which, of course, accounts for the horizontal scar. In younger patients, widening or thickening of the periareolar scar is not unusual and even revision will fail to improve it significantly. For many patients, a moderate or even a longer horizontal scar would have been less conspicuous and would have been a better choice.

25

Ronaldo Pontes

Reduction Mammaplasty: Variations I and II

In the field of mammaplasty, there is a universal trend toward smaller scars and a wider choice of incisions [1–9, 12, 13]. For reduction mammaplasty, tissue should be resected from the basis of the breast, thus preserving the median segment. The rationale presented to the First International Congress of Aesthetic Plastic Surgery in Rio de Janeiro, 1972, and published in 1973 [10] was subsequently developed into two variants in 1983 [11].

In the majority of cases, I have followed my basic technique (Tables 25-1 and 25-2). Nevertheless, I think that surgeons should master different techniques, since one technique does not suit every case.

The two techniques, variation I and II, are easy to perform and allow any type of skin resection. As far as possible, breast reduction should be done in such a way that only a small scar results. In selected cases (young patients with firm skin), variation II is often possible with no skin removal at all (see Fig. 25-29B).

In an attempt to reduce scar size and to obtain a good breast shape, a new type of skin incision was developed (see Fig. 25-6A). Its advantages are marked breast reduction, smaller scar size, and a wide incision-free area between the two submammary scars (see Fig. 25-34). The result is a breast that is firm and stable and that presents a good shape.

Patients' Examination — Surgical Planning

After making sure by either clinical or x-ray examination that no mammary pathologic changes are present, the desired breast size and the unavoidable scars are discussed with the patient. It must be stressed that although their quality is usually good, scars are visible and permanent; they cannot be undone. In addition, how the surgical result may affect her present or future partner cannot be predicted.

Finally, the type of anesthesia, length of hospital stay, number of dressings, time elapsed until removal of stitches, type of bra, and time of return to normal activities are explained.

General anesthesia is used in all cases.

Surgical Technique

A special surgical table is used (Fig. 25-1). The anesthetic tubing must be mobile enough (Figs. 25-2 and 25-3) so that it can be moved to allow access for combined operations (Fig. 25-3; see Table 25-4).

The surgeon must decide on the placement of the nipple and areola, which will be the apex of the new breast cone (Fig. 25-4, point A, and Fig. 25-5). Some thought is needed for determining this point, which is usually projected on the submammary sulcus. This is then marked (E-F, Fig. 25-6) and is purposely short. On the other hand, points E-E should be placed well apart (see Fig. 25-4). The distance from B to C will determine the degree of the conic shape. The more open the angle B-A-C, the more conic will be the new breast. At the same time, the distances D-B and D-C should be adequate to allow the elevation of D to A (see Fig. 25-4).

Points C and B are marked and should be placed 5 to 7 cm from point A. Lines A-B and A-C are curves (see Fig. 25-4). The modification in the markings of the outer breast quadrants are now evident, line A-F being the continuation of curve A-C. Line A-F is curved and uninterrupted, reaching the submammary sulcus at point F. Distance

Table 25-1. Type of incision used in
last 623 patients of 3065 total

Skin marking	Cases	
	Number	Percentage
Inverted T	547	87.9
Lateral curved	63	10.1
Vertical ellipse	2	0.3
Vertical incision without skin resection	4	0.6
Other	7	1.1
Total	623	100.0

Table 25-2. Technique of gland resection
in last 623 patients of 3065 total

Technique of gland resection	Cases	
	Number	Percentage
Variant I	431	69.2
Variant II	192	30.8
Total	623	100.0

E-F is thus remarkably short (see Fig. 25-6).

Marking of point C' is empirical. It is placed 1.5 to 2.0 cm below point C. This is a compensation for what happens when point A is raised for breast mounting. Note in Figure 25-6B that line A-C, formerly exactly the same length as A-B, becomes shorter when the breast is pulled at point A. The measurements are transferred to the opposite side by two reference stitches, one placed on the sternal furcula and the other on the xyphoid. The areolas are marked with a special ring with a 3.5 cm diameter. Skin resection in the area where the areola will be placed is done with a somewhat larger ring (4 cm) (Fig. 25-7).

To simplify Schwarzmann's [13] maneuver, the assistant stretches nipple and areola by compressing the base of the breast with both hands (Fig. 25-8). With the breast suspended from point A, the skin is incised along the entire outline, preserving the dermis on the triangular area A-B-C' (Fig. 25-9). The gland is cut at right angles to the thoracic wall. The incision passes through point C', which is located about 2 cm below the lower margin of the areola, thus following the curved outline of the lateral and medial incisions (Fig. 25-10).

This procedure is repeated on the opposite side; this technique is called variant I.

The remaining glandular masses are compared, and, if necessary, gland and skin are trimmed until

Fig. 25-1. Surgical table ready for surgery. Note the arm rests, which are designed for patient comfort and to avoid nervous compression.

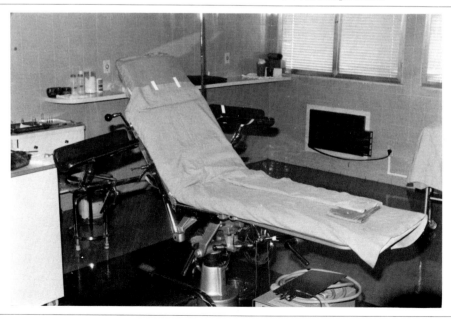

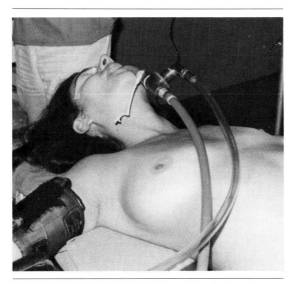

Fig. 25-2. *Patient after intubation. Note the long, mobile tubing, which is of great help for combined surgery.*

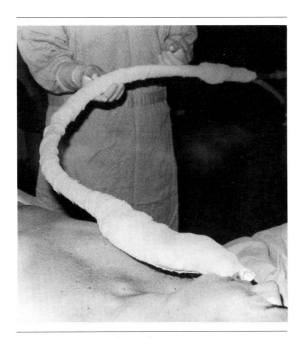

Fig. 25-3. *Tubing with sterile wrapping.*

Table 25-3. *Amount of tissue removed in last 623 patients of 3065 total*

Grams of tissue removed from each side	Cases	
	Number	Percentage
0– 99	80	12.8
100–199	14	2.2
200–299	50	8.0
300–399	65	10.4
400–499	64	10.3
500–599	61	9.8
600–699	50	8.0
700–799	55	8.8
800–899	48	7.7
900–999	23	3.7
1000–1099	26	4.2
1099–1199	30	4.8
1200–1299	9	1.4
1300–1399	13	2.1
1400–1499	10	1.6
1500–1599	6	1.0
1600–1699	6	1.0
1700–1799	4	0.6
1800–1899	3	0.5
1900–1999	3	0.5
2000–2099	1	0.2
2200–2299	1	0.2
2500–2500	1	0.2
Total	623	100.0

identical volumes are obtained. Weighing the amount of resected tissue is useful for this purpose (Table 25-3). The gland is undermined immediately above the thoracic wall so that it can be later rotated in and upward to fill up the superior pole (see Figs. 25-17 and 25-18).

In variant II, one starts by cutting the gland at right angles to the thoracic wall as in variant I. Another incision is then performed along a place parallel to the thoracic wall. The higher this plane, the larger the reduction obtained (see Fig. 25-12). The vertical distance to the plane of horizontal incision is measured (Fig. 25-11) and recorded for the procedure to be repeated at the opposite breast (Fig. 25-12 through 25-16). This technique allows easy reduction of breasts of any size, even huge ones, to any desired size, and breast function is fully retained (see Figs. 25-28 through 25-30).

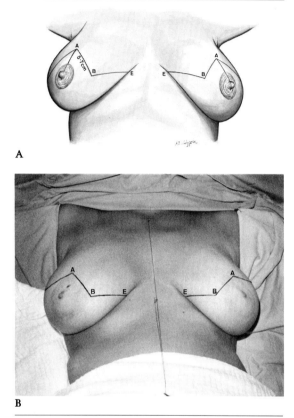

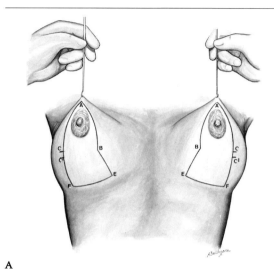

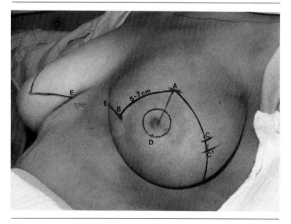

Fig. 25-4. A. Drawing showing demarcation for clarity. B. Patient ready for surgery, showing incision outlines. Note the spacing between points E and E.

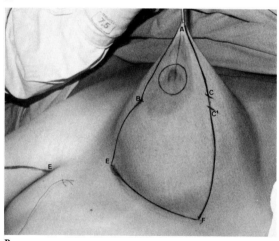

Fig. 25-6. A. Drawing in front view for clarity. B. The breast is raised from point A. Note the curved line A-F and the important point C'. With resting breast, A-C = A-B. With raised breast, A-C becomes shorter than A-B, hence the need of point C' as a compensation.

Fig. 25-5. Same as Figure 25-4 seen from another point of view. Note the curved lateral outline.

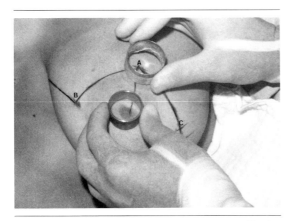

Fig. 25-7. Rings of different diameters—the smaller for initial incision and the larger for later skin excision to accommodate the areola in its new position.

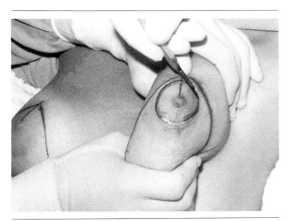

Fig. 25-8. Schwarzmann's maneuver.

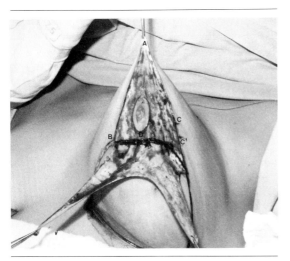

Fig. 25-9. Dermal preservation of the triangle A-B-C'. Outlining the gland incision from B to C', running at about 2 cm from the inferior areolar margin.

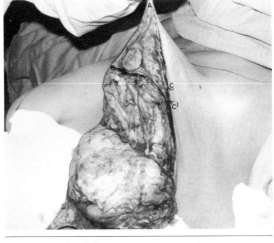

Fig. 25-10. Glandular resection variant I.

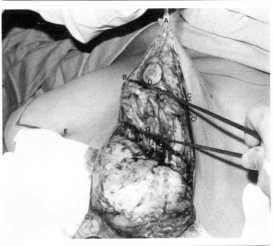

Fig. 25-11. Outlining for variant II. A parallel to B-C' is marked at G. The distance D-G is recorded and transferred to the opposite side. D-G varies according to the intended amount of reduction.

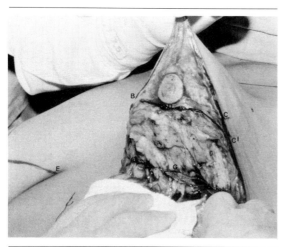

Fig. 25-12. Glandular incision for variant II.

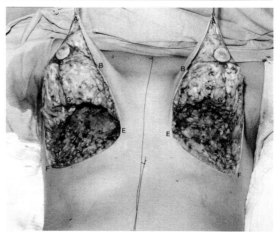

Fig. 25-14. Front view of the mammary stumps for comparison and eventual trimming. This view is common to variants I and II.

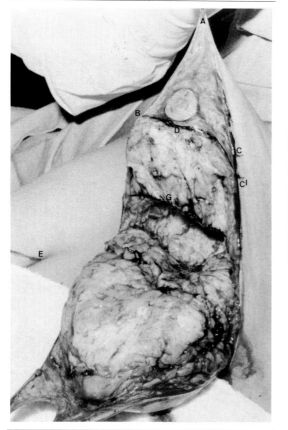

Fig. 25-13. Complete incision for variant II.

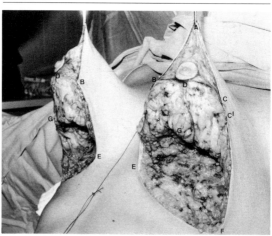

Fig. 25-15. The same as Figure 25-14 from three-fourths view.

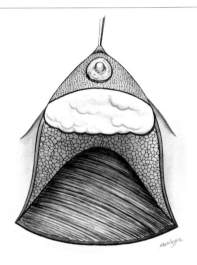

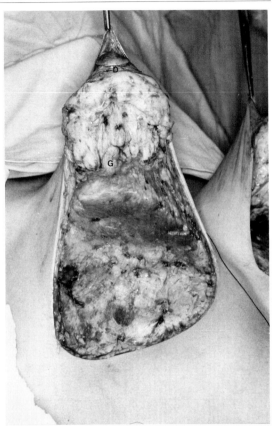

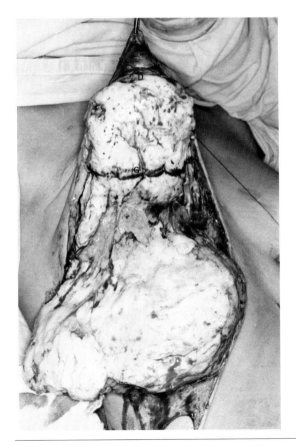

Fig. 25-16. The large amount of glandular tissue that
can be resected by this technique.

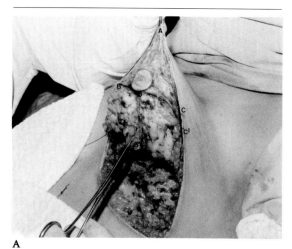

A

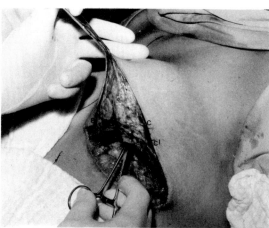

B

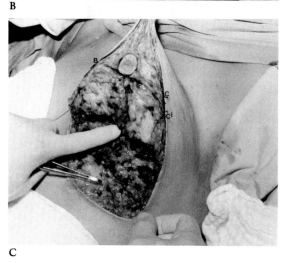

C

Forming the Breast

A Kocher clamp grasps point A while an Allis forceps holds the gland at the lower part of the vertical incision plane (point G, Fig. 25-17A).

The glandular mass is then rotated inward and upward to its new position, which is determined by feeling (Fig. 25-17B). At this point, the gland is anchored to the thoracic wall with one or two Mersilene 3-0 stitches (Fig. 25-17C). A hook is inserted at point D and remains there (together with the Kocher's clamp at point A) until the breasts are molded and the main stitches are placed (see Fig. 25-22).

By raising points A and D and joining C-B, two lateral pillars are formed, and the flat surface is molded into a cone shape (Fig. 25-18). The pillars are joined by one or two 3-0 Mersilene stitches to ensure the conical shape of the breasts. During this procedure, if any difficulty arises in putting the areola in this position, a Z-plasty on the A-B-C dermal segment may be performed. The Kocher clamp and the hook must remain in position until the breast receives the mounting stitches (Fig. 25-19). The glandular tissue is then anchored over the complete extension of the incision with colorless 5-0 nylon stitches (Fig. 25-20).

For shaping the lateral aspect of the breast, the assistant pulls it to a position that reduces the lateral dog-ear (Fig. 25-21), which is then trimmed (Fig. 25-22). At this stage, the advantages of the markings just described become evident. Once finished, the horizontal suture lines are shorter and their ends lie farther apart than with former techniques (Fig. 25-23). This is due to the skin traction caused by the design of the lateral quadrant.

Nowadays, more acceptable scars are obtained by using nonabsorbable material. Such stitches relieve the skin tension on the suture line; they last throughout cicatricial maturation and they do not interfere with wound healing.

Patients sometimes complain that a thin scar becomes wider soon after suture removal. A hypertrophic scar may develop, aggravating the problem. The absorbable material, apart from not

Fig. 25-17. Sequence showing the inward and upward lifting of point G to form the upper pole of the breast. Point G is anchored to its new position with one or two Mersilene 3-0 sutures.

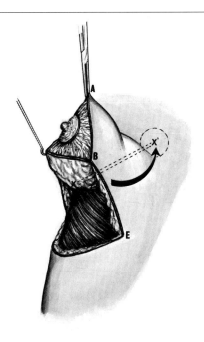

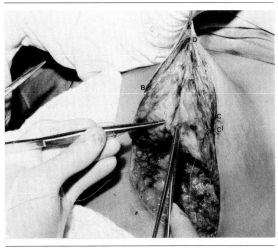

Fig. 25-19. The breast is lifted by a Kocher at point A and a hook at point D; Mersilene sutures pull the two pillars together.

A

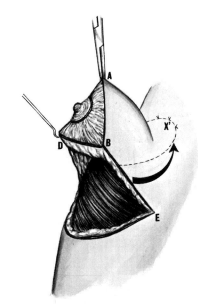

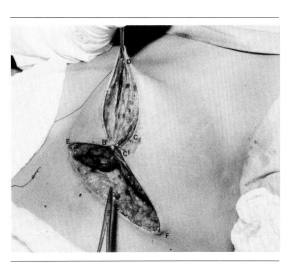

Fig. 25-20. Colorless nylon stitches (5-0) in the dermis on the pillars.

B

Fig. 25-18. Schematic drawings depicting the lifting shown in Figures 25-17 through 25-19.

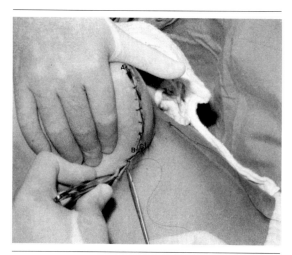

Fig. 25-21. After the main skin stitches are placed, the assistant pulls the breast to a position that reduces the lateral dog-ear.

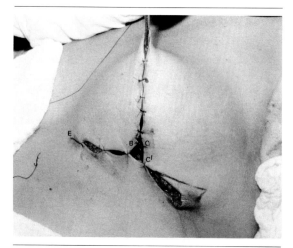

Fig. 25-22. The dog-ear, which must be trimmed.

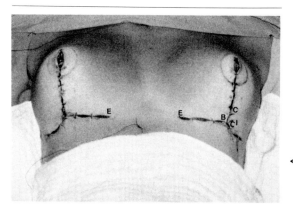

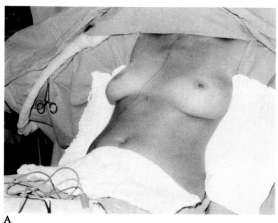

A

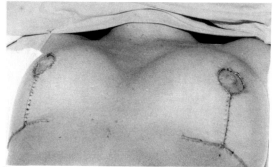

B

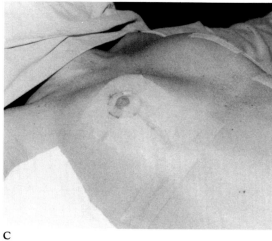

C

Fig. 25-24. Patient before outline (A), after surgery (B), and after dressing with Micropore (C).

Fig. 25-23. Breast mounting completed. Figures 25-4 through 25-15, 25-17, and 25-19 through 25-23 involve the same patient.

Table 25-4. Breast reduction alone and combined
with other operations in 3065 patients

Area	Number
Breast alone	1785
Breast and:	
face	442
abdomen	406
nose	50
liposuction	34
lids	30
scars	4
riding breeches	4
Subtotal	970
Breast, face, and:	
abdomen	182
nose	45
liposuction	3
ears	2
chin	1
Subtotal	233
Breast, abdomen, and:	
nose	7
lids	10
arms	2
ears	1
liposuction	25
thighs	2
Subtotal	47
Breast, face, abdomen, and:	
nose	15
liposuction	8
chin	1
riding breeches	2
Subtotal	26
Breast, face, nose, and:	
chin	1
liposuction	1
thighs	1
Subtotal	3
Breast, abdomen, nose, and:	
liposuction	1
Total	3,065

Table 25-5. Age distribution of last 623
patients of 3065 total

Age (yr)	Cases	
	Number	Percentage
14	2	0.3
15–19	114	18.4
20–24	69	11.1
25–29	45	7.2
30–34	52	8.3
35–39	60	9.6
40–44	73	11.7
45–49	74	11.9
50–54	61	9.8
55–59	35	5.6
60–64	25	4.0
65–69	10	1.6
70–74	3	0.5
Total	623	100.0

lasting as long as necessary, interferes with scar formation. 5-0 nylon is used as intracuticular running suture on the inframammary incision, as isolated stitches on the vertical incision, and as U-shaped stitches on the areola.

The circular skin area excised to accommodate the areola in its new position should be slightly larger than the areola. The sutured area is dressed in Micropore (Fig. 25-24), which is left in place for 1 month and replaced weekly. An adhesive plaster is applied for 24 hours, after which an adequate brassiere is substituted for it, and the patient is discharged. The brassiere may be used immediately after operation, according to the specific procedure and the surgeon's preference.

The patterns of resection in variations I and II are shown in Figures 25-25 and 25-26 (see Table 25-2).

The simplicity of this technique allows the simultaneous performance of other types of surgery (Fig. 25-27; Table 25-4).

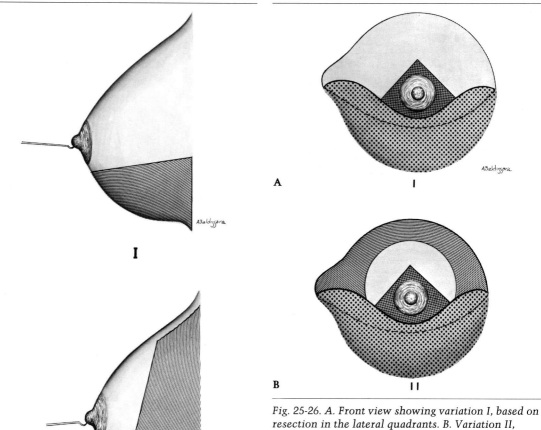

Fig. 25-26. A. Front view showing variation I, based on resection in the lateral quadrants. B. Variation II, called orbital, shows surrounding gland. With this variation, any size breast can be reduced.

Fig. 25-25. Profile showing the dissection in both variations. Hatched area represents resected glandular tissue.

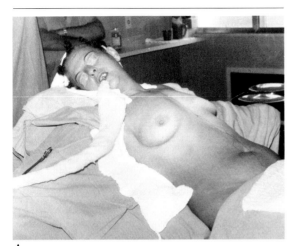

A

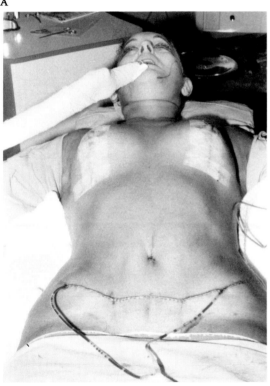

B

Fig. 25-27. Patient before (A) and after (B) combined surgery (face, lids, breast, abdomen). With the described technique, multiple operation becomes feasible.

No blood transfusion, drainage, or prophylactic antibiotics are used. A slight fever is common during the first few postoperative days and is treated with symptomatic medication. Patients are allowed to shower after the third postoperative day, without removing the Micropore placed during surgery. Stitches are removed between the eighth and tenth day. Patients must wear a brassiere continuously for 40 days after surgery, after which they are allowed to perform any kind of activity.

Complications

The technique itself does not seem to lead to any particular complications and can be used for patients of all ages (Table 25-5; Figs. 25-31 through 25-38). Complications are rare. They include hematomas, asymmetry, small residual dog-ears, and hypertrophic scars. The most important complication, however, is the patients' dissatisfaction, caused by either the surgeon's failure to explain the aim of the operation or the patient's own lack of understanding of the limits of surgery. If the skin is too tense, the medial segment of the horizontal scar can slant downward.

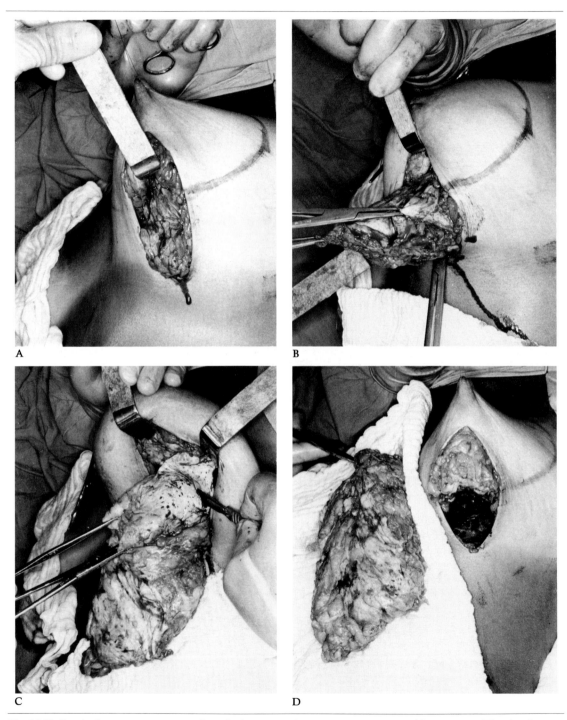

A

B

C

D

Fig. 25-28. Surgical sequence in a case of marked hypertrophy. Variation II glandular resection through vertical incision. Removal of 830 gm and 620 gm of tissue from the breasts. The nipple is pulled upward for easier construction of breast cone. The gland below the circular marking is removed through the vertical incision.

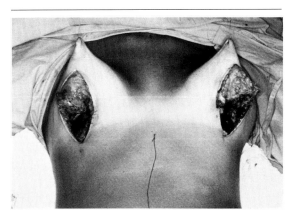

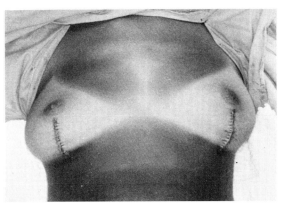

Fig. 25-29. Breast after glandular resection, completed operation.

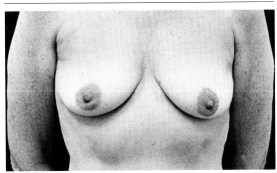

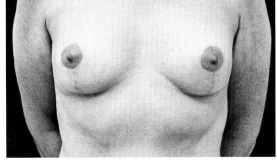

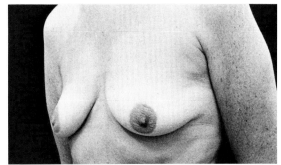

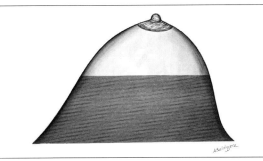

Fig. 25-30. Craniocaudal projection of variation II. The amount to be resected depends on the desired reduction.

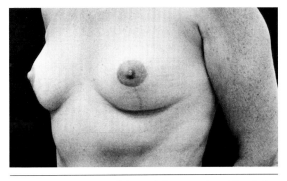

Fig. 25-31. Patient with lateral demarcation. Glandular resection in the medial and lateral quadrants and mastopexia.

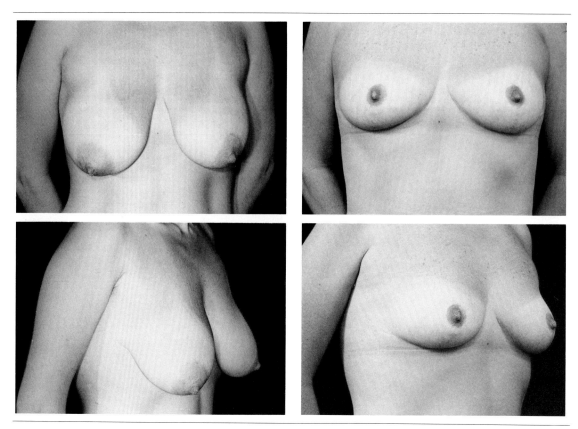

Fig. 25-32. A patient with some degree of hypertrophy and asymmetry, before and 5 years after surgery. Variation I.

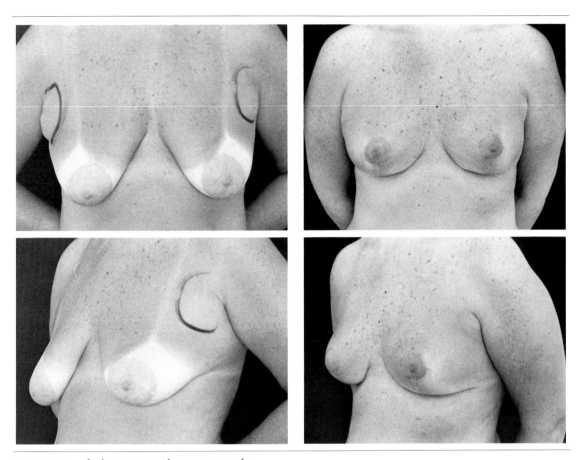

Fig. 25-33. *Marked ptosis provoking great areolar*
displacement. Small scar; variant I glandular resection.
Axilar liposuction.

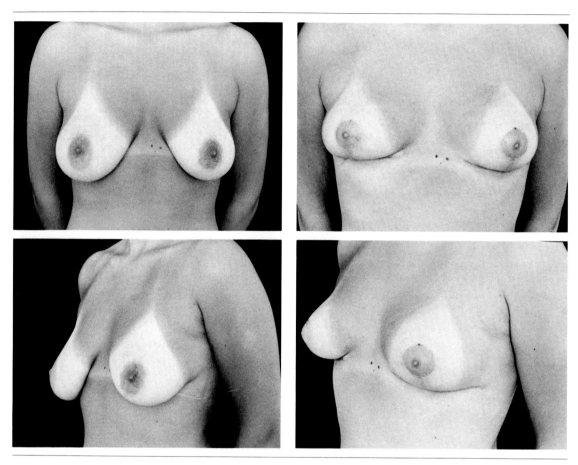

Fig. 25-34. Patient with medium degree of hypertrophy with asymmetry, before and after surgery. Note the wide space between the medial extremes of the horizontal scars.

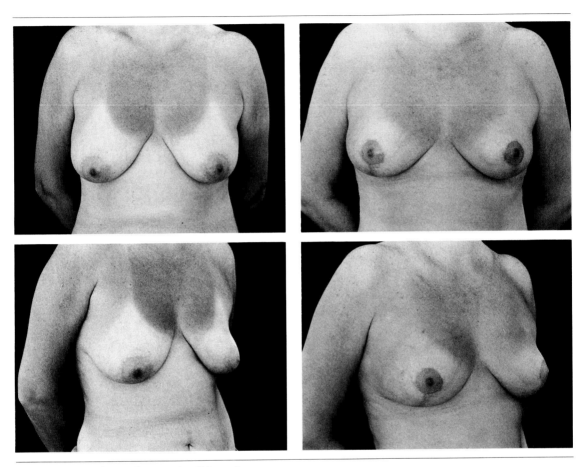

Fig. 25-35. Flaccidity and ptosis. Small lateral scar.
Variant I glandular resection.

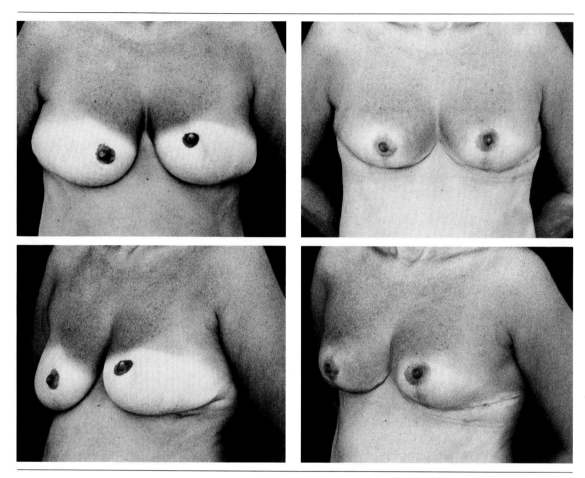

Fig. 25-36. *A difficult case of secondary mammaplasty with convergent and asymmetric areolas. The proposed lateral incision played a decisive role in the good result achieved.*

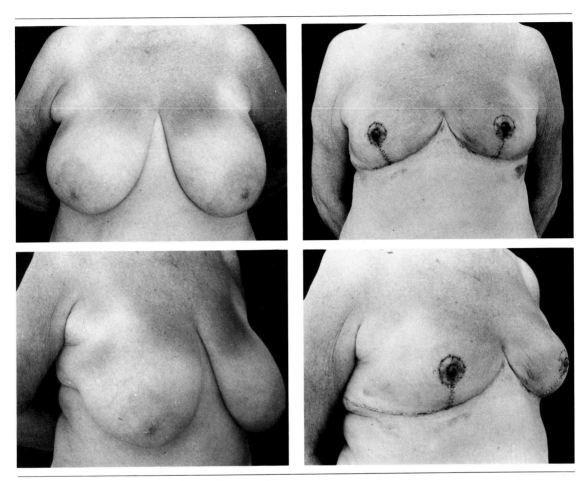

Fig. 25-37. In elderly patients with great hypertrophy,
free transplantation of the areola can be done.
Rationale is the same as that for glandular resection.

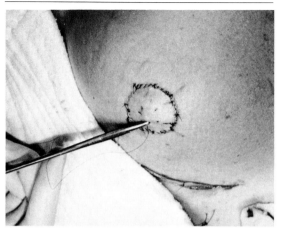

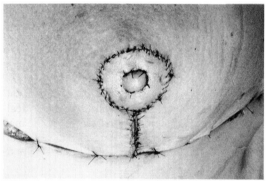

Fig. 25-38. Details of suture. The graft takes perfectly and maintains the anatomical differences between the areola and nipple.

References

1. Arié, G. Una nueva técnica de mastoplastia. *Rev. Latinoam. Chir. Plast.* 3:23, 1957.
2. Cardoso de Castro, C. Mammaplasty with curved incisions. *Plast. Reconstr. Surg.* LVII:619, 1976.
3. Franco, T., and Rebello, C. *Cirurgia estética.* Rio de Janeiro: Livraria Atheneu, 1977.
4. Georgiade, N.G., Serafin, D., Riefkohl, R., and Georgiade, G.S. Is there a reduction mammaplasty "for all seasons?" *Plast. Reconstr. Surg.* 63:765, 1979.
5. Goldwyn, R.M. *Plastic and Reconstructive Surgery of the Breast.* Boston: Little, Brown, 1976.
6. Horton, C.E., Adamson, J.E., Mladick, R.A., and Taddeo, R.J. Reduction mammaplasty. *GP* 40:124, 1969.
7. Marino, H. Plásticas mamárias Editorial Científica. Buenos Ayres: Lopez, 1958.
8. Peixoto, G. Reduction mammaplasty: A personal technique. *Plast. Reconstr. Surg.* 65:217, 1980.
9. Pitanguy, I. Surgical treatment of breast hypertrophy. *Br. J. Plast. Surg.* 20:78, 1967.
10. Pontes, R. A technique of reduction mammaplasty. *Br. J. Plast. Surg.* 26:365, 1973.
11. Pontes, R. Reduction mammaplasty—Variations I and II. *Ann. Plast. Surg.* 6:437, 1981.
12. Ribeiro, L. A new technique for reduction mammaplasty. *Plast. Reconstr. Surg.* 55:330, 1975.
13. Schwarzmann, E. Die Technik der Mammaplastik. *Chirurgie* 2:932, 1930.

COMMENTS ON CHAPTER 25   *Robert M. Goldwyn*

In his first publication describing his method of reduction mammaplasty, Pontes [2] stated that "the most important advance in reduction mammaplasty has been the development of methods which avoid undermining the skin thus simplifying the operation and practically eliminating complications." His basic concept was to preserve "the largest volume of tissue in the median segment of the gland concentrating resection on the internal and lateral sides." This, he noted, was in contrast to the methods of Arié, Pitanguy, Beare, and Strömbeck.

Pontes [2], in 1973, recognized that his original technique was suitable for reducing most breasts except those that were "hard [and] inelastic and very large." In fact, he wrote that in those instances, his method had to "be complemented with immediate wedge resection." To overcome these deficiencies, he evolved his variations I and II [3].

In his present chapter, we note that in 7 of 10 patients for reduction, Pontes utilizes variation I (see Table 25-2). In "selected . . . young patients with firm skin, variation II is often possible with no skin removal at all."

In Table 25-3, Pontes has summarized the grams of tissue removed from each breast in his last 623 patients done by his method. In only 18 percent was the resection per side 1,000 gm or greater. Those patients who have very large breasts and inelastic skin present the greatest problem for techniques that aim for minimal scars — in particular, the avoidance of a large horizontal scar.

In comparing the Pontes technique to the Robbins (inferior pedicle), Freiberg and Boyd [1] recognized that "the markings in the Pontes technique are placed according to the tissue remaining rather than according to the portion to be excised. Thus, emphasis is placed on final contour rather than on reduction in size." However, in removing the breast tissue with the transverse inferior wedge technique of Pontes, the amount of tissue removed must be carefully considered to achieve the size desired by the patient. Pontes' operation requires the surgeon to have the ability of an interior decorator: to view the room as it may look in the future by thinking of it without some of its parts — a subtraction type of mentality.

From their series of 51 patients, Freiberg and Boyd [1] concluded that the Pontes method is better for the "low volume and ptotic breast, whereas the Robbins technique has a more universal application." The Pontes procedure, however, resulted in better nipple projection, especially in the smaller, ptotic breast. According to these authors, both techniques were inadequate to convert a very large breast into a petite one. In this regard and in my experience, the patient depicted by Pontes in Figure 25-37 could be easily done by the inferior pedicle technique in order to obtain the same final volume and result.

I have used Pontes' method for moderate hypertrophy and find it satisfactory. However, my greatest worry was not so much in knowing how much tissue to remove but in worrying whether my excision would decrease nipple-areola sensitivity. This is not so much a problem if one is dealing with breasts that are not very large, but it may become a consideration if one carries the excision too far laterally and too deeply, obvious things to avoid. I have not used the method in enough patients to make any conclusive statement regarding sensation. I do agree, however, that scarring and residual dog-ears are not apparently more or less than in the inferior pedicle technique.

The fact that the Pontes technique does not involve predetermined markings of the new nipple site may give the surgeon more latitude as he claims, but it also imposes on the surgeon the necessity for very accurate determinations intraoperatively. For an inexperienced surgeon or a surgeon inexperienced with this type of technique, that junction of the operation may be the most difficult. Now after almost 20 years of experience with his technique, Pontes has a fluidity in its execution that most of us would like to emulate.

REFERENCES

1. Freiberg, A., and Boyd, J.B. Reduction mammaplasty: A comparison between the Robbins and Pontes techniques. *Plast. Reconstr. Surg.* 78:773, 1986.
2. Pontes, R. A technique of reduction mammaplasty. *Br. J. Plast. Surg.* 26:365, 1973.
3. Pontes, R. Reduction mammaplasty—variations I and II. *Ann. Plast. Surg.* 6:437, 1981.

26

Antonio Roberto Bozola

Reduction Mammaplasty: Preferred Techniques

There is not a single technique of mammaplasty that is capable by itself of solving all aesthetic alterations of the breast. [9, 10]. In this chapter, we will show how a solution can be found for them using similar principles and philosophies for different diagnoses.

The mammaplasty technique that leaves a lateral scar was initially described by Hollander [7] and was later modified and published by several authors [2–4, 8, 13, 17, 19].

The breast can didactically be divided into two components: (1) the skin and subcutaneous tissue, and (2) the glandular cone. One or the other or both can be altered.

Breasts have volume and form with measurements that give them their beauty. Their position and relationships with the body characterize the female form, beauty, and sensuality.

The volume of the breast should be between 200 and 300 ml [6], with a conical or semispherical form, the vertical radius of the base of the cone similar to the posteroanterior projection, the vertical diameter slightly greater or equal to the horizontal diameter. The distance between the apex of the cone and the inferior glandular fold is 6 to 7 cm, and the distance from the apex to the superior glandular edge is one and a half times that distance, or 9.0 to 10.5 cm (Figure 26-1).

The breast is considered without ptosis when it is above an imaginary plane (plane A) that passes through the inferior glandular fold. The glandular cone is slightly concave on its superior aspect and rounded on its inferior aspects. The nipple-areola complex is on the apex of the breast in approximately 83 percent of cases. Taking into account the aspect of the normal breast, we can define the aesthetic alterations in relation to form, volume, ptosis, and nipple-areola complex (form, size, and position).

There can be aesthetic changes even without ptosis. The ratio between skin and subcutaneous tissue versus glandular cone must be one. The greater this ratio, the more the ptosis, and the breast slides under the plane A of the submammary fold.

If we consider another plane M that passes through the apex of the cone, the distance between A and M is the degree of ptosis in centimeters, when M is in a lower position than A (Fig. 26-2). This occurs owing to loss of skin elasticity or reduction in the volume of the breast for any reason. The ratio of container to content will be greater than one.

We can diagnose the probable excess of volume in grams, abolishing the term *hypertrophy*.

Aesthetic alterations of the breast include form (four groups), volume (probable excess in grams), ptosis (*A-M* distance [apex to submammary fold]), and nipple-areola complex (form, position, and size).

It is necessary to remodel the breast cone, and its form and volume, and then to reestablish the ratio of container to content, removing excess skin. After excision and closure the final scar is commonly an inverted T, L, or a vertical one. The less the ptosis or A-M distance, its length is shorter, as will be the amount of glandular tissue resected.

Figure 26-3 shows the possible scars and those that we frequently use. We understand that is not the type of final scar that defines a mammaplasty technique. There are techniques that result in a scar that is a T [9, 11, 12, 14–16, 20, 21], or an L [2, 4, 13, 17, 19], or a vertical [1], lateral [3, 7, 8], or other type of scar.

In 85.5 percent of our cases, we utilize the L as our final scar, but we will show how to remove skin excess using the same philosophy and leaving

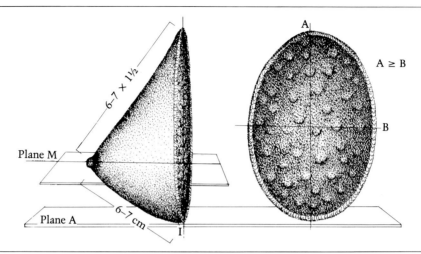

Fig. 26-1. The form of the "normal" breast following a geometric conception with its measurements and ratios, above the horizontal plane that extends to the submammary fold (A), in the meridian of the breast. The plane M is tangential to the apex of the mammary cone.

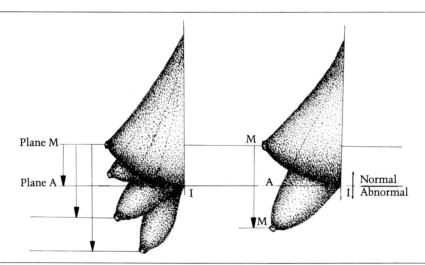

Fig. 26-2. Breast ptosis based on planes A (submammary fold) and M (apex of the cone). If plane M is above plane A, the breast is considered normal. If it is below it, there is a ptosis that will be measured.

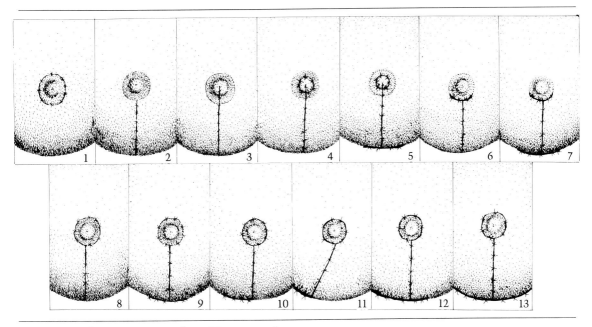

Fig. 26-3. Final scars in mammaplasty. We commonly
use 8, 9, 10, and 12.

other types of scar, all of them designed to reduce
surgical time and morbidity.

We will describe how to treat the mammary
cone and then how we do the marking, the operation, and the suturing with the smallest scar possible.

The positioning of the areola is simple and anatomic, when specific principles and tactics are followed without impairing its circulation and innervation but giving the breast its proper form and
volume.

For some breasts of a certain volume and form
and degree of ptosis, it will not be possible to
shorten the scar beyond a given limit.

There are no miracles, but what happens is that
most of the current techniques remove a greater
amount of skin than necessary, leaving wider and
longer scars because of the tension that exists on
the suture lines.

Classification of the Mammary Cone
Based on Its Form and How to Correct It
If we consider the breast as a cone, the alterations
of its form are in the measurements of its base and
height. The distribution of breast alterations
found is as follows:

GROUP I (13 PERCENT)
There is only ptosis with a normal base, height,
and volume. The ratio between container-content
is greater than one. The A-M distance is greater the
higher the ratio (see Fig. 26-2).

To correct its form, we utilize an inferior pedicle
axial flap [18] with the mammary tissue under
plane A, excluding the areola and its deepithelialized pedicle (Fig. 26-4A, B, and C). This axial flap
is positioned under the undermined breast, raising
it above plane A (Fig. 26-4B). The distal end of the
flap is sutured to the superior edge of the gland and
laterally to the aponeurosis of the pectoralis major
muscle. Sometimes the lateral aspect of the breast
bulges. If this happens, we resect the lateral
quarter of the flap. If the flap is not long enough,
its extremity can be unfolded, obtaining a random
flap from the axial one. This lengthening cannot be
longer than the width of the flap (Fig. 26-4D).

The lateral and medial segments of the breast are
sutured one to each other and placed over the flap,
thereby augmenting the anteroposterior projection. The upper aspect of the gland is increased,
and the inferior aspect is reduced.

We always leave a miniflap of inferior pedicle to
rebuild the subcutaneous fatty envelope of the
breast, so that when the patient raises her arms,

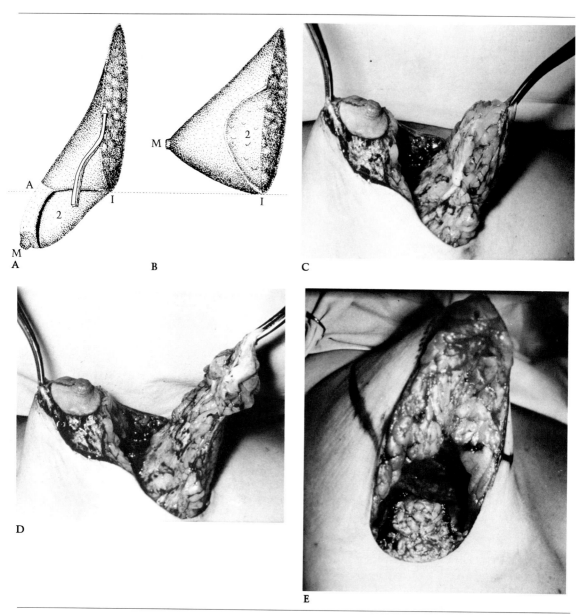

Fig. 26-4. A, B. Glandular correction of breasts of group I. From the excess between planes A and M, we make an inferior pedicle axial flap and place it under the breast. C. The axial flap developed. D. Lengthening of the flap, as described in the text. E. The miniflap kept in all breasts.

there is no concavity above the submammary fold
(Fig. 26-4E).

GROUP II (2 PERCENT)

These breasts have a large base and a normal
height. They project less and have a less ptosis.

To correct its form and to reduce its volume, we
must resect a wedge at the base of the cone and
suture together the lateral and medial portions
(Fig. 26-5A) [1].

If the projection of the breast is too small, the
inferior portion of the wedge is used as an inferior
pedicle and placed under the cone, thus increasing
its projection.

In most cases, there will be associated ptosis,
always smaller, however, than that in groups III
and IV. Along with the wedge we remove excess
tissue under plane A, except for the deepithelialized pedicle, with the nipple-areola complex
raised independently (Fig. 26-5B and C). On the
other hand, if the base is still too large after suturing the lateral to the medial and undermining
them from the thorax, the anteroposterior segments projection will be greater than desired; so
we amputate the base of the cone as will be described for breasts in groups III and IV.

GROUP III (2 PERCENT)

The aesthetic changes of these breasts are due to
the excessive length of the cone; consequently,
they have greater anteroposterior projection and a
tendency to ptosis.

The correction can be made in two ways: First,
amputation of the base of the mammary cone [2,
10, 14] following the curve of the chest, removing
axillary extensions but keeping the subcutaneous
fat with the same thickness over the thorax where
the most important vessels and nerves course (Fig.
26-6A–D). Second, when the extremity of the
cone is too round or deformed, we amputate less of
the base and resect a wedge at the end of the cone
allowing it to be molded better.

GROUP IV (83 PERCENT)

These breasts have alterations of form owing to an
increase in the base and height. These breasts are
the most common.

Reducing the volume and modifying the form
are done by removing the ptotic excess under
plane A, resecting a wedge of tissue to reduce the
base diameter and finally amputating the base of
the cone (Fig. 26-7A–C). These resections can be
made in pieces (Fig. 26-7D) or in a single block
(Fig. 26-7E), the latter being the more difficult.

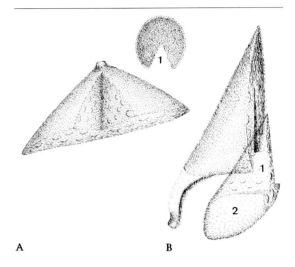

A   B

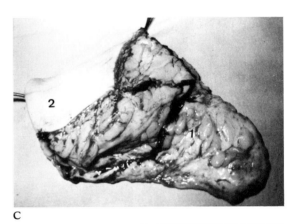

C

*Fig. 26-5. Volume reduction and correction of the
shape of group II breasts as described in the text.*

The amount to be removed depends on the form of
the cone.

All these maneuvers are made easier by placing
traction on the breast at point A, perpendicularly
to the thorax with the patient supine (Fig. 26-7F).

These resections are intended to create a new
cone, with defined volume and dimensions, as
well as removing or moving the ptotic portions,
giving the patient a long-term result without deformity or distortion (Fig. 26-7F).

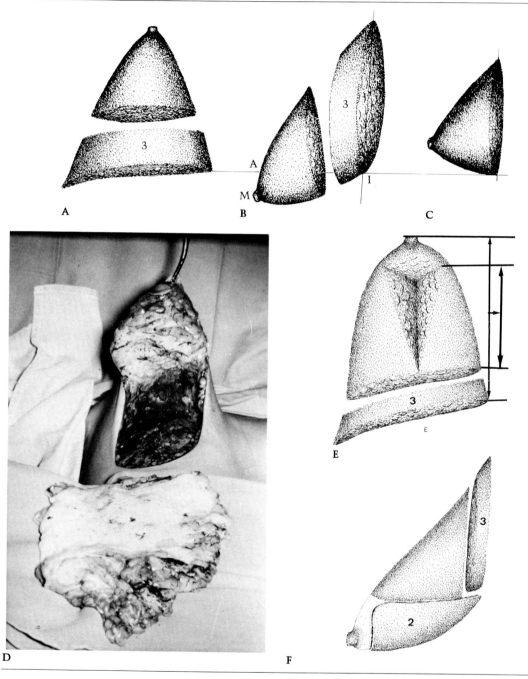

A

B

C

D

E

F

Fig. 26-6. A–D. The first way of "amputating" the
cone, thereby reducing its height and volume. The
portion under plane A is raised, substituting the
portion removed above it. E, F. The second way of
reducing the anteroposterior projection of the breast is
to remove a wedge with subareolar base associated to
an "amputation" of the cone.

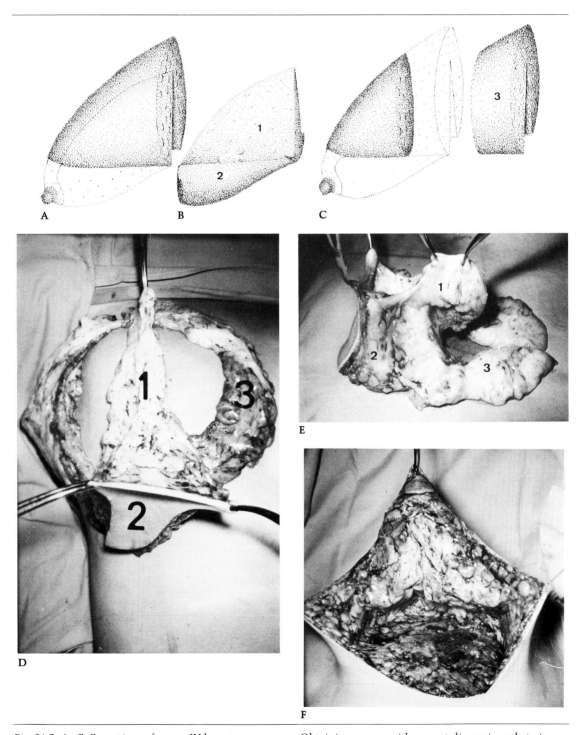

Fig. 26-7. A–C. Resections of group IV breasts, reducing their volume and correcting their form. D. Resections in parts: 1, wedge; 2, excess under plane A; 3, mammary base. E. Resections in a single block. F.

Obtaining a cone with correct dimensions that give a good long-term result; skin elasticity changing with time. The lateral and medial portions are sutured to each other.

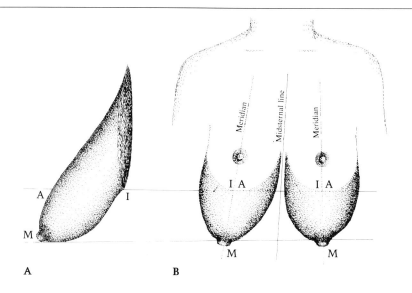

A   B

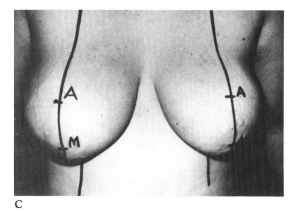

C

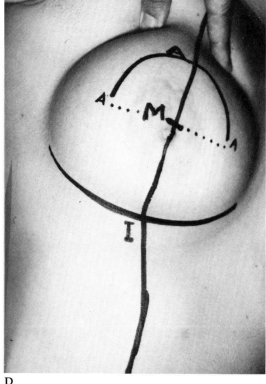

D

Fig. 26-8. A, B. Points A, M, and I with the patient
standing up. C. Marking the mammary meridian, point
A (anterior projection of point I on the breast) and
point M (apex of the cone). D. Marking the superior

semicircle with the pivot point M, the mammary
meridian in a straight line, and the patient supine with
her arms in 90° abduction. E–H. Sequence of the
markings.

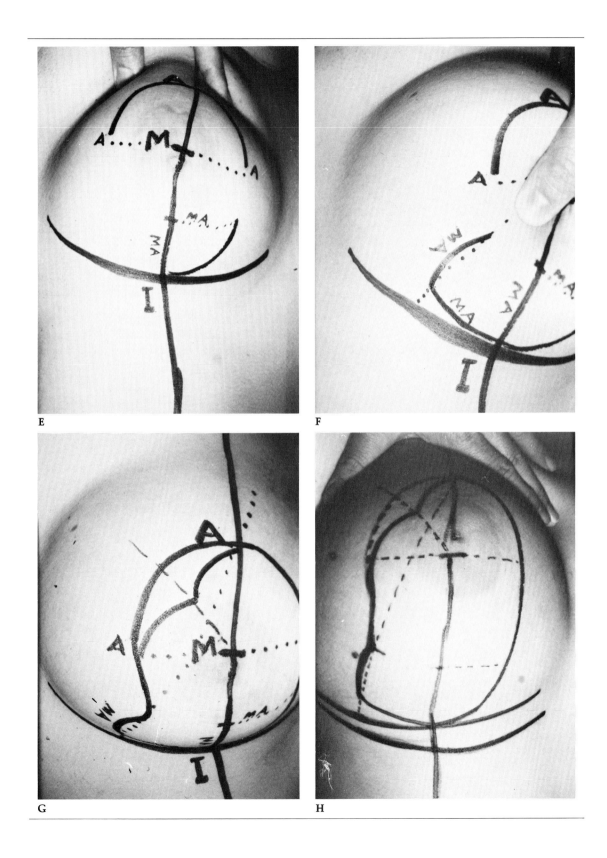

E

F

G

H

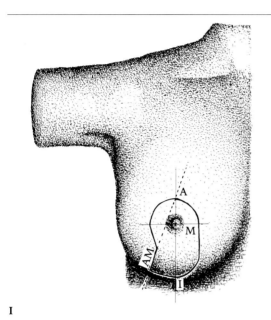

I

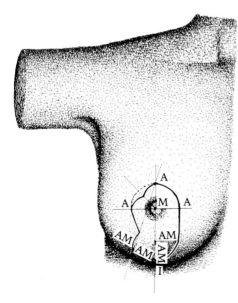

J

Fig. 26-8 (continued). I. Initial marking that is subsequently modified. J. The marking based on the distance A to M that is the amount of ptosis.

Marking and Resectioning the Skin Excess — L Technique

After creating a new breast cone that will provide a good long-term result, we must remove the excess skin; this will result in a variable scar, depending on the ptosis (A-M) and on the position of the areola in relation to point A. Logically, the greater the excess skin in relation to the new glandular cone, the greater the length of the scar will be. It will also be longer if we resect more skin than needed. It is necessary to assess the situation correctly in order to make the required extensions of the scar. These are indispensable factors in obtaining a good result, especially in young patients who more commonly expose their bodies. Wide, hypertrophic, or misplaced scars will cause patients the same unhappiness as did the previous appearance of their breasts.

We initially saw that the normal breast is above plane A of the submammary fold, as determined by measurements (see Fig. 26-1A and B).

We must establish another plane parallel to plane A that passes through the apex of the cone, called plane M.

If we draw a line that divides the breast equally (mammary meridian), its intersection with planes A and M will give us three points: (1) point M on the apex of the cone (greater anteroinferior projection), which, in 83 percent of cases is the site of the nipple; (2) point I on the inferior glandular fold; and (3) point A on the anterior portion of the breast (anterior projection of point I) (Fig. 26-8A and B). The distance A-M measures the amount of skin excess and varies with the amount of ptosis.

In 17 percent of the cases, the apex of the cone is not the nipple; thus, the nipple-areola complex should not be considered when there is ptosis because some breasts bulge at the base, augmenting their inferior portion and hollowing their upper aspect. Other breasts sag down through the apex, taking the areola with them.

The I point is marked on the patient and is equidistant from the midsternal line and from the sternal notch; its distance ranges from 15 to 23 cm. It has the same position on both breasts, even if the breasts have different shapes, volumes, and degrees of ptosis (see Fig. 26-8A and B).

Marking of the mammary meridian and points A, M, and I should be done with the patient standing (Fig. 26-8C). With the patient supine and the arm in 90-degree abduction, we mark the inferior glandular fold. Point I, marked initially on the

submammary fold, will be raised to the prominence of the breast when the patient is supine.

With one hand, we straighten out the breast meridian, and at the pivot point M, we mark a superior semicircle with radius A-M (Fig. 26-8D). On
the breast meridian from point I, we mark a new
point upward, the A-M distance, and from this
point, we draw medially a quarter of a circle on the
inferior quadrant of the marking (Fig. 26-8E).
From point I laterally on the inferior glandular
fold marking, we trace the horizontal distance
A-M. From the end of the horizontal A-M on an
imaginary line that passes through point A, we
also draw the oblique distance A-M (Fig. 26-8H
and I). The superior semicircle is joined to the inferior marking. When we mark the oblique A-M, the
skin of the "imaginary line" should be slightly
pulled in the direction of point A (Fig. 26-8F).

With these basic markings (see Fig. 26-8I), we
obtain good aesthetic results, but with the final
position of the scar, two problems can occur: First,
the vertical scar does not always meet the center of
the areola, sometimes being lateral and tangential
to it; second, the end of the horizontal scar may
not be in the inferior glandular fold but below it.

These problems can be solved by two details in
the marking: First, the end of the horizontal A-M
is raised in proportion to the reduction in the diameter of the base of the mammary cone. This
elevation is of 1 to 2 cm; if the final suture still is
outside the inferior glandular border, we make another correction as will be explained (Fig. 26-8F
and J). Second, on the superior lateral quadrant of
the marking, we draw a skin triangle with equal
arches that join each other at the bisection of the
quadrant.

This triangle, whose height of 1.0 to 2.0 cm, is to
rectify the vertical scar and is made greater than
necessary so that it can be brought under the
subareolar region during skin closure (Figs.
26-8G, H, and J).

All the markings are done keeping in mind the
degree of breast ptosis, having points I and A fixed
and point M variable.

After resection and modeling of the cone, we
begin suturing the skin at the lateral angle formed
by the oblique and horizontal A-M, so that we do
not have dog-ears. When we begin the vertical closure, we do a Z incision on the lateral portion of
the deepithelialized periareolar region in order to
free it to migrate upward (Fig. 26-9A). We distribute the lateral and medial portions equally, stopping 5 to 6 cm beyond the inferior glandular

border, where we do a circular pursestring suture
to compensate, similar to what we do after an ap-
pendectomy (Fig. 26-9B and F). This stitch takes
up the skin excess that traditionally is removed on
the medial side of the submammary fold. If the
breast is flaccid, the amount of skin removed in
this pursestring closure is greater. Sometimes it is
unnecessary or the wound is not totally closed
(Fig. 26-9E).

We mark the areolar diameter as small or as
great as the tension on the pursestring closure. The
pursestring suture is released, and the areolar circles are compared and deepithelialized. The principal sutures are placed.

We generally outline the areola with 3.5-cm diameter and the circle around the pursestring suture with a 2.0-cm diameter. This circle must be
tangential to the apex of the cone superiorly, because after 3 to 6 months, the breast descent will
put it exactly at the apex.

The skin tension around the areola must be similar at the points of fixation and must be equal in
both breasts. It is not important that the deepithelialized circle is not even. There will be pleating on
the medial portion of the periareolar area that disappears in 10 to 60 days; but if it is too accentuated, it will not disappear. In this case, part of
this skin should be returned to the medial submammary fold, transforming the L into a T. This is
the only limiting factor of the L scar and not the
volume removed. Sometimes it is easier to remove
800 gm than 300 gm with the L technique. All depends on the A-M distance.

On the other hand, the diameter of the base of
the cone is almost always reduced.

Notwithstanding the elevation of the angle of
the oblique and horizontal A-M, the suture line
can fall outside the submammary fold.

We can then push the breast in a cephalad fashion, marking the excess above the suture line and
resecting the dog-ear, lengthening the horizontal
scar 1 to 2 cm, but keeping it in or above the submammary fold (Fig. 26-9E).

The breast volume diminishes about 30 percent
during the late postoperative period, after total regression of the edema, absorption of the injured
fat cells, and skin retraction.

All glandular resection and skin sutures have as
their central point the apex of the cone (A), where
the areola will be placed. For this reason, there will
be no problem in elevating it, even with a long
A-M distance, and there will be no traction, tension, compression, or rotation and, therefore, no

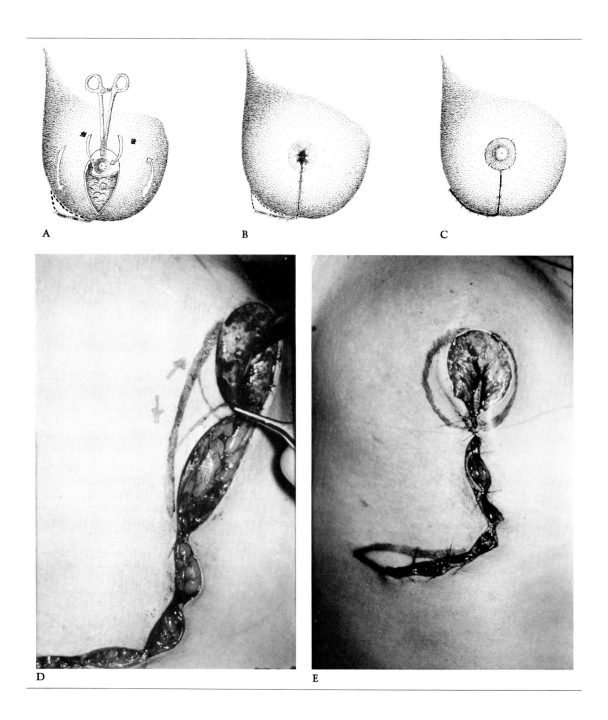

A

B

C

D

E

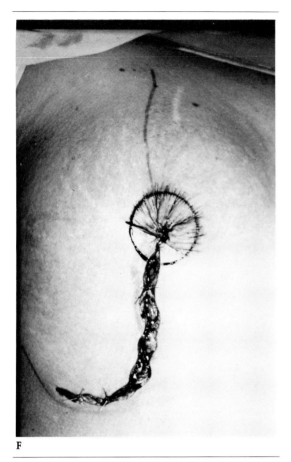

F

Fig. 26-9. A–C. Skin suturing follows the indicated arrows, placing the scars in a less visible position. Z incision in the lateral dermis for areolar release.
D. The lateral skin triangle is adjusted so that its apex meets the midportion of the areola inferiorly.
E. Sometimes the circumareolar pursestring is unnecessary, especially in the breasts with a small A-M distance and not much glandular resection. The horizontal scar is adjusted to the submammary fold, lengthening it 1 to 2 cm with this maneuver.
F. Marking of the deepithelialization circle around the circumareolar purse.

circulatory problems. The compensation from lateral to medial and then finishing upward in a pursestring suture reduces the horizontal scar because it resects skin around the areola, where the scar is traditional. Figures 26-10 through 26-15 show pre- and postoperative views of breasts with an L scar and with reshaping, as we will describe.

Transformation of the L Scar into the Inverted T Scar with a Short Medial Limb

When pleating of the pursestring suture is excessive, generally when the A-M distance is greater than 6 to 7 cm, some skin is returned to the medial submammary fold. All markings for glandular resection and reshaping are equal to the L mammaplasty incision based on the A-M distance. The suture begins at the angle of the oblique and horizontal A-M; the moment that it initiates the vertical closure, a dog-ear forms on the medial side of the wound. We now do the vertical suturing and the pursestring as described. In this case, the superolateral skin triangle is unnecessary and should be removed.

The breast is raised in a craniocaudal direction, marking the resection of the medial and lateral dog-ears, shortening the vertical suture (Fig. 26-16).

The advantage of this procedure is that the medial scar can be the size we want and it will lie under the breast.

Mammaplasty with Vertical Scar— Inverse Arié

With breasts of the same abnormal base, we can accomplish mammaplasty with vertical and periareolar scars if there is hypertrophy or dysmorphy with little ptosis (with generally A-M distance between 2 and 3 cm) and if the skin is elastic, with a thick dermis.

The mammary meridian is marked with the patient standing, as are points A, M, and I. With the patient supine, we mark the superior semicircle with the radius A-M and the pivot point M (Fig. 26-17A).

The lateral and medial extremities of the semicircle join each other at point I. We draw two skin triangles at each side of the marking as we described in the L technique, always greater than necessary. On suturing, we remove skin from one side or the other of the triangle if we want to raise or lower its apex.

The purpose of these triangles is to avoid strangulating the subareolar region, and the apex of the triangle should be at 5 to 6 cm from point I (Fig. 26-17B).

Point I must be elevated in proportion to the reduction of the diameter of the base of the cone or the final scar will be below the submammary fold (Fig. 26-17A, B, and C).

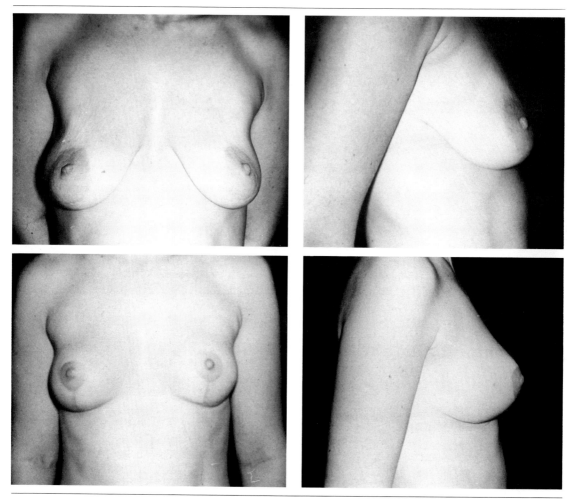

Fig. 26-10. Patient with group I breasts, A-M distance of 4 cm and nipple-areola complex above the point M. The correction is made with an inferior pedicle axial flap, resulting in an L final scar. Six months postoperatively, front view and profile.

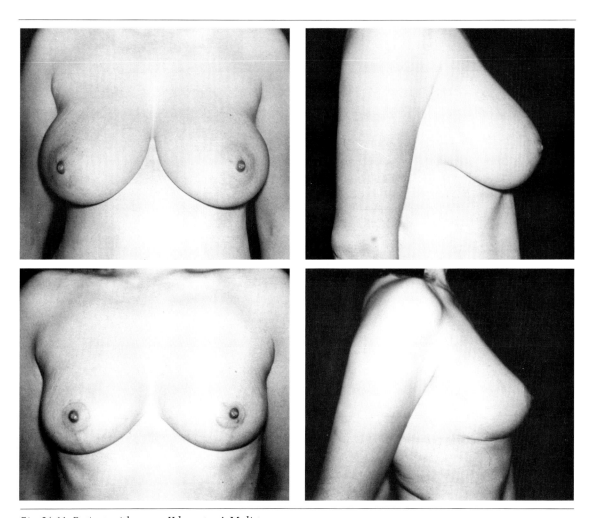

Fig. 26-11. Patient with group II breasts, A-M distance
of 4.5 cm and nipple-areola complex above point M.
Excess tissue was resected under plane A and a wedge
to reduce the laterolateral diameter, removing 380 gm.
Seventeen months postoperatively.

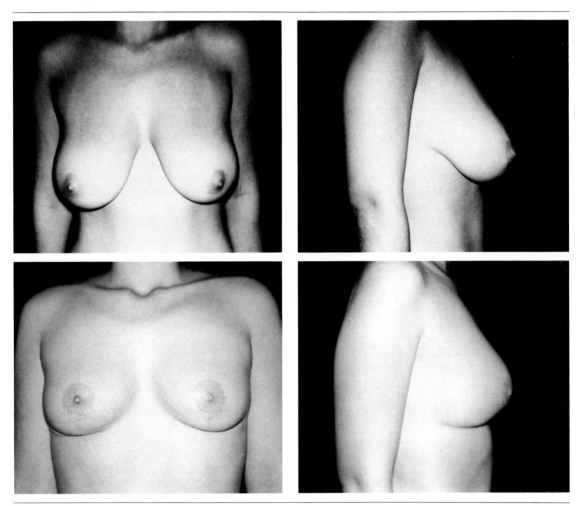

Fig. 26-12. *Patient with group III breasts; ptosis (A-M distance) of 6 cm, coincidence of point M and nipple. The correction is made only with amputation and removal of the base of the mammary cone, resecting 250 gm. Eighteen months postoperatively.*

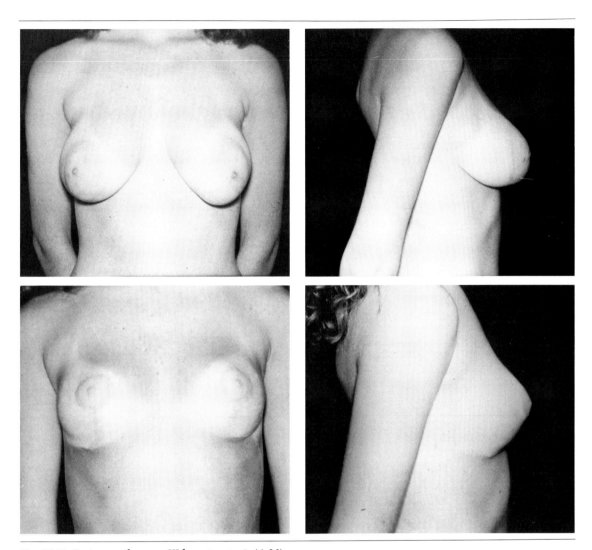

Fig. 26-13. Patient with group III breasts, ptosis (A-M)
of 4 cm. One hundred eighty grams of glandular tissue
was removed. Fourteen months postoperatively.

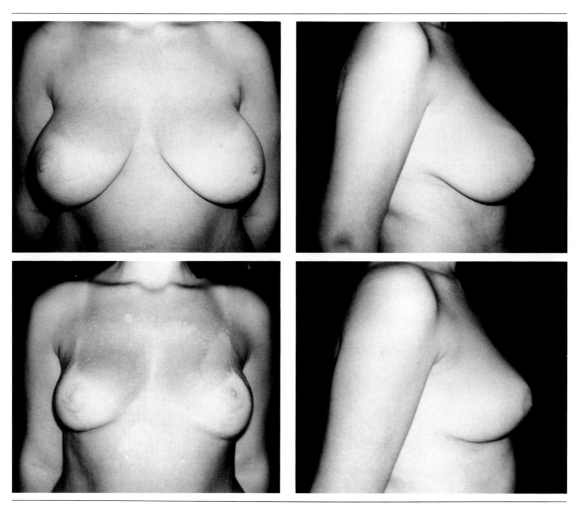

Fig. 26-14. *Patient with group IV breasts, ptosis (A-M) 6 cm. The correction of volume and form was made as described in the text. Resection of 520 gm of tissue from each breast. Eighteen months postoperatively.*

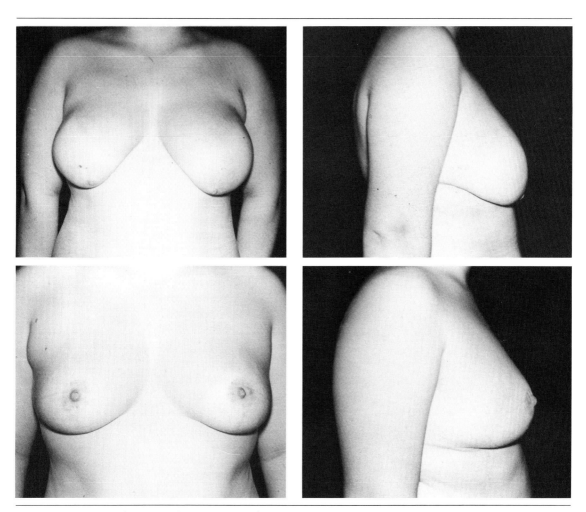

Fig. 26-15. Patient with group IV breasts, ptosis of
5.5 cm, with point M outside the areola — that is,
medial to it. Resection of 450 gm from the left breast
and 300 gm from the right breast. Eighteen months
postoperatively. If we follow the concepts shown,
without considering the areola on the markings, but
the point M, we can put the nipple-areola complex on
the apex of the cone at the end of surgery. Twenty-four
months postoperatively.

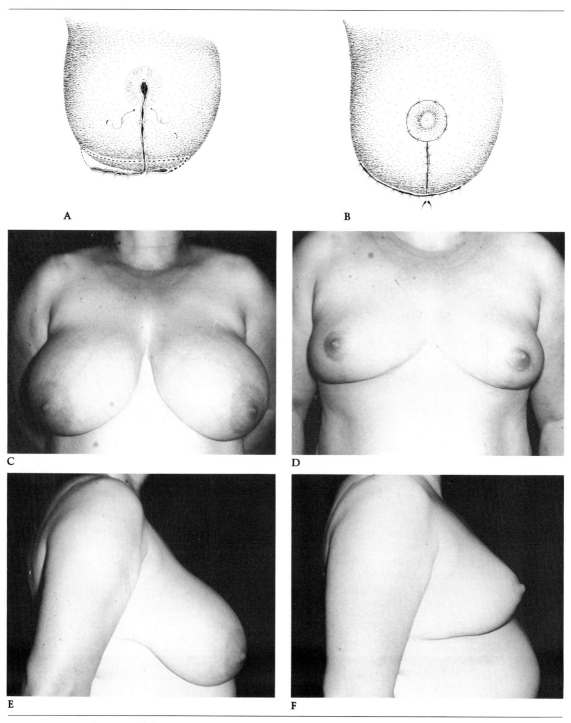

A

B

C

D

E

F

Fig. 26-16. A, B. Changing of the L into an inverted T, transferring part of the excess of skin on the medial side of the breast to the medial portion of the submammary fold. C–F. Pre- and 12 months postoperatively of a patient with group IV breasts, ptosis with A-M distance of 11.5 cm, and tissue resections of 1440 gm from each breast. Seventeen months postoperatively.

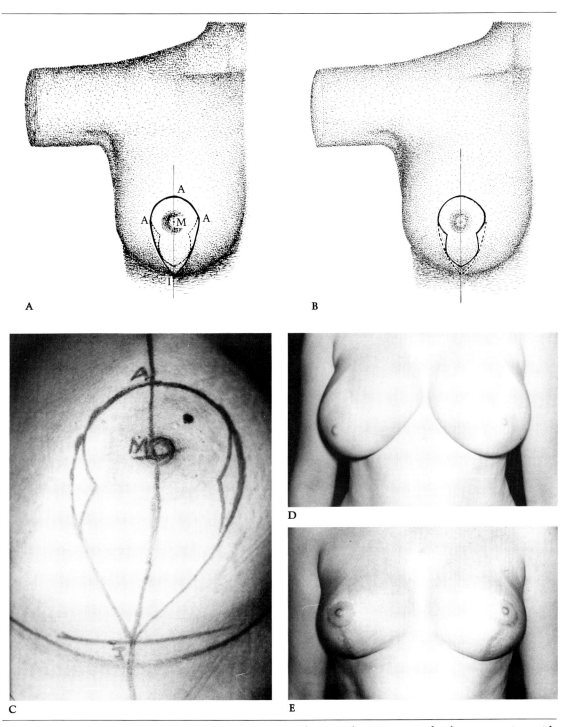

Fig. 26-17. A–C. Skin markings using the mammary meridian and points A, M, and I, which we call the inverse Arié because skin compensation is done upward, finishing in a circumareolar purse. D–G. Pre-

and 18 months postoperatively of a young patient with group IV breasts, A-M distance of 3 cm, glandular resections of 550 gm.

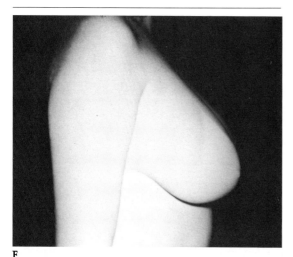

F

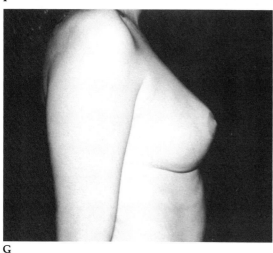

G

Fig. 26-17 (continued).

Glandular resections are done as described according to the alterations of the form and volume of the four groups. We recommend in this technique always to leave an inferior pedicle flap, even with great resections so that point I will not be raised too much and the extremity of the scar will be below it.

We have removed as much as 550 gm of breast tissue with this procedure (Fig. 26-17D to G).

The skin closure is made from down-upward, finishing in a circumareolar pursestring suture to compensate.

The term *inverse Arié* is derived from the fact that the skin closure is made contrary to that conceived by that author [1] because it goes beyond the submammary fold.

Mini T Mammaplasty

Eventually, at the end of the operation, some skin remains on the distal end of the scar, although it can disappear, it usually remains. We always remove it.

If we have made a marking error and the suturing goes beyond the submammary fold, we push the breast in the craniocaudal direction and resect a small transverse fold of skin at the inferior border of the gland (Fig. 26-18).

Mammaplasty with Vertical and Without Periareolar Scar

When the nipple and point A coincide, there will be no skin to be resected over the areola. The form and volume are corrected as described before by a vertical fusiform incision, whose width at its center is twice the distance of A-M, going from the nipple to point I (Fig. 26–19).

If it is difficult to determine point M, the amount of skin to be removed by the fusiform excision can be determined by pinching. Also, here we must raise point I if we reduce the diameter of the mammary base. Sometimes we have to remove some skin around the nipple, reducing the areolar diameter, with the advantage of not losing the natural color transition between the areola and the skin.

The distal end of the incision can be transformed in a "mini T."

On the other hand, we can terminate the fusiform excision at the areolar edge by removing skin on its lower half (Fig. 26-20A–E) [5].

The glandular resection and molding have nothing to do with the form, position, and extension of the scars. These depend on the ptosis (A-M), on the glandular volume removed, and on the position of the areola in relation to point A.

We conclude that a new mammaplasty technique is not only a new design for skin resection, but also a new philosophy of systematization of glandular molding based on the correct appreciation of the morphologic alterations of the breast, along with the appropriate markings for skin resection, thereby obtaining better and smaller scars with good long-term results.

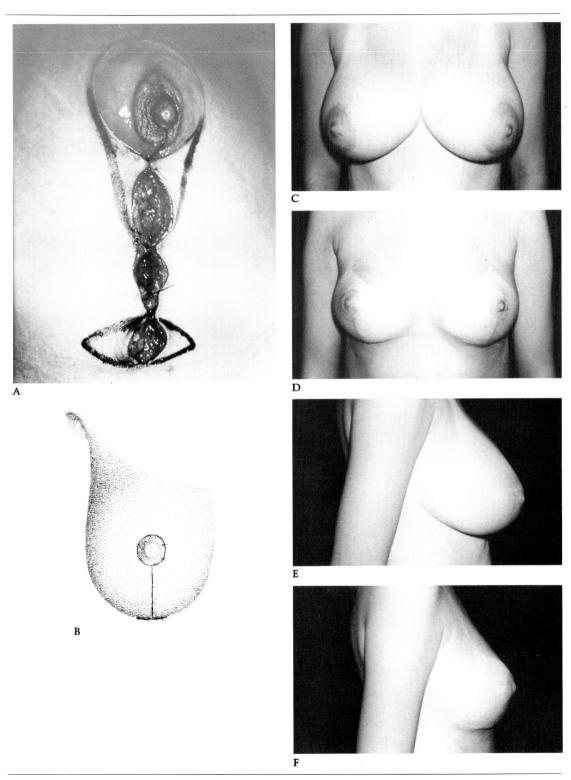

Fig. 26-18. A, B. T mammaplasty similar to the inverse Arié, removing a small tissue excess at the end of the vertical scar. C–F. Pre- and postoperatively of a group IV patient. A-M distance is 3.5 cm, point M is under the nipple; resection involved removal of 580 gm from each breast. Sixteen months postoperatively.

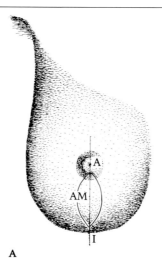

A

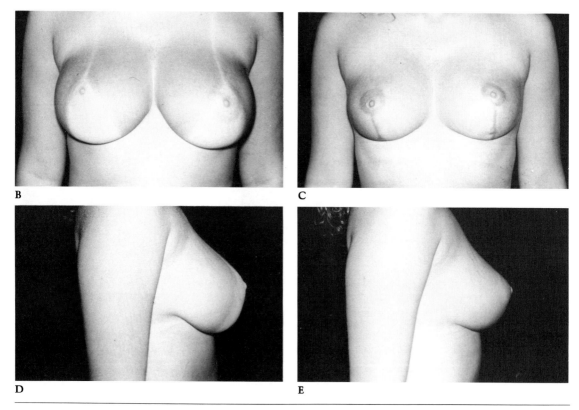

B

C

D

E

Fig. 26-19. A. Fusiform resection from area of the nipple extending to inferior glandular prominence. B–E. Pre- and 6 months postoperatively of a patient with group IV breasts; A-M distance of 2.5 cm, coinciding nipple and point A; tissue resections of 350 gm.

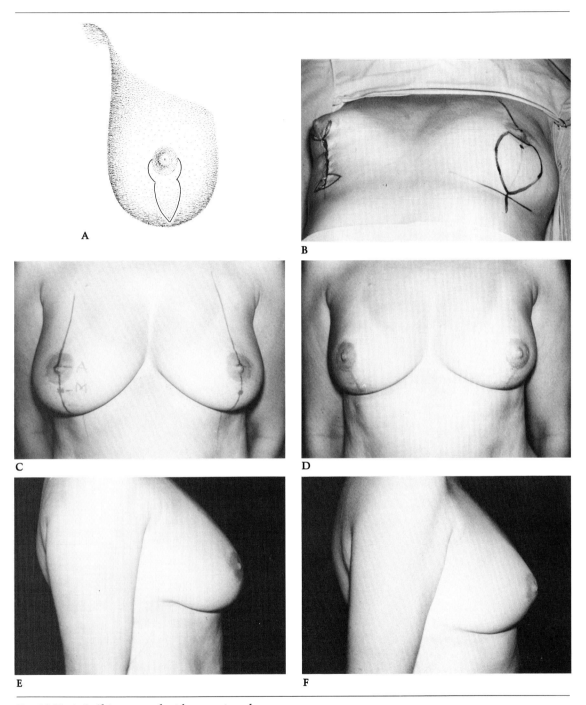

Fig. 26-20. A, B. Skin removed without periareolar resection when point A and nipple are coincident. The possibility of transforming the scar into a mini T. C–F. Pre- and 7 months postoperatively of a patient with group II breasts; A-M distance of 2.5 cm; and tissue resections of 160 gm.

Answers to the Questions	Good	Bad	Acceptable	Very evident	Little evident	Yes	No	Didn't answer	Very pretty	Prettier	Uglier	Didn't answer	Improved	Little improvement	Worsen	Didn't change	I don't know	Disappeared
Your scars are . . .	96.22	3.78		11.32	88.68													
Are your scars totally covered by your bathing suit?						73.58	26.42											
Your scars around the areola are . . .	75.48	1.88	22.64															
Do you like the shape of your breasts?						96.22	3.78											
Is its form similar to those that weren't operated on and are pretty?						75.48	22.64	1.88										
Are your breasts prettier or uglier than those operated on by other techniques?										86.79		13.21						

Did you take off your clothes in the presence of persons of the same and of the opposite sex before the surgery?	37.73	62.27								
Do you now take them off?	91.33	5.67								
Have your intimate and social relationships changed after the surgery?			71.69	28.31						
If you could go back in time, would you like to be operated on by the same technique?	94.34	3.78	1.88							
Those who knew you before and see you now think that . . .			90.00	10.00						
Those who knew your breasts before think that they are . . .					75.48	24.52				
If you had backache previously it has . . .						30.18	30.18	9.46	38.18	
The sensibility of the areola and nipple . . .			13.20			4.90	48.38	35.41	0.02	

Fig. 26-21. Patient questionnaire.

Finally, the objective is to acquire a greater experience, transmit it didactically with honesty, showing the virtues, difficulties, complications, and bad results as well as the good, so that we can correct them in the future, thus depersonalizing the use of the technique.

Results

We utilize the L mammaplasty in 85.5 percent of our patients; in 12 percent, the vertical scar with a periareolar one or mini-T mammaplasty, and, in 2.5 percent, the inverted T.

It is difficult to have a final scar in L if the A-M distance is greater than 6 or 7 cm. In these cases, we generally have an inverted T scar with a medial arm.

The volume removed (in grams) varies from the following:

VOLUME (GM)	PERCENT
0–200 =	5
200–300 =	20
300–400 =	28
400–500 =	32
500–600 =	11
more than 600 =	4

Eighty-one and a half percent of the patients were between 15 and 35 years of age; normal lactation was reported in 13 patients. We sent a questionnaire to 200 patients randomly chosen from 1,103 cases who were at least 6 months postoperative in an effort to evaluate the results from their point of view. An analysis of Figure 26-21 gives us the answers.

COMPLICATIONS AND BAD RESULTS

We had three cases of partial necrosis (one fourth) of the areola, in spite of the absence of traction, torsion, or compression. It was due to the removal of diseased tissue close to or under the nipple-areola complex, leaving it very thin.

Figure 26-21 shows cases with hypoesthesia or anesthesia probably owing to a technical error in the preservation of subcutaneous thickness. Local retraction or depressions occurred more commonly along the horizontal scar because of inadequate thickness of the subcutaneous fat.

An understanding of what is specifically wrong with the breast in terms of form, volume, ptosis,

and position, including the form, size, and position of the nipple-areola complex, makes it easy to understand the causes of bad results so that we can analyze them and not repeat our mistakes.

Mammary Cone

The only alteration that occurs postoperatively is ptosis because of the loss of the skin's elasticity with the passage of time if we have produced a cone with perfect form, having a unitary ratio with the skin and if the scars are well positioned. If the glandular cone is not well made, we will have a poor result.

VOLUME. Errors in resection can occur, leaving volumes greater or smaller than optimal and generally with a wrong form.

FORM. The most common error is to leave the horizontal diameter greater than the vertical one, owing to insufficient wedge resection.

The vertical diameter cannot be too short or flattening of the inferior breast cone will occur.

During resection of the excess tissue under plane A and of the wedge, we place traction on the breast (using a clamp) at point A perpendicularly to the chest wall. Resection is then performed parallel to the skin marking up to point A and not perpendicularly to the chest wall. If this occurs, the inferior portion will look empty, shortening the vertical diameter.

Remember that if an inferior pedicle flap is left, this problem can be solved, even if it is small, because it can fill the empty space on the inferior pole, especially when the patient raises her arms.

Bulging in the inferior portion occurs when amputation of the mammary cone was done incorrectly with measurements: apex to the inferior glandular fold and apex to the superior glandular edge in a proportion greater than the normal 1 : 1.5, with predominance of the first.

Bulging will occur after 12 months postoperatively, even with a short and tight vertical scar. The weight of the breast wins over this resistance, being a common event with the mammaplasty techniques that do not reduce the height of the cone.

Localized bulges appear when we do not follow the chest wall contour during amputation of the lateral slope, leaving the lateral subcutaneous fat thicker than the subcutaneous fat of the thorax. We must thin the upper "oblique A-M flap" when it is positioned over the horizontal A-M, or it will bulge over the inferior flap.

Post-anterior projection occurs when an excessive resection of vertical columns reduces the projection of the breast too much, making it unaesthetic in appearance. A lack of resection overprojects it with a greater chance of ptosis recurrence.

Skin

RESIDUAL PTOSIS. In selected cases, when the patient is young and with a thick dermis, we leave the ratio container-content slightly greater than 1, and the skin will contract [14] over the remodeled gland. This allows us to remove less skin and to have shorter scars, which, without tension on the suture line, will be of good quality. Actually we would rather remove all the excess skin because in observing selected cases, we see some residual ptosis with time. A fatty breast with thin dermis can have residual ptosis after 6 months postoperatively with any resection.

DOG-EARS. Dog-ears generally occur at the end of the horizontal scar in an attempt to keep it short. It is better to have a scar a little bit longer, and well-positioned but without dog-ears.

PERIAREOLAR WRINKLES. To remove the skin excess over the cone, we recommend compensating from lateral to medial and then upward, ending in a circumareolar pursestring suture. By these maneuvers, the skin excess on the medial side of the breast, contrary to what happens in T resections, is directed to the periareolar region. This results in wrinkling in this area in proportion to the ptosis of the breast and to the volume removed. These wrinkles disappear rapidly when they are small; in approximately 2 months, when medium-sized; and, if they are too large, will never disappear. As described, this is the main limiting factor of the L technique — not the volume resected, but the skin excess "container."

Areola

There are three important changes that can affect the areola: position, form, and size.

In the period from 3 to 6 months postoperatively, the areola that was placed tangentially slightly below the apex of the cone when the breast tissue rotates or loosens takes its place on the apex of the cone. The bad positioning of the areola is due to: (1) misplaced deepithelialization of the areolar circle, or (2) wrong amputation of the cone. When the ratio between the measurements from the apex of the cone to the inferior glandular fold and from the apex to the superior glandular edge differs from 1 to 1.5, the areola suffers later positioning. If the first measurement is greater, the areola will "look" upward, and, if the second measurement is greater, it will "look" downward.

If the amputation does not follow the chest wall contour, the areola can medialize or lateralize.

In terms of form, the tension around the areola on the border of the deepithelialized circle must be similar to that on all opposing points. There is a tendency to have more skin excess on the medial side, so that the deepithelialized area can be elliptical, since the sutured areola becomes circular.

The areolar diameter should be between 3.5 and 4.0 cm. Tension on its borders will provoke its enlargement after 6 to 12 months.

Scars

Scars are important in terms of the aesthetic result in relation to their length, position, form, and quality.

LENGTH. They must be the smallest possible, leaving the skin envelope under slight tension, never going beyond the anterior axillary line, because the movements of the arms can pull and enlarge them. If there is a medial scar, it should be only under the breast. Figure 26-21 shows a poor result owing to bad placement of the scars.

FORM. Form depends on the excess of the skin envelope in relation to the molded cone and on the surgeon's preference. The diagnosis is basic to determine the final scar that will result. There are no miracles. Bad results occur when trying to shorten scars more than necessary.

QUALITY. A high rate of good results will occur when the cone is molded correctly and when we cover it with skin and subcutaneous tissue in 1:1 ratio, leaving the smallest scar possible and leaving it well positioned.

If, after these precautions, we still have a hypertrophic scar, it is probably due to the patient's problems with healing.

Figure 26-22 shows some complications attributable to tactical mistakes.

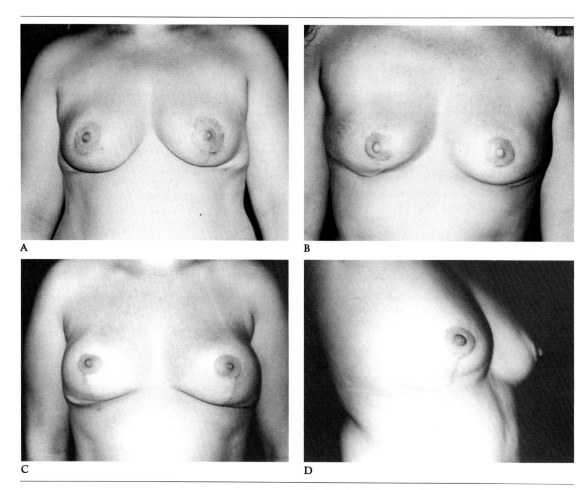

Fig. 26-22. A. Horizontal scars outside the submammary fold, lateral bulging, wrong resection of the cone with an empty laterosuperior portion and asymmetric areolas. B. Excessive tissue removal at the superior pole with irregular and misplaced horizontal scars. C. Lateral dog-ears, irregular areolar contour, and the distance from the apex of the mammary cone to the inferior glandular edge is too great. D. Inferior hollowing when the patient raises her arms owing to absence of the inferior pedicle miniflap. The final scar is like a comma because point I was marked too laterally. When it is marked more medially, the final scar becomes S-shaped.

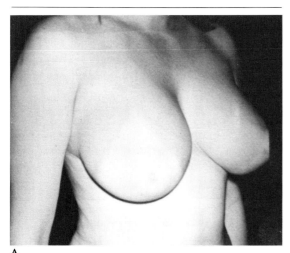

A

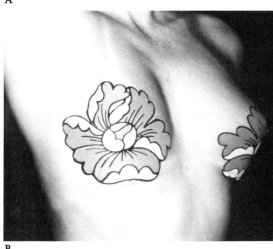

B

Fig. 26-23. Pre- and post operative views of the same patient as in Figure 26-17 in an oblique view using an adhesive paper bra that covers the vertical scar.

It is quite difficult for an operated on breast to stand the close scrutiny of the patient, the surgeon, and of society (Fig. 26-23).

References

1. Arié, G. Una nueva técnica de mastoplastia. Rev. Latinoam.Cir. Plast. 3:23, 1957.
2. Bozola, A.R., et al. Mamoplastia em "L". Contribuição Pessoal. Rev. AMRIGS 26:207, 1982.
3. Dufourmentel, C.Y., and Mouly, R. Plastic mamaire par la mèthode oblique. Ann. Chir. Plast. 6:45, 1961.
4. Elbaz, J.S., and Werheecke, G. La cicatrice em L dans les plasties mamires. Ann. Chir. Plast. 17:283, 1972.
5. Ely, J.F. The devil's incision mammoplasty. Aesth. Plast. Surg. 7:159, 1983.
6. Goldwyn, R.M. Plastic and Reconstructive Surgery of the Breast. Boston: Little, Brown, 1976. P. 16.
7. Hollander, E. Die operation der mamma: Hypertrophie and der Hängebrust. Dtsch. Med. Wochenschr. 41:1400, 1924.
8. Horibe, K., Spina, V., and Lodovici, O. Mammaplastia reductora: Nuevo abordaje del método lateral-oblíquo. Rev. Latinoam. Cir. Plast. 2:7, 1976.
9. Lima, J.C. Breast reduction: New Method and refinements. Transactions of the Seventh International Congress of Plastic Reconstructive Surgery, São Paulo, 1979. Pp. 518–521.
10. Maliniac, J.W. Breast deformities. Anatomical and physiological considerations in plastic repair. Am. J. Surg. 39:54, 1938.
11. Marchac, D., and De Oliarte, G. Reduction mammaplasty and correction of ptosis with a short inframammary scar. Plast. Reconstr. Surg. 69:45, 1982.
12. McKissock, P.C. Correction of Macromastia by the Bipedicle Vertical Dermal Flap. In R.M. Goldwyn (ed.), Plastic and Reconstructive Surgery of the Breast. Boston: Little, Brown, 1976. Pp. 215–229.
13. Meyer, R., and Kesselring, V. Reduction mammaplasty with an L-shape suture line. Plast. Reconstr. Surg. 55:139, 1975.
14. Peixoto, C. Reduction mammaplasty: A personal technique. Plast. Reconstr. Surg. 65:217, 1980.
15. Pitanguy, I. Mammaplastias. Rev. Latinoam. Cir. Plast. 7:139, 1963.
16. Pontes, A. A technique of reduction mammaplasty. Br. J. Plast. Surg. 26:365, 1973.
17. Regnault, P.C.L. Reduction Mammaplasty by the B Technique. In R.M. Goldwyn (ed.), Plastic and Reconstruction Surgery of the Breast. Boston: Little, Brown, 1976. Pp. 269–283.
18. Ribeiro, L., and Backer, E. Mastoplastia con pedículo de seguridad. Rev. Esp. Cir. Plast. 6:223, 1973.
19. Sepúlveda, A. Tratamento das assimetrias mamárias. Rev. Bras. Cir. 71:11, 1981.
20. Skoog, T. A technique of breast reduction: Transposition of the nipple on a cutaneous vascular pedicle. Acta Chir. Scand. 126:453, 1963.
21. Strömbeck, J.O. Mammaplasty: Report of a new technique based on the two pedicle procedure. Br. J. Plast. Surg. 13:79, 1960–1961.

COMMENTS ON CHAPTER 26   *Robert M. Goldwyn*

The preceding chapter by Bozola is noteworthy not just for his technique — really a few techniques — of breast reduction but also for the conceptual thinking and careful analysis that underlie them. Few would dispute that he has studied the female breast in a rational way, taking cognizance of its aesthetics, geometry, and composition. What is particularly important about his view of the breast and his operations of reduction is that he mentally takes apart and rebuilds the major components (soft tissue and glandular cone) of each breast before he actually does it surgically. Only in this way does he feel that one can properly achieve an optimal result. Logically, the surgeon should know what is wrong with the shape and volume of a breast before he or she seeks to change it.

Bozola classifies breasts into four categories, of which his group IV is the most common, constituting 83 percent of all breasts. This type has a greater than normal base and height, and its surgical correction consists primarily of amputating the base to create a new cone and also removing excess skin and subcutaneous tissue not only to give a breast of desired volume and shape that will resist, at least for a while, time and gravity, but to accomplish all this with a minimum of scarring.

Actually, 85 percent of the patients in Bozola's series of 1,103 ended with an L scar, but, as he has written, it would be difficult to have a final scar in an L from the submammary fold to the apex if the cone is greater than 7 cm. Instead of an L, the resultant scar for large breasts is an inverted T.

In his section on results, Bozola has given us information about the amount of tissue removed from his patients: 96 percent had excision of 600 gm or less; only in 4 percent was the amount greater than 600 gm. If, under those circumstances, a T-shaped incision was frequently necessary, one can safely presume that with much larger breasts requiring a much greater volume reduction, the T-shaped scar would be inevitable and likely longer.

In essence, Bozola honestly states what most of us have also discovered — that a large reduction necessitating removal of a large amount of skin generally, but not always (as the reader can see by the descriptions of other techniques in this book),

forces one's hand into an inverted T incision of at least moderate length.

One of Bozola's virtues is to scrutinize without dissimulation of results so that, as he says, one can analyze with objectivity — no interference from the ego — what went wrong in order not to repeat the same error(s). In the spirit of candor, Bozola has written about the common mistakes in planning and executing his procedures as well as how to avoid the pitfalls. Many of the poor results came from faulty amputation of the cone — too little, too much, the wrong area. It is impossible, of course, to give all the results of breast reduction in more than 1,000 patients in only one chapter — even one book. Bozola has presented us with some representative results in a spectrum of breasts, from group I through group IV. Most of the results are excellent, but Bozola has not advertised only perfect outcomes. That the nipple can be placed too high, we note in Figure 26-10 (group I), Figure 26-13 (group III), and Figure 26-14 (group IV), but we also note that many of the postoperative views are longer than 1 year and are intervals sufficient to witness breast descent and nipple elevation or, as was more likely, the nipple had been placed too high at operation because, as Bozola states, the keyhole was sited too high or the cone was incorrectly amputated.

Most of Bozola's 200 patients surveyed by questionnaire were pleased with the outcome as evidenced by the data in Figure 26-21. Only 4 of 200 patients reported asensate nipples, but it is interesting that 70 patients replied that they had no idea about their nipple sensation.

Bozola's techniques — there are more than one — for breast reduction require more analysis of what to do with the hypertrophied breast and more experience in doing it than in other methods, such as the inferior pedicle technique. Although it is true that the purist would argue that any procedure should involve detailed analysis and any procedure can go awry, the operation Bozola has described for his group IV breasts requires considerable judgment and skill in the crucial step of amputating the breast to produce a better cone. Having done resections of the base of the breast in this technique and that of Peixoto (see Chap. 23), I can state frankly that it is not as easy as the diagrams suggest, particularly for the novitiate to know precisely how to resect the breast to give the desired volume and shape. In addition, in the process of resection of the extra skin vertically and around the areola to reduce or eliminate the horizontal scar, there can be undue tension in closure and an unsightly scar can result around the areola or vertically (Fig. 26-17E). This potential problem is not unique to Bozola's method but is also a possibility in other methods that get rid of skin everywhere else but horizontally (except in the volume reduction method of Cloutier, who utilizes a horizontal incision; see Chap. 29).

One reason Bozola's patients generally have good scars around the areola and vertically is that he knows how to resect enough of the cone of the breast either at its base or in its vertical dimension to allow the skin to drape around the new keyhole with minimal tension. True, there may be some puckering, but with time, most of this disappears. Again, knowing where to transect, how much, and at what angle is critical to achieve the pleasing contours Bozola's patients demonstrate. Conversely, an error in amputating a segment of the cone results in an abnormal and displeasing shape. Retaining a portion of the inferior pedicle for use as a miniflap, if necessary, to give fullness or projection is a wise safety maneuver.

Although not every surgeon, for whatever his or her reasons, will switch to Bozola's method, each of us should adopt his thoughtful approach in analyzing every breast for reduction before we operate.

27

Claude Lassus

Personal Method of Reduction Mammaplasty

Durston is said to have been the first person to have performed and described a technique of breast surgery in 1669. From that time, many attempts have been done in the field of aesthetic surgery of the breast to achieve good results. However, we note that the ideal reduction mammaplasty is still to be described. But from the first real description of such a technique in 1923 by the French surgeon Aubert, things have changed and improved considerably. Meanwhile, we can observe that Aubert and others such as Mornard and Hollander in the same period had already performed a safe procedure: wedge resection of the inferior part of the gland by the two first cited authors and a single horizontal scar and a wedge lateral resection of the gland and L-shaped scar by Hollander.

The results obtained by these techniques were not enough, so other methods were developed later. These new methods were less safe because most of them involved wide undermining of the gland and skin, causing, quite often, partial glandular or skin necrosis, and all these methods ended with the huge inverted T scar.

We had to wait until the 1960s for new advances in the field of reduction mammaplasty. In 1957, Arié was first to propose an inferior wedge resection of skin and gland, transposition of the areola on a superiorly based areolar flap, and a single vertical scar. But this technique was suitable only for mildly hypertrophic breasts.

In 1959, Pitanguy adopted the same principles of wedge resection without any undermining but ended up with an inverted T scar; his technique was suitable for all degrees of hypertrophic ptotic breasts. In 1960, Strömbeck brought onto the market another technique allowing a wide and safe glandular resection and a secure transposition of the areola.

In 1963, Skoog, after Schwartzmann, demonstrated the importance of the dermal vascularization for the areola and proposed a transposition of the nipple and areola on a dermopedicle flap while he resected en bloc skin, fat, and gland.

After 1960, plastic surgeons had at their disposal several safe techniques of breast reduction, providing a good reduction of the volume but significant scarring with the classical inverted T scar. When I started my practice in the mid-1960s, I had to look at patients operated on previously and elsewhere and, often, with very poor results: bad shape and prominent scarring. I immediately became aware that reduction mammaplasty had to (1) be a safe procedure, (2) give a good lasting result, (3) preserve sensibility and function, and (4) leave minimal scarring. That is why I soon developed a procedure combining the principles of Skoog and Arié. My procedure included:

1. Resection en bloc of skin, fat, and gland.
2. Transposition of the areola on a dermoglandular pedicle.
3. A single vertical scar, even in huge hypertrophic ptotic breasts (Fig. 27-1).

In these latter cases, there was an inconvenience: 2 or 3 cm of the vertical incision was visible below the inframammary fold (Fig. 27-1). Thus, I modified the technique. The addition of a short horizontal scar eliminated this drawback in 1977. I was, it seems, the first to describe such a technique. Later, others proposed reduction mammaplasty finishing with a short horizontal scar.

From the 1980s, however, evolution of the mores and the development of topless fashion on the beaches have made candidates for breast reduction more demanding about the residual scar. That is why, to me, the last challenge in reduction

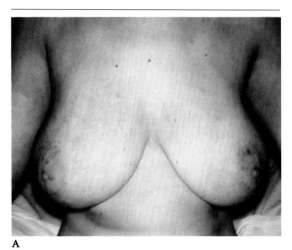

A

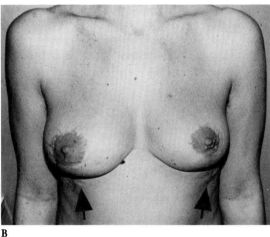

B

Fig. 27-1. A. Before. B. After 12 years.

mammaplasty is the scarring. This is why I decided to go back to my first method and to end every breast reduction with a single vertical scar, staying above the brassiere line, all the more so because looking at patients operated on 10, 15, or 20 years previously, I appreciated the persistent satisfactory volume and shape obtained with this procedure (Fig. 27-2).

I know now that there is not and probably never will be one method that is best for all cases for breast reduction in spite of the fact that some surgeons (and I am one of them) will use one method to the exclusion of all others. I wish to demonstrate my method, which is suitable for all types of hypertrophic and ptotic breasts.

Why a Single Vertical Scar?

After a surgical procedure, it would be ideal to have no scar. Since this is impossible to achieve, we have to use procedures providing minimal scarring because the quality of the scar does not depend on the quality of the surgeon or the surgery and because even the best scars never become invisible. We can treat small ptotic hypertrophic breasts with a single periareolar scar, of course, but in my hands, the average-sized or large breast will need longer incisions and therefore more scarring, and, again in my hands, the vertical scar is the least and the best, with time, its visibility diminishes. Even in patients who heal with good scars, a vertical scar is better, so much more so in patients who develop hypertrophic scars or keloids or in patients who already have scars in the mammary area, mainly those having undergone a breast cancer operation who need reconstruction on one side and reshaping of the contralateral side to achieve symmetry.

In almost all cases, it is possible to finish with a single vertical scar. If we measure the distance between the inferior border of the areola and the inframammary crease in young breasts, we generally find that it is about 8 cm. I do not agree with those who say that the vertical scar must not exceed 5.5 cm. This is true in small breasts but is not so for all cases; it depends on breast volume. It can be 5 or 5.5 cm, but it can also be 8.5 or 9.0 cm and stay above the inframammary fold in bigger breasts (Fig. 27-3).

Sometimes, at the end of the operation, the vertical scar seems to be 1 or 2 cm too long, but a few weeks later, because of the descent of the breast, this is no longer the case (Fig. 27-4).

Technique
PREOPERATIVE DRAWINGS
All the drawings are done while the patient is upright.

1. First, two key points are marked: point A and point B. Point A is the new nipple position. It is where a vertical line coming from the existing nipple crosses a horizontal line coming from a point located 2 cm below the midpoint between the acromonion and the olecranion (Fig. 27-5). Point B is 3, 4, or 5 cm (depending on the amount of the ptosis and of the hypertrophy) above the crossing of the inframammary fold

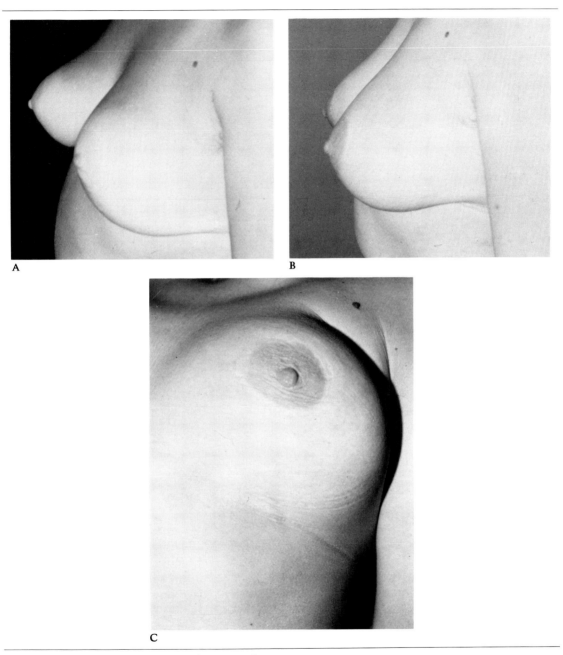

Fig. 27-2. A. A patient 3 years after a reduction with
the Lassus technique (first manner). B. Fifteen years
postoperatively. C. The scar is quite inconspicuous 15
years later.

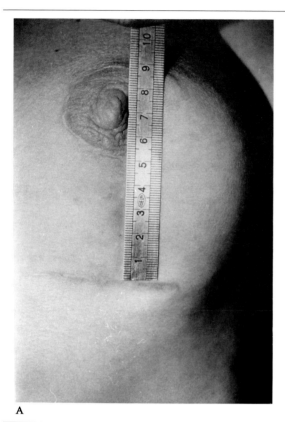

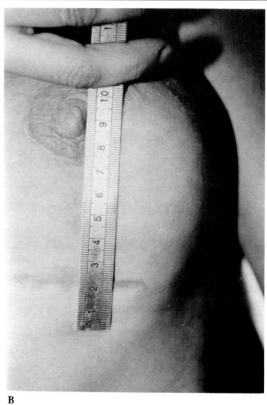

A

B

Fig. 27-3. A. Result of a short horizontal scar technique. The vertical position is 5.5 cm. B. We see that the new inframammary fold is well below the horizontal scar.

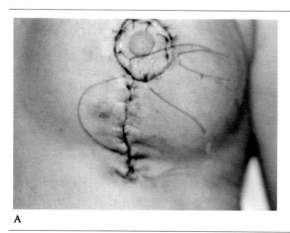

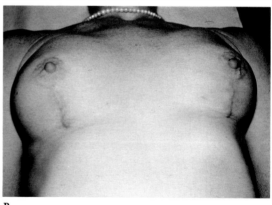

A

B

Fig. 27-4. A. In the immediate postoperative period, the vertical scar looks too long. B. A few weeks later, it fits perfectly.

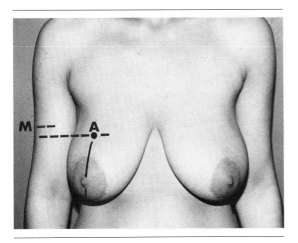

Fig. 27-5. The new nipple position: point A.
(M = midhumerus.)

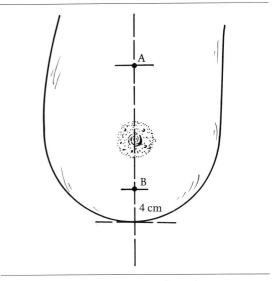

Fig. 27-6. Point B is 3, 4, or 5 cm above the
inframammary fold depending on the amount of ptosis.

with a vertical line coming from the nipple (Fig.
27-6).

2. Between these two points, the area for resection
   is determined by shaping the breasts with one's
   hands (Fig. 27-7). Where the fingers touch each
   other, a point is marked below (Fig. 27-8). After
   the pinch is released, point A is now joined to
   point B with an external and an internal line
   passing through the points marked. The drawing shows approximately the amount of resection to be done (Fig. 27-9). An adjustment is
   generally necessary at the end of the procedure.
3. A superiorly based areolar flap is then fashioned. It must go 5 cm beyond the existing nipple as advocated by Skoog (Fig. 27-10). If the
   distance between point A and the existing nipple is more than 9 cm, a laterally based nipple
   pedicle is created, which contains the sensory
   nerves. This will be demonstrated later.

Before starting the operation, one pinches the
breasts again to check the adequacy of the markings (Fig. 27-11).

OPERATION
The semisitting position is preferred. First, the
markings are incised superficially to avoid their
disappearance from the bleeding during the procedure. A 40-mm circle is incised superficially
around the nipple (Fig. 27-12).
Deepithelialization of the nipple pedicle is then

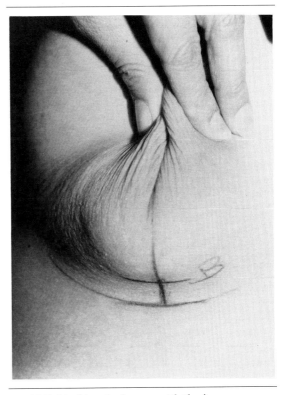

Fig. 27-7. Pinching the breasts with the fingers.

446

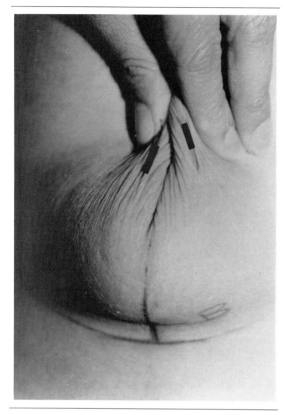

Fig. 27-8. Marking the width of the resection area.

done as usual taking care to avoid leaving epithelium (Fig. 27-13).

The next step is to incise down to the pectoralis fascia along the lateral borders of the resection wedge (Fig. 27-14). The breast is then elevated from the fascia, starting from point B and moving upward a little above point A (Fig. 27-15).

Afterward, the inferior border of the nipple-bearing pedicle is separated from the surrounding skin (Fig. 27-16).

The breast is now resected beneath the flap, leaving a 5-mm glandular lining (Fig. 27-17). The resection can be carried out higher if necessary. It can also be extended more laterally on one or both sides to avoid any excessive bulging in the lateral areas (Fig. 27-18). We therefore are performing an en bloc resection of skin, fat, and gland in the lower portion (Fig. 27-19B) and a resection of fat and gland in the upper portion (Fig. 27-19A).

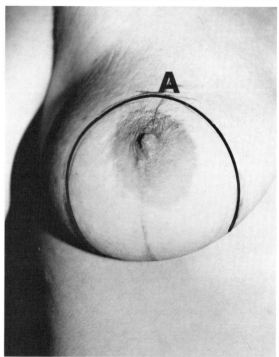

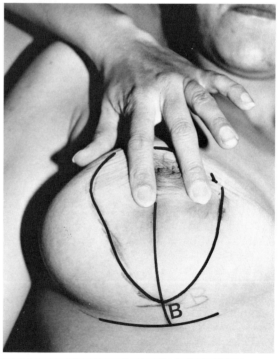

Fig. 27-9. Drawing of the resection area.

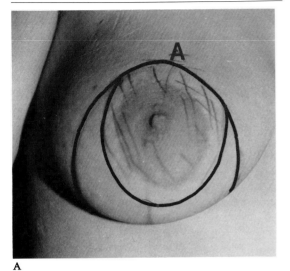

A

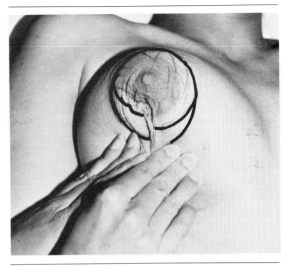

Fig. 27-11. Rechecking adequacy of the drawings.

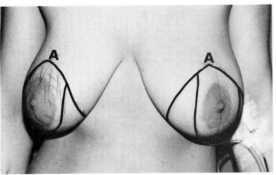

B

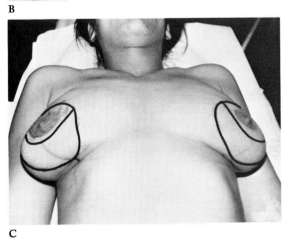

C

Fig. 27-10. A. The superiorly based areolar flap. B. All the drawings are completed. C. The patient supine.

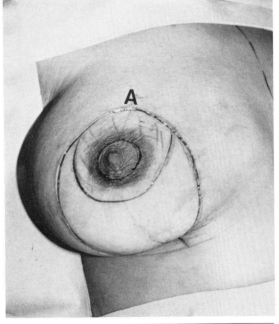

Fig. 27-12. Superficial incision of the drawings.

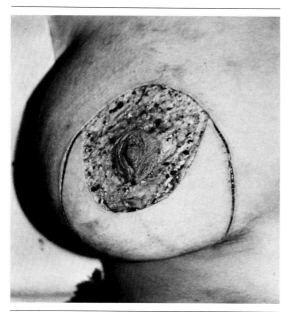

Fig. 27-13. The areolar flap is deepithelialized.

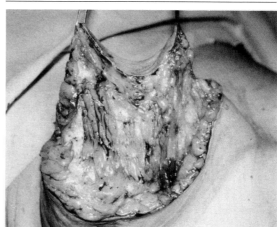

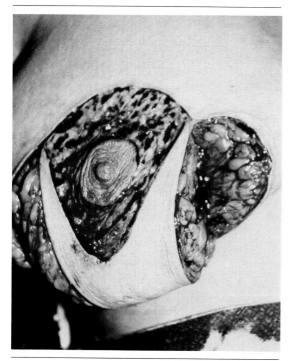

Fig. 27-14. Lateral borders of wedge resection are incised down to the pectoralis fascia.

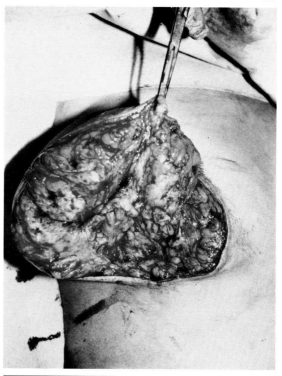

Fig. 27-15. Elevation of the gland from the pectoralis fascia.

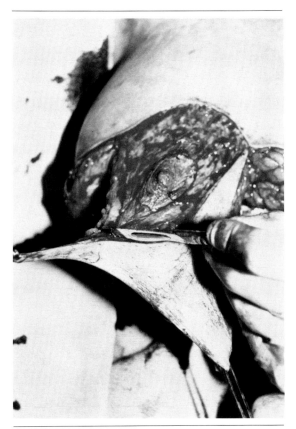

Fig. 27-16. *Inferior border of the nipple pedicle being separated from surrounding skin.*

It is now time for bringing together skin edges with a few temporary interrupted sutures starting from point B and working upward (Fig. 27-20). We can then check the volume and the shape. They are rarely satisfactory at this time. Generally it will be necessary to correct one or both of them. If the resection has been insufficient, after releasing the holding stitches, it will be easy to excise more where it is needed.

After that, skin edges are drawn together again until the desired shape is obtained. Methylene blue is then applied along the new suture line; three or four horizontal lines are drawn on both sides, each of them having a number, the same on the left as on the right (Fig. 27-21). Stitches are then cut and the outline of the new area to be excised appears clearly (Fig. 27-22) and is easily done (Fig. 27-23). The breast is reconstructed uniting 1 to 1, 2 to 2, 3 to 3, and so on.

The operation is completed with subcutaneous stitches and an intradermal running suture (Fig. 27-24).

No drainage is used because no undermining has been done and there is almost no risk of bleeding.

VARIATION

When the distance between point A and the nipple is more than 9 cm (Fig. 27-25), a laterally based areolar pedicle is used (Fig. 27-26).

Then the procedure is done in the same way as before (Fig. 27-27).

Postoperative Care

The patient is discharged the next day. She has to control her temperature. She is told to restrict movements of her arms for 2 weeks. The intradermal running suture is left for 14 days. Steri-Strips are applied for another week after its removal. The shape is rarely satisfactory in the immediate postoperative period (Fig. 27-28). Two months are necessary to get the final shape and volume since the breast will diminish in volume by approximately one fourth during this period.

Results and Indications

This procedure gives the best results in young patients with an elastic skin and a firm glandular breast. For a beginner using this technique, I recommend starting with small hypertrophic ptotic breasts in young patients (Fig. 27-29). When one has become familiar with the method, it is possible to extend the indication to larger breasts (Fig. 27-30 and 27-31), even when more than a 1-kg resection (Figs. 27-32 and 27-33) is necessary.

In older patients (older than 60 years of age), the final result is generally less beautiful because the skin has lost part of its elasticity and because the glandular tissue has been replaced mostly by adipose tissue. We get acceptable results anyway (Fig. 27-34) with a single vertical scar.

Complications

Complications are few and rare. Occasionally secondary procedures are necessary to correct these difficulties. Additional reduction may be necessary if there is an inadequate resection because of either a new desire of the patient or a weight gain. The additional revision is done through the original incisions, and the scar can also be revised.

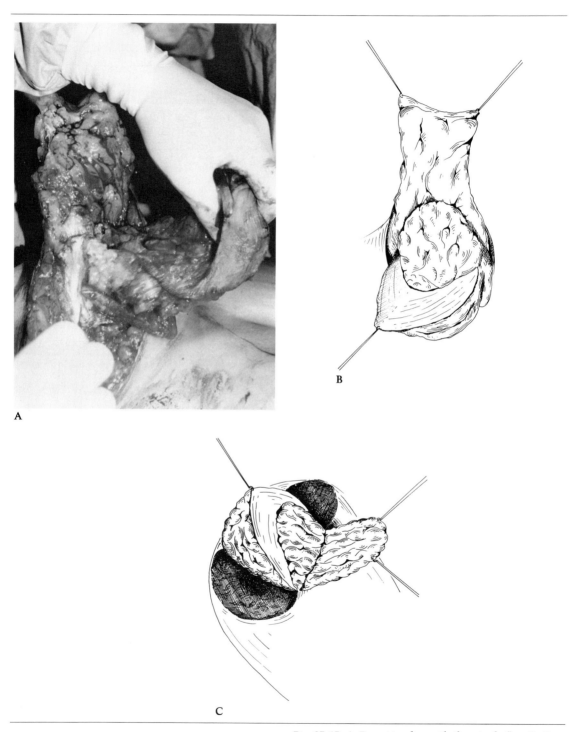

Fig. 27-17. A. Resection beneath the nipple flap. B, C.
The resection.

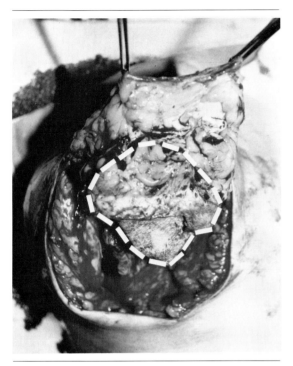

Fig. 27-18. Outlining a new portion of resection.

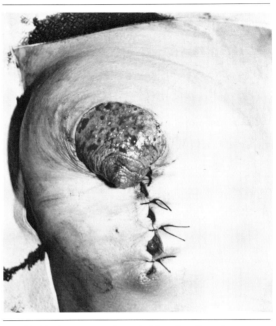

Fig. 27-20. Approximation of skin edges by a few temporary interrupted sutures.

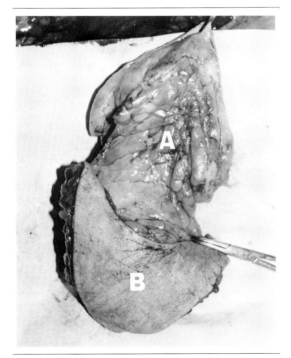

Fig. 27-19. En bloc resection of fat and gland in the upper portion (A) and skin, fat, and gland in the lower portion (B).

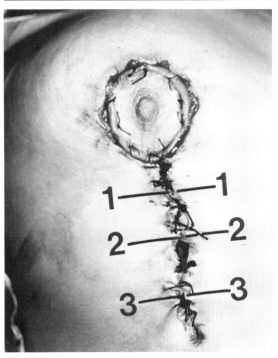

Fig. 27-21. A nice mold has been done with new skin sutures. Methylene blue has been applied on the new suture line. Horizontal lines have also been drawn.

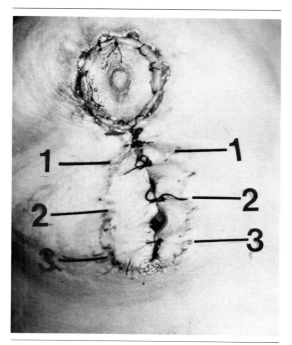

Fig. 27-22. *Drawing of the new resection to be done.*

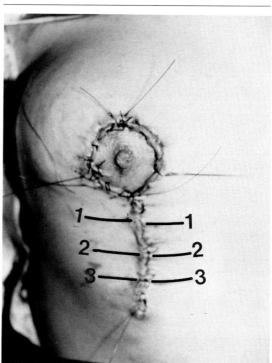

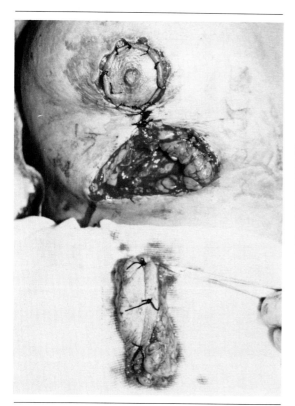

Fig. 27-23. *The new resection is completed.*

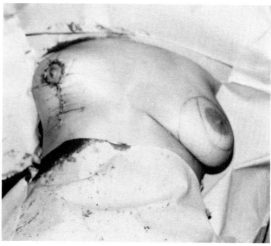

Fig. 27-24. *One side is finished.*

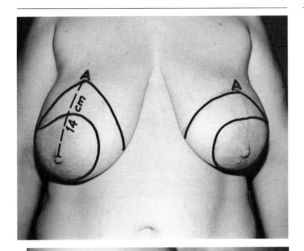

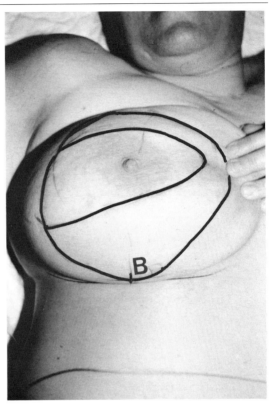

Fig. 27-26. Laterally based nipple flap.

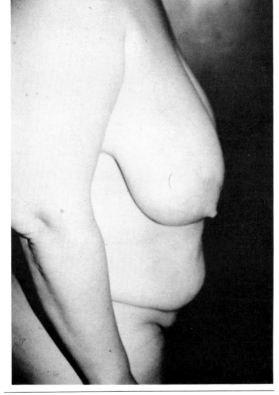

Fig. 27-25. Distance between A and the nipple is 14 cm.

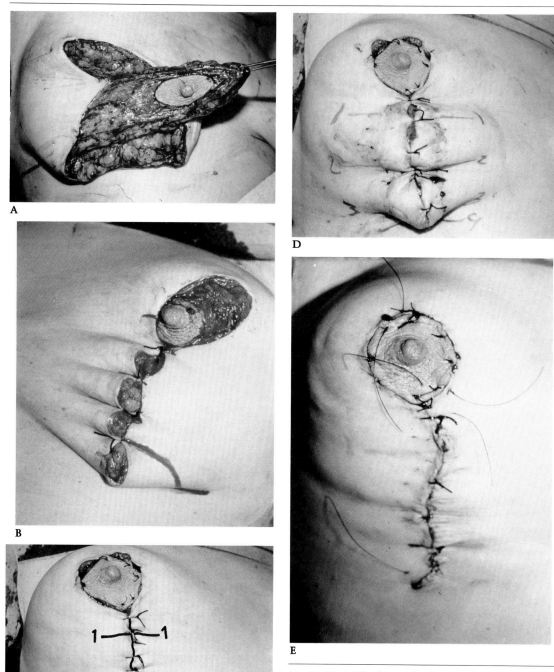

A

B

C

D

E

Fig. 27-27. A. The lateral flap is raised. B. Unsatisfactory mold. C. A new breast cone is shaped according to the trick described. D. New resection to be done. E. End of the operation on one side.

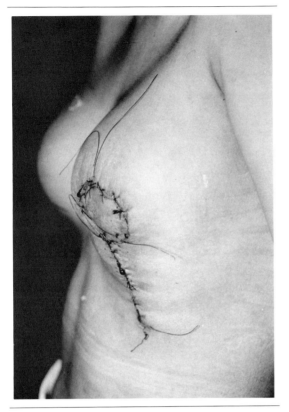

Fig. 27-28. Appearance of the breast 10 days postoperatively. Weight of tissue removed is 140 gm from each breast.

INFECTION

We have never had any case of infection because the most common cause is fat necrosis and, with the resection en bloc of skin, fat, and gland, eliminating any undermining, this complication is avoided.

HEMATOMA

For the same reason, no hematoma has ever occurred in spite of the fact that no drainage is used.

NIPPLE-AREOLA LOSS

Surprisingly we never had a single impending nipple-areola necrosis with the vertical technique. We got some with the short scar procedure. If the nipple-areola complex is blue at the end of the operation, I recommend, as I did several years ago, making holes in the areola with a No. 11 blade to help the veinous drainage. If this is not sufficient, I advocate releasing the areola and leaving it alone for 5 or 6 days; this period of time allows it to

recover nicely. It is then possible to resuture under local anesthesia (Fig. 27-35).

SCARS

Wide and hypertrophic scars are the most common problems seen postoperatively. That is why the patient must be informed precisely in her preoperative visit of the fact that she will have scarring and of the possibility of poor scars, particularly if the candidate already has bad ones. It is my firm opinion that this technique does not produce worse scars than other techniques because skin tension is not greater and because skin resection is not done entirely in the areolar area.

If necessary, scar revisions may be done 1 or 2 years after the initial reduction; generally, a nice improvement can be attained. On the other hand, we can understand why a single vertical scar is preferable in a patient with hypertrophic scars (Fig. 27-36). We may get some improvement with scar revision, but we never can shorten an existing long horizontal scar.

INADEQUATE SHAPE

An improper shape can be improved by additional tightening of the skin and even more glandular resection in the inferior part of the breast. This can be done adequately using the maneuver described in Figure 27-21. The result is shown in Figure 27-37.

SCAR TOO LONG

A scar that is too long may still occur, but this usually occurs only when the surgeon is first learning this technique. It is always easy to eliminate the excess length of the scar with a triangular skin resection performed either at the time of the operation (Fig. 27-38) or a few months later. In fact, sometimes on the table, the scar looks too long, but after a few weeks, it corrects itself (see Fig. 27-4).

In conclusion, with this procedure, complications are rare and results are satisfactory. But because of the lack of exact accurate preoperative planning, it is more difficult to avoid the problems of asymmetry and inadequate shape after a breast reduction. However, with the patient in a sitting position and the surgeon using the steps I have recommended in Figure 27-21, the results of this à la carte operation can be gratifying to both the patient and the surgeon.

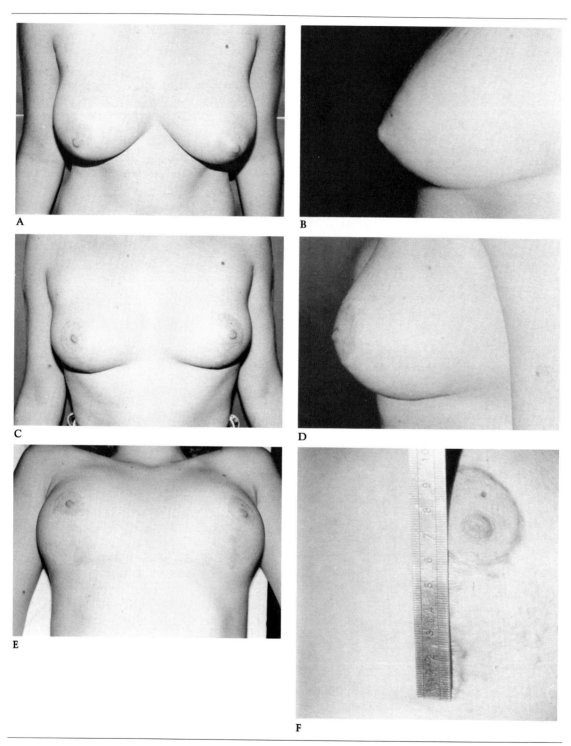

Fig. 27-29. A, B. Before. C–E. After 1½ years. F. The
length of the scar is 6 cm. Weight of tissue removed is
300 gm from each breast.

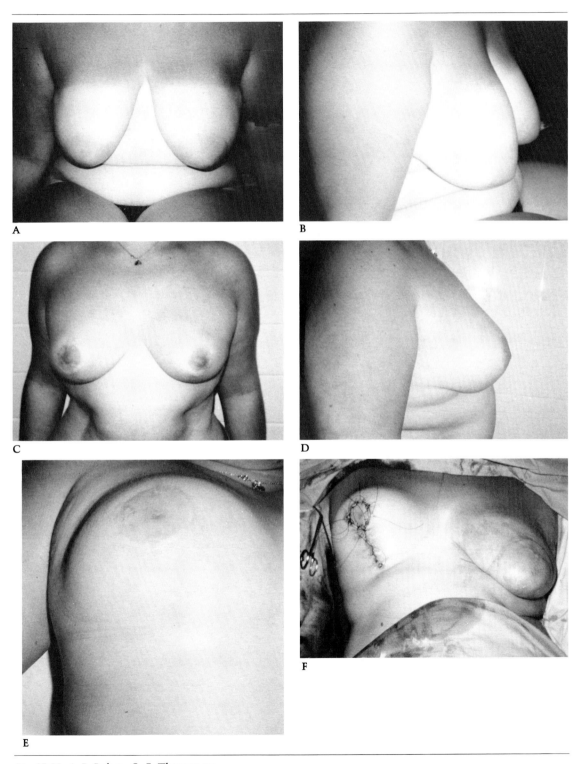

Fig. 27-30. A, B. Before. C–E. Three years
postoperatively. F. On the operating table. Weight of
tissue removed is 350 gm from each breast.

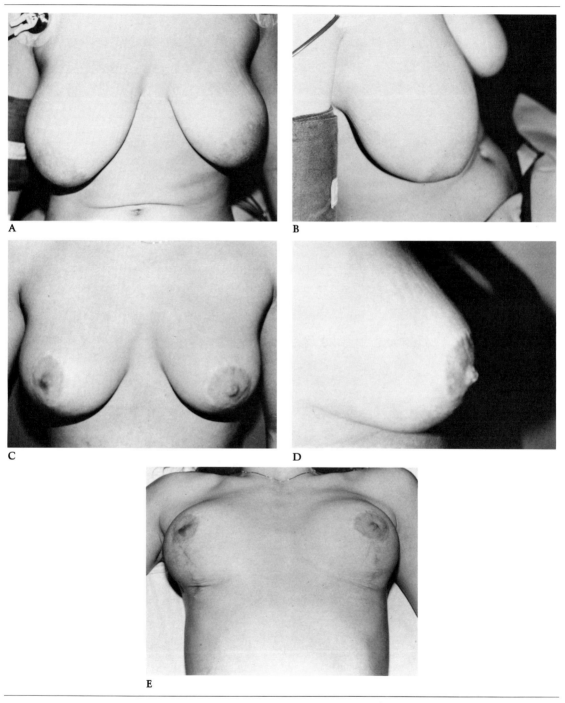

Fig. 27-31. *A, B. Before. C–E. After. Weight of tissue removed is 500 gm from each breast.*

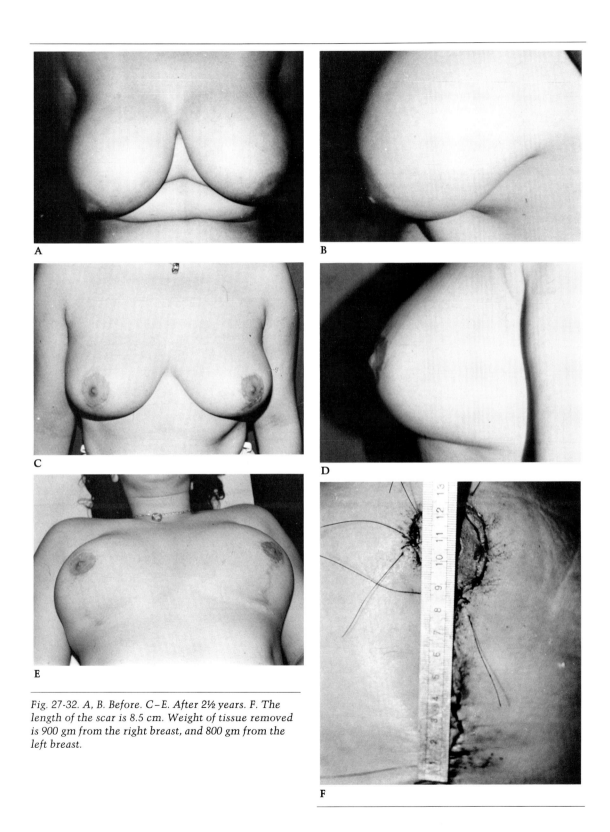

Fig. 27-32. A, B. Before. C–E. After 2½ years. F. The length of the scar is 8.5 cm. Weight of tissue removed is 900 gm from the right breast, and 800 gm from the left breast.

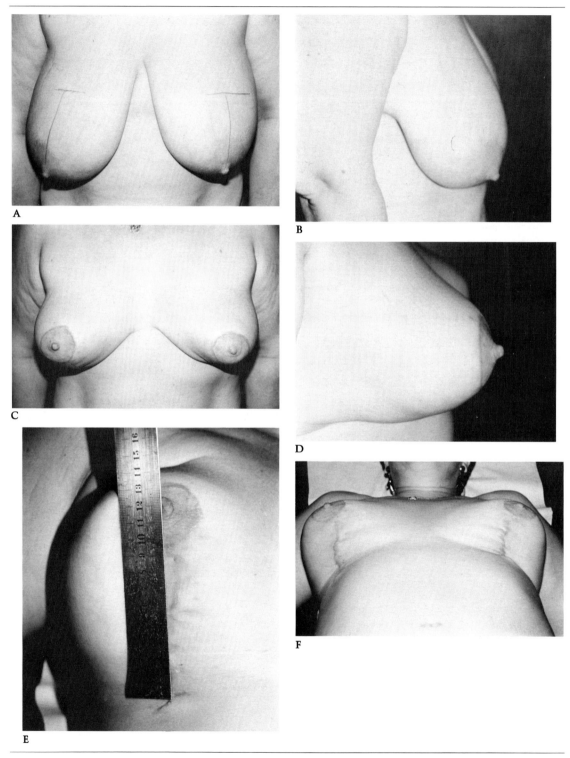

Fig. 27-33. A, B. Before. C, D, F. After. E. The length of the scar. Weight of tissue removed is 650 gm from the right breast, and 550 gm from the left breast.

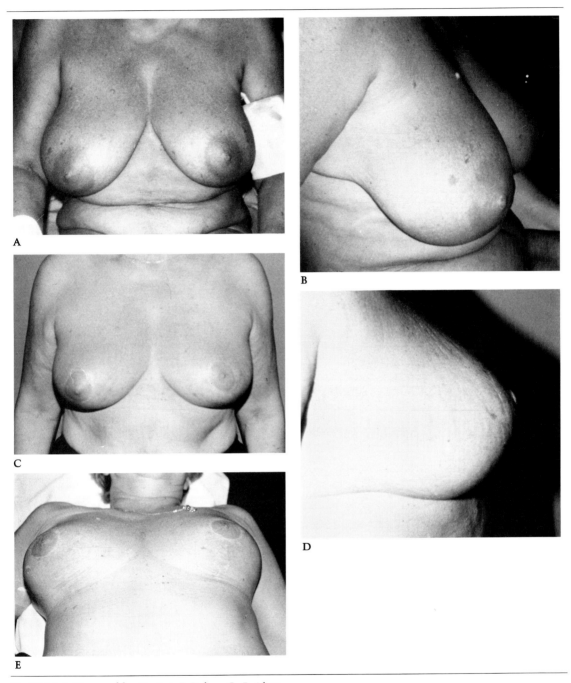

Fig. 27-34. A 68-year-old patient. A, B. Before. C–E. After.

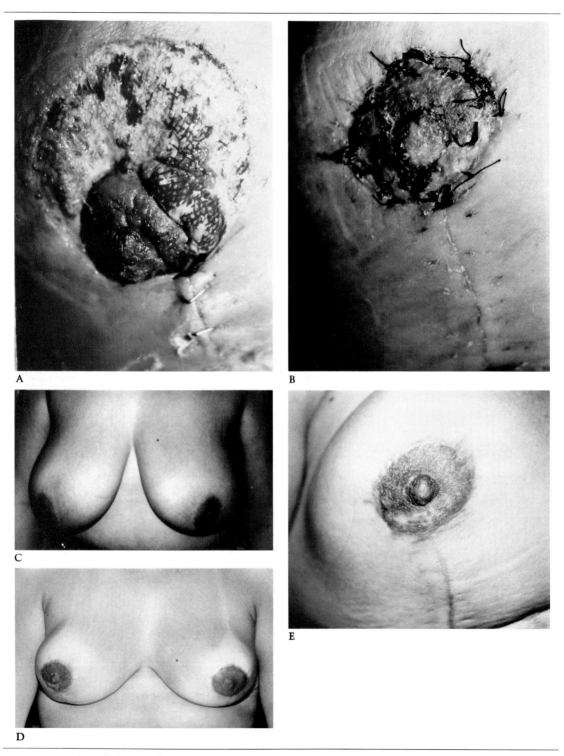

Fig. 27-35. A. The suffering areola has been released. B.
Six days after, it is resutured. C. Before. D. One year
postoperatively. E. On a close view, we can notice a
light discoloration of the inferior part of the areola.
Weight of tissue removed is 500 gm from the right
breast, and 420 gm from the left breast.

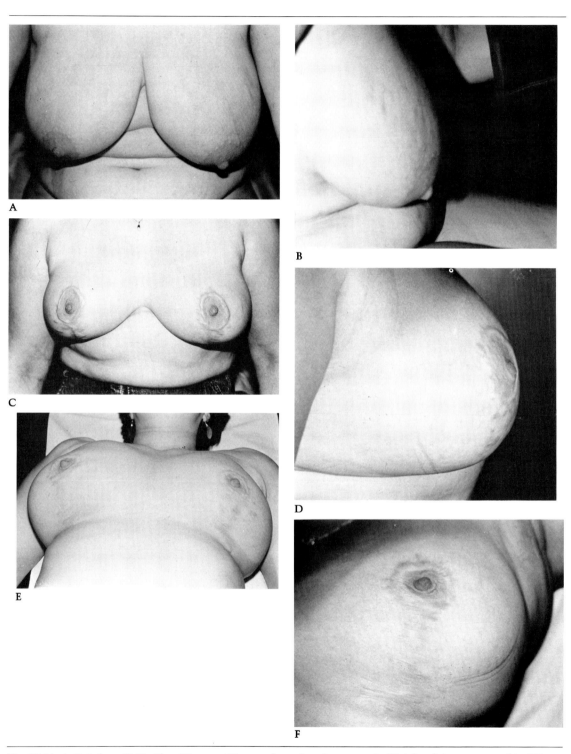

Fig. 27-36. A, B. Before. C, D. After 2½ years. The result is impaired by the hypertrophic scar. E, F. Appearance of the scar at that time. Such a single vertical scar is already too much. Weight of tissue removed is 450 gm from each breast.

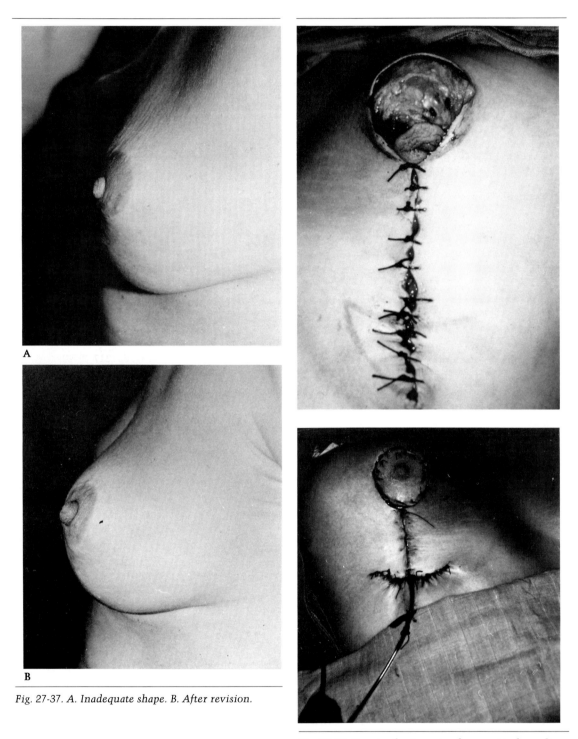

Fig. 27-37. A. Inadequate shape. B. After revision.

Fig. 27-38. How to shorten a too long vertical scar by
the addition of a short horizontal one.

Selected Readings

Arié, G. Una nueva tecnica de mastoplastica. *Rev. Latin-oam. Chir. Plast.* 3:23, 1957.

Aubert, V. Hypertrophie mammaire de la puberté. Résection Partielle Restauratrice. *Arch. Franco-Belges de Chir.* 3:284, 1923.

Balch, C.R. The central mound technique for reduction mammaplasty. *Plast. Reconstr. Surg.* 67:305, 1981.

Bostwick, J., III. *Aesthetic and Reconstructive Breast Surgery.* St. Louis: Mosby, 1983.

Courtiss, E.H., and Goldwyn, R.M. Reduction mammoplasty by the inferior pedicle technique and alternative to free nipple and areola grafting for severe macromastia or exterme ptosis. *Plast. Reconstr. Surg.* 59:507, 1979.

Durston, W. Sudden and excessive swelling of a women's breast. Philos. Transactions of the Royal Society of London IV:1069, 1670.

Georgiade, N.G., and Georgiade, G.S. Hypermastia and Ptosis. In N.G. Georgiade et al (eds.), *Essentials of Plastic, Maxillofacial and Reconstructive Surgery.* Baltimore: Williams & Wilkins, 1987. P. 694.

Georgiade, N.G., Georgiade, G.S., Riefkohl, R., and Barwick, W.J. (eds.), *Essentials of Plastic, Maxillofacial and Reconstructive Surgery.* Baltimore: Williams & Wilkins, 1987.

Georgiade, N.G., Serafin, D., Riefkohl, R., and Georgiade, G.S. Is there a reduction mammoplasty for "all seasons"? *Plast. Reconstr. Surg.* 63:765, 1979.

Goldwyn, R.M. (ed.). *Plastic and Reconstructive Surgery of the Breast.* Boston: Little, Brown, 1976.

Hallock, G.G., and Cusenz, B.J. Salvage of the congested nipple during reduction mammoplasty. *Aesth. Plast. Surg.* 10:143, 1986.

Hauben, D.J. Experience and refinements with the supero-medial dermal pedicle for nipple areolar transposition in reduction mammoplasty. *Aesth. Plast. Surg.* 8:189, 1984.

Hester, T.R., Jr., Bostwick, J., Miller, L., and Cunningham, S.J. Breast reduction utilizing the maximally vascularized central breast pedicle. *Plast. Reconstr. Surg.* 76:890, 1985.

Hoffman, S. Recurrent deformities following reduction mammaplasty and correction of breast asymmetry. *Plast. Reconstr. Surg.* 78:55, 1986.

Hollander, E. Die operation der mammahypertrophie und der Hängebrust. *Munchen Med Wochnschr.* 70:672, 1923.

Lassus, C. A technique for breast reduction. *Int. Surg.* 53:69, 1970.

Lassus, C. New refinements in vertical mammaplasty. Presented at the 2nd Congress of the Asian Section of International Plastic Reconstructive Surgery. Tokyo, 1977.

Lassus, C. Minimal scarring in mammaplasty. 9 Tag. Ver. Deutsch Plast. Chir. Cologne, 1978.

Lassus, C. New refinements in vertical mammaplasty. *Chir. Plast.* 6:81, 1981.

Lassus, C. Treatment of impending nipple necrosis — a technical note. *Chir. Plast.* 8:117, 1985.

Lassus, C. An "all season" mammaplasty. *Aesth. Plast. Surg.* 10:9, 1986.

Lassus, C. Breast reduction: Evolution of a technique — a single vertical scar. *Aesth. Plast. Surg.* II:107, 1987.

Marchac, D., and Olarte, G. Reduction mammoplasty and correction of ptosis with a short inframammary scar. *Plast. Reconstr. Surg.* 69:45, 1982.

Mathes, S.J., Nahai, F., and Hester, T.R. Avoiding the flat breast in reduction mammaplasty. *Plast. Reconstr. Surg.* 66:63, 1980.

Mornard, P. La mastopexie esthétique du prolapsus mammaire par le procédé de la transposition du mamelon. *Presse - Mod.* 33:317, 1925.

Moufarrege, R., et al. Reduction mammoplasty by the total dermoglandular pedicle. *Aesth. Plast. Surg.* 9:227, 1985.

Peixoto, G. Reduction mammaplasty: A personal technique. *Plast. Reconstr. Surg.* 65:217, 1980.

Peixoto, G. The infraareolar longitudinal incision in reduction mammoplasty. *Aesth. Plast. Surg.* 9:1, 1985.

Pitanguy, I. *Breast Hypertrophy.* Transactions of the Second International Congress of Plastic and Reconstructive Surgery. London: Livingstone, 1959. P. 509.

Regnault, P. Breast reduction B technique. *Plast. Reconstr. Surg.* 65:840, 1980.

Schwartzmann, E. Uber eine neue Methode der Mammoplastic. *Wien. Med. Wochnschr.* 51:1103, 1925.

Schwartzmann, E. Die technik der Mammoplastic. *Chirurgie* 2:962, 1930.

Skoog, T. A technique of breast reduction. *Acta Chir. Scand.* 126:453, 1963.

Strömbeck, J.O. Mammaplasty: Report of a new technique based on the two-pedicle procedure. *Br. J. Plast. Surg.* 13:79, 1960.

Strömbeck, J.O. Reduction mammoplasty: Some observations, some reflections. *Aesth. Plast. Surg.* 7:249, 1983.

COMMENTS ON CHAPTER 27 *Robert M. Goldwyn*

Lassus has recounted his 30-year experience with minimal scar methods for reduction mammaplasty. It is obvious that the search for the Holy Grail procedure is an arduous one. Although Arié [1] advanced reduction mammaplasty by his technique, which involved inferior wedge resection, a superiorly based nipple-areola flap, and a vertical scar, this procedure was not well suited for extremely large breasts. In those instances, the scar extended visibly onto the chest. Pitanguy [5], as Lassus relates, modified Arié's method with a short horizontal incision that eliminated the objectionable scar below the inframammary fold. Lassus, however, wanted a technique that could reduce "huge" breasts and leave the patient only a vertical scar in addition to the perioareolar scar. This can be done; however, it is not easily done, which is evident from Figures 27-20 through 27-24 and Figure 27-27B, C, and E. This *all season*, to use his term, mammaplasty embodied, as was also stated, the ideas of Hollander [3] and Elbaz [2] of a short scar, the concept of Arié of a vertical scar, and the principals of Skoog [6] for transposition of the areola by a pedicle superiorly based flap and en bloc resection of skin, fat, and gland. The excess tissue that would be removed in other procedures with a T-shaped incision (horizontal scar) is taken away, as it is in almost every other short scar procedure, by resecting more tissue around the nipple-areola and the vertical incision. After having done all this, a horizontal scar with the Lassus procedure may still be necessary, although it will likely not be long.

In a fairly recent article, Lassus [4] stated that his technique "can solve the many different types of breast deformities," which he classifies as follows:

Class 1. Small breast plus mild degree of ptosis. Usually a single vertical scar, or at most a short horizontal one, is all that is left . . .

Class 2. Normal volume plus moderate ptosis. A single vertical scar is all that is necessary but it may be easier to add a short horizontal scar.

Class 3. Normal volume or moderate hypertrophy plus severe ptosis. Once again a vertical scar and a short horizontal one result from surgery but it is more difficult in these cases to keep the scarring above the brassiere line.

Class 4. Average hypertrophy plus moderate ptosis. Once again the vertical scar and a short horizontal one are left.

Class 5. Massive hypertrophy and severe ptosis. A vertical scar and a short horizontal scar result.

Class 6. Gigantomasty. A vertical scar plus an acceptable horizontal one. . . .

Therefore, even for Lassus, for most categories except class 1 (small breast plus mild degree of ptosis) it is possible to end up *easily* without any kind of horizontal scar. In the other situations, a short horizontal scar is helpful (classes 2 and 3) or necessary (classes 4, 5, and 6).

Without obviously having the vast experience of Lassus, I tried his technique on a few occasions and found it completely satisfactory with all the advantages he states for what he has described as classes 1 and 2. For a patient in class 4, it is more difficult for me to avoid a moderately long horizontal scar, and for class 5, my horizontal scar was only slightly shorter than it would have been had I used the inferior pedicle technique. I am sure that Lassus would have done much better on each of those occasions.

Again, the personal question for the reader is how much he or she will do operatively to avoid the horizontal scar. In reality, it is not so much the existence of that scar that is objectionable but its length and, in that regard, especially the segments that extend medially and laterally beyond the confines of the breast, where, in younger patients, their visibility is always displeasing and, if hypertrophic, the appearance is deforming. Therefore for younger patients, whose breasts fall into what Lassus has called class 1, 2, or 3, his short scar procedure or one of the many others described elsewhere in this book should be considered and possibly done. However, for patients who have massive hypertrophy (class 5) or actual gigantomastia (class 6), these procedures that attempt to reduce or eliminate the horizontal scar are difficult for most of us who are used to techniques where the horizontal scar is intrinsic, such as the inferior pedicle method, the Skoog procedure, and the McKissock technique.

The lesson to be learned perhaps not only from this chapter but from the entire book is that the surgeon must be flexible in treating a patient for breast hypertrophy and should tailor the procedure to the patient and not the patient to the procedure because the surgeon has only one technique in his or her repertoire.

REFERENCES

1. Arié, G. Una nueva tecnica de mastoplastia. *Rev. Latinoam. Cir. Plast.* 3:23, 1957.
2. Elbaz, J.S. Traitement des hypertrophies mammaires avec ou sans ptose avec la methode dite "oblique externe." A propus de 114 cas operes. Paris: These Med, 1963, P. 546.
3. Hollander, E. Die Operetion der mammahypertrophie und der Hängebrust. *Dtsch. Med. Wochenschr.* 50:400, 1924.
4. Lassus, C. An "all-season mammoplasty." *Aesth. Plast. Surg.* 10:9, 1986.
5. Pitanguy, I. *Breast Hypertrophy.* Transactions of the Second International Congress of Plastic and Reconstructive Surgery. London, 1960. Edinburgh: Livingstone, 1960. Pp. 509–522.
6. Skoog, T. A technique of breast reduction. *Acta. Chir. Scand.* 126:453, 1963.

28

Gaston-François Maillard

A Z-Mammaplasty with Minimal Scarring

In this chapter, I describe an improved technique for reduction mammaplasty that has the advantage of giving a satisfactory final shape to the breast while producing a minimal scar. The method involves periareolar deepithelialization with displacement of the nipple-areola complex, partial subcutaneous mastectomy at the base of the mammary cone, and a Z-plasty to interlock two triangles of skin left after the removal of a little excess skin in the region above the inframammary fold. The Z-plasty adds skin vertically to the inferior pole, resulting in a better final shape and reducing tension around the areola. Any further excess skin is left to retract spontaneously.

The best indication for this operation is in young women with elastic skin free of striae "gravidarum." Our experience now covers 115 patients aged 14 to 30 years with reductions of up to 900 gm per breast, and we have encountered no major complications over a 6-year follow-up period.

With classic techniques of reduction mammaplasty like those of McKissock [9] Skoog [16], or Strömbeck [17], the reduced breast has a satisfactory shape but bears a large scar along the entire inframammary fold. This may be the method of choice for middle-aged women, but problems can arise with younger patients, such as teenagers, because they may develop serious hypertrophic scarring, and we are confronted more and more with very early mammaplasty. It is very sad to see gross hypertrophic scarring after an apparently satisfactory "classic" operation. Young breasts tend to be less pliable than older ones, and the rigidity of the tissues of the flap bearing the nipple-areola complex sometimes renders the procedure hazardous.

The first successful attempt to create a new concept of mammary reduction was by Peixoto [12, 13]. He converted a large pyramid into a smaller one by removing its base, claiming that the final aspect of the operated breast was mainly due to the shape and amount of the remaining glandular adipose tissue. This was perhaps the first time that it was stressed that the skin could be allowed to retract spontaneously. Another important point is that the glandular function is preserved. Marchac [8] published the next step in the same direction with a mammaplasty involving a short transverse scar. To minimize the transverse scar, the excess skin is resected along a vertical axis, but the lower margin of the excision remains 4 to 5 cm above the inframammary fold. This allows the skin of the lower part of the breast to be converted into thoracic-wall skin. These two techniques were important steps in the difficult search for a "perfect" reduction mammaplasty. It is attractive to use the inherent elasticity of the skin to reduce the scar on the inferior aspect of the new breast. It also seems logical to remove the base of the cone and avoid cutting the lactiferous ducts just below the nipple-areola complex. The technique is really an adaptation of a partial subcutaneous mastectomy, leaving only what is necessary to give a good residual volume.

Arié [1] described the first useful technique with a single vertical scar, but since the scar often extended beyond the inframammary fold, this technique did not gain wide acceptance, except for small ptotic breasts. The oblique method of Dufourmentel and Mouly [2] utilizes practically the same principle of a single "pinch," but it is restricted to the lateral quadrant. To diminish the

Substantial portions of this chapter and all figures are reproduced with permission from G.F. Maillard. A Z-mammaplasty with minimal scarring. *Plast. Reconstr. Surg.* 77:66, 1986.

encroachment of the scar onto the thoracic wall, Elbaz and Verheecke [3] and Meyer and Kesselring [10] made the scar L-shaped, using a "dog-ear" resection. The same effect is achieved, but in a more sophisticated way, in the B technique of Regnault [14]. We described a form of Z-plasty [7] developed from the oblique techniques like those previously mentioned but that offers certain advantages (in our book *Plastic and Reconstructive Breast Surgery*).

One problem is the vertical displacement of the nipple-areola complex; it can be accomplished by means of a periareolar Schwarzmann deepithelialization procedure [15]. Unfortunately, even if one avoids a too long transverse scar in the inframammary fold in these original techniques, one cannot avoid too much tension around the areola, also a problem in the dermal vault technique of Lalardrie and Jouglard [5].

Advantage can be taken of the skin elasticity in young patients prior to the development of striae gravidarum. If one compares the hypertrophic breast of a teenager and a middle-aged woman lying down, one can see that in the former, the nipple-areola complex moves upward, whereas the breast that has lost its elasticity stays laterally on the thoracic wall and the distance from the sternal notch to the nipple-areola complex stays about the same as in the upright position. In addition, younger patients tend to have been less exposed to vascular damage owing to smoking, so that careful, limited dermoglandular dissection will be relatively free of risk.

When reviewing a first series of pure Peixoto [12] and Marchac [8] or mixed procedures (42 breasts), we were faced with enlarged scars or even distortion and secondary enlargement of the nipple-areola complex. One other point of dissatisfaction was the flatness of the breast owing to incomplete narrowing of the base of the cone. Many reduced breasts ended with a too short nipple-areola complex–inframammary fold distance, and the breast mound looked as though it was partially amputated at its inferior pole.

We now propose the addition of a small Z-plasty at the inferior pole of the breast to a combination of the two aforementioned methods for the following reasons:

1. By interlocking the two triangular flaps of a Z-plasty, we add more skin vertically in the area of the inferior pole, resulting in a better shape (*le Galbe* in French).

2. The upper triangle acts like the diaphragm of a camera, reducing the tension around the inferior part of the areola and avoiding, at least partially, a secondary widening of the scars and of the nipple-areola complex.

3. The lower triangle provides some transverse tension to help reduce the width of the base of the cone and fix the inframammary fold, thus avoiding any tendency for a secondary downward luxation of the inferior pole.

4. The Z-plasty is in essence a plastic procedure with wide application. In our method, it is used as a rotation advancement, similar to that used by Millard [11] in his cleft lip closure.

Technique

With the patient standing, the vertical axis of the breast is drawn, joining the midclavicular point to the nipple (Figs. 28-1 and 28-2). By gently displacing the breast laterally and then medially, an "arched gateway" [7] is drawn, as in Marchac's procedure [8], but the amount of deepithelialization can also be estimated by gently pinching the skin, as suggested by Peixoto [13] (Fig. 28-1). The base of the arched gateway is drawn about 5 cm above the inframammary fold, and its length is 5 cm on the unstretched skin. Then two oblique lines are drawn to join the periareolar deepithelialization. Thus, the skin to be removed at the inferior pole forms an isosceles triangle pointing upward (see Figs. 28-1 and 28-2). Laterally and medially are two other triangles that will be used for the Z-plasty at the end of the operation.

The breast is hooked firmly up and a tourniquet is applied at its base (Fig. 28-3) to facilitate the Schwarzmann procedure [15]. Then the skin to be removed is incised together with the underlying subcutaneous tissue until the glandular substance is reached. Traction is exerted on the base of this triangle by two strong Lahey clamps. At this stage, a wide subcutaneous dissection is performed at the level of the ligaments of Cooper up to the 3 and 9 o'clock positions (Fig. 28-4). Pulling the two clamps upward permits a downward subcutaneous dissection reaching and widely undermining the inframammary fold (Fig. 28-5). After the first purely subcutaneous dissection, a complete undermining of the retromammary space is performed, first by sharp and then by blunt dissection. It is important to preserve as many perforating branches of the internal mammary ar-

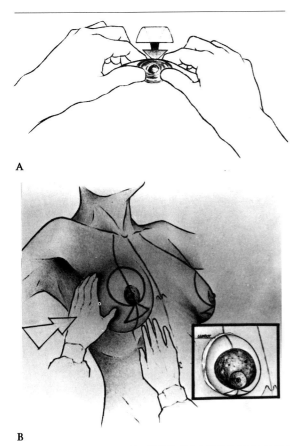

A

B

Fig. 28-1 A. A periareolar deepithelialization is estimated on the vertical axis of the breast by gently pinching the skin (Peixoto 5). B. A 5 × 5 cm isosceles triangle is drawn, the base of which is 5 cm above the mammary fold.

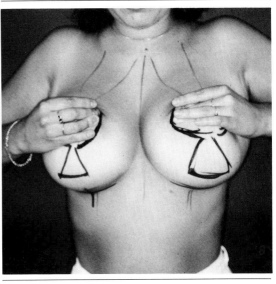

Fig. 28-2. An ideal candidate for the Z-plasty technique: a 20-year-old patient with firm skin and mammary tissue and no striae. The triangles are marked below the round periareolar deepithelialization area.

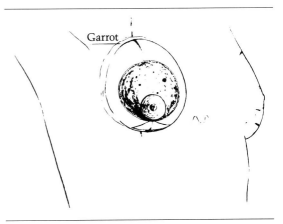

Fig. 28-3. A tourniquet (garrot) is applied to the base of the breast to facilitate the deepithelialization.

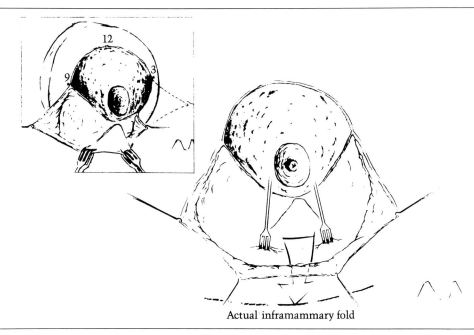

Actual inframammary fold

Fig. 28-4. A wide subcutaneous dissection is performed at the deepest level of the ligaments of Cooper as far as the 3 and 9 o'clock positions. By pulling upward on two clamps fixed to the isosceles triangle, the dissection is extended to the inframammary fold, which is widely undermined. Beginning with an initial purely subcutaneous approach, the retromammary space is finally completely dissected.

tery as possible.* The tourniquet is then removed.

The breast is again pulled up by a skin hook so that the glandular reduction can be performed horizontally at the base of the cone, if possible in one piece, and the weight determined. The operative specimen resembles that from a subcutaneous mastectomy with a small triangle of skin attached to its inferior pole. It has the shape of a disk, of which the thickness depends on the amount of resection (Fig. 28-6). The hook is removed and the remaining volume estimated visually and by palpation. At this stage, the breast looks somewhat flat, so we follow the technique of Marchac [8] and place a single suture between the gland, just above the areola, and the pectoralis fascia in the infraclavicular region (Fig. 28-7). This produces a fullness in the upper quadrant. After hooking up the breast again, the lateral and medial glandular remnants are gently approximated to reconstruct the infe-

rior pole. The hook is removed, and a first key stitch is placed to move the areola to the top of the denuded area. Excess skin is left to allow for retraction by its natural elasticity. If this does not occur satisfactorily, one must attempt a better defatting of the skin, but without endangering its vascularization. A perfect atraumatic dissection using only scalpel, scissors, and skin hooks is essential. Next, the two skin triangles are interlocked horizontally in the form of a Z-plasty (Fig. 28-8). First, the lateral triangle is sutured down into the new inframammary fold; this exerts some horizontal tension and helps to narrow the base of the cone. Then the medial triangle is gently pulled to produce a rotation-advancement and diminish the tension around the areola like the diaphragm of a camera (Fig. 28-8). Clinical judgment and estimation of skin viability are essential at this stage, bearing in mind that, as Gillies and Millard [4] emphasized, beauty is a constant battle between vascularization and necrosis. This exchange of the two triangles adds tissue vertically and gives a better shape to the inferior pole (Fig. 28-9).

The mammary gland is a purely cutaneous appendage like other exocrine or apocrine glands. By

---

* Now, we carefully use blunt dissection along the lateral border of the pectoralis muscle to preserve the fourth, fifth, and sixth intercostal nerve branches to the nipple-areola complex for better sensibility.

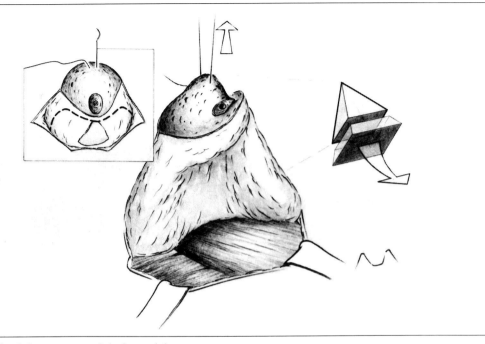

Fig. 28-5. Glandular resection of the base of the
mammary cone using Peixoto's method that converts a
large pyramid into a small one.

respecting most of the medial perforating
branches of the internal mammary artery and part
of the vascularization of the external mammary
artery, there is little risk of ischemia if the surgery
is performed correctly. Skin sutures present few
problems because of the shortness of the scars. Because very little skin is removed, there is no tension on the inframammary Z-shaped scars. We
have encountered only a few rare cases of periareolar tension, depending on the degree of reduction and the width of the deepithelialization. Now
we increase the *diameter* of the areola up to *50 or
52 mm** to diminish this tension. Inverted dermal
sutures are inserted first and then completed by a
continuous subcuticular suture and Steri-Strips. A
suitable self-adhesive dressing that is, however,
not stuck to the skin is fashioned and changed
every week for 4 to 6 weeks. This is an important
technical detail to help skin retraction around the
smaller breast cone and the thorax itself. Suction
drainage is utilized for 2 days. In other words, the

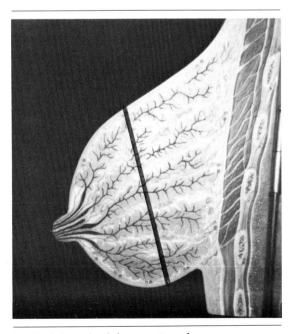

Fig. 28-6. The glandular resection plane.

*New finding.

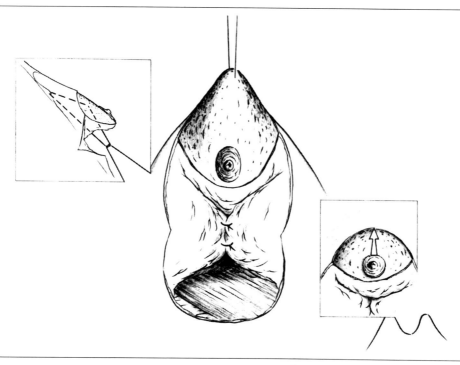

Fig. 28-7. Placing a single suture between the gland just above the areola and the pectoralis fascia in the infraclavicular region produces a fullness in the upper quadrant.

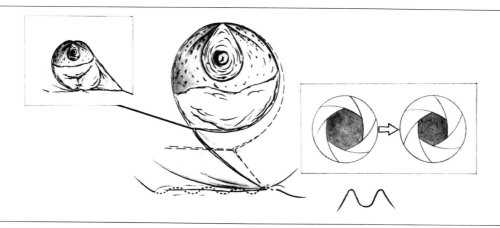

Fig. 28-8. After moving the areola up, the two triangles are interlocked horizontally in the form of a Z-plasty. First, the lateral triangle is sutured into the new inframammary fold; then the medial one is gently advanced and rotated to diminish the tension around the areola, like the diaphragm of a camera.

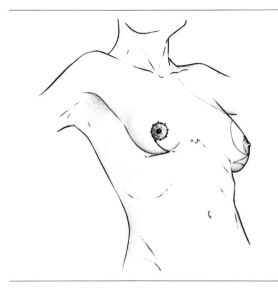

Fig. 28-9. Result at the end of the procedure.

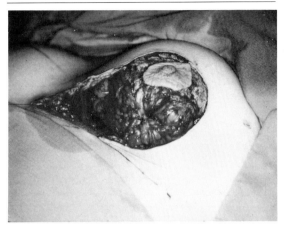

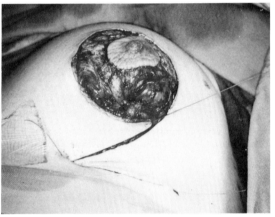

Fig. 28-10. The interlocking of the two Z-plasty triangles at operation, demonstrating the minimal tension on the skin because practically no skin is resected.

principal work is performed on the gland itself; there is very little skin suturing, but a good immobilization dressing is very important.

Indications

Although technically not easy, the method is a great challenge in the quest to avoid long scars on the young thorax and breast. The best indications are in young women, under 30 years of age, with good, thick, elastic skin. Patients with striae gravidarum, indicating the rupture of elastic fibers, are no longer candidates for this surgery. An interesting but rare indication is the adjustment of the healthy side contralateral to a Poland syndrome reconstruction. It can also be attempted to adapt the breast opposite a postmastectomy reconstruction, providing that the breast fulfills the requirements of good elasticity of the skin and firmness of the gland. One other indication is a ptotic change after pregnancy with glandular atrophy but with a good thick skin.

Results

We have used this new technique on about 200 breasts in 115 patients aged 14 to 40 years, with an average age of 28 years, over a period of 7 years (Figs. 28-10 through 28-15). The first candidates were chosen for moderate hypertrophy, with 300-gm reductions on each side. These are the best indications, with uniformly good results and shape. More recently, we have extended the procedure up to 900 gm per breast, but it is more difficult and the periareolar subcuticular suture often results in some temporary wrinkles that disappear with time (Figs. 28-16 through 28-21).

No hematomas or skin sloughs were encountered. Three early patients required secondary revision of the defatting below the site of the new inframammary fold, all done under local anesthesia. In cases of large glandular resection, more than 600 gm on each side, we noticed some enlarge-

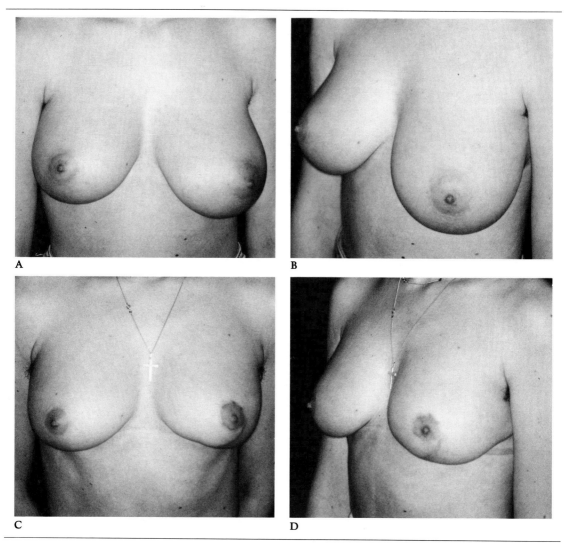

A

B

C

D

Fig. 28-11. Young patient with unilateral hypertrophy before (A and B) and 6 months after (C and D) reduction to show the minimal Z-shaped scar.

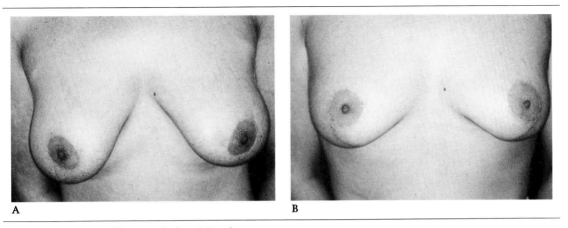

Fig. 28-12. A 20-year-old patient before (A) and 1 year
after (B) a 250-gm resection on each side. Note the
natural-looking breast with minimal scarring.

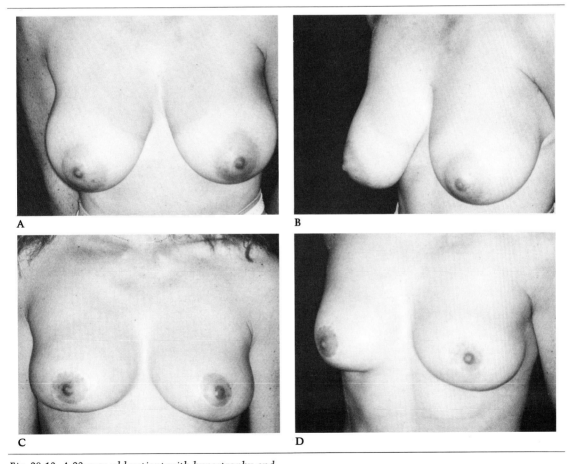

Fig. 28-13. A 23-year-old patient with hypertrophy and
ptosis before (A and B) and 13 months after (C and D) a
300-gm reduction on each side.

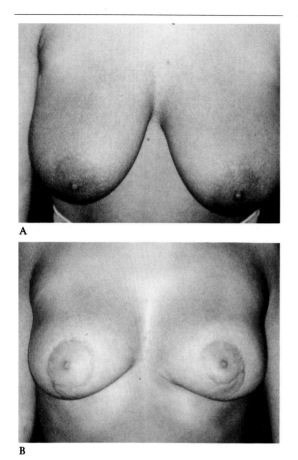

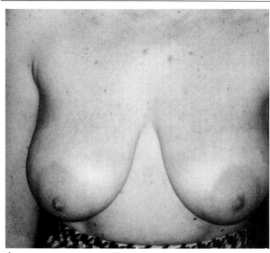

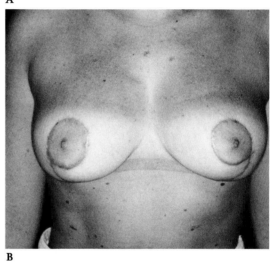

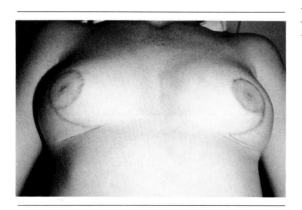

Fig. 28-14. *A 19-year-old patient with hypertrophy before (A) and 3 years after (B) a 350-gm reduction on each side.*

Fig. 28-16. *A 20-year-old patient, with virginal hypertrophy (A) and one year after (B) a 500-mg reduction on each side.*

Fig. 28-15. *Same patient as in Figure 28-14 to show the minimal Z-shaped scar.*

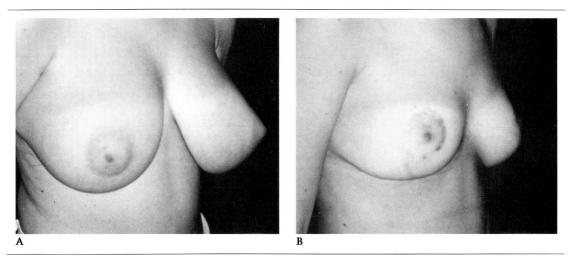

A   B

Fig. 28-17. Oblique view: preoperative (A) and
postoperative (B).

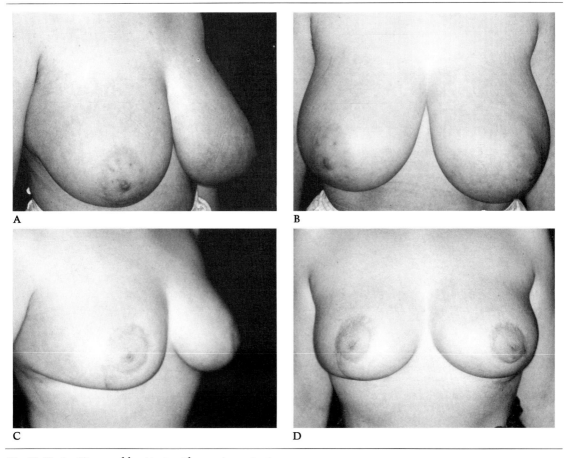

A   B

C   D

Fig. 28-18. An 18-year-old patient with very important
virginal hypertrophy (A and B) and one year after (C
and D) a 900-mg reduction on each side.

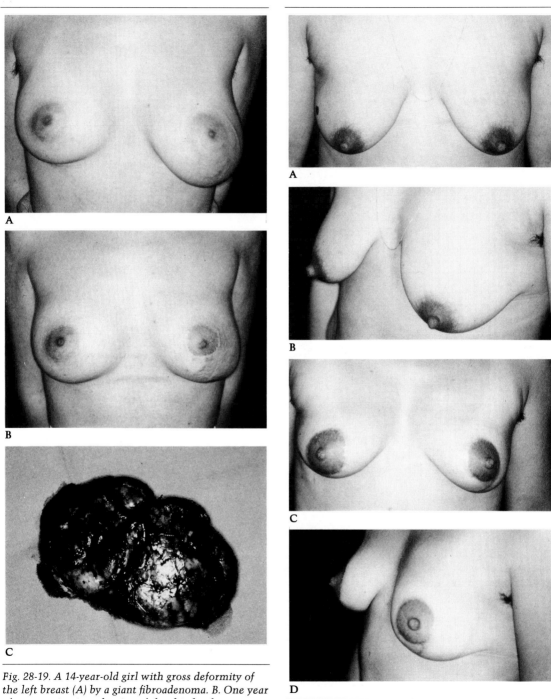

Fig. 28-19. A 14-year-old girl with gross deformity of the left breast (A) by a giant fibroadenoma. B. One year after resection in redraping of the skin by the same Z-procedure. C. The 400-mg giant fibroadenoma after resection.

Fig. 28-20. A, B. Ptotic breasts after pregnancy but with good firm and elastic skin. C, D. One year after the Z-procedure in a ptosis case.

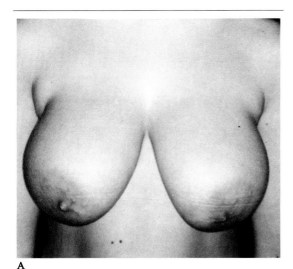

A

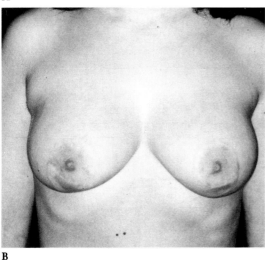

B

Fig. 28-21. A. A 16-year-old girl with distorted upper pole of the breast owing to ptosis of the virginal hypertrophy. B. Two years after the Z-procedure. Note the slight discoloration around the areola but the excellent natural shape and the very short scar.

ment of the nipple-areola complex but very much less than with the original Peixoto [12, 13] or Marchac [9] techniques. The Z-shaped scar is minimal within a few weeks after operation (see Figs. 28-10 and 28-11) and virtually invisible after 3 years (see Fig. 28-15). Because the horizontal scar disappears

completely, the only slight visible oblique scar can be referred by the patient to a possible "breast biopsy." Sensitivity of the nipple-areola complex was objectively and subjectively slightly reduced at the beginning but improved during the 6-year follow-up period and was never a real complaint. To date, some of our patients have become pregnant. We have proof that their reduction mammaplasty constitutes no contraindications to breast-feeding because the lactiferous ducts are not cut deep to the nipple-areola complex as in older methods.

References

1. Arié, G. Una nueva tecnica de mastoplastia. *Rev. Latinoam. Chir. Plast.* 3:23, 1957.
2. Dufourmentel, C., and Mouly, R. Plastie mammaire par la méthode oblique. *Ann. Chir. Plast.* 6:45, 1961.
3. Elbaz, J.S., and Verheecke, G. La cicatrice en L dans les plasties mammaires. *Ann. Chir. Plast.* 17:283, 1972.
4. Gillies, H., and Millard, D.R. *The Principles and Art of Plastic Surgery.* Boston: Little, Brown, 1957.
5. Lalardrie, J.P., and Jouglard, J.P. *Chirugie Plastique du Sein.* Paris: Masson, 1974.
6. Maillard, G.F. A Z-mammaplasty with minimal scarring. *Plast. Reconstr. Surg.* 77:66, 1986.
7. Maillard, G.F., Montandon, D., and Goin J.L. *Plastic and Reconstructive Breast Surgery.* Paris: Masson, 1983.
8. Marchac, D. Mammaplasty with a short transverse scar. In H.B. Williams (ed.), Transactions of the International Congress of Plastic and Reconstructive Surgery. Montreal, 1983.
9. McKissock, P.K. Reduction mammaplasty with a vertical dermal flap. *Plast. Reconstr. Surg.* 49:245, 1972.
10. Meyer, R., and Kesselring, U.K. Reduction mammaplasty with an L-shaped suture line. *Plast. Reconstr. Surg.* 55:139, 1975.
11. Millard, D.R. *Cleft Craft. The Evolution of Its Surgery* (Vol. 1). Boston: Little, Brown, 1976.
12. Peixoto, G. Reduction mammaplasty: A personal technique. *Plast. Reconstr. Surg.* 65:217, 1980.
13. Peixoto, G. Reduction mammaplasty. *Aesth. Plast. Surg.* 8:231, 1984.
14. Regnault, P. Reduction mammaplasty by the "B" technique. *Plast. Reconstr. Surg.* 53:19, 1974.
15. Schwarzmann, E. Die Technik der Mammaplastik. *Chirurgie* 2:932, 1930.
16. Skoog, T. A technique of breast reduction. Transposition of the nipple on a cutaneous vascular pedicle. *Acta Chir. Scand.* 126:453, 1963.
17. Strömbeck, J.O. Mammaplasty: Report of a new technique based on the two-pedicle procedure. *Br. J. Plast. Surg.* 13:79, 1961.

COMMENTS ON CHAPTER 28   *Robert M. Goldwyn*

Maillard has described in detail the rationale and the technique of the Z-mammaplasty, which he has adapted from the methods of Elbaz, Mayer, Regnault, and, principally, Peixoto, the last having popularized resecting the mammary cone so that a large pyramid becomes a small one (see Chap. 23). The principle of the Z-mammaplasty is the removal of the inferior pole of the breast and, if necessary, a segment from the periareola area. The nipple-areola complex is generally safe, being carried on what Maillard has described as a "vast internally based dermoglandular flap."

It should be emphasized that Maillard's earlier Z-shaped mammaplasty that appeared in a book [1] of which he was one of the authors is not the same as the procedure he has detailed in this chapter [2]. The former technique was a Z-shaped modification of the oblique method and was abandoned because of the medialization of the nipples as a result of what Maillard calls the "lateral pinch."

The patients that Maillard has shown in this chapter illustrate his versatility with his later method. In my experience, however, this Z-shaped mammaplasty is best used, as he himself has written, in young women with good skin turgor, in whom the expected amount of tissue to be resected per breast does not exceed 500 gm, and in whom one need not raise the nipple-areola more than 10 cm. It is true that Maillard has also described and shown patients who successfully had 900 cm removed. Undoubtedly, the more experience one has with a particular method, the easier it is to perform and apply it to a greater variety of situations. The author of the technique is not only its proponent but also becomes its virtuoso.

The skin of a younger patient is generally but not always more elastic. It will shrink to the new contour created by glandular resection. In fact, this phenomenon underlies the success of many other techniques, especially the volume reduction method of Cloutier (see Chap. 29). As we know, the ability of skin to contract is a regular occurrence after subcutaneous mastectomy. Maillard correctly recognized that he is performing a "partial subcutaneous mastectomy."

The younger patient for whom the Z-mamma-

plasty is best intended is also the one who particularly merits a procedure with minimal scarring because of the tendency of that age group to thickened scars, a point that Maillard stresses.

The problem with all short scar techniques lies not so much in resecting tissue but in eliminating excess skin. In Maillard's technique, extra skin is managed by generous periareolar deepithelialization, by spontaneous retraction of the skin after removing breast tissue, and by resecting skin in a limited fashion in a vertical direction while keeping the lower margin of the excision 4 to 5 cm above the inframammary fold, a key point in the Marchac technique (see Chap. 22). Although the primary purpose of the Z-plasty is to add skin vertically to the inferior pole of the breast to give the whole breast a better shape while also reducing periareolar tension, the Z does get rid of extra skin laterally by bringing it in centrally so that ultimately, little skin has to be resected because of the interlocking of the two large limbs of the Z-plasty.

Despite the Z-plasty, however, considerable tension may remain on the areola, and widening of the scar is not uncommon. In fact, one can see this readily in Figure 28-18.

Widening of the periareolar scar can be lessened by revision, but the younger the patient, the less the success of revision, especially if the scar has hypertrophied. Yet, it is the younger patient for whom the procedure of the Z-mammaplasty is especially beneficial. With regard to spreading of the scar, the use of permanent intradermal sutures may be helpful but may not always be so; this is still a matter of controversy.

In summary, the Z-mammaplasty is a safe technique for mild to moderate hypertrophy, particularly in a younger patient whose nipple-areola transfer will not exceed 10 cm and in whom the amount of tissue resected will be no greater than 500 to 600 gm, even though with experience, larger resections, up to 900 gm, are possible.

REFERENCES
1. Maillard, G.F., Montandon, D., and Goin, J.L. *Plastic and Reconstructive Breast Surgery.* Paris: Masson, 1983.
2. Maillard, G.F. Personal communication, 1988.

29

A. MacLeod Cloutier

Volume Reduction Mammaplasty

For one reason or another, I have had a few patients requesting removal of their mammary prostheses. In every case, the breast returned to its original size and shape in a matter of days after the operation. This fact led me to believe that it might be possible to reduce the breast by removing a prosthetic-shaped mass of breast tissue with a resultant decrease in size without breast distortion. However, I surmised that this procedure would work only on a breast that was covered by skin without stretch marks and on a breast that was not overly pendulous. Because there are many young women who want a breast reduction with minimal scarring, I soon had likely candidates.

The operation performed on the first few patients behaved exactly as though a prosthesis had been removed. The areola shrank on the operating table, and as long as a good thickness of breast tissue was left attached to the skin, no dimpling occurred. The transverse incision made in the inframammary fold was, in most cases, hardly noticeable at the end of a year.

The operation worked extremely well in the relatively young patient and exceptionally well in patients with asymmetric breasts. There is no other operation that I know of that can so readily match one breast to the other (Figs. 29-1 and 29-2).

In the properly selected patient, the appearance of the breast after volume reduction is normal. In the rare instance that breast size has increased and where it appears that for whatever reason volume reduction is not applicable, a standard reduction mammaplasty can be performed but with the use of a medial pedicle.

Since developing this procedure, I learned that in 1669, Durstan performed the same one, with minor variations [2]. Morestin and Guinard [1], in 1907, Velpeau [3] in 1857, and Thorek [2] in 1942 described removing breast tissue alone in cases of mammary hypertrophy. Efforts to completely remodel the breast by more complicated operations soon came into vogue, and the simple procedure was forgotten. However, the advantages of simply removing breast tissue alone make the method worthwhile.

Method

With the patient under general anesthesia, the breast is completely detached from the pectoral fascia through an inframammary incision about 10 cm long. Breast tissue is then removed, leaving at least 4 cm of breast tissue under the areola and 2 cm under the surrounding skin (Figs. 29-3 through 29-5). All bleeders are clamped and cauterized, a drain is inserted, and the skin is closed with a continuous 4-0 plain catgut suture. After the other breast has been reduced, dry dressings are applied, and a brassiere is used to hold the breasts and dressings in place. Drains are removed the following day.

This procedure has been used in 216 patients on a total of 401 breasts. Adequate volume reduction was achieved in all cases. Breasts of DD cup size were reduced to a D and often a C cup, and D cup size breasts were reduced to size B.

The operation has four main advantages for the patient: (1) scarring is minimized by using an inframammary incision; (2) the distal ducts are undisturbed; (3) there is little or no interference with blood supply to the breast; and (4) the resulting appearance is natural (Figs. 29-6 through 29-9). These advantages make the operation particularly attractive in cases of virginal hypertrophy.

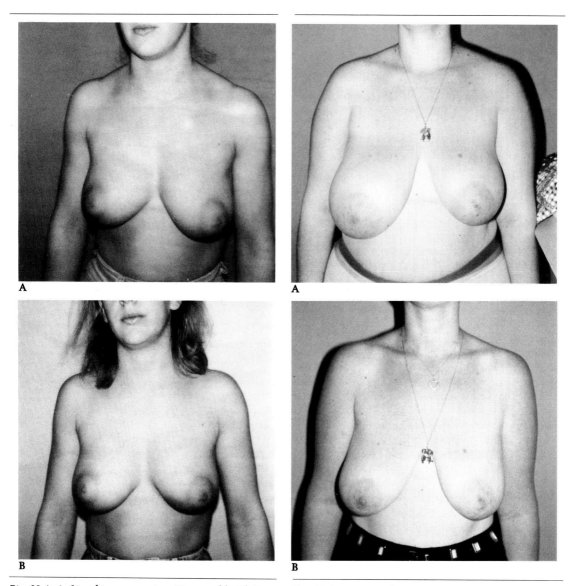

Fig. 29-1. A. Size discrepancy in a 17-year-old girl. B. Postreduction left breast 6 months later.

Fig. 29-2. A. Breast discrepancy in a 35-year-old woman. B. Postreduction right breast.

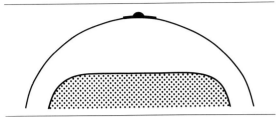

Fig. 29-3. Theoretical outline of tissue resection.

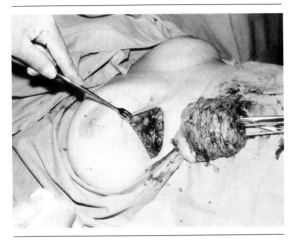

Fig. 29-4. Breast mass excised.

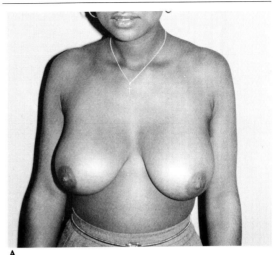

A

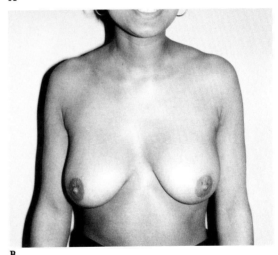

B

Fig. 29-6. A. Mild hypertrophy in a 25-year-old woman.
B. Postreduction 1 year later.

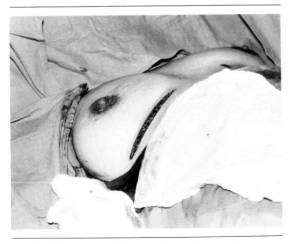

Fig. 29-5. Incision and breast shape after excision.

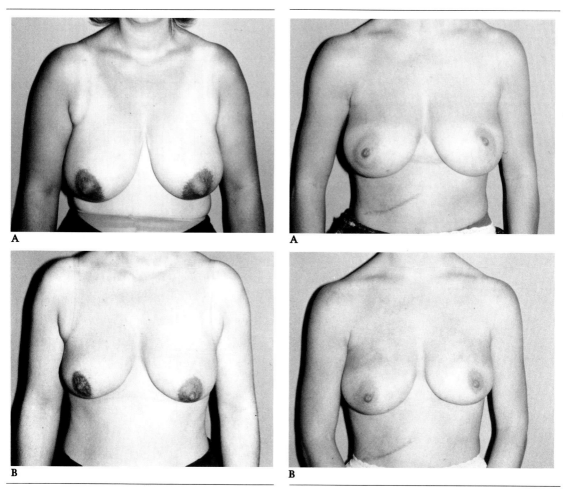

Fig. 29-7. A. Hypertrophy in a 34-year-old woman. B. Postreduction 1 year later.

Fig. 29-8. A. Mild hypertrophy in a 20-year-old woman. B. Postreduction. Slight discrepancy in the left breast.

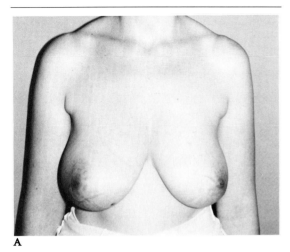

A

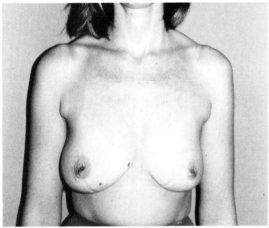

B

Fig. 29-9. A. Hypertrophy in a 27-year-old woman. B. Postreduction 9 months later.

References

1. Morestin, H., and Guinard, A. Hypertrophie mammaire traitée par la résection discoide. *Bull. Soc. Chir. Paris* 33:649, 1907.
2. Thorek, M. *Plastic Surgery of the Breast and Abdominal Wall.* Springfield, IL: Thomas, 1942. Pp. 1–398.
3. Velpeau, A. *Traité des Maladies du Sein et de la Région Mammaire.* Paris: Masson, 1854.

COMMENTS ON CHAPTER 29   *Robert D. Midgley*

I have performed the volume reduction mammaplasty technique as described by Cloutier for 13 years with high patient satisfaction. My strict criteria for selection of patients for this procedure are the following:

1. Moderate bilateral virginal hypertrophy of the breasts.
2. Breast asymmetry of one cup size difference.
3. Maximum amount of breast reduction to be under 300 gm per breast.

Having performed this operation on 66 breasts, I have found the following advantages:

1. Normal nipple sensation.
2. Ability of the breast to lactate satisfactorily.
3. Minimal internal scarring, allowing more precise mammogram interpretation.

4. No need for operative blood transfusion.

Disadvantages in properly selected cases are uncommon and include:

1. Slightly higher incidence of hematoma (5%). To minimize this, I routinely use a suction hemovac.
2. Unpredictable failure of elastic take-up of the skin brassiere (10%). This is less in patients younger than 21 years of age. My patients wear a snug brassiere day and night for 6 weeks postoperatively.

Provided that there is strict adherence to the selection criteria, Cloutier's simple time-saving yet effective operation is highly recommended.

30

Gordon Letterman and
Maxine Schurter

Reduction Mammaplasty and Free Composite Nipple-Areolar Grafts

Breasts of massive proportions and those of great pendulosity can be safely and dramatically reduced and a satisfactory facsimile of the breast can be created using a free composite nipple-areolar graft.

Reduction is accomplished by amputating an unlimited but desirable quantity of adipose tissue, mammary gland, and skin, including the nipple and areola. A likeness of the breast is structured by using the remaining tissue to create a conical mound on which, at an appropriate site, a free full-thickness graft of the nipple and areola is fixed to a dermal bed [46].

Background

The first incontrovertible description of a reduction mammaplasty with subtotal amputations of the breasts and restructuring using free nipple-areolar grafts must be credited to Thorek [39, 41, 42, 44, 49, 50, 78, 85].

In 1921 at a meeting of the North Shore Branch of the Chicago Medical Society, Thorek [77] read a paper entitled "Possibilities in the Reconstruction of the Human Form." The paper, which was published the following year, gives the case history accompanied by the pre- and postoperative photographs of the patient on whose breasts Thorek had done subtotal amputations and reconstructions with free grafts of the nipples and areolae (Figs. 30-1 and 30-2).

Thorek wrote: "In a careful search of the available literature no record is found of the deliberate attempt to transplant the nipple. This experimen-tal study proved that that may be accomplished for cosmetic reasons."

He gave the following description of the operative procedure. "Under general anesthesia (scopolamine-morphine supplemented by ether), the breasts were amputated, leaving sufficient tissue for remodeling. The breasts were then remodeled. The great pendulosity caused the nipples to occupy a lower-most position of the pendant breasts and were therefore removed during the ablation. The nipples were then transplanted from the ablated breasts to the newly constructed ones."

Over a period of 25 years, Thorek wrote a variety of papers on reduction mammaplasty and free grafting of the nipple and areola [78–82, 84, 85]. Thorek's [83] comprehensive book entitled *Plastic Surgery of the Breast and Abdomen* contains a detailed description of the preoperative preparation, measurements, patient's position, anesthesia, and 12 steps of his own operative procedure (Figs. 30-3 through 30-6).

In 1928, Dartiques [21] challenged Thorek's claim of priority in the successful use of the free nipple graft when he published his operation for the correction of fourth-degree ptosis in *Le Monde Medicale.* Thorek [78] totally rejected Dartiques' claim on the basis of an historical review that Dartiques [20] himself had published in the *Archives Franco-Belges de Chirurgie,* April 15, 1925. Writing of free nipple grafts, Dartiques said "En 1922 Max Thorek (de Chicago) representait ce procede New York Medical Journal et Medical Record."

Later papers by Thorek reinforced his claim to priority in the use of free nipple grafts and fur-

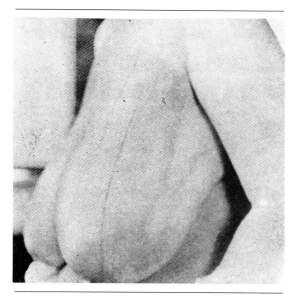

Fig. 30-1. Preoperative view of Thorek's patient with virginal hypertrophy of the breasts on whom he operated in 1921. (From M. Thorek. Possibilities in the reconstruction of the human form. N. Y. Med. J. Med. Rec. 116:572, 1922.)

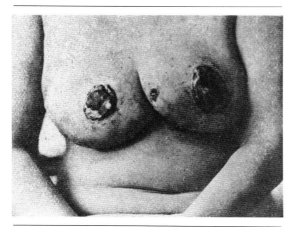

Fig. 30-2. Thorek's patient as she appeared "two weeks after amputation and remodeling of the breasts." (From M. Thorek. Possibilities in the reconstruction of the human form. N. Y. Med. J. Med. Rec. 116:572, 1922.)

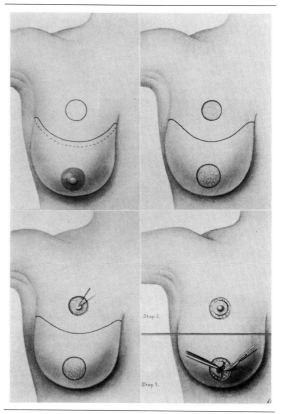

Fig. 30-3. (Top left) Thorek's operation. Solid line on anterior surface of the breast shows incision and new nipple-areolar site. Dotted line indicates posterior incision. (Top right) Thorek's operation. The nipple-areolar graft has been obtained. Above a circular dermal bed has been prepared to receive the transplant. This circle is slightly smaller in circumference than the donor site. "This, for allowing retraction and harmonious coaptation between transplant and margin of circular area for reception of the nipple." (Bottom left) Nipple and areola in new site. Cambric needle passing through the nipple and into the breast substance steadies the graft during subsequent manipulations. (Bottom right) "Wrong method of grafting." Step 1: Nipple-areolar graft obtained. Step 2: Recipient dermal circular area is too large for retracted graft. No consideration has been given to retraction. (This figure and Figs. 30-4 through 30-7 are from M. Thorek. Plastic Surgery of the Breast and Abdominal Wall. Springfield, IL: Thomas, 1942.)

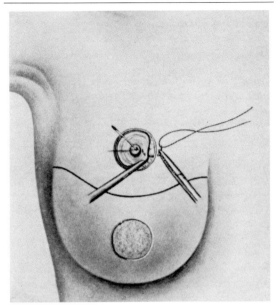

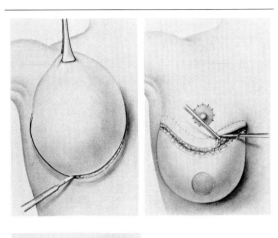

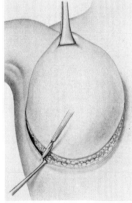

Fig. 30-5. (Upper left) Posterior incision being made slightly above the submammary sulcus. (Upper right) Anterior incision being undermined. (Lower left) Undercutting of posterior incision.

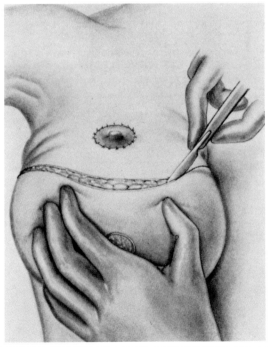

Fig. 30-4. (Top) Thorek's operation. Nipple steadied by cambric needle. Nipple-areolar graft and recipient margins apposed by interrupted sutures. (Bottom) Transplanted nipple-areolar graft sutured in position. Incision across the anterior surface of the breast for removal of the bulk of breast by sharp dissection.

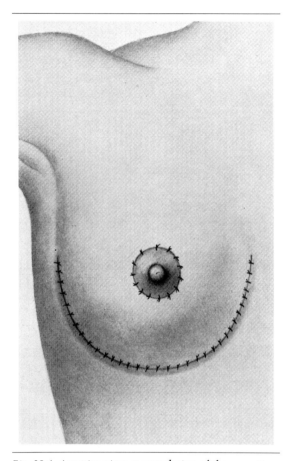

Fig. 30-6. Anterior view at completion of the operation.

nished microscopic proof of survival of transplanted nipples.

In his book concerned with the breast and published in 1942, he wrote: "Thus priority for this operation unreservedly belongs to me because my detailed operation antedates that of any other author by at least five years. A thorough study of the literature establishes that fact definitely" [83].

Adams [1–5] popularized reduction mammaplasty with nipple transplantation and described his own modifications of Thorek's technique. He [6] presented his last paper on this subject entitled "Mammaplasty with Free Transplantation of the Nipples and Areolae: A Thirteen-Year Follow-up Report" at the First Congress of the International Society of Plastic Surgeons meeting in Stockholm in 1955.

The experience of Thorek, Dartiques [20–24], Lexer [52], Updegraff [87], Adams [1–6], Bames

[8], May [62–65], Malbec [53], and Marino [59] established the value of the free nipple graft in reconstruction of the breast.

Maliniac [54–58] provided critical analyses of free transplantation of the nipple. Moreover, Gupta [29] provided us with a critical review of contemporary procedures for mammary reduction.

Indications for Operation

Partial amputation of the breast and its reconstruction using a free composite nipple-areolar graft is clearly the procedure of choice when the breast is of such extreme pendulosity that elevation and repositioning of the nipple by any other modern method of mammaplasty might result in necrosis of the nipple, areola, mammary gland, adipose tissue, or skin.

Free nipple grafts are indicated for the patient who has been accepted as a candidate for reduction mammaplasty but who is obese, possibly hypertensive, or diabetic or has other conditions that are not compatible with a long anesthetic. It is expedient for the patient whose massive breasts cause or contribute to neurogenic, pulmonic, or musculoskeletal problems. Indeed, it is a comparatively easy operation that can be completed in a relatively short period of time with a minimal loss of blood. Conway [12] summarized his argument for the use of the procedure in patients whose breasts are of such size and weight as to constitute a handicap to respiration as follows:

Attention is called to the importance of the weight of the female breasts as a handicap to respiratory physiology. The breasts act as the resistance point in a lever of the third kind, which means that their actual weight exerts the greatest possible mechanical disadvantage to inspiration. This consideration emphasizes the physiological benefit of reduction mammaplasty in those persons in whom the mammary glands are significantly overweight. Preliminary physiologic studies have shown that persons with large breasts exhibit increased work of breathing.

The effects of hypertrophic breasts on the musculoskeletal system have been detailed by Letterman and Schurter [45, 51]. There is an anatomic basis for these symptoms, and reduction mammaplasty is usually curative. The skeletal and postural relationships to reduction mammaplasty have also been considered by Pitanguy [69]. "Neurologic changes with excessively large breasts" have been described by Kaye [30].

There are many other indications for mammaplasty and free nipple grafts. It is the operation of choice and often the only choice for relieving the patient inflicted with true gigantomastia [32, 47, 70, 73, 88].

The nipple being carried on a dermal pedicle or bridge that for any reason shows evidence of impending avasularity may be saved by removing it as a free composite nipple-areolar graft and transplanting it on an appropriately located dermal bed of a newly created conical breast mound.

Free nipple-areolar grafts can be useful in reconstruction of the breasts following subcutaneous mastectomy [35–38, 40, 43, 59, 71] and mastopexy, as well as the correction of certain asymmetries and other congenital anomalies [58, 72, 83].

Preoperative Discussions, Studies, and Planning

The surgeon must have a thorough understanding of the patient and her expectations. The patient must be fully informed of the functional and structural limitations of the reconstructed breast. Possible unfavorable results and complications must be understood before the operation. A careful medical history should be taken and a complete physical examination done with particular attention to the breasts. Photographs, measurements, and a study of body contour are important. Appropriate hematologic, radiologic, and electrocardiographic studies should be obtained. Preoperative mammography is used to detect small nonpalpable lesions and to investigate the nature of nodularity. Postoperative mammography provides a source for comparison with future films. Since some blood loss must be anticipated (usually minimal), scheduling should allow the healthy patient to bank her own blood in case an intraoperative transfusion becomes advisable.

PREOPERATIVE DESIGN

Preoperative measurements and markings are made on the patient's chest and breasts prior to her receiving any medications. They are made with the patient in an erect sitting or standing position. However, the patient must stand if the breasts rest on the thighs when seated. Moreover, the patient should be capable of remaining in a fixed position throughout the period required for marking. Even minor movements of the upper portion of the

body may alter measurements by 1 or 2 cm, and such deviations can prove critical to achieving a symmetric reconstruction. The patient's head should face directly forward with the eyes looking straight ahead. The neck-chin angle should be approximately 90 degrees, with the shoulders back (Fig. 30-7).

The midline of the chest and upper abdomen is marked downward from the center of the suprasternal notch. At the level of the xiphoid process, the midline frequently deviates to one side as it continues on toward the umbilicus. Therefore, the midchest line is marked from the midsternal notch as though a plumb line were dropped from that point. The clavicles are measured from their medial (sternal) ends to the lateral (acromial) ends. In our experience, this distance has generally been 14 to 16 cm regardless of the body build, and there is little variation in the length of the two bones. One half of the length of the clavicle is measured from the medial end. A line is drawn downward from the midclavicle to the nipple. This line has been referred to as the breast axis or meridian. Since the sizes of the two breasts are rarely if ever equal, these lines will not necessarily be equidistant from the midline. It is better, however, to form a normally shaped reconstructed breast on each side than to alter the line passing from the midclavicle to the nipple on one side and thus create an ill-formed breast on that side (Fig. 30-8).

Along the midclavicular-nipple line, a point (a) is chosen, which will be the apex of the newly formed breast. It is rarely above the level of the inframammary crease (Fig. 30-9). Furthermore, it must be a point that "looks right" when the surgeon manually molds a potentially new breast of desired size from the superior portion of the existing breast. This point (a) is usually 22 to 27 cm from the suprasternal notch. It is important that points (a) on each breast are level, because they are later involved in selecting the new nipple sites. For this reason, the points are measured from the suprasternal notch rather than the clavicles, because one clavicle is often higher than the other.

From each apical point (a), an inverted V (a-b and a-c) is marked out on the breast surface. Each limb of the V is 7 cm in length—i.e., (a-b) and (a-c) are each 7 cm. The angle of the V varies with the amount of tissue to be removed and the degree of projection and conicity desired for the forthcoming reconstruction. The distance between the inferior extent of the two limbs (b and c) is usually 9 to 13 cm (Fig. 30-10).

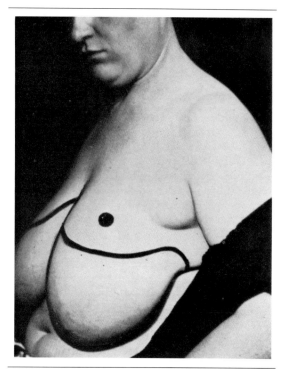

Fig. 30-7. A patient of Thorek's sitting erect for preoperative "outlines on the anterior surface of the breast."

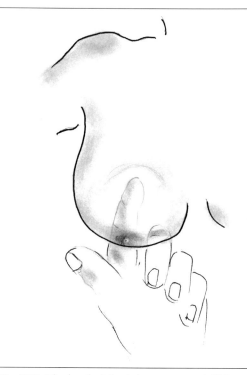

Fig. 30-9. The level of the inframammary fold is noted on the anterior surface of the breast.

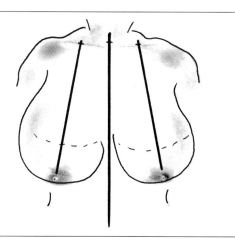

Fig. 30-8. The midclavicular line is dropped downward from the suprasternal notch. A line is drawn from the middle of the clavicle to the nipple. The inframammary fold is shown as a dotted line.

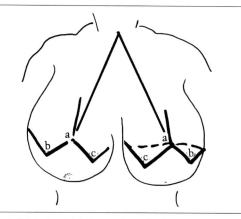

Fig. 30-10. Point (a) is located on the breast axis on each side, and the distances are checked from the suprasternal notch for symmetry. Lines a-b and a-c are each 7 cm in length. The angle b-a-c is variable.

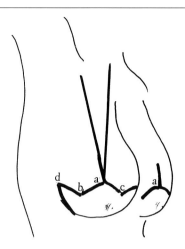

Fig. 30-11. With the arm elevated, (d) is marked at the lateral extent of the inframammary fold. Point (b) is connected to (d).

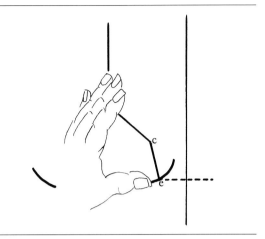

Fig. 30-12. A point (e) is marked on each inframammary fold 6 cm from the midsternal line. The lines c-e and d-e are drawn, completing the delineation of skin to be resected.

With the arm elevated, the lateral end of the inframammary fold is marked (d) on the breast; this is usually at the anterior axillary line. This point (d) is connected to point (b) on the anterior surface of the breast (Fig. 30-11). With the breast elevated and displaced laterally, a point (e) is marked 6 cm from the midline within the submammary fold. This is an arbitrary point since it will be altered in the final closure, but it does help to prevent scars from crossing the midline. In that area they tend to contract or form keloids. Point (c) is joined to point (e). The entire extent of the inframammary crease is marked out connecting points (d-e) (Fig. 30-12).

Finally, all measurements and points are doubly checked to be certain that the final closure will be easily and accurately accomplished without undue tension [7]. To ensure this, the points (b) and (c) at the lower extremes of the inverted V are held together and approximated to a midportion of the inframammary line. If the point (a) of the V has been marked out too high, closure will certainly be too tight; the point should be lowered. If the point (a) has been marked out too low, the reconstructed breast will prove pendulous. As a final test of the validity of the markings, the lateral (b-d) and the medial (c-e) lines on the anterior surface of the breast should be manually approximated to their corresponding segments of the inframammary line (d-e). Difficulty in approximating these lines

is indicative of an impending tight closure and poor healing.

The future nipple sites are not predetermined.

SITTING POSITION

For the past 35 years, we have used the sitting or semisitting position for reduction mammaplasty and reconstruction with free nipple-areolar grafts with general anesthesia (Fig. 30-13). For us, it has proved mandatory since the new nipple-areolar sites are not precisely chosen as part of the preoperative measurements and design. Indeed it is most difficult, if not impossible, to select a new nipple site and ensure symmetry of the nipples with the patient supine. Furthermore, in the sitting position, the preoperative markings can again be easily verified, and if found necessary, intraoperative adjustments in size, shape, and position can be made and thus a greater degree of symmetry can be achieved (Figs. 30-14 and 30-15).

When we first used the sitting position, some complications were encountered. These prompted a detailed analysis of the entire problem. As a result of this study, preventive measures were instituted. Thus, a simple routine for positioning the patient evolved. Special precautions are taken to ensure the integrity of the cardiovascular, respiratory, and musculoskeletal systems. The peripheral nerves and soft-tissue structures are well protected (see Fig. 30-13). We have described these

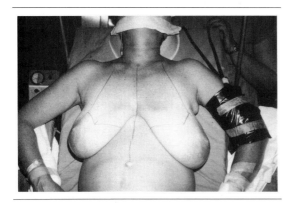

Fig. 30-13. The patient has been centered on the operating table, which has then been slowly elevated to the sitting position. The shoulders must be level. The elbows are padded. The blood pressure cuff is in place with its plastic covering. A drool pad is secured beneath the chin. The intravenous cannula is on the dorsum of the forearm, so that flexion of the elbow will not displace it.

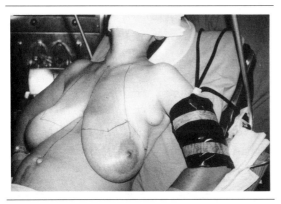

Fig. 30-14. A support is placed under the head to prevent pressure on the occiput and also to prevent hyperextension of the neck. An ether screen keeps the drapes off the face.

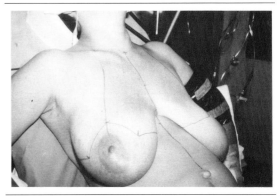

Fig. 30-15. Oblique view of the patient in the sitting position.

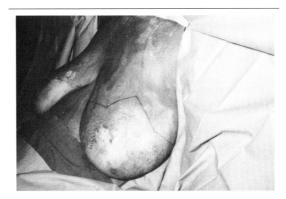

Fig. 30-16. Patient in the sitting position prepared for surgery.

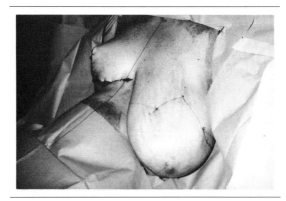

Fig. 30-17. Same patient as in Figure 30-16 after removal of desired amount of breast tissue on the right side. The sitting position provides the opportunity to view both breasts at the same time.

precautionary measures elsewhere in great detail [48]. If proper care is taken, the sitting position for mammaplasty is safe and can be of great advantage to the surgeon (Figs. 30-16 and 30-17).

Since the final aesthetic result achieved by a reduction mammaplasty is judged primarily on the size, shape, and position the breasts assume with the individual standing, the sitting position represents the optimum operative position for the patient with tremendously large breasts.

The semisitting position was Thorek's choice for his mammary reduction and reconstruction (Fig. 30-18). Later, it was graphically described and endorsed by Lamont [33, 34]. Biesenberger [9] used it when doing his transposition mammaplasty.

Operation

After careful preoperative planning, painstaking measurements, and accurate markings, the patient is brought into the operating room and centered on the table in the dorsal recumbent position.

After preparing the patient for the semisitting position, a general anesthetic is initiated, followed by oral endotracheal intubation. While all vital signs are monitored, the patient is gradually brought into a semisitting or sitting position (Fig. 30-19) [60]. Frequent blood pressure readings are the guide to safety during this change in position. The breasts, chest, neck, shoulders, arms, and abdomen are prepared with an antiseptic solution. Drapes are applied in a sterile manner, leaving the patient exposed from the clavicles to the upper abdomen and laterally to the table. In some cases of extreme gigantomastia, it is advisable to place the patient on a sterilely draped operating table.

Attention is first directed to the right breast. Skin incisions following the lines (a-b) and (a-c) of the inverted V are made superficially on the anterior surface of the breast, thus delineating the inverted V and encompassing the nipple and areola. Next, an incision is made connecting the inferior end (b) of the inverted V to the lateral-most point (d) of the inframammary line. The point (c) of the inverted V joins point (e) in the medial submammary fold. The area of skin to be excised is thus outlined by these cutaneous incisions and the inframammary crease (d-e). The superficial skin incisions are next deepened into the subcutaneous tissue.

A large hook is positioned at the apex of the inverted V (a). This is used to elevate the breast

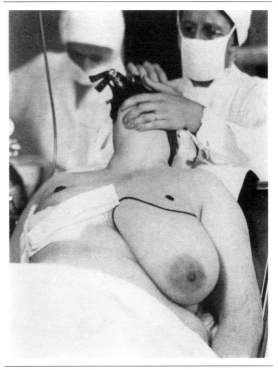

Fig. 30-18. Thorek's patient in the sitting position. The right breast has previously been operated on; the left breast is prepared for operation. (From M. Thorek. Plastic Surgery of the Breast and Abdominal Wall. Springfield, IL: Thomas, 1942.)

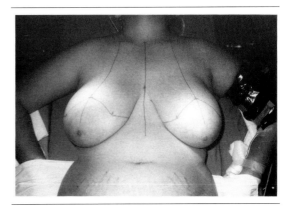

Fig. 30-19. A 21-year-old girl with preoperative markings in the sitting position on the operating table.

thus facilitating the resection. The incision now traversing the entire anterior surface of the breast (d-c-a-b-e) is deepened perpendicularly to the skin down through the gland to the level of the fascia of the pectoralis major muscle. The cutting cautery facilitates this procedure. Hemostasis is obtained as the operation progresses. Care is taken not to undermine the skin of the breast. The desired amount of breast is then resected off the pectoralis fascia down to the inframammary fold. Finally, an incision is made connecting the extremes of this fold (d-e).

This last incision, when deepened to the fascia, completes the partial amputation of the breast with its nipple and areola. After clearly labeling the specimen "right," it is transferred to a sterile back table [17–19]. There, the surgeon or an experienced member of the surgical team circumscribes the new nipple-areolar complex. To do this, the specimen must be held under suitable tension (Fig. 30-20). The size of the areola is best determined preoperatively. The nipple and areola are removed as a free full-thickness, smooth muscle–carrying graft (Figs. 30-21 and 30-22). The undersurface of the graft is freed of subcutaneous tissue (Fig. 30-23). More important, the smooth musculature is left intact, thus preserving the contractibility of the areola and the erectile function of the nipple.

Meanwhile, at the operating table, the breast tissue is molded into a conically shaped mound. The distal ends (b and c) of the inverted V are approximated with a guide suture. A small single hook now replaces the larger instrument at the apical angle (a) used during the resection. With tension on this hook, the opposing sides (a-b and a-c) are accurately approximated; thus, the vertical portion of an inverted T closure is completed.

The opposing transverse skin edges (d-b-c-e and d-e) are aligned and temporarily sutured at strategic intervals. The underlying subcutaneous tissues are then approximated with a limited number of sutures. At this phase of the operation, it is necessary to direct attention to the lateral and medial aspects of the inframammary closure. Laterally, it may become necessary to resect additional tissue. Indeed, it may be necessary to angle the excision from the perpendicular to include even more breast tissue. Routinely, a surplus of skin and subcutaneous tissue must be excised medially to obtain a pleasing conical mound. In doing so, however, every effort should be made to extend the

incision the shortest possible distance beyond point (e) and to avoid crossing the midline. Additional subcutaneous sutures may be needed to provide medial and lateral apposition of the tissues. Finally, the transverse skin edges are closed with an intracutaneous running wire suture to avoid stitch marks and to provide a secure closure.

Attention is now directed to the left breast, on which a similar operation is done. Bearing in mind that very large breasts are usually unequal in size, shape, and weight, great effort may be needed to achieve symmetry. It helps to compare the weight of the two resected specimens, but this is not a substitute for the judicial observations of the experienced surgeon. Palpation and critical comparisons of the two breasts are of the utmost importance.

New nipple sites for the breasts are confirmed only after all reasonable symmetry of the conical mounds has been obtained (Fig. 30-24). The new sites must be verified by comparative measurements and visual observations.

A circular marker is used that is the same size as that used to obtain the grafts. This allows the grafts to be placed under the same tension as they were in the donor sites. In reviewing postoperative results in the literature, both for the transposed and grafted areolae, it seems that there is a tendency to make the new areolae too large. The size of the marker should, therefore, be carefully considered. A marker larger than 4.5 cm would rarely be used (Fig. 30-25).

The circle marker should be centered on the mound. There, it is usually over the top of the vertical suture line. It should not be so low as to leave the upper portion of the suture line showing; this would result in a scar above the areola. It should be low enough to permit some postoperative elevation if the final location should prove too high.

The tops of the grafts must always be level. This is judged by eye, and it is also carefully measured from the suprasternal notch. Two other measurements are made: one from the medial edge of the circle to the midsternal line, and one from the inframammary fold to the bottom edge of the circle. If there was significant preoperative asymmetry, it will be necessary to compromise on these two measurements.

After the sites are finally chosen and marked with a dye, incisions are made along the markings through the epidermis. The epidermis is then re-

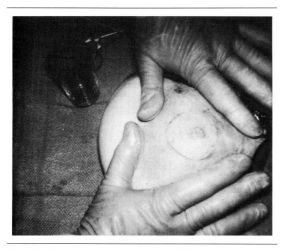

Fig. 30-20. Amputated specimen held under tension with new areolar size marked.

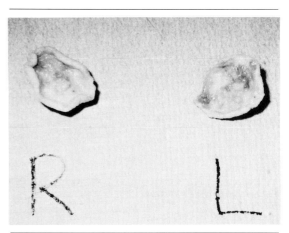

Fig. 30-23. Undersurface of nipple-areolar grafts.

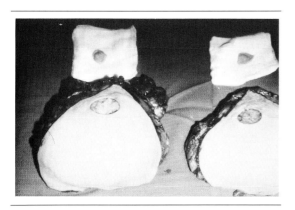

Fig. 30-21. Amputated specimens with nipples and areolae removed.

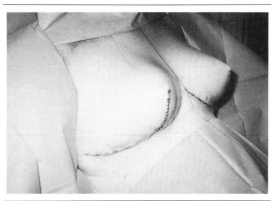

Fig. 30-24. Same patient after reduction and reconstruction of conical-shaped breasts. New nipple sites are yet to be selected.

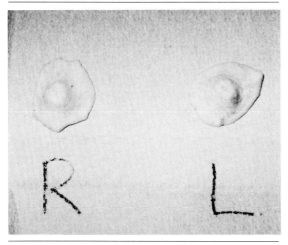

Fig. 30-22. Nipple and areolar full-thickness composite grafts marked right and left.

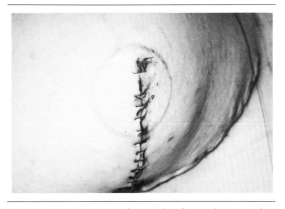

Fig. 30-25. The new areolar site has been chosen and marked on the breast. Temporary sutures.

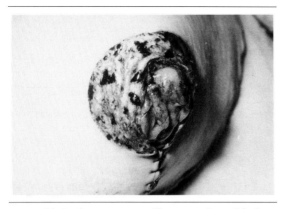

Fig. 30-26. Epidermis removed leaving a dermal bed. The bed is disrupted after removal of silk sutures.

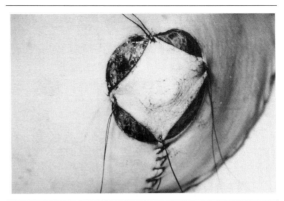

Fig. 30-28. Nipple-areolar graft secured with four sutures placed in the dermis of the recipient site.

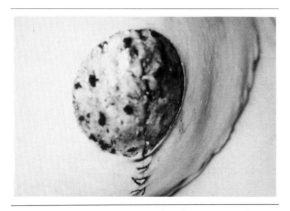

Fig. 30-27. Dermal bed repaired with interrupted inverted fine absorbable sutures.

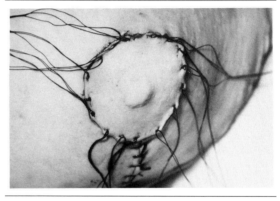

Fig. 30-29. Graft sutured in position with silk sutures left long.

moved, leaving a clean dermal bed for reception of the graft. As the epidermis is removed, the underlying portion of the vertical suture line is disrupted. The sutures are removed, and a defect is created in the dermal bed (Fig. 30-26). This defect is closed with very fine interrupted inverted absorbable sutures cut on the knots (Fig. 30-27). The least possible foreign body material should be left beneath the grafts.

The grafts themselves have had the undersurfaces trimmed of all subcutaneous tissue, leaving dermis and its smooth muscle fibers. However, the nipples may require tailoring. If the nipples are very thick, some of the undersurface of the ducts is removed. If the nipples are aesthetically too large in diameter for the shape and size of the new breasts, central cores can be removed and the cut

edges closed with a few fine catgut sutures. Healing resembles a normal central nipple depression.

The grafts are placed on the dermal beds and sutured there with 4-0 silk sutures through the graft and the subcuticular recipient site; these sutures never pierce the bordering skin. Thus, periareolar skin stitch marks are eliminated. Four equidistant sutures (Fig. 30-28) are placed and each quadrant is then bisected until the edges of the grafts are well approximated to the recipient skin edges. This usually requires 16 to 32 sutures on each side. The sutures are left long to tie over a stent (Fig. 30-29). The nipples and areolae are covered with fine mesh grease gauze, and a dry gauze bolus is superimposed; the silk sutures are tied over this bolus, providing even pressure on the grafts (Fig. 30-30). Steri-Strips are placed over the

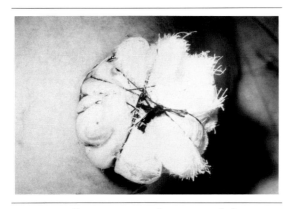

Fig. 30-30. Silk sutures are tied over gauze bolus as a stent.

suture lines. A light compression dressing is applied and held in place with a wraparound gauze. Drains are rarely necessary.

At the conclusion of the operative procedure, the return to the supine position demands the same gentle care and attention to details as were exercised in the initial maneuvers necessary to establish the sitting position. Martin [61] has cautioned: "Postural changes made later in the course of an anesthetic or at the termination of the surgery can easily be more homeostatically threatening than was the initial establishment of the surgical position."

Advantages

There are several advantages of this modification of Thorek's procedure for partial amputation of the breast and reconstruction using free nipple-areolar grafts:

1. The preoperative design is not based on a fixed pattern. Rather, it is individualized [66, 75, 89, 92].
2. The new nipple sites are not determined preoperatively. A conical mount is completed, and only then are the new nipple sites selected. This is a real advantage in achieving final symmetry of the reconstructed breasts. A 25- to 30-year follow-up of a limited number of patients who had free grafts surprisingly revealed that the position of the nipple had changed relatively little over the years, reemphasizing the importance of the initial site selected for the graft.
3. The free nipple-areola complex is taken as a true

composite graft of nipple, areola, and muscle in an effort to preserve erectility, sensitivity, and sensuality in the transplant.
4. The shape of the breasts at the completion of the procedure is pleasing. A conical breast mound of desired size and suitable projection is readily achieved with a midwedge resection. The flat broad reconstructed breast that has neither a conical shape nor adequate projection is unacceptable [68]. The natural contour that can be obtained persists for many years (see Figs. 30-39 and 30-40).
5. Proper care and precautionary measures are taken to ensure that the sitting position is safe for mammaplasty.
6. There are no flaps to be undermined, and the procedure takes a relatively short time.
7. Patient satisfaction is long-lasting. They are our most grateful group of patients.

Results

Partial amputation mammaplasty and reconstruction using free nipple-areolar grafts is a satisfying operation for those properly selected and prepared. The procedures can solve the many aesthetic, social, and economic problems created by gigantomastia and can relieve the physical disabilities and psychological stress suffered by these patients. Preoperative and postoperative photographs of patients of various ages illustrate the results of the procedure (Figs. 30-31 through 30-44).

COMPLICATIONS AND UNFAVORABLE RESULTS

The complications and unfavorable aesthetic results obtained with modern methods of reduction mammaplasty have been well documented by McKissock [67], who has given much thought to this aspect of the procedures. In an introductory paragraph, he writes:

The nature of surgery for breast reduction, with all its attendant vascular risks, makes it a fertile field for complications, beyond which, moreover, there lies a vast minefield of potential errors that are hazards to the unwary surgeon. These potential errors should not properly be categorized as complications, yet they underlie the great majority of unfavorable results seen in reduction mammaplasty. Some of them should be considered as inherent drawbacks to the operation which are beyond the surgeon's control and which both surgeon and patient are obliged to accept if they elect to undertake the

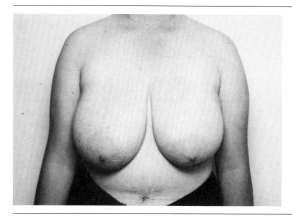
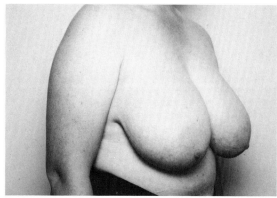

Fig. 30-31. Frontal and oblique preoperative views of a patient shown in operative series.

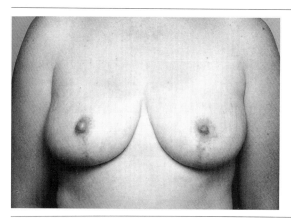
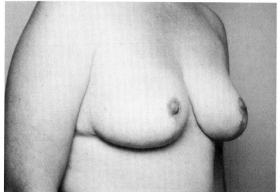

Fig. 30-32. Frontal and oblique views of patient in Figure 30-31 14 months after surgery.

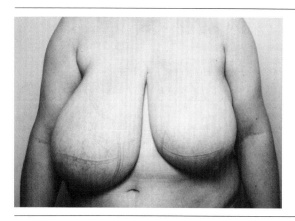
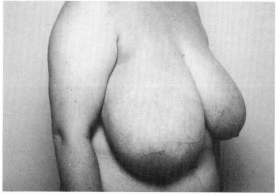

Fig. 30-33. Frontal and oblique preoperative views of a 56-year-old patient.

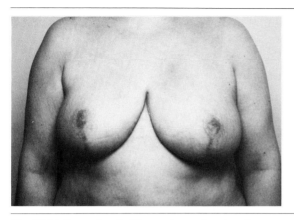
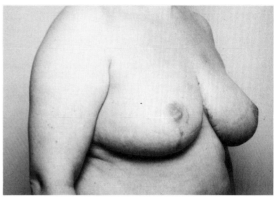

Fig. 30-34. Frontal and oblique views of patient in
Figure 30-33 1 year after surgery.

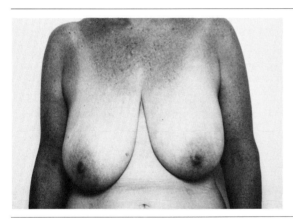
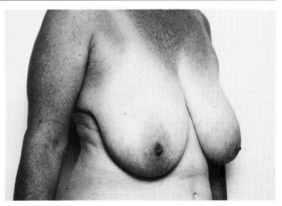

Fig. 30-35. Frontal and oblique preoperative views of a
27-year-old patient.

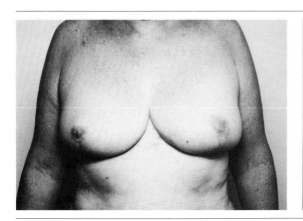
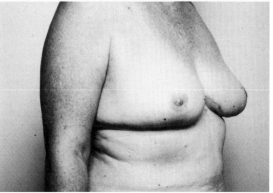

Fig. 30-36. Frontal and oblique views of patient in
Figure 30-35 18 months after surgery.

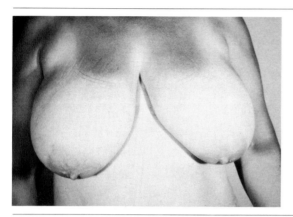
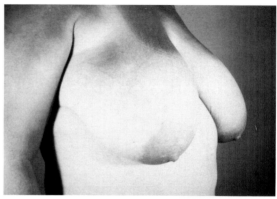

Fig. 30-37. Frontal and oblique preoperative views of a 35-year-old patient.

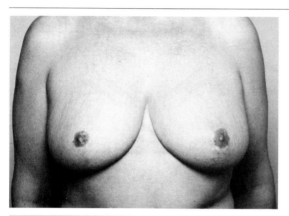
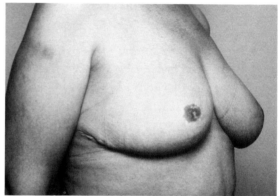

Fig. 30-38. Frontal and oblique views of patient in Figure 30-37 5 years after surgery.

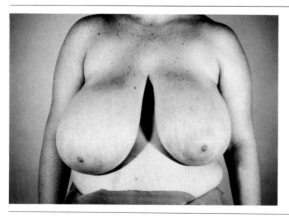
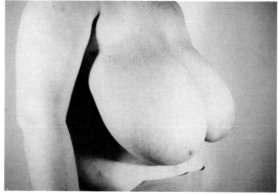

Fig. 30-39. Frontal and oblique preoperative views of a 37-year-old patient.

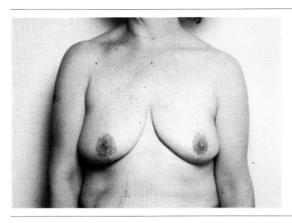
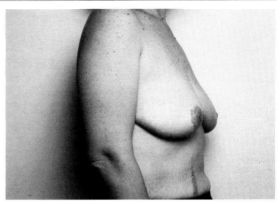

Fig. 30-40. Frontal and oblique views of patient in
Figure 30-39 10 years after surgery.

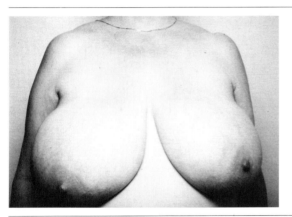
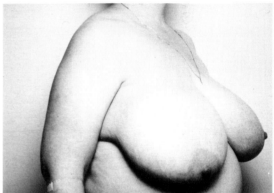

Fig. 30-41. Frontal and oblique preoperative views of a
40-year-old patient.

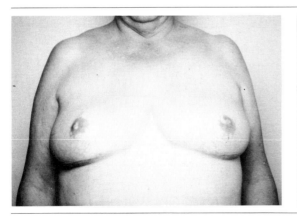
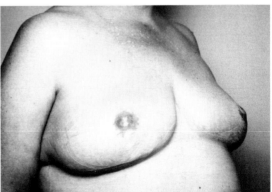

Fig. 30-42. Frontal and oblique views of patient in
Figure 30-41 3½ years after surgery.

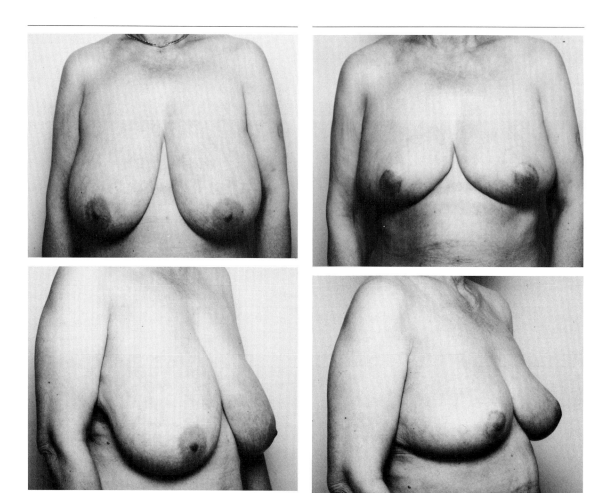

Fig. 30-43. Frontal and oblique preoperative views of a 60-year-old patient.

Fig. 30-44. Frontal and oblique views of patient in Figure 30-43 6 months after surgery.

surgery. Other factors that affect the quality of the result should come under the heading of artistic errors in craftsmanship, these are under the control of the surgeon and relate more to his or her understanding of the operation.

McKissock considers the complications and causative factors of avascular necrosis, partial and total loss of the nipple, skin loss, and fat necrosis. Among the inherent drawbacks, he discusses scarring, interference with lactation, changes in nipple-areolar sensibility, and the alterations with time in size and shape. Symmetry, breast shape, nipple position, and nipple-areolar deformities are

discussed as "artistic errors in craftsmanship." He mentions infection, poor wound healing, and hematoma for completeness.

Gigantomastia corrected by a partial amputation and reconstruction using free nipple-areolar grafts fortunately is a procedure relatively free of complications. There are no pedicles or undermined skin flaps with which to contend. The resection avoids the possibilities of an inadequate blood supply with loss of breast tissue, pedicles, flaps, nipples, and areolae. A desirable amount of tissue can be safely and expeditiously excised. Successful nipple-areolar grafts are the rule. Even partial loss of the nipple or areola is most unusual. With proper but easy planning, satisfying symmetrical facsimiles of the breasts with properly placed nipple-areolar grafts can be created.

Unfortunately, the inverted "T" scars of this procedure share the inherent drawback of the other modern methods of mammaplasty using this configuration. Hypertrophic scars and keloids may mar an otherwise pleasing result. Any variation in areolar pigmentation is amenable to tattooing.

Although the skillful surgeon will encounter a minimum of unfavorable results, McKissock admonishes that "if no one has ever said 'There has never been performed a mammoplasty completely free of any imperfections,' then I will say it now."

Goldwyn [27] has provided an excellent commentary on McKissock's thoughtful treatise.

In 1952, Conway [11] published his experience with 110 consecutive cases of mammaplasty. Various techniques of transposition of mammary gland were applied in 22 cases of macromastia with major complications in 6 cases (27%) and satisfactory results in only 12 cases (54.5%). Sixty-eight cases of macromastia were treated by partial breast amputation with free composite nipple grafts. With this technique of operation, there were no major complications. The nipple grafts were completely successful in 65 cases (95%). Transplanted nipples regained sensation and erectility. The result of operation was satisfactory in all cases. Eight patients who became pregnant following free transplantation of nipples exhibited no complications as a result of this technique of mammaplasty for macromastia.

Six years later, Conway [13] wrote that in 135 cases of macromastia, the operation used was "partial amputation of the breast (reduction mammaplasty) with construction of a mammary eminence and transplantation of the nipple as a free composite graft consisting of skin, erectile tissue and mammary ducts." Twenty-two minor complications were encountered, including "hypertrophic scars, hematoma, crusting of the central part of nipples with scarring, wound abscess, wound infection requiring drainage and subsequent secondary closure, and minor disruption of the suture line requiring secondary closure."

Importantly, there were no cases in which the free composite nipple grafts failed.

Loss of Lactation

The greatest disadvantage and the most often sited criticism of free nipple grafts is the loss of the ability to breast-feed. "The first which may be of great importance, is the complete loss of function of the breast as an organ of lactation. The disadvantages in the nipple transplant operation are the interruption of the lactiferous ducts, rendering lactation impossible . . . " [68].

Responsible and highly respected surgeons have reported cases of lactation following free nipple grafts, however. Curiously, Townsend [86] has reported that in a series of 23 patients in whom the nipple and areola were removed by sharp dissection and transplanted to a deep dermal bed, "only one patient had a baby after operation. She was seen six weeks postpartum and, although she had been warned that she would be unable to breast feed the baby, she reported vast quantities of milk in the left breast. Even after six weeks without any attempt at breast feeding, milk could be expressed from at least 7 ducts in the nipple." Townsend writes that "Strömbeck studied a number of mammograms after injecting 30 percent Urografin into the milk ducts. This revealed cross-connections between the lobes that had occurred following his operation" [76]. Townsend found it "interesting to speculate on the number of anastomotic cross-connections that must have occurred" following this patient's operation. However, he does not offer an explanation for the anastomosis of the lactiferous ducts.

Clarkson and Jeffs [10] in their paper on modern mammaplasty called attention to the fact that Gillies and Millard [26] reported a patient operated on by Clarkson who lactated after a free graft transplant in a breast reduction.

In The Principles and Art of Plastic Surgery by Gillies and Millard [26], Sir Harold Gillies wrote:

One would not expect the free-grafted nipple to lactate, but incredible as it may seem, here it is. Following an abdominal reduction, this case was turned over to P.C. to carry out a mammaplasty. He free-grafted the nipples. Two years later a note arrived from the patient stating she was in the National Maternity Hospital, Dublin, and that milk was flowing from her nipples. A letter was immediately sent to Dr. Barry, master of the hospital, pre- and postoperative photographs were enclosed, along with an explanation of the nipple free graft method that had been used. A request was made for his confirmation that milk was actually escaping through the nipples. Here is Dr. Barr's answer: "I can assure you that Mrs. X was making no mistake when she said that milk came out of her nipples. In view of the operation, I had advised that she should not feed her baby, and gave her stilboestrol. Much to my surprise, on the fourth day of the puerperium the breasts became active, secreting milk, which gained access to the outside world through the nipples."

Thorek [85], in the course of providing microscopic proof of the survival of the transplanted nipple, offers this report and translation of Professor Antonio Prudente [85] of Buenos Aires:

I think that it is of utmost importance to note certain observations made upon one of my patients who became pregnant shortly after the operation. During pregnancy, her physician observed colostrum coming from the transplanted nipple. After delivery, about 30 grams of milk came from the nipple each day.

There was enlargement of the new breast which could be the more readily appreciated through pictures sent me by the husband. In the beginning, I thought this impossible, but after meditating upon the question and listening to the opinion of Prof. Carmo Lordy, a noted embryologist, I came to the conclusion that I was confronted with true glandular regeneration. In the case in question, this regeneration was possible because of the transplantation of the nipple reestablishing communication with the lactoferous canals.

After further microscopic studies of the transplanted nipple in pregnant patients, Prudente [85] concluded:

When the terminal portions of the lactoferous canals are transplanted with the areola, the cells, having embryologic characteristics, have power to regenerate the glandular acini, which may be observed as regeneration of the mammary gland tissue; this being more pronounced in the presence of a pregnancy following the operation.

It is prudent and mandatory to emphasize to the patient that in obtaining a free composite nipple-areolar graft, the lactiferous ducts are completely severed; thus, lactation becomes theoretically impossible. But never, never say never!

Nipple Projection and Erectility

Reports concerned with nipple projection and erectility following free nipple-areolar transplants are found scattered through the literature. Craig and Sykes [16] state that in 13 cases (26 nipples), no patient had experienced erection of the nipples following operation. However, in Townsend's [86] series of 23 patients, "59 percent experienced

an erectile response and if one compares this with the objective findings where 72 percent had some muscle present it seems that even a small amount of muscle left in the transplanted nipple gives in most cases an erotic sensation." Indeed, these many differences may be attributed in large part to the presence or absence of smooth muscle in the nipple-areolar graft.

Sensitivity and Sensuality

Courtiss and Goldwyn [15] have made an extensive study of breast sensation before and after plastic surgery. Concerning reduction mammaplasty and free nipple-areola transplantation, they write:

When reconstruction was performed by using free nipple/areola grafts, no breast (even as long as two years after surgery) had normal sensation in the nipple and areola. However, some sensation (notably crude touch and light pressure, patchy and decreased at best) returned in all patients. Sensation in the peripheral skin was similar to that in those patients operated upon by the transposition methods.

Sensuality was reported as being normal, or even increased, by many patients — even when they could not perceive the painful stimulus and had a minimal response to crude touch and light pressure.

Craig and Sykes [16] reported that in techniques involving separation of the nipple from the mammary gland, six patients noticed no differences in sensitivity, and only one reported that postoperative sensation was impaired. Objectively, responses to cotton, wool, and pinprick were normal in seven nipples, but two-point discrimination was no less than 1 inch in any case. Six nipples gave a 50 percent response to cotton, wool, and pinprick. Finally, no sensitivity could be elicited in 13 nipples.

Townsend [86] studied the sensation in 46 transplants. There was no return of sensation in 8 grafts. In the remaining, sensation was enhanced in 2, normal in 11, and diminished in 23. Thus, sensation was felt in 82 percent of the breasts. The return of sensation varied over a period of 2 months to a year. He states:

The results are not quite so good as the overall figures suggest. Thus, of the 65 percent who had sensation to pin-prick, about half responded in only a moderate or patchy fashion. On the other hand, 2 of the transplanted nipples showed 2 point discrimination of ¼ inch; the best recorded for the controls was ½ inch, but it may well be that this was due to the stretched state of the nipple and areola.

Grenabo [28] tested the sensitivity of 80 grafted nipples. Among these 80 nipples, the sensitivity was totally lost in 1; in 35 nipples, the sensitivity was less than that on the skin of the breast; in 25 nipples, it was the same; and, in 16 nipples, it was better than in the skin over the breast.

Reduction and free nipple grafting is preferred by some plastic surgeons to methods using a pedicle-carried nipple and areola. It is believed that a better reconstructed facsimile of the breast can be obtained. Therefore, the patient is given the choice of a better shaped breast using a free graft or an increased chance of retaining sensation with transposition of the nipple and areola.

Conclusions

Professor Skoog, in his monumental work *Plastic Surgery* [74], directs attention to Sir Astley Cooper's eloquent comments on the beauty of the female breast and the functional significance of its shape. Almost 150 years ago (1840) Sir Astley Cooper [14] wrote:

The natural obliquity of the mamilla, or nipple, forwards and outwards, with a slight turn of the nipple upwards, is one of the most beautiful provisions in nature, both for the mother and the child. To the mother, because the child rests upon her arm and lap in the most convenient position for sucking, when the child reposes upon its mother's arm, it has its mouth directly applied to the nipple, which is turned outward to receive it; whilst the lower part of the breast forms a cushion upon which the chest of the infant tranquilly reposes.

After a reduction mammaplasty with free nipple-areolar grafts, it is impossible to reconstruct a breast of eloquent beauty that is endowed with the sensibilities and functional capabilities of the ideal breast. However, any appropriate amount of breast tissue may be safely and expeditiously resected. Reconstruction results in an aesthetically satisfying facsimile of the breast.

Furthermore, the procedure provides ready answers to the numerous aesthetic, social, and economic problems that have their source in breasts of gigantic proportions, and it relieves the physical disabilities and psychological distress imposed on the "big-breasted woman" [25–27, 29–39]. There is an extremely high degree of patient satisfaction.

References

1. Adams, W.M. Free transplantation of the nipples and areolae. *Surgery* 15:186, 1944.
2. Adams, W.M. One stage mammaryplasty, with free transplantation of the nipples. *Memphis Med. J.* 22:127, 1947.
3. Adams, W.M. Free composite grafts of the nipples in mammaryplasty. *South. Surg.* 13:715, 1947.
4. Adams, W.M. Technique of the operation for free composite grafts of the nipples in mammaryplasty. *Postgrad. Med.* 2:375, 1947.
5. Adams, W.M. Labial transplant for correction of loss of the nipple. *Plast. Reconstr. Surg.* 4:295, 1949.
6. Adams, W.M. Mammaplasty with free transplantation of the nipples and areolae: A thirteen-year follow-up report. In T. Skoog (ed.), Transactions of the First Congress of the International Society of Plastic Surgeons. Stockholm and Uppsala: 1955. Baltimore: Williams & Wilkins, 1957.
7. Aufricht, G. Mammaplasty for pendulous breasts; Empiric and geometric planning. *Plast. Reconstr. Surg.* 4:13, 1949.
8. Barnes, H.O. Gigantomastia; two-stage operation for reduction of extremely large breasts versus one-stage technic. *Plast. Reconstr. Surg.* 4:352, 1949.
9. Biesenberger, H. *Deformitäten und kosmetische Operationen der weiblichen Brust.* Vienna: Wilhelm Maudrich, 1931.
10. Clarkson, P., and Jeffs, J. Modern mammaplasty. *Br. J. Plast. Surg.* 20:297, 1967.
11. Conway, H. Mammaplasty: Analysis of 110 consecutive cases with end-results. *Plast. Reconstr. Surg.* 10:303, 1952.
12. Conway, H. Weight of breasts as handicap to respiration. Argument for reduction mammaplasty in selected cases. *Am. J. Surg.* 103:674, 1962.
13. Conway, H., and Smith, J. Breast plastic surgery: Reduction mammaplasty, mastopexy, augmentation mammaplasty, and mammary construction: Analysis of 245 cases. *Plast. Reconstr. Surg.* 21:8, 1958.
14. Cooper, A.P. *On the Anatomy of the Breast.* London: Longman, Orine, Green, Brown & Longmans, 1840.
15. Courtiss, E.H., and Goldwyn, R.M. Breast sensation before and after plastic surgery. *Plast. Reconstr. Surg.* 58:1, 1976.
16. Craig, R.D.P., and Sykes, P.A. Nipple sensitivity following reduction mammaplasty. *Br. J. Plast. Surg.* 23:165, 1970.
17. Crikelair, G.F., and Malton, S.D. Mammaplasty and occult breast malignancy: Case report. *Plast. Reconstr. Surg.* 23:601, 1959.
18. Crikelair, G.F., and Malton, S.D. Addendum to: Mammaplasty and occult breast malignancy. *Plast. Reconstr. Surg.* 31:176, 1963.
19. Crikelair, G.F., Richey, D., and Symonds, F.C. Histologic studies of the female breast before and after free nipple transplant. *Plast. Reconstr. Surg.* 34:590, 1964.
20. Dartigues, L. Traitement chirurgical du prolapsus mammaire. *Arch. Franco-Belg. Chir.* 28:313, 1925.
21. Dartigues, L. Etat actuel de la chirurgie esthetique mammaire. Les differentes procedes de mastoplastie en general et de la greffe areolomammelonnaire en particulier. *Monde Med.* 38:75, 1928.

22. Dartigues, L. Mammectomie totale et autogreffe libre areolo-mamelonnaire; mammectomie bilaterale esthetique. *Bull. Mem. Soc. Chir. Paris* 20:739, 1928.

23. Dartigues, L. De la greffe autoplastique libre areolo-mamelonnaire combinee a la mammectomie bilateral totale: Les raisons de sa prise. *Paris Chir.* 21:11, 1929.

24. Dartigues, L. Mammectomie bilateral totale avec greffe areolo-mamelonnaire libre. *Bull. Mem. Soc. Chir. Paris* 25:289, 1933.

25. Durston, W. Concerning the death of the big-breasted woman. *Philos. Trans. R. Soc. Lond.* IV:1068, 1670.

26. Gillies, H., and Millard, D.R., Jr. *The Principles and Art of Plastic Surgery.* Boston: Little, Brown, 1957.

27. Goldwyn, R.M. Comments on McKissock, P.K. Complications and Undesirable Results with Reduction Mammaplasty. In R.M. Goldwyn (ed.), *The Unfavorable Result in Plastic Surgery.* Boston: Little, Brown, 1984.

28. Grenabo, K-J. Discussion in W. M. Adams. Mammaplasty with free transplantation of the nipples and areolae: A thirteen-year follow-up report. In T. Skoog (ed.), Transactions of the First Congress of the International Society of Plastic Surgeons, Stockholm and Uppsala, 1955. Baltimore: Williams & Wilkins, 1957.

29. Gupta, S.C. A critical review of contemporary procedures for mammary reduction. *Br. J. Plast. Surg.* 18:328, 1965.

30. Kaye, B. Neurologic changes with excessively large breasts. *South. Med. J.* 65:177, 1972.

31. Kendall, H., Kendall, F., and Boynton, D. *Posture and Pain.* Baltimore: Williams & Wilkins, 1952.

32. Lalardrie, J.P., and Jouglard, J.P. *Chirurgie Plastique du Sein.* Paris: Masson & Cie, 1974.

33. Lamont, E.S. Plastic surgery in reconstructing enlarged breasts. *Surgery* 17:379, 1945.

34. Lamont, E.S. Plastic surgery in mammoth breasts. *Surgery* 25:276, 1949.

35. Letterman, G.S., and Schurter, M. Total mammary gland excision with immediate breast reconstruction. *Am. Surg.* 21:835, 1955.

36. Letterman, G.S., and Schurter, M.A. Experiences with Adenomammectomy and Immediate Breast Reconstruction. In T.R. Broadbent (ed.), Transactions of the IV International Congress of Plastic Surgery, International Congress Series No. 174:1023. Amsterdam: Excerpta Medica Foundation, 1967.

37. Letterman, G.S., and Schurter, M.A. Experiences with adenomammectomy and immediate breast reconstruction. *Panminerva Med.* 9:467, 1967.

38. Letterman, G., and Schurter, M. Reconstruction of the breast following subcutaneous simple mastectomy. *J. Am. Med. Wom. Assoc.* 23:911, 1968.

39. Letterman, G., and Schurter, M. Will Durston' "Mammaplasty." *Plast. Reconstr. Surg.* 53:48, 1974.

40. Letterman, G., and Schurter, M. Inframammary-based dermofat flaps in mammary reconstruction following a subcutaneous mastectomy. *Plast. Reconstr. Surg.* 55:156, 1975.

41. Letterman, G., and Schurter, M. A comparison of modern methods of reduction mammaplasty. *South. Med. J.* 69:1367, 1976.

42. Letterman, G., and Schurter, M.A. A History of Mammaplasty with Emphasis on Correction of Ptosis and Macromastia. In R.M. Goldwyn (ed.), *Plastic and Reconstructive Surgery of the Breast.* Boston: Little Brown, 1976.

43. Letterman, G., and Schurter, M. Adenomammectomy. *Surg. Clin. North Am.* 57:1035, 1977.

44. Letterman, G., and Schurter, M. History of Reduction Mammaplasty. In J.G. Owsley, Jr. and R.A. Peterson (eds.), *Symposium on Aesthetic Surgery of the Breast.* St. Louis: Mosby, 1978.

45. Letterman, G., and Schurter, M. The effects of mammary hypertrophy on the skeletal system. *Ann. Plast. Surg.* 7:425, 1980.

46. Letterman, G., and Schurter, M. Suggested nomenclature for aesthetic and reconstructive surgery of the breast. Part I: Breast reduction. *Aesth. Plast. Surg.* 7:187, 1983.

47. Letterman, G., and Schurter, M. Free nipple-areolar grafts in reduction mammaplasty. Presented at the Seventeenth Annual Meeting of the American Society for Aesthetic Plastic Surgery. Washington, D.C., 1984.

48. Letterman, G., and Schurter, M. A sitting position for mammaplasty with general anesthesia. *Ann. Plast. Surg.* 20:522, 1988.

49. Letterman, G., and Schurter, M. Reduction Mammoplasty with Free Nipple Grafts. In M. Gonzalez-Ulloa, R. Meyer, J.W. Smith and G. Zaoli (eds.), *Aesthetic Plastic Surgery* (Vol. 4). Padova: Piccin, 1988.

50. Letterman, G., and Schurter, M. History of Aesthetic Breast Surgery. In J.R. Lewis, Jr. (ed.), *The Art of Aesthetic Plastic Surgery.* Boston: Little Brown, 1989.

51. Letterman, G., and Schurter, M. Effects of Mammary Hypertrophy on the Skeletal System. In J.R. Lewis, Jr. (ed.), *The Art of Aesthetic Plastic Surgery.* Boston: Little, Brown, 1989.

52. Lexer, E. Hypertrophie bei der Mammae. *Munch. Med. Wochenschr.* 59:2702, 1912.

53. Malbec, H. Glandular mastectomy: Immediate reconstruction. *Plast. Reconstr. Surg.* 10:204, 1952.

54. Maliniac, J.W. Pendulous hypertrophic breast: Comparative values of present-day methods of repair and procedure of choice. *Arch. Surg.* 31:587, 1935.

55. Maliniac, J.W. Critical analysis of mammectomy and free transplantation of the nipple in mammaplasty. *Am. J. Surg.* 65:364, 1944.

56. Maliniac, J.W. Amputation versus transposition of gland and nipple in mammaplasty. *Plast. Reconstr. Surg.* 3:37, 1948.

57. Maliniac, J.W. Evaluation of principal mammaplastic procedures. *Plast. Reconstr. Surg.* 4:359, 1949.

58. Maliniac, J.W. *Breast Deformities and Their Repair.* New York: Grune & Stratton, 1950.

59. Marino, H. Glandular mastectomy: Immediate reconstruction. *Plast. Reconstr. Surg.* 10:204, 1952.

60. Martin, J.T. The Head Elevated Position. In J.T. Martin (ed.), *Positioning in Anesthesia and Surgery.* Philadelphia: Saunders, 1978.

61. Martin, J.T. General Requirements of Safe Positioning for the Surgical Patients. In J.T. Martin (ed.), *Position in Anesthesia and Surgery.* Philadelphia: Saunders, 1978.

62. May, H. Mammaplastic procedures in the female. *Pa. Med.* 53:609, 1950.

63. May, H. Breast plasty in the female. *Plast. Reconstr. Surg.* 17:351, 1956.

64. May, H. *Reconstructive and Reparative Surgery* (2nd ed). Philadelphia: F.A. Davis, 1958.

65. May, H. Breast plasty in hypertrophy of the female breast. *J. Germantown Hosp.* 6:65, 1965.

66. McKissock, P.K. Reduction mammaplasty. *Ann. Plast. Surg.* 2:321, 1979.

67. McKissock, P.K. Complications and Undesirable Results with Reduction Mammoplasty. In R.M. Goldwyn (ed.), *The Unfavorable Result in Plastic Surgery.* Boston: Little, Brown, 1984.

68. Morris, W.J. Reduction Mammaplasty with Free Nipple and Areolar Grafts. In J.Q. Owsley, Jr., and R.A. Peterson (eds.), *Symposium on Aesthetic Plastic Surgery of the Breasts.* St. Louis: Mosby, 1978.

69. Pitanguy, I. *Aesthetic Plastic Surgery of Head and Body.* Berlin/Heidelberg/New York: Springer Verlag, 1981.

70. Schurter, M., and Letterman, G. Amputation mammaplasty with free nipple grafts. *J. Am. Med. Wom. Assoc.* 16:854, 1961.

71. Schurter, M., and Letterman, G. Subcutaneous mastectomy. *J. Am. Med. Wom. Assoc.* 27:463, 1972.

72. Schurter, M., and Letterman, G. Breast deformities and their surgical repair. *J. Invest. Dermatol.* 63:138, 1974.

73. Schurter, M., and Letterman, G. Comment on Personal Preferences for Reduction Mammaplasty by I. Pitanguy. In R.M. Goldwyn (ed.), *Plastic and Reconstructive Surgery of the Breast.* Boston: Little, Brown, 1976.

74. Skoog, T. *Plastic Surgery.* Stockholm: Almquist & Wiksell International, 1974.

75. Strömbeck, J.O. Mammaplasty: Report of a new technique based on the two-pedicle procedure. *Br. J. Plast. Surg.* 13:79, 1960.

76. Strömbeck, J.O. Macromastia in women and its surgical treatment. *Acta. Chir. Scand.* 341[Suppl.]:1, 1964.

77. Thorek, M. Possibilities in the reconstruction of the human form. *N. Y. Med. J. Med. Rec.* 116:572, 1922.

78. Thorek, M. Esthetic surgery of the pendulous breast, abdomen and arms in the female. *Ill. Med. J.* 58:48, 1930.

79. Thorek, M. Histological verification of the efficacy of free transplantation of the nipple. *N. Y. Med. J. Med. Rec.* 134:474, 1931.

80. Thorek, M. The possibilities of surgical esthetic remodeling of the human form. *Tri-State Med. J.* 3:621, 1931.

81. Thorek, M. Simplicity versus complicated methods in the reconstruction of pendulous breasts. *Ill. Med. J.* 69:338, 1936.

82. Thorek, M. Plastic reconstruction of the female breasts and abdomen. *Am. J. Surg.* 43:268, 1939.

83. Thorek, M. *Plastic Surgery of the Breast and Abdominal Wall.* Springfield, IL: Thomas, 1942.

84. Thorek, M. Twenty-five years' experience with plastic reconstruction of the breast and transplantation of the nipple. *Am. J. Surg.* 67:445, 1945.

85. Thorek, M. Plastic reconstruction of the breasts and free transplantation of the nipple. *Int. Surg.* 9:194, 1946.

86. Townsend, P.L.G. Nipple sensation following breast reduction and free nipple transplantation. *Br. J. Plast. Surg.* 27:308, 1974.

87. Updegraff, H.L. Reconstruction of the breast. *Calif. West. Med.* 46:28, 1937.

88. Winkler, E. Subtotale Mammektomie mit freier Mamillen-transplantation bei chronischer Mastopathie und Mammahypertrophie. *Langenbecks Arch. Chir.* 286:14, 1957.

89. Wise, R.J. A preliminary report on a method of planning the mammaplasty. *Plast. Reconstr. Surg.* 17:367, 1956.

90. Wise, R.J. Surgical Management of the Hypertrophic Breast. In F.W. Masters and J.R. Lewis, Jr. (eds.), *Symposium on Aesthetic Surgery of the Face, Eyelid, and Breast.* Phoenix, 1970. St Louis: Mosby, 1972.

91. Wise, R.J. Breast Reduction with Nipple Transplantation. In R.M. Goldwyn (ed.), *Plastic and Reconstructive Surgery of the Breast.* Boston: Little, Brown, 1976.

92. Wise, R.J., Gannon, J.P., and Hill, J.R. Further experience with reduction mammaplasty. *Plast. Reconstr. Surg.* 32:12, 1963.

31

Gilbert P. Gradinger

Reduction Mammaplasty with Nipple Graft

Every woman seeking reduction mammaplasty wants smaller, comfortable, attractive breasts. Every reduction mammaplasty technique involves removal of excess breast tissue, excess skin, reshaping the breast, and elevating the nipple-areola complex to a natural position, either as part of a pedicle or as a free graft. The two most important factors in deciding which nipple-moving technique to be used is establishing whether or not it is important to the patient to maintain the ability to breast-feed and to retain pleasurable nipple sensation.

There is probably no other elective plastic surgical procedure that has as widespread or as equal a distribution in age as reduction mammaplasty (Fig. 31-1).

Having already stated that the major advantage of nipple transposition procedures are the retention of the ability to breast-feed and the preservation of nipple sensation, one must ask, "What are the advantages of the free nipple graft?" In my opinion, the most important advantages are simplicity and safety. It is simpler to shape the breast because it is unnecessary to fashion a separate pedicle of tissue to transport the nipple-areola complex. In the free nipple graft procedure, the skin and breast tissue are treated as a single entity [7]. It is safer because there is no folding of pedicle tissue; thus, the risk of nipple or fat necrosis within the pedicle is eliminated.

Patients Who Undergo Nipple Graft

We utilize the nipple transposition technique (usually inferior pedicle) in approximately 80 percent of our patients. The free nipple graft group (20%) is comprised of the following categories of

patients: (1) postmenopausal women with very large breasts who have little or no pleasurable nipple sensation; (2) patients with large, painful, tender, lumpy breasts that are difficult to examine; (3) patients with hypertrophy and nipple inversion; (4) postmastectomy patients whose remaining breast is hypertrophied; and (5) patients with gigantomasty (i.e., over 1,000 gm to be removed per breast). It has been noted in the literature that the larger the breasts, the less likely it is that there will be normal sensuality preoperatively [8], and, regardless of which transportion procedure is performed, the greater the amount of tissue removed, the greater the disturbance in postoperative sensation [4]. The same authors made several pertinent and important points viz-a-viz nipple-areola grafting:

1. If the smooth muscle is removed, as in thinned nipple and areolar grafts, normal erection will be lost.
2. Response to crude touch, light pressure, and painful stimuli is uniformly diminished postoperatively.
3. Sensuality was reported as being normal or even increased postoperatively by many patients.

They concluded that "diminished sensation of the skin of the breast, areola, or nipple is not synonymous with impaired sensuality."

This chapter is based largely on G.P. Gradinger. Reduction mammoplasty utilizing nipple-areola transplantation. *Clin. Plast. Surg.* 15:641, 1988.

Patient Counseling

All patients are advised that they are considering trading large, uncomfortable breasts without scars for smaller, comfortable breasts with scars. When the transposition procedure is recommended, the patient is advised that she may be unable to breast-feed and that there will probably be some alteration in nipple sensation. She is also advised of the remote possibility of having to convert the nipple transposition procedure to a nipple graft if there are circulatory disturbances to the nipple observed during or soon after surgery. Patients undergoing nipple-areola graft are told that they will not be able to breast-feed and that there will probably be little, if any, feeling in their nipples, but that they will most likely regain nipple projection and erectility [9]. Adams [1] presented two cases of nipple-areola transplantation at the American Society of Plastic and Reconstructive Surgeons meeting in 1942. In both, there was return of erectility, elevation, normal tactile sensation, and constriction of the areola. Anderson [2], reporting on 25 patients, found no failure of graft take, noting that slough of the tip of the nipple was not uncommon; he thought that the literature was full of misinformation regarding the results of nipple grafting and that virtually all his patients developed a reasonable sensitivity and erectility. Our findings closely parallel the findings of these earlier authors.

Preoperative Evaluation, Planning, and Marking

When the attractive breast is viewed in profile, the nipple is the most prominent point. The breast shape is not truly conical, but there is or should be a definite apex. If the nipple-areola complex is to project properly, it needs to rest on an elevated platform that resists settling. Regardless of which reduction mammaplasty procedure is used, the breast mass settles relatively more than the nipple-areola. The best platform for the nipple-areola (whether transposed or transplanted) is provided when medial and lateral skin and breast tissue flaps are brought together in a near-conical manner. Planning for accomplishing this is described and illustrated. Evaluating and premarking the patient's breast while she is sitting comfortably is the most accurate method in my hands. Because the appearance of the breast is judged with the patient upright, it seems logical that the surgery should be planned with the patient upright. With proper planning, no intraoperative adjustments in skin incisions or nipple location are necessary [10, 11].

Determining Nipple Location

In the attractive female breast, the lower border of the areola is just above the level of the submammary fold (Fig. 31-2). Armstrong [3] demonstrated that marking this point on the hypertrophied breast is greatly simplified by the use of a tape measure or flexible ruler (Fig. 31-3). This level can also be determined with the use of an obstetric caliper or by holding the breast with a finger in the fold and the thumb on the anterior breast skin at the level of the fold. Arbitrary measurements, such as the distance from the midclavicular line or suprasternal notch, are used as verifying points of reference. The midhumeral point is not used because it is almost always too high for nipple location. The nipple should rarely be planned less than 20 cm from the midclavicular or midsternal point. The upper areola point is marked 2.5 cm above the nipple, and the lower areola point 2.5 cm below the nipple. Five centimeters below the lower areola point is the point where inferior edges of the medial and lateral flaps will be brought together postoperatively (Fig. 31-4A). The medial extent of the submammary incision should end 2 to 3 cm from the midline to avoid a visible scar in that area. The posterior end of the incision should not extend beyond the anterior axillary line. The length of the inframammary line and the length of the anterior surface of the breast (Fig. 31-4B) are measured. The difference in these two lengths will determine how wide the keyhole pattern will be spread. The length of the medial and lateral flaps when added together equal the length of the submammary line (Fig. 31-4C). Figure 31-4D demonstrates that with asymmetric breasts, the markings are similarly asymmetric to achieve the same final result. Figure 31-4E illustrates the geometric principles that the more obtuse an angle is, the greater the coning effect of closing that angle and reconstituting a circle. This emphasizes the importance of not only spreading the arms of the keyhole pattern, but also opening the portion of the pattern that is to become the circle that will accommodate the nipple-areola graft.

Breast Contour

After the marking has been completed, it is necessary to evaluate the thickness of the skin and breast flaps. Planning postoperative breast volume is less complicated and more accurate than in the transposition procedure in which the flap that carries the nipple and areola contributes significantly

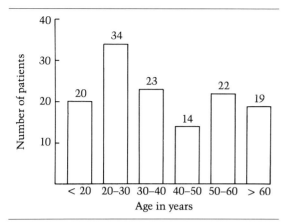

Fig. 31-1. This graph shows the age distribution of 132 consecutive patients in a 3-year period undergoing reduction mammaplasty.

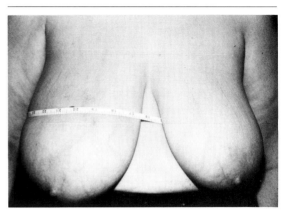

Fig. 31-3. A method of locating the lower edge of the nipple-areola at the inframammary fold. (The use of obstetric calipers or the thumb on the anterior surface of the breast and the index finger in the fold are equally effective.)

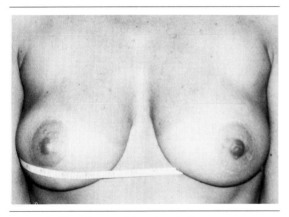

Fig. 31-2. This 36-year-old patient is 2 years postmastopexy. The lower border of the areola is properly located at the level of the inframammary line.

Surgical Procedure

The patient's preoperative photographs are placed in an easily visible position in the operating room. With the patient under general anesthesia, the previously made skin markings are scratched prior to final skin preparation. Final markings with dye-impregnated needles are carried out after preparation and drape (Fig. 31-5). The nipple-areola is excised, preserving its full thickness as a composite graft. It is not thinned; it is only defatted (Fig. 31-6). It is important to preserve the smooth muscles to achieve postoperative nipple projection and areola contractility.

It is most important to leave breast tissue between the medial and lateral flaps to augment breast projection and to produce a rounded or conical look. The amount of tissue to be retained varies in different patients (Fig. 31-7A, B). After resection of the lower portion of the breast, medial and lateral flaps are temporarily sutured and the submammary line is sutured from its medial and lateral aspects toward the center (Fig. 31-8A). Accurate preoperative planning eliminates the need for any adjustment of these flaps. No glandular or subcutaneous sutures are used. The procedure is performed with running subcuticular absorbable suture (Fig. 31-7B). At this point, there is good projection of the dermal bed on which the nipple-areola graft will be placed (Fig. 31-7C). The nipple graft is then sutured in place (Fig. 31-7D). Jackson-Pratt drains are placed through small separate stab

to the breast bulk. By evaluating the skin and the underlying breast tissue preoperatively with the patient in the sitting position, a decision can be made as to how thick the flaps should be and how much breast tissue is to be retained between the edges of the medial and lateral skin flaps. In almost every case, the greatest amount of tissue is removed from the lateral flap. It is seldom necessary or advisable to significantly thin the medial flap. Because of asymmetry, in addition to markings being different, the amount of breast tissue retained in the flaps must be adjusted.

516

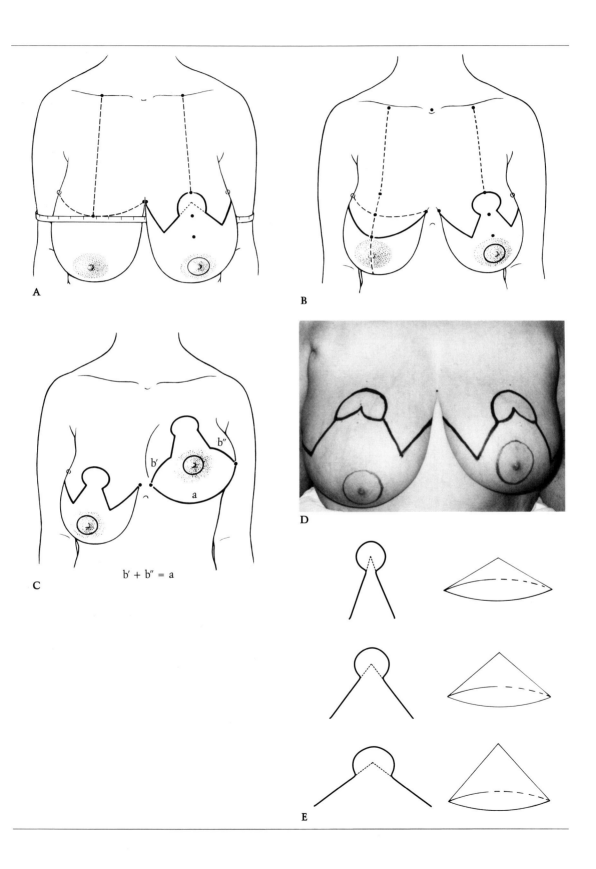

$b' + b'' = a$

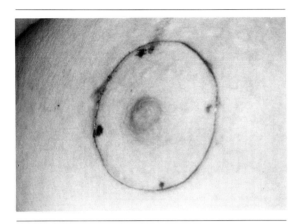

Fig. 31-5. The 5-cm areola circle is marked with methylene blue containing needles at four equidistant points prior to excising the nipple-areola graft. Two dots are placed at 12 o'clock for proper orientation when suturing the graft.

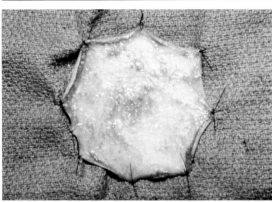

Fig. 31-6. The deep surface of the nipple-areola graft shows intact dermis and nipple base. The smooth muscle fibers are retained in this composite graft.

Fig. 31-4. A. The lower areola point being marked on the right breast at the lowest point on the curved submammary line and in proper relation to the breast meridian. The marking of the left breast is complete. The upper point of the keyhole is not less than 18 to 19 cm below the midclavicular line and is 5 cm above the lower areola point. The inferior border of the medial and lateral flaps will be brought together 5 cm below the lower areolar point. B. This demonstrates the convex line drawn on the anterior surface of the right breast and the dotted inframammary line. The length of the inframammary line is subtracted from the length of the convex line on the anterior surface of the breast. The numerical difference then indicates how widely the keyhole pattern needs to be opened at its lowest point. That is how the pattern on the left breast was determined. C. The length of the medial and lateral flaps when added together equals the length of the submammary line. The 5 cm circle has been drawn on the areola with the nipple in the center. D. Asymmetric breasts will have different-shaped patterns; the keyhole is more widely open on the larger breast. Note that the planned nipple site on the right breast is not on the same meridian as the patient's nipple preoperatively. It is necessary that this change be planned to avoid placement of the nipple too far medially. E. This shows that the more obtuse the angle of the pattern (that is, the wider open the keyhole pattern), the greater the coning effect when the pattern is closed. This is true of the projected nipple site, as well as the limbs of the medial and lateral flaps. This is very important in providing a projecting platform on which to suture the nipple-areola graft.

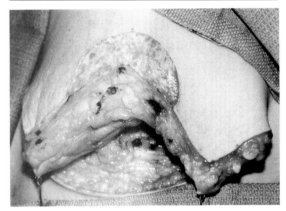

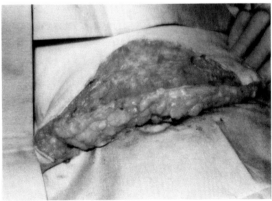

Fig. 31-7. Different amounts of breast tissue will be retained between the medial and lateral flaps, depending on the thickness of the breast and the amount of bulk necessary to properly shape the breast.

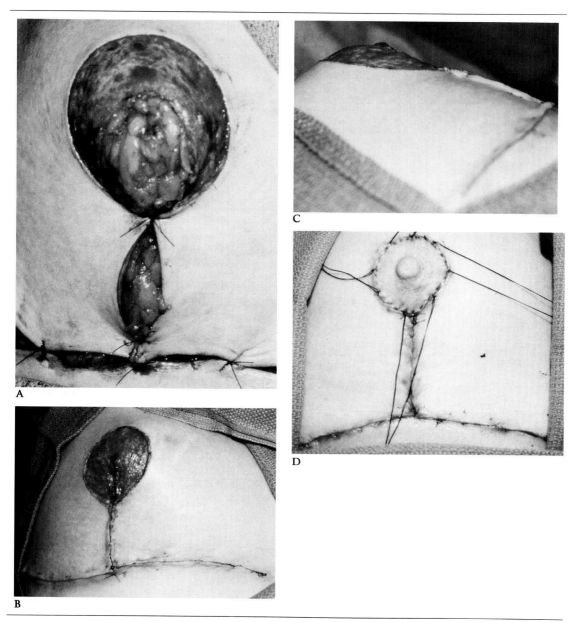

Fig. 31-8. A. The temporary sutures for reconstituting the breast have been placed. Note the coning effect. If more bulk is needed, the breast tissue between the flaps is preserved or an inferior central mound of tissue is left as demonstrated in Figure 31-9. B. The single-layer closure with subcuticular absorbable suture is completed. C. With the patient supine, this lateral photograph shows the projection of the dermal platform on which the graft will be placed. D. The silk sutures are left long to be used for tying a bolster of fine-mesh gauze and polyfoam sponge over the graft. Sutures are full thickness on the areolar side and dermis only on the skin side. Sutures that penetrate the areola do not leave suture marks postoperatively.

wounds in the skin below the inframammary fold prior to closure. Steri-Strips are used on the skin, and a circumferential bandage is put in place. A patient technique adapted to give even, better rounding in the lower portion of the breast is illustrated in Figure 31-9. The mound of breast tissue that is left after deepithelialization closely simulates the lower portion of the inferior pedicle in the transposition technique. It helps to overcome any flattening that may appear when one is using relatively thin flaps.

Postoperative Course

The patient is typically hospitalized 1 or 2 days, and the drains are removed before the patient is discharged in a soft cotton brassiere. At 10 days, the typical patient shows evidence of areola take and necrosis of the surface of the nipple (Fig. 31-10A, B). This necrosis is expected. It is the only procedure in plastic surgery of which I am aware that the surgeon anticipates partial necrosis of a graft. If there is no superficial necrosis, it is probably evidence that the graft was thinned too much and final projection and erectility will be absent. Figures 31-10C through F demonstrate the 3-year follow-up on the patient presented with the 10-day postoperative superficial nipple necrosis.

Long-Term Follow-up

A pleasing breast shape is achieved and maintained (Fig. 31-11). The shape of the breast does not change appreciably over many years. This is true even in patients who demonstrate poor dermal elasticity and skin resiliency. There is a natural settling owing to stretching of the skin with time. One of the major advantages of the nipple-areola graft is that the scar at the junction of the skin and areola is less likely to show either widening or hypertrophy than with transposition procedures. This is probably because there is no pull of the pedicle or tension in the suturing.

Postoperative Problems and Complications

Scars are the most frequent consequence of reduction mammaplasty. The quality of scars following reduction mammaplasty is unpredictable. Regardless of the procedure, scars in the submammary fold may hypertrophy. The vertical scar from the lower border of the areola to the submammary fold rarely hypertrophies. If the breasts are extremely heavy medially, it may be necessary to join the skin and breast resection from the two sides. One way of doing this without leaving scars that are visible in any form of clothing is illustrated in Figure 31-12. It is very important that this midline excision be in the form of a V, as either a transverse or vertical excision will result in a midline scar hypertrophy.

GRAFT NIPPLE CIRCULATORY PROBLEMS

Figure 31-13 demonstrates a technique that can be utilized intraoperatively or probably in the first 24 hours postoperatively if the patient develops signs of inadequate circulation to the nipple-areola complex. Conversion of a nipple-areola transposition procedure to a nipple-areola free graft is simple in a superior pedicle or a vertical bipedicle procedure. It is probably also possible to do it in an inferior pedicle procedure by placing the graft on the dermal bed of the inferior pedicle at a distance 6 to 8 cm from its base.

LONG-TERM POSTOPERATIVE PROBLEMS

Nipple position and settling are common postoperative problems. One of the most common problems seen in long-term follow-up in reduction mammaplasty patients is the appearance that the "bottom has fallen off." This is most often because the nipple was placed too high on the chest wall. The second cause is that the bulk of the breast tissue from a horizontally oriented bipedicle flap or from an inferior pedicle flap tends to go back to its original dependent position and descend while the nipple stays in its new elevated location. The tendency for this to happen in a nipple-areola graft procedure is greatly reduced. The explanation for this is the fact that breast tissue and skin are a single entity. Only one patient in our series demonstrated a significant appearance of nipples riding too high on the breast mass postoperatively (Fig. 31-14). Surgical correction was accomplished by excising skin and breast tissue from both the vertical and horizontal directions from the lower areolar point to the submammary fold (Fig. 31-14).

NIPPLE-AREOLA DEPIGMENTATION

None of the Caucasian patients in our series demonstrated significant depigmentation in the nipple-areola graft. Any patient with dark pigmented nipple-areola may demonstrate depigmentation postoperatively (Fig. 31-15A, B). Repigmentation can be achieved by punch-graft from the areola

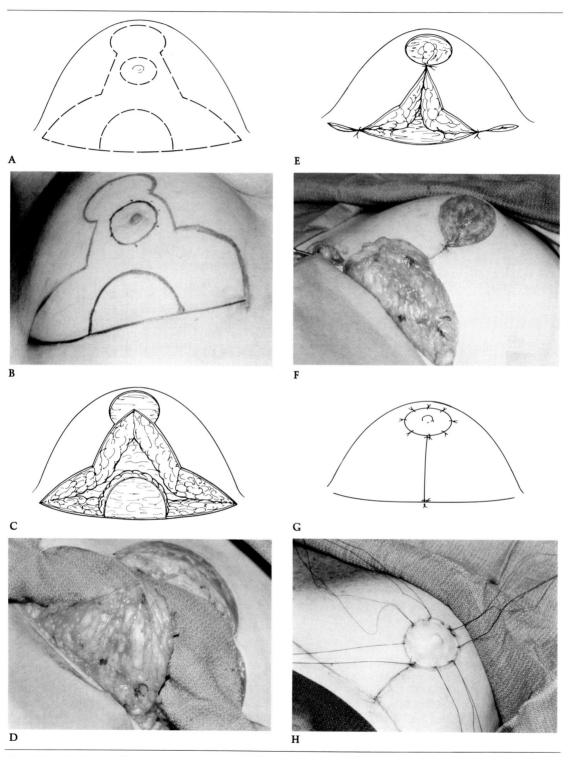

Fig. 31-9. A, B. A centrally located inferior mound of breast tissue that is retained to form a pleasing, rounded appearance to the inferior aspect of the breast. This mound is approximately 8 cm in length and 7 cm in height. C, D. The centrally located mound and the breast tissue that has been resected. E, F. The breast having been partially reconstituted and the central mound still not having been placed deep to the skin. G, H. The completed closure.

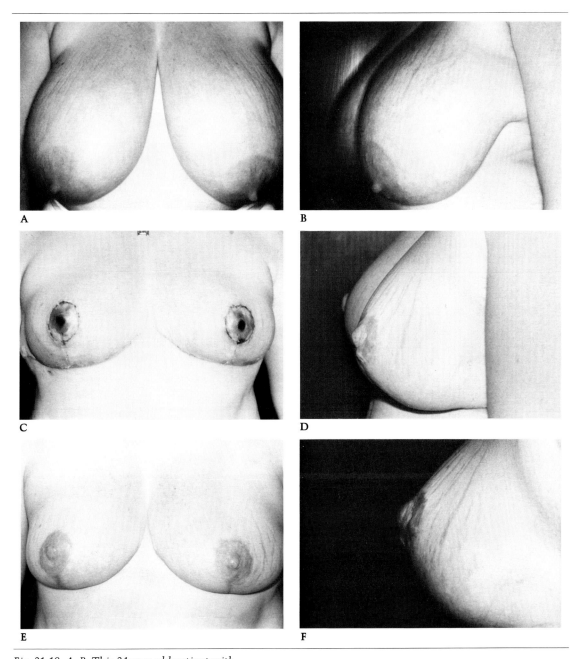

Fig. 31-10. A, B. This 34-year-old patient with
symmetrical hypertrophy had 2500 gm of tissue
excised. C. On the tenth postoperative day, the typical
appearance of the superficial portion of the nipple
graft undergoing avascular necrosis is seen. D–F. The
close-up of the nipple-areola graft at 3 years. This graft
shows good contractility and erectility.

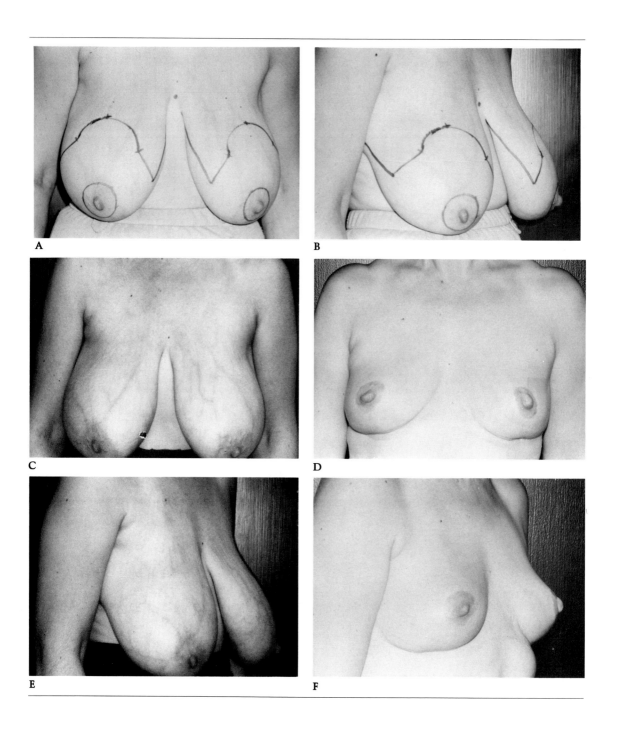

A

B

C

D

E

F

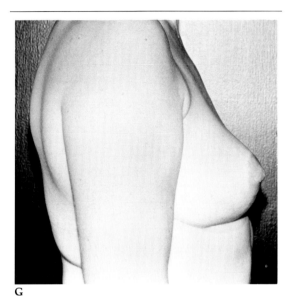

G

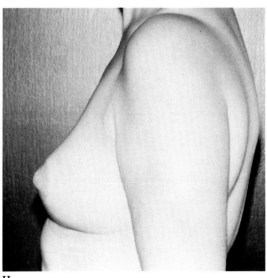

H

Fig. 31-11. A 33-year-old patient who underwent resection of 800 gm of tissue from each breast and a nipple-areola transplantation type of reduction mammaplasty. A. Preoperative markings. Note especially the wide spread of the keyhole pattern. This can also be noted in B. C. Preoperative view with the distended superficial veins and the marked ptosis. D. Eight-year follow-up frontal view. E. Oblique preoperative view. F. Oblique postoperative view. G. Right lateral view. H. Left lateral eight-year follow-up view. These photographs demonstrate the maintenance of the projection of the nipple at the apex of the breast without elongation of the height of skin and breast tissue between the nipple and the inframammary fold.

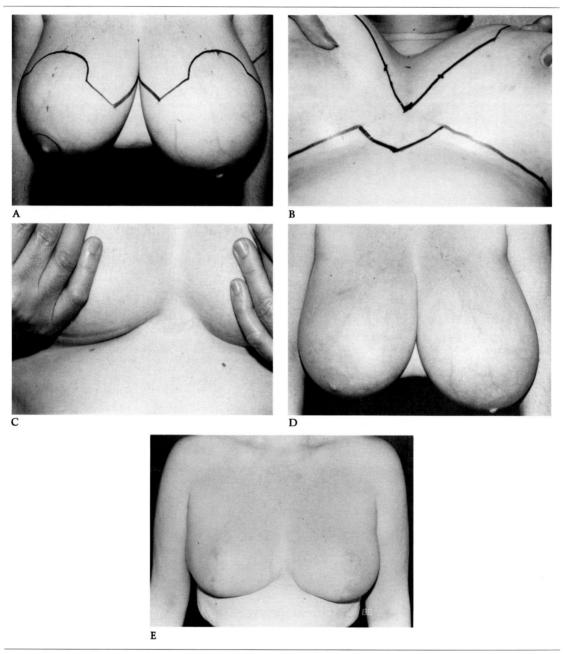

Fig. 31-12. These photographs demonstrate excision of the midline skin in an inferior direction in a patient who has very broad, full breasts medially. A. A 45-year-old patient with very heavy breasts and midline overlap. B. V-excision of skin, subcutaneous tissue, and breast tissue to aid in contouring the midline. Note that the scar is directed inferiorly to avoid a scar that would be visible in any type of clothing. C. The scar is of good quality 5 years postoperatively. D. Preoperative view. E. Five-year postoperative view.

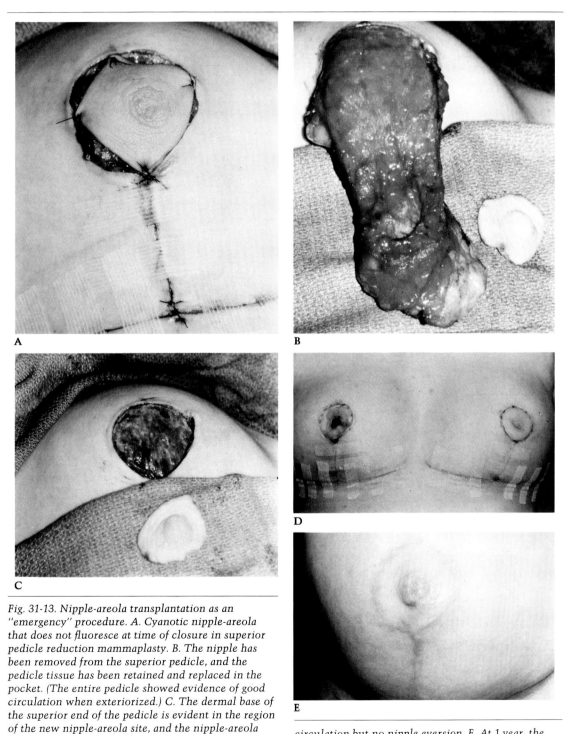

Fig. 31-13. Nipple-areola transplantation as an "emergency" procedure. A. Cyanotic nipple-areola that does not fluoresce at time of closure in superior pedicle reduction mammaplasty. B. The nipple has been removed from the superior pedicle, and the pedicle tissue has been retained and replaced in the pocket. (The entire pedicle showed evidence of good circulation when exteriorized.) C. The dermal base of the superior end of the pedicle is evident in the region of the new nipple-areola site, and the nipple-areola graft is ready for suturing. D. At 10 days, the nipple-areola graft of the right breast shows a superficial necrosis. The left nipple-areola complex has good circulation but no nipple eversion. E. At 1 year, the nipple-areola complex appears quite normal. The breast contour shows that the ability to retain the bulk of the pedicle glandular tissue resulted in a nicely shaped breast.

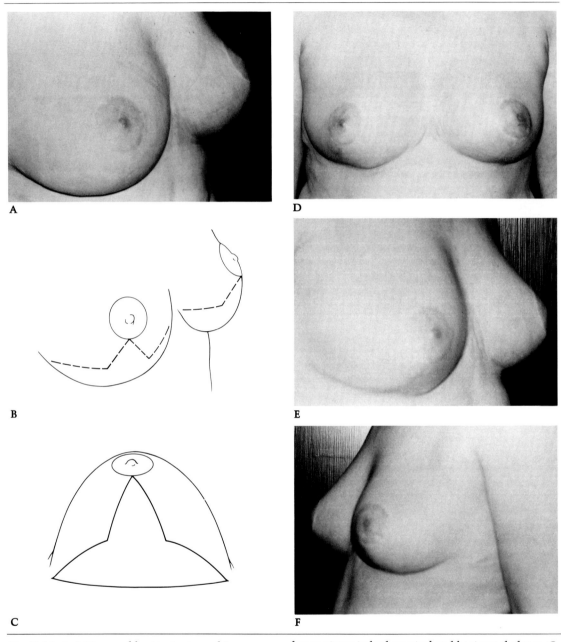

Fig. 31-14. A. A 55-year-old patient returned 2 years after resection of 2200 gm of tissue and noted that her "nipples were too high." B. Diagrammatic representation of skin excision with small amount of breast tissue in both vertical and horizontal planes. C. Gland excision viewed from undersurface of breast. D–F. Frontal and bilateral oblique views 1 year after revision was performed.

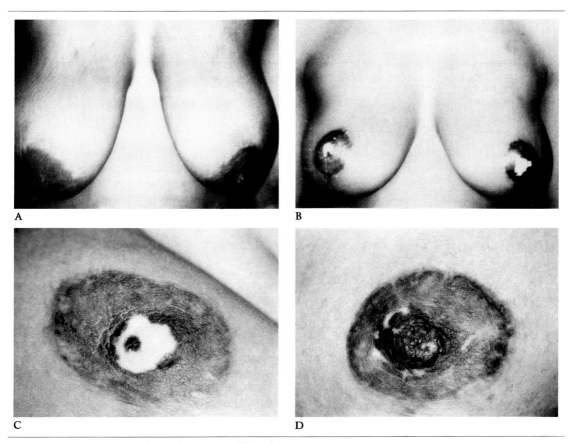

Fig. 31-15. A. Preoperative photo of a 45-year-old black
patient. B. Extensive depigmentation 1 year
postoperatively. It is most apparent in the nipple
where the greatest degree of necrosis occurs. C. A
close-up of the nipple-areola prior to punch grafting
from areola to the nipple. D. One year following
grafting, demonstrating pigment and projection. Also
note the healed donor sites. (Courtesy of Dr. Roger
Friedenthal)

528

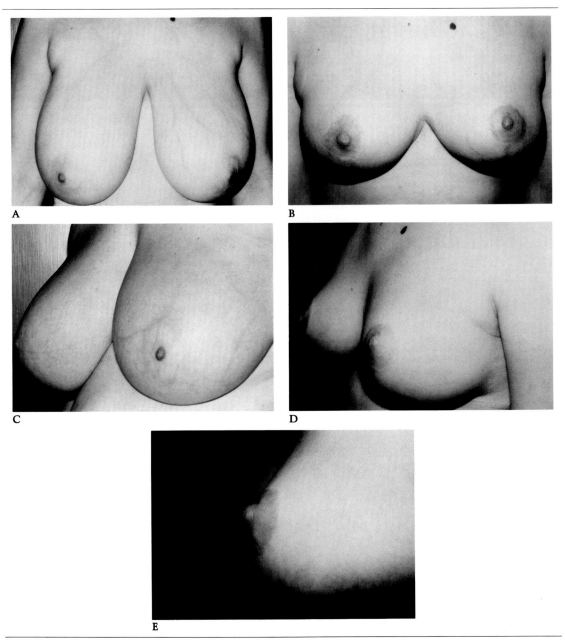

A

B

C

D

E

Fig. 31-16. A 23-year-old woman who had total 2100-gm resection. A. Minimal nipple projection existed preoperatively. B. Two years postoperatively, with good nipple projection. C. Oblique preoperative view. D. Two-year postoperative oblique view. E. Close-up of nipple-areola complex 2 years postoperatively.

(Fig. 31-15C, D) or by pigment tattooing. It is wise to advise deeply pigmented patients about this potential complication.

FAILURE OF GRAFT TAKE

Only 1 of 156 consecutive nipple-areola grafts failed to "take." In this case, at 9 days, the graft was removed, and 2 days later, a full-thickness graft from the groin was successfully transplanted.

There were no cases of significant hematoma, infection, or fat necrosis, although occasionally there was delayed healing with drainage and healing by secondary intention at the junction of the vertical and horizontal suture lines and the areola and vertical suture lines.

Conclusion

Reduction mammaplasty utilizing nipple-areola graft is a good procedure and should be considered for patients in any age group who fit the criteria stated earlier (Fig. 31-16). It offers the following advantages:

1. A well-shaped breast is achieved.
2. Breast shape may be maintained better than with other pedicle procedures.
3. Complications are fewer because there is no unnatural folding of tissue nor is there concern for preservation of blood supply to the nipple and areola.
4. There is less scarring at the junction of the skin and areola.
5. Accurate preoperative planning with no intraoperative adjustment is simply accomplished.

6. Postoperative breast examination is facilitated because the breast is uniformly smooth without irregularities caused by folded pedicles or flaps.

This procedure has proved to be satisfactory. It will probably be performed on an increasing number of patients undergoing reduction mammaplasty.

References

1. Adams, W.M. Free transplantation of the nipples and areolae. *Surgery* 15:196, 1944.
2. Anderson, R. Free nipple graft. Presented at Meeting of Canadian Society of Plastic Surgery, 1977.
3. Armstrong, D.R. The submammary fold as the key to simplified planning in reduction mammaplasty. Presented at Meeting of the Society for Clinical Aesthetic Surgery, 1982.
4. Courtiss, E.H., and Goldwyn, R.M. Breast sensation before and after plastic surgery. *Plast. Reconstr. Surg.* 58:1, 1976.
5. Friedenthal, R. Personal communication.
6. Gradinger, G.P. Reduction mammaplasty utilizing nipple-areola transplantation. *Clin. Plast. Surg.* 15:641, 1988.
7. Penn, J. Breast reduction. *Br. J. Plast. Surg.* 7:357, 1955.
8. Thorek, M. Plastic reconstruction of the breast and free transplantation of the nipple. *J. Int. Coll. Surg.* 9:194, 1946.
9. Townsend, P.L.G. Nipple sensation following breast reduction and free nipple transplantation. *Br. J. Plast. Surg.* 27:308, 1974.
10. Wise, R.J. Preliminary report on a method of planning the mammoplasty. *Plast. Reconstr. Surg.* 17:367, 1956.
11. Wise, R.J., Gannon, J.P., and Hill, J.R. Further experience with reduction mammaplasty. *Plast. Reconstr. Surg.* 32:12, 1963.

COMMENTS ON CHAPTERS 30 AND 31

Robert M. Goldwyn

With their characteristic thoroughness and historical sense, Letterman and Schurter have described a procedure that is still useful and often preferable, especially with "breasts of massive proportions and those of great pendulosity," to quote them. No other method of reduction mammaplasty provides the surgeon with comparable latitude to cut where necessary and to mold where desirable.

Rubin [4] summarized the criticisms of free nipple grafting: loss of nipple sensation; loss of nipple erection; duct blockage with cyst formation after severing duct-nipple continuity; possible cancer formation; inability to nurse; failure of nipple and areola grafts; and poor cosmetic results.

The preceding two chapters have answered many of those criticisms: reasonable nipple sensation can return, a fact that they have observed and that Townsend [5] also described in two thirds of his cases; nipple erection is possible if the smooth muscle is taken with the graft, something that Letterman, Schurter and Gradinger try to do; duct blockage and cyst formation is extremely rare after nipple-areola grafting; reduction by nipple-areola transplantation is not associated with an increase in breast cancer; the ability to lactate and nurse is definitely decreased but, as the authors have said, "never say never," since some women are able to nurse even though the prospective patient should be told that it is an unpredictable event; and poor cosmetic results are most apt to occur when the operation is not done optimally. As Rubin [4] has also stated, some of the results shown by Thorek and by Conway did produce flat breasts, but the modifications suggested by Letterman and Schurter as well as those by Rubin [4] and Gradinger can give a patient breasts of very pleasing shape and volume as well as of almost perfect symmetry.

To many surgeons unfamiliar with reduction by nipple-areola transplantation, a major disadvantage is the requirement of grafting the nipple-areola and the possibility of graft loss. However, as Letterman and Schurter have noted, complete necrosis of the nipple and areola rarely occurs, and in their own series, it did not happen. Of 156 nipple-areola grafts reported by Gradinger, only one was lost, the patient then requiring a full-thickness graft from the groin.

With regard to failure of the nipple-areola transplant, the alternative of using a pedicle in breasts that are enormous carries a strong likelihood of nipple-areola necrosis, either partial or total. Too often, the surgeon who is trying to utilize a transposition method in a patient with gigantomastia will be forced to compromise in the amount of tissue to be removed in order not to devascularize that pedicle. The patient then has breasts whose volume is excessive and whose shape is displeasing.

I must confess that in my enthusiasm to demonstrate to myself and possibly others, such as residents, that the inferior pedicle technique has universal applicability, I have attempted it under circumstances that logically suggested the alternative of nipple-areola transplantation.

Rubin [4] has pointed out that the need to mobilize the nipple on a pedicle that is extremely long often requires sacrificing the fourth intercostal nerve, thereby decreasing or eliminating nipple-areola sensation, an objective that might have lent the surgeon to choose a transposition technique. If, then, the patient has a breast that is large and a shape that is ugly as well as a nipple-areola without sensation, what has the surgeon accomplished? The older patient, glad to be relieved of her weighty burden, may not be critical of the result; a younger patient will be much less sanguine.

Gradinger, who uses the transplantation technique in approximately 20 percent of his patients, reserves it for those who are postmenopausal with very large breasts without much sensation; for those with large, painful, tender lumpy breasts that are difficult to examine; for those with hypertrophy and nipple inversion; for the postmastectomy patient whose opposite breast is hypertrophied; and for those with gigantomastia, where more than 1,000 gm of tissue per breast ought to be removed. He has stated that "any patient who anticipates the possibility of breast feeding her baby or who has pleasurable nipple sensation is advised to have a transposition procedure" [2].

A patient of mine in whom nothing but a transplantation procedure could have been used, except bilateral mastectomy, was a 32-year-old woman with massive breast enlargement in the twenty-first week of pregnancy [1]. A total of 6,895 gm of tissue was removed from the right side, and 6,700 gm of tissue from the left side. She later delivered a normal, healthy baby at term.

Letterman and Schurter and Gradinger have described their modifications of Thorek's procedure. Letterman and Schurter, unlike Gradinger, do not base their preoperative design on a fixed pattern but, rather, they individualize it; the new nipple sites are not determined preoperatively but only after the "conical mount is completed"; the nipple-areola is taken as a true composite of nipple, areola, and muscle in an effort "to preserve erectility, sensitivity and sensuality in the transplant"; a midwedge resection is utilized to eliminate the flat breast and to achieve a conical one; a sitting position is used to give a true idea of the eventual shape, volume, and symmetry of the breasts.

A problem that I have found with the nipple-areola grafting technique in black patients is the hypopigmentation, about which the authors have commented. Tattooing can rectify the situation as can tanning with ultraviolet or artificial rays or naturally. Punch grafts from the pigmented areola to the nipple is another way of restoring relatively normal pigmentation, an alternative used by Friedenthal, whom Gradinger cites.

In conclusion, since its first description by Thorek about 70 years ago, breast reduction by nipple-areola transplantation continues to be a useful alternative [3] and sometimes the only treatment for certain patients because of the simplicity, safety, and predictability.

REFERENCES

1. Gargan, T.J., and Goldwyn, R. Gigantomastia complicating pregnancy. *Plast. Reconstr. Surg.* 80:121, 1987.
2. Gradinger, G.P. Reduction mammoplasty utilizing nipple-areola transplantation. *Clin. Plast. Surg.* 15:641, 1988.
3. Hawtof, D.B., Levine, M., Kapetansky, D.I., and Pieper, D. Complications of reduction mammaplasty: Comparison of nipple areolar graft and pedicle. *Ann. Plast. Surg.* 23:3, 1989.
4. Rubin, L.R. The Surgical Treatment of the Massive Hypertrophic Breast. In N.G. Georgiade (ed.), *Aesthetic Breast Surgery.* Baltimore: Williams & Wilkins, 1983. Pp. 322–333.
5. Townsend, P.L.G. Nipple sensation following breast reduction and free nipple transplantation. *Br. J. Plast. Surg.* 27:308, 1974.

32

Unilateral Reduction Mammaplasty

Saul Hoffman

Reduction mammaplasty is usually performed on both breasts simultaneously, but there are occasions when unilateral reduction is indicated. The techniques normally used for bilateral reduction may need to be modified to obtain the best possible symmetry.

This chapter discusses the indications, techniques, and complications of unilateral reduction mammaplasty.

Indications

CONGENITAL AND DEVELOPMENTAL PROBLEMS

Severe breast asymmetry can be very disturbing to a young woman (see Case 1). Even a slight deviation from normal can have significant psychological effects with body image disturbances in adolescents [12].

Since it is not unusual for breasts to develop at different rates, it would be preferable to wait until full development before performing surgery. On the other hand, these young women are often so unhappy with their condition that they pressure their parents to seek early correction.

In severe cases, it may be advisable to proceed with an operation with the understanding that additional surgery may be necessary if further changes occur (see Cases 2 and 3). The psychological benefits of early surgery can outweigh the disadvantages of a possible second operation. Naturally, the patient must be prepared for the possibility of changes and revisional surgery.

Maliniac [7] classified breast asymmetries into four groups. Simon et al [13] expanded the classification into six categories:

Category I: One breast hypoplastic, the other normal size, with or without ptosis.

Category II: Both breasts hypoplastic, but unequal in size.

Category III: One breast hypertrophic, the other normal; either or both may be ptotic.

Category IV: Both breasts hypertrophic and unequal in size; either or both may be ptotic.

Category V: One breast hypoplastic, the other hypertrophic.

Category VI: Unilateral hypoplasia of thorax, pectoral muscles, and breast.

ACQUIRED CONDITIONS

Cystosarcoma phylloides (giant fibroadenoma) may cause a dramatic enlargement of a breast. Removal of the tumor usually corrects the problem, but when breast tissue has been replaced by tumor, augmentation may be necessary (see Case 4).

Trauma (burns), infection, or radiation may create a situation in which the affected breast is smaller than the contralateral breast. Cases have been reported in which the developing breast has been destroyed by surgery or radiation. Management may involve reduction of the large breast or augmentation of the smaller, or a combination of both.

POSTMASTECTOMY

Postmastectomy is now by far the most common indication for a unilateral reduction, which is often necessary for symmetry (see Case 5). Occasionally, patients who have had a mastectomy request reduction of a large contralateral breast, even though they do not desire reconstruction. Several patients have complained that the remaining breast has increased in size following the mastectomy. They are likely to feel unbalanced and uncomfortable (see Case 6).

Planning the Operation

Techniques normally used for bilateral reduction mammaplasty may need to be modified. The surgeon should be familiar with several methods so that he or she can select the operation that will provide the best symmetry.

When one breast is small, a decision must be made to either reduce the larger breast to the size of the smaller one or augment the hypoplastic side. A careful evaluation of the patient's desires and expectations must be made, and the limitations of the procedure must be explained in detail. An explanation of the appearance of the scars is mandatory. Photographs may be helpful to demonstrate the scars and provide the patient with a proper informed consent (see Chap. 7). When the contralateral breast is ptotic, a mastopexy will provide better symmetry, but some women may prefer to accept some residual asymmetry than live with the scars of a mastopexy.

When planning a simultaneous augmentation of one breast and reduction of the other, consideration must be given to the changes that will occur postoperatively (see Case 2). Although one cannot accurately predict these changes in everyone, a general pattern can be expected and allowances made. In the reduced breast, the distance from the nipple to the inframammary fold will increase with a concomitant change in the nipple-to-breast relationship so that the nipple will appear higher. In severe cases, this has been referred to as "bottoming out." To compensate for this tendency, the nipple should be placed slightly lower on the breast mound (see Chap. 7). Although changes in the augmented breast are less likely, there may be descent with time. For this reason, Radlauer and Bowers [10] recommend a two-stage procedure for optimal symmetry.

It is more difficult to obtain symmetry when reducing only one breast. Fischl et al [3] have described the use of a pattern similar to that devised by Wise [16], but made from the smaller breast. The nipple-to-clavicle and nipple-to-inframammary fold distances are measured and duplicated on the larger breast (see Case 7).

Other important considerations are the shape and volume of the breast, as well as the diameter of the areola.

Most plastic surgeons have a preference for a certain type of reduction mammaplasty. The McKissock technique and the inferior pedicle technique appear to be the most popular methods [8, 11]. In unilateral reduction mammaplasty, however, the technique that will most clearly match the smaller breast should be the one selected. In general, the inferior pedicle technique is preferred because it is the most versatile. The pedicle can be sculpted to match the contour of the contralateral breast while preserving sensation and nipple function. Breasts reconstructed with silicone implants tend to be firmer and fuller superiorly. By advancing the inferior pedicle superiorly and suturing it to the fascia, the superior portion of the breast is augmented to obtain better symmetry with the reconstructed breast. This principle has also been utilized with a free nipple graft. When a large reduction is necessary, particularly in older women, an amputation reduction with free nipple graft gives good results (see Case 6).

The reconstructed breast often lacks projection. In these cases, the type of reduction described by Pitanguy [9] can be utilized for the contralateral breast. Tissue is removed from the posterior portion of the mammary gland, thus reducing the amount of projection. When a smaller reduction is required, the superior pedicle technique is preferred.

Recently, Berrino et al [1] described a technique for unilateral reduction that sculpts the breast from the undersurface, utilizing a short incision. The authors claim this method is more versatile than standard techniques and therefore is more useful when only one breast requires reduction. They use four types of incisions, depending on skin elasticity and the amount of breast tissue to be resected. The mammary gland is separated from the underlying fascia and sculpted from the undersurface to match the contralateral breast. They claim satisfactory to excellent results in more than 77 percent of cases.

Determining the amount of breast tissue to be removed in a unilateral reduction mammaplasty can be challenging. Estimates are made preoperatively, but there is no accurate method of measuring breast volume. Bouman [2] described measuring breast volume by water displacement. Tegtmeier [15] developed an instrument based on this principle.

Kirianoff [5] used hollow templates, which he placed in a brassiere and filled with water to measure the volumes of asymmetric breasts. Grossman and Roudner [4] devised a simple but practical method for measuring volume, which consists of a calibrated plastic cone that fits around the breast. I find this to be the easiest and most useful method.

Preoperative measurements and markings are made with the patient in the standing position. Photographs are available for viewing in the operating room, and the specimens of breast tissue are weighed. During the operation, the patient is placed in a sitting position in order to check for symmetry [6, 14].

Category VI of Simon et al's classification includes hypoplasia of the thorax, pectoral muscles, and breast, as in Poland's syndrome. Correction is difficult, and symmetry is almost impossible to achieve. Occasionally, a unilateral reduction mammaplasty is indicated, but more often, the hypoplastic side must be augmented.

Case Reports

CASE 1

C.S., a 16-year-old girl, consulted about the possibility of corrective surgery on her breasts. She gave a history of lack of development of the left breast and overdevelopment of the right breast. She had been under psychiatric care for 2 years. Her psychiatrist advised against plastic surgery. She was extremely shy, embarrassed, and apprehensive during the initial examination. There was marked hypertrophy of the right breast and hypoplasia of the left breast (Fig. 32-1A). Pigmentation of the skin over the left breast had been present since birth.

Reduction of the hyperplastic right breast was clearly indicated. Simultaneous augmentation of the left breast was recommended to obtain the best possible symmetry. The patient consulted another psychiatrist, who agreed that surgery was advisable. Reduction mammaplasty of the Strömbeck type and augmentation with a 275-ml oval silicone prosthesis were performed (Fig. 32-1B–F).

A marked personality change was noted soon after surgery. The patient was no longer shy and embarrassed; she began dating and was able to terminate her psychiatric care. She has since married.

CASE 2

This patient was first seen at age 13, complaining of lack of development of the right breast and enlargement of the left breast (Fig. 32-2A,B). She was very unhappy and anxious to have correction as soon as possible. Since she was only 13, she was advised to wait a year to see whether any further development would occur. Since there was very little change during that time, it was decided to reduce the left breast and augment the right breast in one operation. At 1 year, the implant remained soft and symmetry was good (Fig. 32-2C–E). At 2 years, the areola had stretched and there was some recurrence of the tubular deformity (Fig. 32-2F). At 6 years, with some weight loss, the left breast became smaller and the right breast slightly ptotic (Fig. 32-2G–I).

CASE 3

J.F., a 15-year-old girl, complained of breast asymmetry of 3 to 4 years' duration. She had been treated for scoliosis with a brace 1 year before but otherwise was in good health.

On examination, the left breast was hypertrophic and ptotic, with the nipples measuring 21 cm from the clavicle. The right breast was normal, with the nipple at 17 cm (Fig. 32-3A).

Although she was young, it was considered unlikely that further changes in her breasts would occur. She was most anxious to have surgery since her appearance distressed her and dressing was a problem.

A left reduction mammaplasty was performed with a satisfactory early result (Fig. 32-3B,C). She returned 5 years later, complaining that the right breast was now larger. Her appearance at that time was almost a mirror image of her original deformity (Fig. 32-3D).

CASE 4

A 13-year-old girl complained of rapid growth of her right breast over a 4-year period. On examination, a large tumor could be palpated, and biopsy confirmed the presence of a giant fibroadenoma (Fig. 32-4A).

Preoperatively, the patient was marked as for a unilateral reduction mammaplasty (Fig. 32-4B). The excess skin and the fibroadenoma were removed (Fig. 32-4C,D). Since the tumor had replaced almost the entire breast, a silicone implant was required for volumetric symmetry (Fig. 32-4E,F). This was covered by an inferiorly based dermal flap. The nipple was replaced as a full-thickness graft (Fig. 32-4G,H).

Note the higher position of the nipple postoperatively, in spite of the lower placement at surgery owing to some bottoming out. The nipple should have been placed closer to the inframammary fold to compensate for this.

CASE 5

A 39-year-old woman underwent a right modified

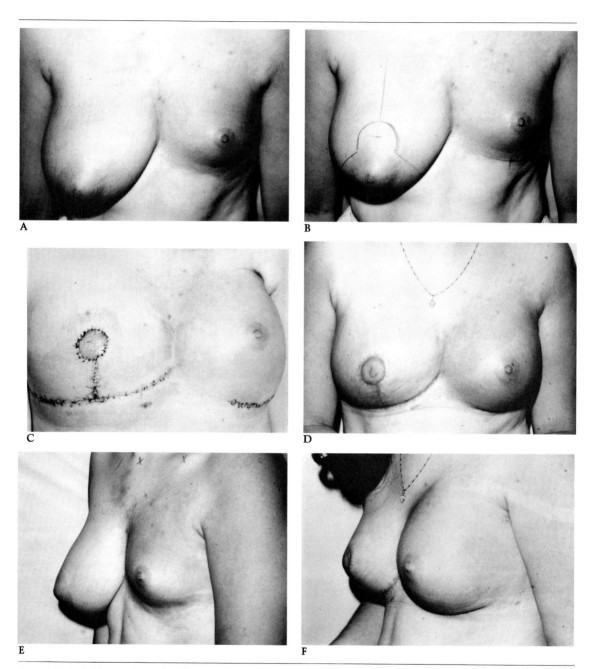

Fig. 32-1. A. A 16-year-old girl with severe breast asymmetry. Note hypoplasia of the left breast with pigmentation of the overlying skin and hypertrophy of the right breast. B. Preoperative plans for right reduction and left augmentation. Note the lower right nipple position to allow for descent of the left nipple and ascent of the right nipple. C. Immediate postoperative view. D. Three months postoperatively. E. Oblique preoperative view. F. Oblique postoperative view. (From B.E. Simon, S. Hoffman, and S. Kahn. Treatment of asymmetry of the breasts. Clin. Plast. Surg. 2:375, 1975.)

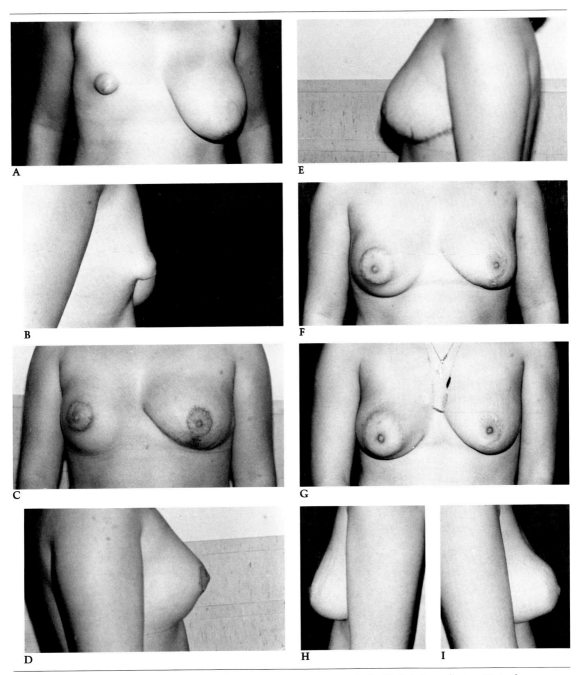

Fig. 32-2. A. A 13-year-old girl with severe breast asymmetry. Note the left tubular breast. B. Lateral view. C. One year postoperatively. D. Right lateral view 1 year postaugmentation mammaplasty. E. Left lateral view 1 year postreduction mammaplasty. F. Two years postoperatively. G. Six years postoperatively. H. Left lateral view. Note the reduction in size of the breast with slight ptosis but good nipple position. I. Right lateral view. Note the mild capsular contracture, attenuation of the areola with slight recurrence of the tubular deformity.

538

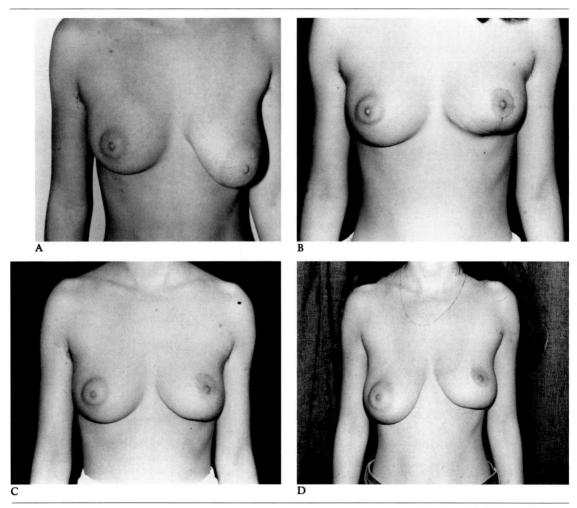

A **B**

C **D**

Fig. 32-3. A. A 15-year-old girl with left breast hypertrophy. B. Immediate postoperative result. C. Two years postoperatively. D. Five years postoperatively. Note hypertrophy of the right breast—mirror image of the original deformity.

Fig. 32-4. A. A 13-year-old girl with a rapidly growing fibroadenoma of her right breast. B. Preoperative plan—markings with a 20 percent solution of silver nitrate. Note the nipple position on the right side is lower than that on the left side. C. Preoperative plan with amount of skin to be resected and nipple circumscribed for removal as a full-thickness graft. D. Skin and nipple-areolar complex excised. E. Resected specimen. F. Inflatable silicone implant in place—contains 80 ml of saline. G. Postoperative appearance. Note the change in position of the grafted nipple. H. Oblique view. (From S. Hoffman. Giant fibroadenoma of the breast: Immediate reconstruction following recision. Br. J. Plast. Surg. 30:170, 1978.)

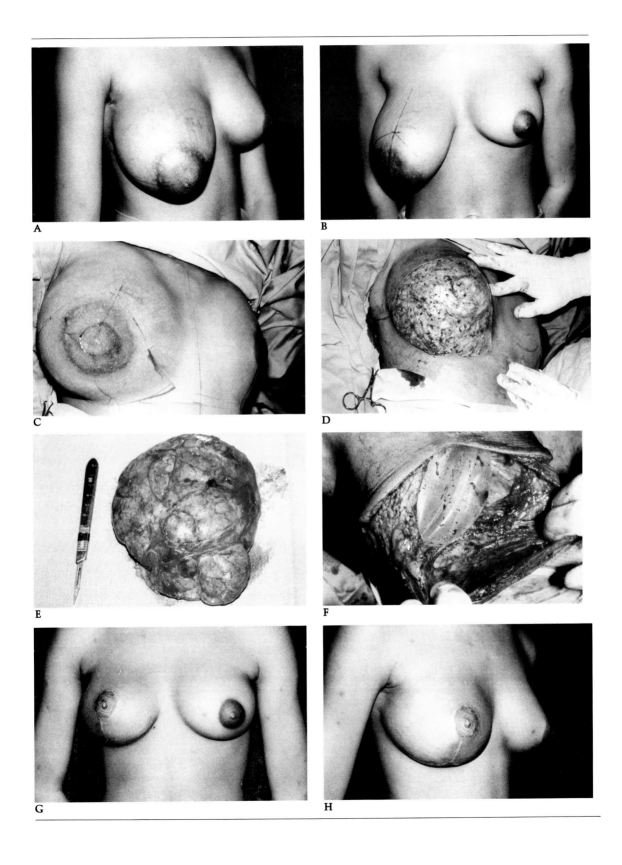

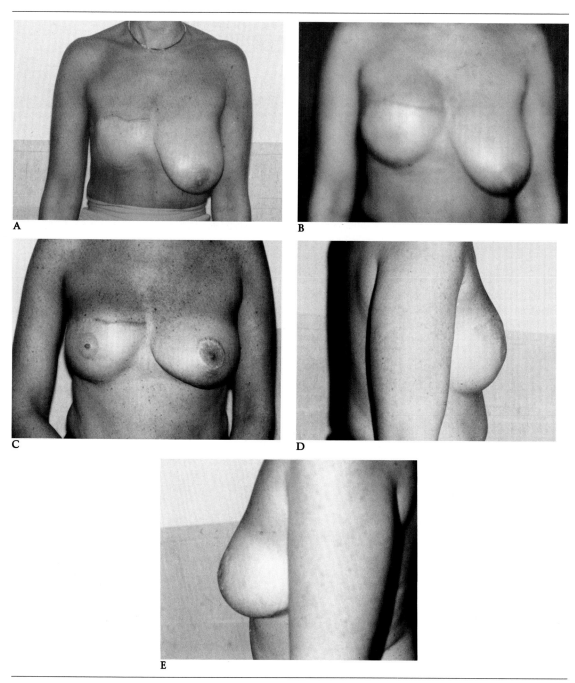

Fig. 32-5. A. A 39-year-old woman 1 year post–right
modified radical mastectomy. B. Three months
post–first stage reconstruction with a silicone implant.
C. Nine years postoperatively. D, E. Lateral views.
Note the good nipple position and symmetry but
slightly less projection of the reconstructed breast.

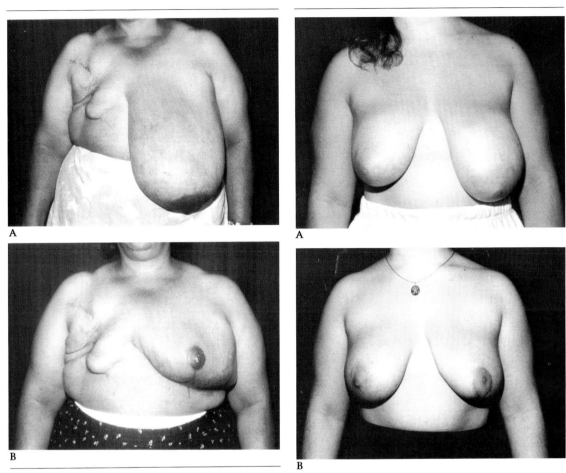

Fig. 32-6. A. A 64-year-old obese woman with marked hypertrophy of her left breast. B. Three months postoperatively. (Courtesy of Dr. E.D. Altchek).

Fig. 32-7. A. An 18-year-old woman with left breast hypertrophy and bilateral ptosis. B. Six months after a reduction of 530 gm of tissue using the inferior pedicle technique. (Courtesy of Dr. E.D. Altchek).

radical mastectomy for a small infiltrating intraductal carcinoma (Fig. 32-5A). One year later, a first-stage reconstruction was performed with a 360-ml silicone implant (Fig. 32-5B). Three months later, a left reduction mammaplasty, using the superior pedicle technique was performed; 250 gm of breast tissue were removed.

The nipple was reconstructed with a composite graft from her left nipple and the areola from a full-thickness medial thigh graft.

A 9-year follow-up study revealed good symmetry (Fig. 32-5C – E).

CASE 6
A 64-year-old woman underwent a right modified radical mastectomy for carcinoma. She com-

plained that her breasts had always been large and uncomfortable but that the remaining breast enlarged after her mastectomy (Fig. 32-6A). She was not interested in breast reconstruction. A left reduction mammaplasty of the amputative type with a free nipple graft was performed (Fig. 32-6B).

CASE 7
An 18-year-old woman complained that her left breast was much larger than her right breast (Fig. 32-7A). She had difficulty with her clothing and was embarrassed by her appearance. Although both breasts were ptotic, she did not want scars on

her right breast and elected to have only the left breast reduced.

The reduction was planned according to the technique described by Fischl et al [3] using an inferiorly based pedicle. Five hundred and thirty grams were removed (Fig. 32-7B).

References

1. Berrino, P., Galli, A., Rainero, M.L., and Santi, P. Unilateral reduction mammaplasty: Sculpturing the breast from the undersurface. *Plast. Reconstr. Surg.* 82:88, 1988.
2. Bouman, F.G. Volumetric measurement of the human breast and breast tissue before and during mammaplasty. *Br. J. Plast. Surg.* 23:263, 1970.
3. Fischl, R.A., Rosenberg, V.I., and Simon, B.E. Planning unilateral breast reduction for asymmetry. *Br. J. Plast. Surg.* 24:402, 1971.
4. Grossman, A.J., and Roudner, L.A. A simple means for accurate breast volume determination. *Plast. Reconstr. Surg.* 66:851, 1980.
5. Kirianoff, T.G. Volume measurements of unequal breasts. *Plast. Reconstr. Surg.* 54:616, 1974.
6. Letterman, G., and Schurter, M. A sitting position for mammaplasty with general anesthesia. *Ann. Plast. Surg.* 20:522, 1988.
7. Maliniac, J.W. *Breast Deformities and Their Repair.* Baltimore: Waverly Press, 1950. P. 153.
8. McKissock, P.K. Reduction mammaplasty with a vertical dermal flap. *Plast. Reconstr. Surg.* 49:245, 1971.
9. Pitanguy, I. Surgical treatment of breast hypertrophy. *Br. J. Plast. Surg.* 20:78, 1967.
10. Radlauer, C.B., and Bowers, D.G., Jr. Treatment of severe breast asymmetry. *Plast. Reconstr. Surg.* 47:347, 1971.
11. Robbins, T.H. A reduction mammaplasty with the areola-nipple based on an inferior dermal pedicle. *Plast. Reconstr. Surg.* 59:64, 1977.
12. Schonfeld, W.A. Body image disturbances in adolescents with inappropriate sexual development. *Am. J. Orthopsychiatry* 34:493, 1964.
13. Simon, B.E., Hoffman, S., and Kahn, S. Treatment of asymmetry of the breasts. *Clin. Plast. Surg.* 2:375, 1975.
14. Smoot, E.C., Ross, D., Silverberg, B., et al. The sit-up position for breast reconstruction. *Plast. Reconstr. Surg.* 77:60, 1986.
15. Tegtmeier, R.E. A quick accurate mammometer. *Ann. Plast. Surg.* 1:625, 1978.
16. Wise, R.J. A preliminary report on a method of planning the mammaplasty. *Plast. Reconstr. Surg.* 17:367, 1956.

COMMENTS ON CHAPTER 32   *Robert M. Goldwyn*

In this chapter, Hoffman makes several important points.

1. *Importance of operating soon in patients with significant asymmetry.* Women with such asymmetry have to endure a severe psychological burden. In my practice, I have had several adolescents who have been sexually promiscuous and a few have even become pregnant as an unconscious way of asserting themselves, their own femininity, and their capacity for motherhood. The timing of the operation cannot be precise and fixed since it will necessarily vary with the degree of asymmetry and the patient's desires and physical and emotional development. In general, it is better to err on the early side and make adjustments later that may be necessary as growth continues, a point that Hoffman has well illustrated with a few of his own patients. It would be far worse to delay the procedure and have the patient suffer low self-esteem and possibly engage in self-destructive behavior.

2. *What does the patient want?* The adage of "listen to the patient" is never wrong, and with these patients, it is mandatory. Frequently, a patient will prefer her very large breast and will think that the smaller one can be successfully augmented to match it. Occasionally, achieving symmetry to accommodate the patient's wishes will require reducing one breast and augmenting the other. These patients must understand that firmness can occur, even using an expander as a prelude, and the asymmetric breast may possess the same volume, but rarely the same shape, as the other breast.

3. *Selecting the right operation to fit the patient.* Hoffman, with common sense, advises not to be inflexible in our choice of technique for unilateral reduction. Several methods, which are mentioned, are available. The choice depends on the size and shape of the opposite breast and specifically the amount and location of the extra tissue to be removed.

For modest breast asymmetry requiring a *small* reduction, Schulman and Westreich [2] have found that excising a wedge of breast tissue via a circumareolar incision is simple and effective. This technique works best in women without ptosis or with only mild ptosis.

I agree with Hoffman that the inferior pedicle technique or the Pitanguy method (see Chap. 10) is useful in patients needing unilateral reduction. Whatever the method, the surgeon's task is easier if the preoperative markings are done very carefully in a sitting or standing nonmedicated patient (if that method of reduction requires preoperative markings) and if the design corresponds to the shape and volume of the opposite breast.

It should be noted that the inframammary fold may be lower on the heavier breast and may rise as weight is removed. Using the inframammary fold to measure the new nipple-areola site is still more reliable in case of asymmetry than is using the sternal notch or the midhumerus as reference points because the weight on the larger side stretches the anterior breast skin downward correspondingly [1]. Again, one should be careful to place the new nipple-areola location lower rather than higher, a caveat repeated throughout this book.

During operation, the patient should be sitting vertically. The surgeon should check continually that the nipple-areola is not too high and that it corresponds to the opposite side. Placing the nipple-areola too high will be aggravated by gravity and time, a point well demonstrated by Hoffman in one of his patients (see Fig. 32-4).

Another point to emphasize in addition to those given by Hoffman is to avoid removing too much tissue. This unfortunate error will produce a situation opposite to what the patient had previously. Now, a once too large breast will be too small. It is better to underdo and rectify later with a small procedure on an outpatient basis than to augment the breast just reduced or to make the opposite breast too small as a desperate move to attain symmetry. These alternatives should not be done in the operating room without discussion with the patient.

Immediately after operation and for a few weeks thereafter, the patient will continue to show asymmetry. She should be reassured that after the swelling disappears and healing occurs, she will look less asymmetric. It is hoped that in the future, computer imaging will take the guesswork out of this procedure.

REFERENCES
1. Dowden, R.V., Dinner, M.L., and Labandter, H.P. Breast reduction for asymmetrical hypertrophy. *Plast. Reconstr. Surg.* 73:928, 1984.
2. Schulman, Y., and Westreich, M. Treatment of mild breast asymmetry. *Plast. Reconstr. Surg.* 67:31, 1981.

33

John G. Kenney and
Milton T. Edgerton, Jr.

Reduction Mammaplasty in Gender Dysphoria

Before undertaking breast reconstruction in transsexual patients, a plastic surgeon needs to understand the nature and diagnosis of this condition.

Cross Gender Identity

Cross gender identity, one form of which is known as transsexualism, is a pediatric neuropsychiatric disorder of profound magnitude. It affects an individual's total concept of self. Transsexualism has been defined by Money and Gaskins [8] as "a disturbance of gender identity in which the person manifests, with constant and persistent conviction, the desire to live as a member of the opposite sex and progressively takes steps to live in the opposite sex role full time."

It is estimated that there are approximately 10,000 patients in the United States and at least 50,000 patients worldwide who can be classified by the American Psychiatric Association *Diagnostic and Statistical Manual of Medical Disorders* (3rd ed.) (DSM-III) [4] as transsexuals. The psychological phenomenon known as *transsexualism* is cross-cultural and has been documented as present throughout human written history. The reported worldwide incidence is approximately one in 50,000 individuals [2].

During the 1960s and 1970s, the ratio of male to female transsexual patients seeking surgical treatment was approximately 4–5:1. However, by the late 1980s, in some clinics, this ratio has approached 1:1. Transsexual patients who are biologic females are referred to as female (or "female to male") transsexuals. These patients request surgical and hormonal affirmation of their male identity and habitus. The patient population represents diverse socioeconomic and racial backgrounds without any one group predominating.

Despite professional controversy, there are many patients whose needs and symptoms meet this diagnosis of transsexualism. When patients are carefully selected, surgical treatment in conjunction with continuing psychiatric support has become the standard of care. As surgical techniques have improved, more psychiatrists and psychologists have encouraged their patients to pursue surgical treatment as a means to bring their lives into harmony. No other treatment approach (e.g., psychotherapy, analysis, electric shock therapy, hormone regulation) has offered even modest relief for transsexualism.

Etiology

How an individual develops gender identity is a complex phenomenon. It begins in early childhood and becomes a summation of cultural, genetic, psychological, and social influences, which evolve and mature throughout adolescence and adulthood. How an individual perceives his or her own sex and projects that sexual role image is also a complex phenomenon. Genetic biologic sexual determination is only one small piece of the final gender identity.

Clinical transsexualism produces a profound disturbance in the way a patient views his or her body image. The term *sex reassignment* is probably a misnomer. A better term may be *gender affirmation.* Even before surgery, these patients are convinced that they *are* already members of the "opposite" sex. They wish merely to have their true sexual identity confirmed surgically and hormonally.

The vast majority of transsexuals are of normal, and some possess superior intelligence. Most have absence of major mental illnesses. Laboratory studies such as computed tomography (CT) scans, electroencephalogram (EEG), chromosome analysis, and routine endocrine function studies are within normal limits. However, ongoing endocrinologic research suggests that there may be subtle abnormalities seated within the hypothalamus producing alterations in the usual cyclic pattern of releasing hormones. There may also be abnormalities in end-organ responses to these hormones. Even slight chemical abnormalities or imbalances may play a significant role in the pathogenesis and expression of transsexualism.

Often, a transsexual will state that he or she feels "trapped" in his or her existing body framework. Their genitalia, breasts, and gonads seem totally foreign to them. These opposite gender organs are repulsive to the patient; they are viewed as a mistake of nature. Surgical and hormonal therapy in conjunction with psychiatric counseling offers much by affirmation of the patient's sexual identity.

In the past, professional controversy, faintheartedness, and unreasoned bias left many patients without access to reputable professional help and guidance. Misunderstanding by health care professionals and general social intolerance of persons with gender problems have forced many transsexual patients to endure severe psychological hardships. Transsexual patients experience ridicule, alienation from friends and family, and social isolation at the workplace. These are extreme burdens for any individual to bear.

A multidisciplinary team of professionals is the most efficient and effective means to evaluate transsexual patients. This allows for objectivity in patient evaluation and treatment. The potential for making a diagnostic error, such as might be made by a solo practitioner, is minimized. The expertise of various health care professionals in a gender identity team can be combined to provide maximum patient benefit. The team used for the evaluation, screening, and treatment of transsexual patients may include a psychiatrist, psychologist, gynecologist, urologist, endocrinologist, and plastic surgeon who is experienced in genitourinary reconstruction. This also allows for various patient treatment programs to be evaluated objectively by the team during follow-up. Careful patient screening and selection improves diagnostic accuracy, ethical objectivity, and scientific long-term follow-up.

Diagnosis of Transsexualism

Diagnostic criteria for transsexualism defined by the American Psychiatric Association [4] include the following:

1. The patient feels a sense of discomfort and inappropriateness about his or her anatomic sex.
2. The patient wishes to be rid of his or her own genitalia and live as a member of the opposite sex.
3. The disturbance has been continuous (not limited to periods of stress) for at least 2 years.
4. There is no physical intersex or genetic abnormality.
5. There is no mental disorder such as schizophrenia.

Requisites Before Surgery for Transsexualism

The University of Virginia Gender Identity Team follows the general guidelines adopted by the Harry F. Benjamin Society for the standard of care in the treatment of transsexual patients. These are:

1. The gender dysphoric must demonstrate that the desire for sexual reassignment has existed for more than 2 years.
2. The diagnosis of gender dysphoria must be initially made by an independent clinical behavioral scientist with experience in the field.
3. That therapist must have a psychotherapeutic relationship with the patient for more than 1 year.
4. With the advice and consent of the clinical behavioral scientist, the patient must participate in a program of hormonal sex reassignment for a period of at least 6 to 12 months prior to surgery.
5. The patient fulfills the "real life test" — that is, he or she lives and works exclusively in the cross gender for a period of not less than 1½ to 2 years.

In addition to fulfilling these requirements, each patient is individually interviewed and evaluated by all members of the gender identity team. Their professional evaluations allow the formulation of a comprehensive treatment program.

Pivotal in the diagnostic and treatment process of transsexualism is the psychiatrist's role. If a patient receives surgical treatment as a result of improper or hasty diagnostic criteria, a postoperative crisis may occur.

Subsets of Gender Disorders

Subsets of gender disorders exist that may complicate proper diagnosis. The differentiation between transsexualism, homosexuality, and transvestism is critical. At times, the differences may be subtle. A true homosexual does not find his biologic genitalia foreign or objectionable. He would feel mutilated if penectomy and castration were performed. This sharply contrasts with the expressions of relief and appreciation consistently reported postoperatively by true transsexuals.

The adult female-to-male transsexual routinely gives a history of psychosexual conflict dating back to early childhood. This is manifested by extensive and pervasive feelings of masculinity as a child. Parental and sibling interviews confirm these reports. Not surprisingly, a stressful parent and child relationship is also common. Despite prolonged psychiatric counseling, medical testing, peer ridicule, and family pressure, cross gender emotions and feelings intensify. These feelings continue unabated into adolescence and adult life, manifesting themselves in true female-to-male transsexualism.

Considerations Before Operations

Prior to any surgical treatment on breasts or genitalia, a number of individual psychological and social issues must be addressed. Psychiatric support plays a critical role pre- and postoperatively. While enrolled in preoperative therapy, topics for discussion include:

1. Exploration of the patient's gender identity in relationship to parent-child interaction during infancy, childhood, and adolescence.
2. Exploration of internal motivational patterns for surgery.
3. The social ramifications for living in the gender of conviction as well as the ways of informing family members, friends, and associates at work.
4. Legal issues such as name change, change of birth certificate, driver's license, and other legal documents.

5. The other ramifications of permanent sterilization.

The patient must be cross living and cross dressing full time. This should include social and work activities. This "real life test" of gender confirmation is the most important single requirement for patient selection and preparation for surgical therapy!

Presurgical Hormone Therapy

Prolonged preoperative hormonal therapy is important to both the patient and the treating health care professionals. Prior to initiating hormonal treatment, liver function tests, complete blood counts, serum lipid profile, and glucose tolerance tests should be performed. Psychological changes during hormone therapy commonly accompany the physical changes. Female-to-male transsexual patients generally receive Depo-Testosterone, 300 mg intramuscularly every 3 weeks. This is continued indefinitely postoophorectomy and hysterectomy. Androgenic hormones suppress ovarian function and produce significant physical changes, such as:

1. Increase in body mass and muscle bulk.
2. Deepening of voice and thickening of the vocal cords.
3. Development of generalized body hair, which in some individuals may be substantial.
4. Development of male pattern baldness in genetically predisposed individuals.

Psychiatric treatment needs to be intensified perioperatively. The psychological stresses of surgery can have a tremendous impact on the patient's emotional equilibrium.

Ill-Suited Candidates

Even when all diagnostic therapeutic requisites have been fulfilled, certain individuals are not suitable as candidates for operation. These include the following:

1. Those with emotional sexual ambiguity—that is, patients who waver in their sexual role or have unrealistic expectations of surgery.
2. Those patients who legally cannot give informed consent.
3. Those patients with severe psychiatric dis-

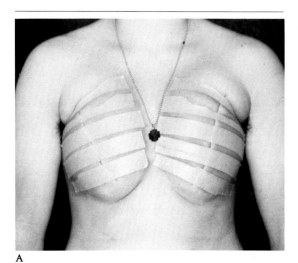

A

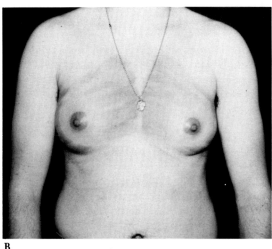

B

Fig. 33-1. A. Taping technique used to bind the breasts. B. Chronic dermatitis resulting from taping technique.

Once the DSM-III criteria of female-to-male transsexualism have been met and a thorough preoperative evaluation has been completed, surgical treatment will often be indicated. Long-term results and patient satisfaction with surgical treatment have been excellent in our clinic (and *all* other clinics with long-term experience with gender surgery). No patient that we have treated at the Virginia Gender Clinic has ever regretted undertaking surgical therapy. The senior author has been treating and following the surgical results on gender dysphoric patients for more than 29 years. Surgical treatment continues to be the only effective alternative for most transsexuals. There is still no demonstrated effective long-term nonsurgical therapy. Surgical gender reassignment procedures are supplemented with hormonal therapy and psychiatric counseling. This triple approach allows the patient to resume a relatively normal and more comfortable role in society.

Order of Surgery in the Female-to-Male Transsexual

The female-to-male transsexual patient presents with a predictable hierarchy of surgical requests. Hysterectomy removes only one remnant of feminization. Oophorectomy removes another. In addition, oophorectomy stops estrogen production. This allows exogenously administered testosterone to be more effective. Prior to phalloplasty, breast reduction and chest wall contouring remove the last external vestiges of body contour feminization. Prior to chest wall contouring, patients typically bind their breasts or wear very loose clothing to minimize or camouflage a female chest wall appearance. These efforts may be very elaborate (Fig. 33-1). Sometimes a hygiene problem may result with the development of chronic dermatitis and intertriginous infections. Frequently, breast reduction and chest wall contouring are performed prior to phalloplasty. There are several distinct advantages in contouring the breasts and chest wall first:

1. Chest wall contouring produces a predictable surgical result with less potential for complications or morbidity than phallourethroplasty.
2. Patients report immediate satisfaction with the procedure.
3. Total hospital costs are less. Frequently, chest wall contouring can be performed on an outpatient basis.

orders such as paranoia or a history of delusions.
4. Those patients who refuse presurgical psychotherapy. (This inflexibility usually reflects more deep-seated problems.)
5. Those patients who exhibit antisocial behavior such as uncontrollable alcoholism or criminal behavior.
6. The effeminate homosexual who believes surgery might allow him to escape the stigma of homosexuality.

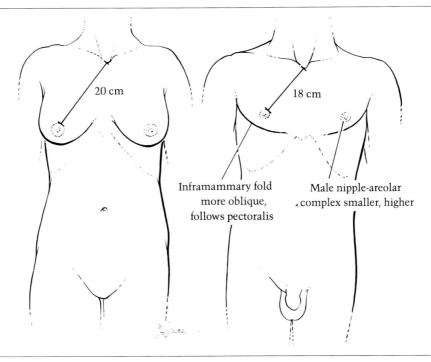

Fig. 33-2. Compared with the female chest wall pattern, in a male chest appearance, the nipple-areola complex is smaller and higher in position in the chest wall. The inframammary fold is also more oblique, following the inferior margin of the pectoralis major muscle.

Objectives of Chest Wall Contouring

The goals of chest wall contouring in the female transsexual patient are:

1. Removal of the breast tissue and excess skin, creating an aesthetically pleasing male-contoured chest wall with breast mounds appropriate in size for the male.
2. Obliteration of the inframammary crease.
3. Reduction of the diameter of the female nipple-areola complex to a diameter appropriate for men.
4. Placement of surgical incisions to simulate the valleys of the inferior margins of the pectoralis major muscle — or other natural lines.

The key to obtaining satisfactory results in chest wall contouring in patients with gender dysphoria is the proper matching of each patient with the most appropriate surgical technique. Individual considerations must be taken into account. The basic principles of reduction mammaplasty in

women provide the background for planning a chest wall contouring procedure for female-to-male transsexuals. The anatomic elements such as the nipple-areola complex, the skin envelope, the amounts of breast tissue and fat, and the depth of the inframammary crease should be considered individually in planning the operative procedure. In virtually all female-to-male transsexual patients, the nipple-areola complex must be reduced in diameter. The normal diameter of a male pattern nipple-areola complex should never exceed 25 to 30 mm. The female nipple-areola complex is generally much larger. The female areola must therefore be reduced to a male pattern diameter. This is readily accomplished by direct circular incision within the nipple-areola complex (Fig. 33-2). The projection of the nipple must also be reduced in most patients. A female nipple as prominent as that in a normal female is unacceptable to female-to-male gender dysphoric patients. These patients find that a low profile (male-appearing) nipple is an important aspect of breast reduction. It is even more important than preserving erogenous sensation to the nipple, which they tend to equate with femininity. The nipple is easily reduced either by direct horizontal or vertical resection (and downfolding of the remainder) of approximately one

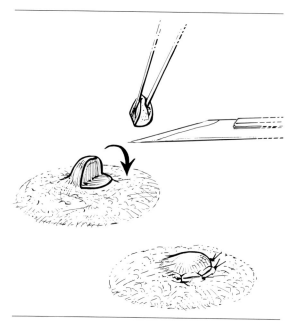

Fig. 33-3. *Nipple reduction performed by the vertical wedge technique.*

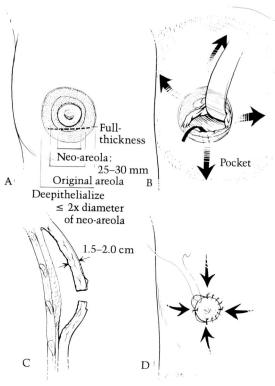

Fig. 33-4. *See text for description.*

half of the existing nipple (Fig. 33-3). This will produce a male pattern appearance of the nipple. The next goal in chest wall contouring is to remove any excess of breast tissue, skin, or subcutaneous fat to produce an aesthetically acceptable male pattern chest wall with minimal scarring.

Vascular Supply to the Breast

A detailed description of the arterial supply of the breast was given by Jacques Maliniac [7]. He described the variations of the blood supply to the breast. These included contributions from the lateral thoracic artery, internal mammary artery, and intercostal arteries. There was no consistent predominant blood supply that could be determined preoperatively. He also noted a superficial and deep periareolar plexus of vessels. These anatomic descriptions have become the basis for the variety of parenchymal and dermal pedicle flaps that have been described for successful reduction mammaplasty. In general, the blood supply of the female breast and nipple-areola complex is robust. Aufricht [1], in 1949, stated, "avoidance of a particular branch of the mammary arterial tree has no practical value. From the surgical point of view, all breast tissues are well vascularized. There is a sufficient blood supply from any direction of the breast hemisphere to nourish the corresponding tissue."

Obtaining a Male Chest

The procedure selected to reduce the breast mound and skin envelope depends on the size of the breast to be reduced. To produce a male pattern chest wall, significantly more breast tissue must be removed than when performing a standard reduction mammaplasty in female patients.

The Small Female Breast

When the breast is relatively small (an A cup) and the preoperative position of the nipple-areola complex is adequately high on the chest, a concentric periareolar skin reduction technique can be used (Fig. 33-4). We have found this technique very useful in contouring the chest wall in patients with small breasts. Our technique is a modification of a procedure described for the treatment of massive gynecomastia described by Davidson [3]. Initially, the size of the nipple-areola complex is measured. The areolar diameter selected is approximately 30 mm. A concentric circle is drawn around this on the breast skin. The circumference of the outside of the excised skin doughnut should not exceed *twice* the circumference of the areola. The concentric circle of skin around the nipple-areola complex is then deepithelialized circumferentially (Fig. 33-4A). A full-thickness incision from the 9 o'clock to the 3 o'clock position is then made within the deepithelialized area. The breast and the fatty tissues are then resected in a radial fashion down to the chest wall, leaving 1.5 to 2.0 cm of breast and fatty tissue beneath the skin envelope as well as beneath the nipple-areola complex (Fig. 33-4B,C). The breast tissue beneath this soft tissue mound is resected to the anterior axillary line, subclavicular area, medially to the sternum, and inferiorly over the margins of the rectus sheath and serratus fascia. It is important to break up the inframammary fold. This can be done by either direct incision of existing subdermal attachments or by disrupting them by using the suction-assisted lipectomy technique. It is also important to taper the periphery of the excised breast tissue and fat. This will avoid a peripheral "step off" deformity. Feathering and tapering is readily accomplished by suction-assisted lipectomy technique.

Once the breast tissue has been resected and the periphery "feathered," the dermal margins of the nipple-areola complex are sutured to the dermal margins of the breast skin. Serial closure begins with sutures placed at the 12, 3, 6, and 9 o'clock positions. Suturing continues until the wounds are closed (Fig. 33-4D). Careful preoperative planning is important. When the circumference of the deepithelialized concentric circle is more than twice the circumference of the desired nipple-areola complex, concentric closure tends to produce dermal "puckering" around the margins. This "pleating" or "puckering" of the margins may be unacceptable. If, in the preoperative planning session, severe "pleating" is to be expected, an alternative method of chest wall contouring should be selected. The concentric periareolar skin reduction technique for reduction mammaplasty produces consistent, acceptable results in properly selected female-to-male transsexual patients who do not need removal of large amounts of breast skin. When the breast size is greater than an A cup or when the entire nipple-areola complex

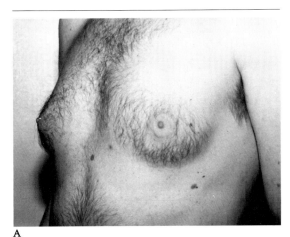

A

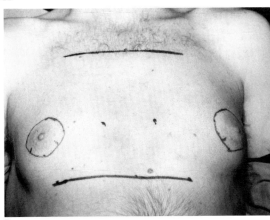

B

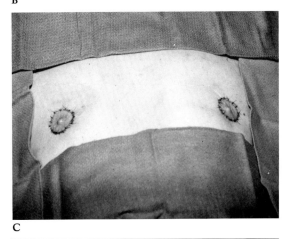

C

Fig. 33-5. A. Preoperative A-cup breast. B. Intraoperative markings for concentric reduction. C. Concentric closure technique completed.

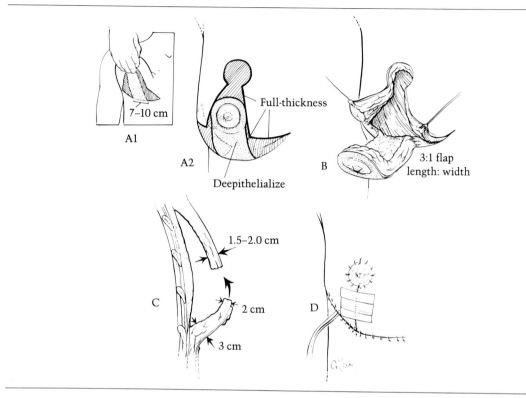

Fig. 33-6. See text for details.

must be repositioned, alternative techniques of breast reduction should be used. With concentric reduction, scarring is minimal and is confined to the periareolar area (Fig. 33-5).

The Larger Female Breast

When the breast size is a B cup or greater, either a nipple-areola complex pedicle technique or breast amputation with free nipple grafting must be chosen. In reducing the larger breast, the nipple-areola complex must be reduced and repositioned in the cephalad direction. This allows for the nipple-areola complex to be positioned at the level of the midhumeral line. This level is consistent with a normal male pattern chest wall appearance.

Nipple-areola complex–pedicled transposition techniques are generally confined to dermal pedicles. Parenchymal pedicles are of limited value in contouring the chest wall in the female transsexual patient. To achieve an acceptable contour, breast and fatty tissue must be resected beneath the nipple-areola complex down to the chest wall.

This requirement limits any parenchymal pedicle technique for breast reduction. Specific nipple transposition techniques are based on an anticipated pedicle length. The safe length-width ratio when the nipple-areola complex is transposed by a dermal pedicle technique is approximately 3:1. The primary disadvantage of pedicle reduction techniques is scarring. An inverted T-incision— that is, some component of a horizontal incision with a vertical limb—is unavoidable.

Inferior Pedicle Technique For Movement More Than 3 cm

Of the dermal techniques available, we have found the inferiorly based dermal pedicle to be the most useful and versatile (Fig. 33-6). This technique is especially useful when the nipple-areola complex must be moved more than 3 cm.

Our technique is a modification of the technique described by Georgiade [6] used to reduce hypertrophied breasts when it is necessary to re-

move large amounts of breast tissue. The patient is
marked preoperatively in a standing position. The
reduction of the nipple-areola complex position is
marked in a new position before the nipple-areola
complex is selected. The central vertical segment
of the dermal flap is marked for deepithelialization (Fig. 33-6). The flap's length-width ratio is
3:1. Lateral to the deepithelialized pedicle, full-
thickness skin and breast excisions are performed.
A subcutaneous pedicle of tissue approximately
1.5 to 2.0 cm in thickness is left over the breast
apron. The remaining breast tissue is removed.
Approximately 1.5 cm of parenchymal tissue is
left on the posterior aspect of the deepithelialized
inferiorly based dermal flap. The inferior aspect of
the pedicle should not be thinned to less than 3 cm
in order to maintain adequate blood supply. Pedicle length varies but is generally from 10 to 18 cm.
Once the nipple-areola complex has been secured
into its new position, the skin margins are redraped and the redundant skin is excised. The vertical scar segment is generally 3 to 5 cm in length.
The horizontal incisional length varies depending
on the size of the breast being reduced. It is important not to cross the midline sternal area with the
horizontal incision. Incisions in this area produce
unsightly scars or webbing. Meticulous attention
to skin redraping avoids a lateral dog-ear deformity.

The inferior dermal pedicle technique has both
advantages and disadvantages. The advantages are
preservation of the blood supply to the nipple-areola complex as well as preserving sensation. The
overall contour of the chest wall is good with the
reconstructive goals achieved. This technique,
however, is more time consuming than other techniques, and blood loss may be greater than with
other techniques. There is a vertical segment of
scarring that may not be acceptable to some patients. In addition, the inframammary crease is
not disrupted. This is especially important in
some patients who have a well-defined inframammary crease. In certain patients, the vertical pedicle technique may produce an unacceptable fullness in the lower portion of the new breast. In
addition, contracture of the vertical scar segment
tends to distort, with time, the nipple-areola complex into an elliptical configuration (Fig. 33-7).

Superior Pedicle Technique
Another alternative in dermal pedicle flaps for repositioning the nipple-areola complex in patients

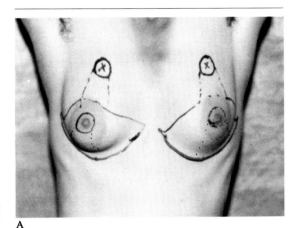

A

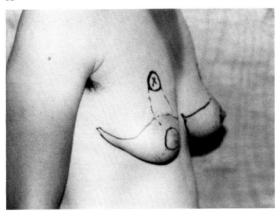

B

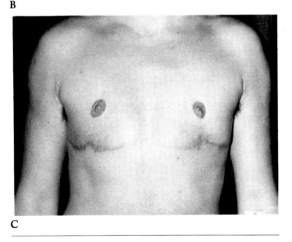

C

Fig. 33-7. A,B. Preoperative markings for the vertical
dermal pedicle technique. This technique is useful for
reducing the modest breast. C. Postoperative
appearance. Note the distortion of the nipple-areola
complex.

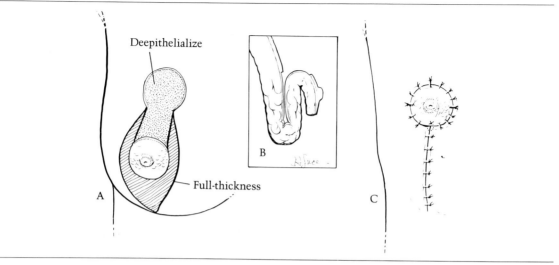

Fig. 33-8. See text for details.

with modest breast size is the superiorly based dermal pedicle technique (Fig. 33-8). This technique is useful when the nipple-areola complex is to be moved only 3 to 5 cm cephalad. Initially, the nipple-areola complex is reduced concentrically within a keyhole pattern. The superior margin of the keyhole pattern is the upper edge of the new nipple-areola complex position on the chest wall. Full-thickness vertical incisions are made at the deepithelialized margins adjacent to the nipple-areola complex (Fig. 33-8A). A full-thickness horizontal incision is made just beneath the inframammary crease. The breast tissue and subcutaneous tissue are excised radially until a male pattern chest wall contour is obtained. The blood supply to the nipple-areola complex is based superiorly. The dermal flap is then folded in a cephalad direction and sutured to its new position on the chest wall (Fig. 33-8B). The remaining skin envelope is tailored and contoured to avoid any skin redundancy. The remaining wounds are then closed in a standard fashion (Fig. 33-8C). An inverted T-incision often results with a vertical limb of approximately 2 to 4 cm. This technique has advantages in reducing the moderate-sized breast. The vertical limb incision is short, and the inframammary crease can be obliterated. The horizontal limb of the incision can be placed to conform to the lateral and inferior margins of the pectoralis fascia. Blood loss is usually less than that for a formal vertical pedicle technique, and operating time is reduced.

Necrosis of the nipple-areola complex is a potential complication. This has not occurred in our series of patients in whom raising the level of the areola by the superiorly based dermal pedicle technique has been no greater than 4 or 5 cm (Fig. 33-9).

Nipple-Areola Grafting

Another excellent technique for chest wall contouring in gender dysphoric patients is breast amputation with free nipple grafting. This technique is similar to one described by Lexer [9] in 1912 for reduction of large breasts in normal females. It was one of the earliest techniques used to reduce pendulous breasts. The technique's most recent description was in 1972 by Farina and Vallano [5]. We have modified these previously described techniques so that they may be adapted to contouring the chest wall in the female-to-male transsexual patient. We refer to this technique as the chest wall apron flap. Amputation and free nipple grafting can produce consistently good cosmetic results. It is a relatively simple operation to perform. The nipple may be placed at any level, and no vertical scar below the nipple is produced. It also allows the surgeon to address the individual anatomic concerns during the operation. This technique allows for accurate intraoperative placement of the nipple-areola complex. In addition, the inframammary fold may be directly ex-

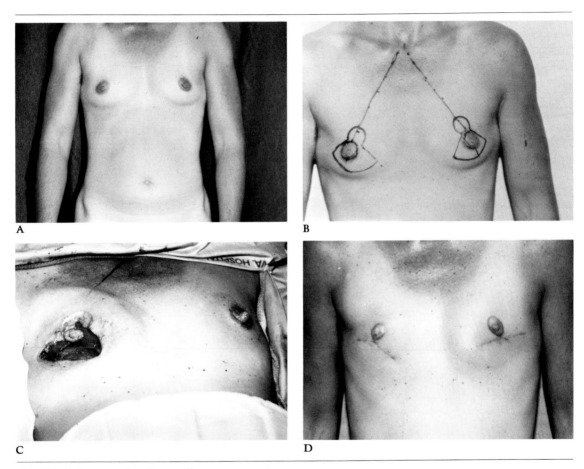

Fig. 33-9. A. Preoperative chest wall appearance prior
to reduction mammaplasty—superior pedicle
technique. B. Preoperative markings. Note that the
distance for cephalad repositioning of the nipple-
areola complex is small. C. Intraoperative view of
superior dermal pedicle technique. D. Early
postoperative appearance.

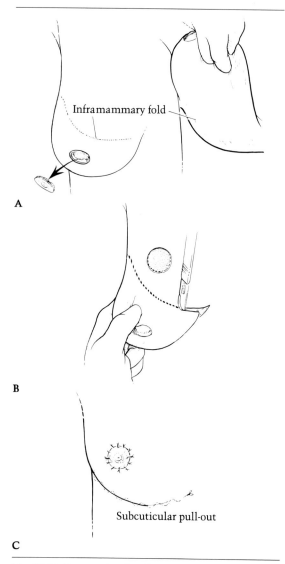

Fig. 33-10. *See text for details.*

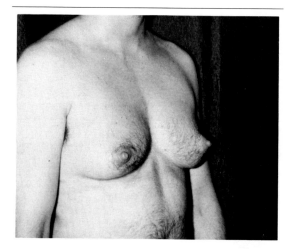

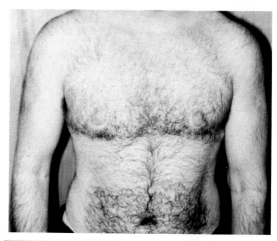

Fig. 33-11. A. Preoperative photo prior to chest wall apron flap reconstruction. Note the deep inframammary fold present. B. Postoperative appearance at 4 years. Note the obliteration of inframammary fold and accurate positioning of nipple-areola complex.

cised to improve the overall chest contour. The skin is excised in such a manner as to simulate the subpectoralis muscle valley. This technique is applicable to breasts of all sizes and avoids any vertical scars.

The operative procedure is as follows: The nipple-areola complex is circumscribed at a diameter of 25 mm, removed as a full-thickness graft, and carefully defatted (Fig. 33-10A). The inframammary crease is excised (Fig. 33-10B). The excision is carried laterally to the anterior axillary line with a slight inferior curve to parallel the lower border

of the pectoralis major muscle. A relatively thin subcutaneous apron flap is raised to a level just inferior to the clavicle. This apron flap should be approximately 2 cm in thickness to ensure a good blood supply as well as to adequately contour fullness of the chest wall (Fig. 33-10C). The remaining breast tissue is then removed down to the level of the pectoralis fascia, extending laterally to the anterior axillary line and medially to the lateral border of the sternum. The superiorly based composite skin and breast apron flap is drawn inferi-

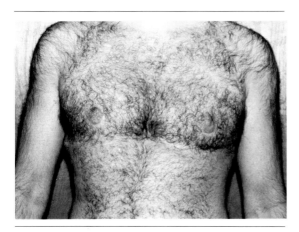

Fig. 33-12. Reduction mammaplasty by chest wall apron flap technique.

orly, and the excess skin is marked for excision. This level is always cephalic to above the defect left by the earlier excision of the nipple-areola complex. The redundant skin margins are tailored and contoured at an appropriate level. A lateral dog-ear deformity is avoided by careful skin excision and planning. The wound margins are then approximated and closed in layers. An intradermal pull-out suture is recommended. The positions of the nipple-areola complexes are then selected. The two marked circles of skin in these locations are deepithelialized and the nipple-areola full-thickness grafts are sutured into position with a bolus tie-on type of dressing (Fig. 33-10D and 33-11). One criticism of this technique is the potential for permanent loss of nipple-areola sensation. However, this has not been a problem for any of our patients. Areola sensation is a low priority in female-to-male transsexual patients (much less important than breast symmetry, contour, or appearance of scars). Approximately 50 percent of our patients with free graft areola reconstruction report a return of significant sensation within 2 years postoperatively. Return of sensation has been reported to be as high as 82 percent in one series of patients [10]. Hypopigmentation of the nipple-areola complex can occur when a graft take is incomplete. Incomplete graft take, however, is unusual. This complication has occurred in 3 percent of our patients. However, this potential complication is minimized and is camouflaged by hair development on the chest wall in patients receiv-

ing testosterone therapy (Fig. 33-12). Tattooing is also quite effective to blend areas of areola vitiligo.

Complications

Complications of reduction mammaplasty in gender dysphoric patients can be kept to a minimum. Early complications such as wound infection, hematoma, necrosis of skin flaps, and necrosis of the nipple-areola complex are infrequent in the hands of plastic surgeons who handle tissue gently. Of 100 consecutive female-to-male transsexual patients undergoing chest wall contouring at the University of Virginia Medical Center (several surgeons) between 1980 and 1988, early complications were as follows:

1. Wound infection — 2 percent.
2. Hematoma — 4 percent.
3. Partial necrosis of skin flaps — 2 percent.
4. Partial or complete necrosis of the nipple-areola complex — 2 percent.

Minor complications such as unsightly scars or minimal asymmetry occurred in 3 percent of patients. Five percent of the patients required a secondary surgical procedure.

In gender dysphoric patients, reduction mammaplasty is an integral part of surgical therapy. Almost all female-to-male transsexuals have breasts of sufficient size to require surgical correction. The correction provides a great deal of satisfaction to the patients. Breast reduction enables the patients to experience a freedom of dress and personal confidence that they lacked preoperatively. No female transsexual patient treated by the University of Virginia Gender Identity Team who has undergone reduction mammaplasty has ever regretted the procedure. Not one of these patients has ever asked for subsequent breast reconstruction. The scars and expense of surgery were more than offset by the reduced sense of deformity.

There are a number of techniques available to the female-to-male transsexual patient who seeks breast reduction and contouring of the chest wall to a more masculine appearance. Selection of the proper technique for each individual patient is critical to an optimum outcome. In general, small-breasted individuals may be treated by the concentric reduction technique. Moderate breast size may be adequately contoured by a vertical dermal pedicle technique or superiorly based dermal pedi-

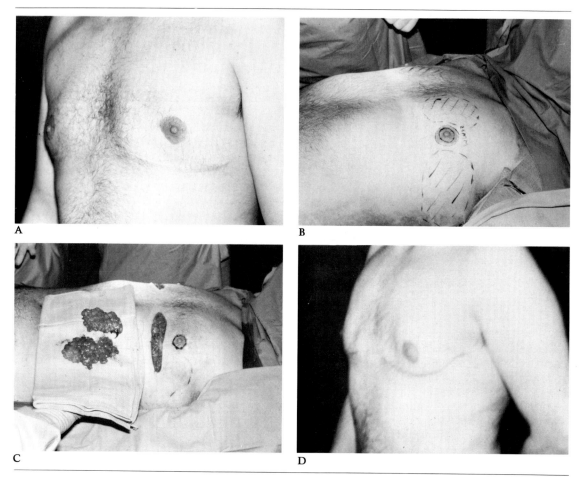

A

B

C

D

cle technique. When breast size is substantial, the most useful and versatile technique to achieve a male pattern chest wall is the chest wall apron flap – free nipple grafting technique, modified to place scars along the pectoral muscles. Breast reduction and chest wall contouring help bring the anatomic and psychological genders into harmony.

Unfortunately, at the University of Virginia Gender Clinic, we continue to see a number of patients who have had breast reduction operations by plastic surgeons who are unfamiliar with the nuances of female-to-male breast reduction methods. Sometimes it is impossible to salvage these postoperative deformities. This chapter constitutes a plea for more sophisticated surgical management of these patients (Figs. 33-13 and 33-14).

If the neuropsychiatric disorder known as transsexualism can be clearly identified during child-

Fig. 33-13. A. Preoperative photo of a patient dissatisfied with previous chest wall contouring. The nipple-areola complex was too large, and substantial amounts of breast tissue remained. B. Intraoperative markings demonstrating planned nipple-areola concentric reduction and the amount of residual breast tissue to be resected. C. Intraoperative view demonstrating concentric nipple-areola reduction, scar revision, and the amount of residual breast tissue resected. D. Postoperative appearance. Note the inframammary incision parallels the lateral and inferior pectoralis margins in a natural fashion.

hood, early psychiatric intervention may yet produce satisfactory treatment. Only time will tell. If discreet abnormalities in the central nervous system's releasing factors and hormones are identified, medications may be developed that can alter psychosexual behavior. Earlier intervention into this disorder may someday allow transsexual pa-

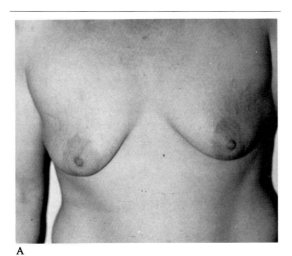

A

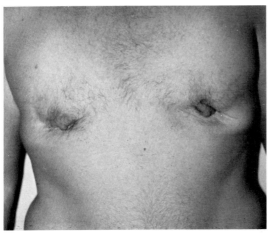

B

Fig. 33-14. A. Preoperative view of a 42-year-old patient. B. Postoperative view 12 months after reduction (subcutaneous mastectomy via semicircular periaerola incision). Note the displeasing concavity under the areola as well as fullness laterally. For contouring, the patient will return for liposuction, which, in retrospect, would have been wiser to have been used at the original operation.

tients to live comfortable lives with their original biologic sex. Until such a breakthrough occurs, female and male transsexual patients will still require surgical therapy. Female-to-male transsexualism is a complex psychosocial disorder requiring long-term therapy. An increasing number of these patients are coming to plastic surgeons for help. Treatment involves extensive psychiatric and surgical therapy integrated through gender identity teams and guided through the talents of a variety of health care specialists.

References

1. Aufricht, G. Mammaplasty for pendulous breasts — empiric and geometric planning. Plast. Reconst. Surg. 4:13, 1949.
2. Benjamin, H. The Transsexual Phenomenon. New York: Julian Press, 1966.
3. Davidson, B.A. Concentric circle operations for massive gynecomastia to excise the redundant skin. Plast. Reconst. Surg. 63:350, 1979.
4. Diagnostic and Statistical Manual of Mental Disorders (3rd ed.). Washington, D.C.: American Psychiatric Association, 1980.
5. Farina, R., and Vallano, J. B. Reduction mammaplasty with free grafting of the nipple and areola. Br. J. Plast. Surg. 25:393, 1972.
6. Georgiade, N.G., et al. Reduction mammaplasty utilizing an inferior pedicle nipple-areolar flap. Ann. Plast. Surg. 3:211, 1979.
7. Maliniac, J.W. Arterial blood supply of the breast. Arch. Surg. 47:329, 1943.
8. Money, J., and Gaskins, R. Sex reassignment. Int. J. Psychiatry Med. 9:249, 1970–1971.
9. Serafin, D. History of breast reconstruction. In N.G. Georgiade (ed.), Reconstructive Breast Surgery. St. Louis: Mosby, 1976.
10. Townsend, P.L.G. Nipple sensation following breast reduction and free nipple transplantation. Br. J. Plast. Surg. 27:308, 1974.
11. Walker, P.A., et al. Standards of care: The hormonal and surgical sex reassignment of gender dysphoric persons. Ann. Plast. Surg. 13:476, 1984.

COMMENTS ON CHAPTER 33 *Robert M. Goldwyn*

What Kenney and Edgerton have written reflects their considerable compassion for and extensive experience with transsexual patients. If ever the injunction of "treating the patient as a whole" has validity, it is in the setting of helping those whose anguish about their sexual identity has been excruciating and long-standing. Changing one's gender requires commitment and courage, qualities that those who do transsexual surgery must also possess to some degree. For many years before our society had even a minimal understanding of the plight of sexual identity problems, Edgerton devoted his notable talent and energy to improving their lives. Only someone of his stature could have pioneered and continued this type of surgery in an academic setting in full view of colleagues and staff who undoubtedly perceived, at least initially, these special patients and their operations as odd and even distasteful.

That the authors have apportioned much of the chapter to giving the reader a comprehension of the transsexual patient emphasizes the fact that no aspect in their medical or surgical management should be undertaken without considerable thought concerning each person's past history; emotional, social, and physical health; and future plans. No surgeon should engage in cross identity procedures without the aid of a gender identity team to evaluate each prospective patient in detail and over a sufficient length of time. That none of the patients in the authors' series regretted their sex change is testimony to the wise selection of patients.

My experience with transsexual surgery has been limited to the breast, mostly female to male. Perhaps my castration anxiety has restricted my surgical activities to above the umbilicus.

My experience with reduction mammaplasty in transsexuals is much less than that of the authors. Perhaps it is my persistent naiveté that makes me try, still, to avoid scars outside the areola, even in those patients who seek reduction for very large breasts. In patients with a bra cup size of A or B, it is relatively easy to achieve male configuration with a standard subcutaneous mastectomy. In patients who are very large, however, the surgical treatment is difficult because not every patient, even the most hirsute as a result of taking testosterone, can completely hide a horizontal or a T-shaped scar or one that extends medially at either end of a central incision through the areola.

In large-breasted transsexuals, I do a bilateral subcutaneous mastectomy and depend on tissue contraction for shrinkage. The second stage, 6 to 9 months later, involves reducing the diameter of the areola and the projection of the nipple, if required, as well as resecting remaining breast tissue or excess skin and folds — the approach being via the areola, utilizing concentric deepithelialization. Liposuction is useful for the final contouring. I admit that the chest contour in most of my patients (Fig. 33-14) is inferior to what Kenney and Edgerton have shown in their illustrations, but my patients do not have telltale chest scars that might become hypertrophic in some instances. Obviously, reducing large breasts is a problem that still awaits a better solution.

34

Robert M. Goldwyn

Complications and Unfavorable Results of Reduction Mammaplasty

Although reduction mammaplasty is associated with a high rate of patient satisfaction, many things can go wrong. The fact that the breast has sexual significance makes misfortune especially difficult for the patient. Problems can range from being relatively minor, such as stitch reaction, to distinctly major, such as nipple loss. This chapter will attempt to bring together these mishaps, several of which have been described or mentioned elsewhere in this book.

Preoperative Concerns
THE WRONG PATIENT
Operating on a patient physically or emotionally ill-suited can be catastrophic. Proper patient selection is mandatory in every elective procedure (Fig. 34-1). I detailed guidelines for screening patients in Chapter 8. The patient to be avoided is the one who has unrealistic expectations, particularly about scars — the person who does not truly comprehend emotionally, perhaps only intellectually, that she could have hypertrophic scarring. Telling a prospective patient that scars "tend to fade" may mistakenly convey the idea that all the scars will eventually disappear, not merely lessen. As mentioned earlier (Chap. 8), a good way, I have found, of getting the patient to be realistic is to show her a postoperative photograph of someone with very bad scars. Incidentally, if this is done, it should be noted in the record since it could be useful later in discussions with her or her attorney.

The patient with an emotional illness or systemic disease may be unfit for reduction mammaplasty at the time that she has the initial consultation. Careful history taking, physical examination, and laboratory investigation (to detect co-

agulopathy, for example) should be done. One should also communicate, of course, with those whom she is consulting for other problems.

INADEQUATELY EXAMINED BREASTS
It is surprisingly easy to examine a patient for reduction mammaplasty without actually thinking about each breast, both breasts, and those areas of the breast that will require modification to produce an excellent result. Seeing without observing and examining without thinking characterize medicine by rote — unfortunately, a particularly comfortable pattern to lapse into when one is fatigued. To prevent operating without thinking, one should plan the procedure before doing it, not at the operating table. The surgeon should study the patient's photographs the day before and immediately prior to operation and should thoughtfully examine the patient again just prior to operation even if the method planned does not necessitate preoperative marking.

The breast should be adequately examined to rule out malignancy, as was emphasized earlier (see Chap. 8).

WRONG BREAST SIZE
The surgeon should never guarantee a patient a specific cup size, yet the surgeon must be aware of the breast size that the patient wants (see Chap. 8) (Fig. 34-2).

POOR RAPPORT
If the surgeon and the patient have good rapport, the course of treatment will be much easier and

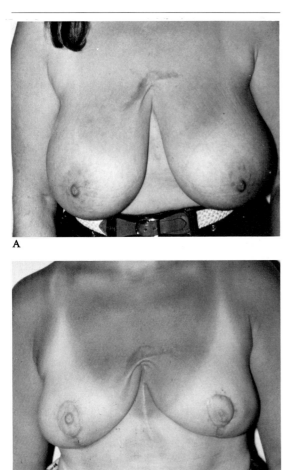

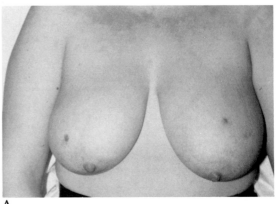

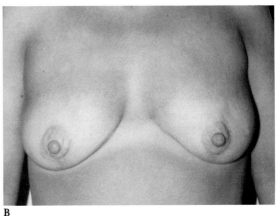

Fig. 34-1. A. Preoperative 33-year-old patient who had had correction of congenital heart defect as a baby. The fact that she already had scars made her "not concerned," she said, about additional scarring. B. Ten months postoperatively the patient was very happy with the results, which were good but not superb. Her outcome matched her expectations.

Fig. 34-2. A. Preoperative view of a 22-year-old patient who wants a large B or a C cup size. B. Postoperative at 2 years. The patient feels that her breasts are too small. Although she says she is not "very unhappy" with the results, she is certainly not happy.

satisfying to each. This is not just a matter of good public relations but is the essence of medicine and surgery: caring truly about the patient. If the patient rightfully perceives her surgeon to be uncaring, she will not do well emotionally if a complication arises.

Preoperatively, the patient should not feel inhibited about calling and asking lingering questions. Failure to return a call or to respond to a letter is a serious mistake and one that is easily avoidable. If the surgeon senses that the patient wants another appointment, she should receive it speedily. It is better to facilitate communication prior to the operation than afterward.

FAILING TO CANCEL OR POSTPONE AN OPERATION

Any patient who develops a significant medical or emotional problem near the time of or even on the day of operation should not have the procedure. Because the anesthesiologist usually examines the patient and screens her is no reason for the surgeon to abrogate responsibility about deciding whether and when to operate. If, for example, the patient has an acute infection elsewhere — conjunctivitis, cystitis — her surgery should be canceled.

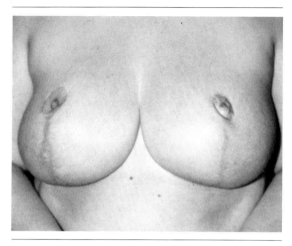

Fig. 34-3. A 40-year-old woman 5 years after reduction by another surgeon. The patient is extremely unhappy with her high nipples. She complains also of persistent pain in her scars and breasts and is clinically depressed. I referred her to a psychiatrist for therapy before I would undertake corrective surgery. She never returned to me.

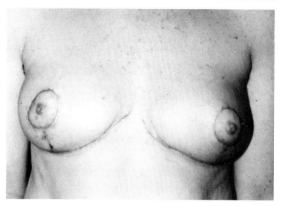

Fig. 34-4. Faulty incisions in a 23-year-old patient 3 weeks postoperatively. She later had revision of medial scars so that they would fit into the submammary sulcus.

The decision becomes more difficult when the patient calls a day prior to her procedure to report symptoms of a cold. If she has a fever or is sneezing or coughing, or says that she has been extremely fatigued for the past few days, my advice would be to postpone her surgery. I would not want the patient to become febrile postoperatively without knowing whether the fever was due to a viral infection or an infection in the wound or elsewhere.

Under the best circumstances, complications can occur with any procedure. Why increase that risk for the patient having a completely elective operation?

PLACING THE NIPPLES TOO HIGH IN THE PREOPERATIVE MARKING

I have stressed at length in Chapter 8 the common and unfortunate error of siting the nipple-areola too high (Fig. 34-3). When in doubt, place it lower. I will repeat here that proper marking is better done with the patient upright and not premedicated.

Improper Positioning of the Patient

Improper positioning of the patient on the operating table can result in pressure sores, musculoskeletal strains, and brachioplexus injuries (see Chap.

8). Another point to remember is that the electrocautery, if used, must be working safely and the patient appropriately grounded.

Errors of Anesthesia

Every surgeon should be aware of what is happening to the patient in a general way from the point of view of the anesthesia she is receiving. Has she been properly intubated? One can observe the movement of her chest with ventilation. One should also check the color of her lips and her blood for oxygen saturation and pay attention to the monitors giving arterial oxygen readings, blood pressure, electrocardiographic tracings, and pulse rate. This does not mean that the surgeon should neglect what he or she is doing on the field, but it does mean that he or she should be generally aware of what others are doing to the patient.

Technical Errors

Cutting the wrong thing or not cutting the right thing can obviously cause a poor surgical result. Inattention, carelessness, fatigue, or ignorance could be responsible. When an operation becomes "routine," the patient becomes more at risk.

FAULTY INCISION

Even though the incisions may have been marked preoperatively, it is advisable to check their location during operation, with regard especially to the medial extension of the inframammary incision to avoid going outside the fold. Care taken

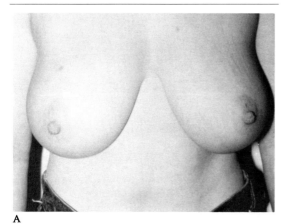

A

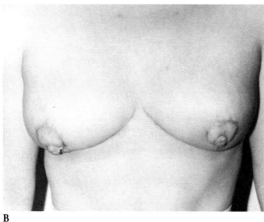

B

Fig. 34-5. A. Preoperative view of a 32-year-old woman. B. Postoperative view at 10 months. Nipples point displeasingly downward. Patient did not request correction.

now will eliminate a problem that will likely require revision (Fig. 34-4).

ASYMMETRY

In teaching centers, a cause of asymmetry can be the fact that not only were the breasts asymmetric prior to operation, but the same surgeon is not operating on both breasts. This is not the place to argue the merits of the various methods of training residents. The point here is that reduction mammaplasty usually involves two breasts; therefore, symmetry is not an easy objective to achieve. If the patient's surgeon has another surgeon doing part of the operation, the primary surgeon must carefully supervise his or her helper.

Throughout the operation, the surgeon must be alert not only about the amount of tissue removed but also from where it is taken. Periodically weighing the tissue and raising the patient into a sitting position are helpful in attaining symmetry.

As mentioned in Chapter 8, the surgeon should judge symmetry from the foot of the table and elicit the opinion of others present, although he or she is responsible for the result.

FAULTY PLACEMENT AND ASYMMETRY OF THE NIPPLES

No matter what the preoperative markings or how they were done, either before or during operation, the location of the nipple must be checked to be certain that it is correct (Fig. 34-5) and that both nipple-areola complexes are symmetric and of equal diameter and shape. A few minutes spent in measuring the position of the nipple can avoid hours of anguish for the patient and the surgeon later, including the need for another operation. It is critical to measure the distance of each nipple from the midline and from the submammary sulcus.

IMPENDING NIPPLE-AREOLA NECROSIS

The nipple-areola must be periodically inspected during operation to determine its apparent viability by noting its color and by testing its capillary filling. If the nipple-areola does not appear healthy, it is necessary to open the incision to rule out torsion or bleeding. Perhaps the wound must be closed differently to avoid tension or, indeed, more tissue resected to decrease the bulk that has produced the tension. Occasionally, it is necessary to refrain from completely closing the wound around the nipple-areola and along the vertical incision. Secondary healing proceeds with surprising rapidity, and delayed suturing may not be required.

If one has doubt about the viability of the nipple or areola after all these maneuvers, intravenous fluorescein in conjunction with a Wood lamp should be administered. A surgeon who does many reduction mammaplasties should be sure that the operating room or pharmacy stock this substance.

In a black patient, the epidermis should be removed by abrasion or as a split graft to see the uptake of the fluorescein. In my experience, the fluorescein test is seldom wrong. If the nipple-areola and part of its pedicle fail the test, the nipple-areola should be removed as a graft and the avascular segment of the pedicle amputated [20]. The nipple-areola must then be placed on a vascular bed, where it almost always survives. In grafting the nipple-areola, it is necessary to be sure that the nipple is in contact with the substrate by stitching it down using pressure to ensure maximum attachment.

DOG-EARS

At the end of this procedure, most surgeons become slightly fatigued, and it is easy not to take special care to eliminate dog-ears. One commonly used method is to close the wound from the ends toward the midline. This maneuver has additional advantages of decreasing tension centrally so that there is less chance for necrosis at the junction of the inverted T. The other advantage is that it decreases the length of the inframammary incision if it has not already been fully made. However, one disadvantage is that as more tissue is brought centrally, the nipple-areola distance to the inframammary fold can lengthen — another reason to check the distance to be sure that it does not exceed 6.5 to 7.0 cm.

From a technical point of view, it is easier to eliminate dog-ears by turning the patient slightly to the opposite side and by sitting down. One must also be sure that the extension of the incision, if necessary, to eliminate the dog-ear does not rise too high or extend too far and that it matches as much as possible that of the opposite side (Fig. 34-6).

EXCESSIVE BLOOD LOSS

Careful dissection and the punctilious use of electrocautery will decrease blood loss. In the last 20 years, I have not needed to transfuse a patient having a reduction mammaplasty.

Infiltration with epinephrine is also effective in minimizing blood loss. Although this technique has the theoretical disadvantages of interfering with pedicle vascularity and causing the "rebound phenomenon" (brisk bleeding after the epinephrine effect has passed), these do not usually happen.

Autologous blood transfusion is discussed in Chapter 8.

NIPPLE-AREOLA INVERSION AND DISTORTION

In Chapter 18, nipple-areola inversion and distortion are discussed, as are measures to prevent their occurrence. The surgeon should not attempt to correct preexisting nipple inversion at operation;

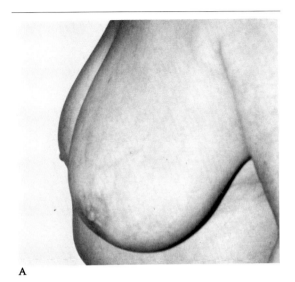

A

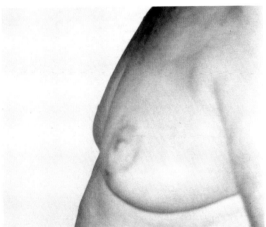

B

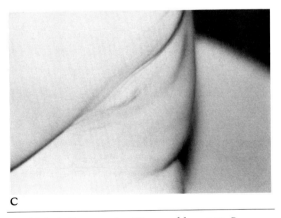

C

Fig. 34-6. A. Preoperative 68-year-old woman. B. Postoperative at 1 year after removal of 1150 gm. C. Dog-ear visible.

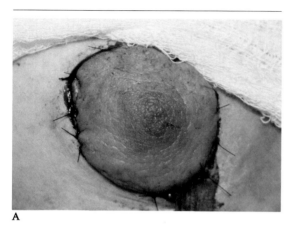

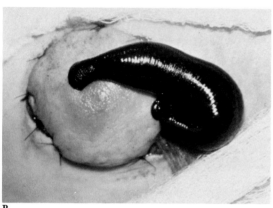

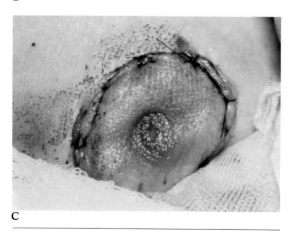

Fig. 34-7. A. Venous engorgement of areola and nipple 5 hours after operation. B. Leech applied at 5½ hours postoperatively. C. Four days after operation. Leeches had been stopped 24 hours before this photograph. The nipple-areola complex regained normal vascularity and healed uneventfully with normal sensation.

otherwise, blood supply to the nipple-areola may be compromised.

Concerns Immediately Postoperative
AREAS OF GENERAL MANAGEMENT
Many things can go awry postoperatively. Here, I will emphasize only a few. The first is incomplete or faulty orders. The surgeon should write orders or check those that someone else has written. For example, one must be certain that the patient, in the recovery room has received her antibiotics if desired, her proper diabetic regimen if required, and cortisone, if needed, for a prior condition.

Orders concerning voiding should be explicit. I do not routinely use an indwelling catheter. However, a catheter should be considered for a patient who is unable to urinate despite having received adequate intravenous fluids, as well as having gone through the ritual of getting up to void, hearing running water, and possibly receiving bethanachol chloride (Urecholine). Prior to inserting a catheter, the patient's bladder should be percussed by someone experienced in this procedure. Suprapubic drainage by needle aspiration is also an alternative.

Postoperative orders must include instructions for examining the nipple-areola to detect necrosis. Dressings should be loose and permit easy access for that purpose.

IMPENDING NIPPLE NECROSIS
Impending nipple necrosis is the dread of every surgeon [30]. If the nipple-areola appears to be extremely blue and engorged, the surgeon should remove a few stitches. If this produces no change in color, the patient may have to return to the operating room to rule out pedicle torsion or underlying hematoma. If, despite these measures, the nipple-areola complex still shows venous obstruction, medicinal leeches may help (Fig. 34-7) [2]. I have utilized these measures with success in two memorable cases. Because the leech (Hirudo medicinalis) carries Aeromonas hydrophila, the patient can develop an infection and should prophylactically receive tetracycline or another antibiotic to which the leech is sensitive [29]. Aeromonas is resistant to penicillin and ampicillin.

INFECTION
Wound infection in the immediate postoperative period is unusual but can occur [18]. In most instances, the causative organism is Streptococcus.

As mentioned in Chapter 8, the value of prophylactic antibiotics for breast reduction has not yet
been proved. However, if a patient becomes febrile and the wound looks erythematous, she
should be given penicillin intravenously if she is
not already on an antibiotic to which *Streptococcus* is sensitive. Although the wound should be
cultured, antibiotics should not be withheld.

Ransjo et al [16] showed that cultures taken during reduction mammaplasty in 25 patients (49
breasts) grew predominantly *Staphylococcus epi-
dermidis* and anaerobic *Propionibacterium acnes.*
It is assumed, although not definitely known, that
these bacteria are normal inhabitants of the mammary ducts of most women [26].

Rand and Bostwick [15] reported pyoderma gangrenosum in a 19-year-old student 4 days after reduction mammaplasty. She had been on oral ce-
phalosporin but developed a fever; cultures were
negative, perhaps reflecting the effect of the previously administered antibiotics. She eventually
needed debridement; tissue samples showed only
nonspecific inflammation. She was managed successfully with intravenous globulin (because of
hypogammaglobulinemia) and with prednisone.

Cruse and Foord [7], in a prospective study of
22,649 wounds, determined that electrocautery
doubled the incidence of wound infection in four
varieties of wounds: clean, clean-contaminated,
contaminated, and dirty. This adverse effect of
electrocautery has not been a consistent finding in
other studies.

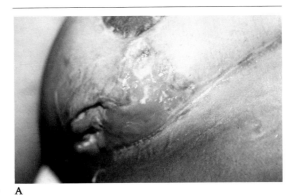

A

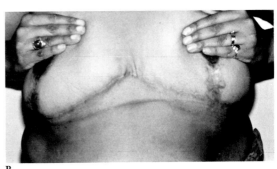

B

Fig. 34-8. A. A 38-year-old woman referred because of a
dehiscence. The surgeon stated that closure was under
excessive tension. The patient and family were very
displeased and angry that the surgeon, according to
them, did not see her daily in the hospital and "ran
away." Reassurance, wet to dry dressings, and frequent
visits to the office were the treatment. B. Three
months later, the wounds have healed but the patient
is still angry at the surgeon.

HEMORRHAGE AND HEMATOMA

Hemorrhage is always possible after any operation. It is rare after reduction mammaplasty, and if
it occurs, it is apparent.

Perpere et al [14] reported severe bleeding in a
28-year-old woman 2 hours after an uneventful
reduction mammaplasty. The cause was "acute fi-
brinolysis," without the specific factor responsible mentioned.

Strömbeck [22], in reviewing 671 patients, reported the incidence of hematoma to be 2.7 percent; McKissock's [12] incidence was 2.21 percent
in 360 patients having an average resection of
724 gm.

Although most hematomas occur in the first 24
hours, McKissock [11,12] noted that infrequently
hemorrhage can occur up to 9 days following operation and even consecutively in the same patient.
Possible causes for late bleeding are extreme phys-

ical exertion, aspirin ingestion, or an unrecog-
nized clotting disorder.

One should be quick to drain an expanding hematoma before it causes pressure and necrosis of
the skin with loss of tissue and possibly loss of
nipple-areola viability.

The presence of a hematoma, even if evacuated,
increases the likelihood of infection. For this reason, the patient should be given antibiotics if she
has not already been receiving them.

Early Complications and Unfavorable Results

WOUND DEHISCENCE

Frequently, a suture line will disrupt at the junction of the inverted T if stitches are removed too
early, before the twelfth to fourteenth postopera-

568

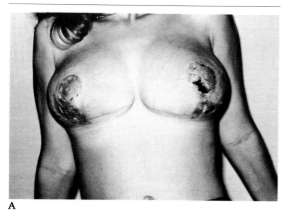

A

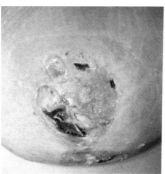

B

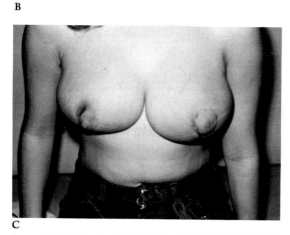

C

Fig. 34-9. A. An 18-year-old patient referred 2 weeks after reduction because she was a student in Boston and wanted to return to school. B. Left nipple-areola at the time of the initial visit. C. Three months later, she was healed. Daily dressings were done by the patient using soap and water. Three to four times per week she visited my office for reassurance, and I had weekly communication with the referring doctor to preserve that relationship. The patient later returned to her original surgeon for revision.

tive day [27] (Figs. 34-8, 34-9). Intradermal Vicryl helps to maintain coaptation after the sutures have been removed from the skin and dermis (intradermal pull-out suture).

A patient may call to say that during the night the wound has "split open." This is more likely to occur if the closure has been tight. She should be seen immediately and sutured if wound separation is significant. Otherwise, a prominent scar may result.

OCCULT CANCER

Rarely, fortunately, does a young patient without a worrisome family history or suspicious mammogram and physical examination have an unsuspected malignancy detected microscopically during or soon after operation [17]. The patient should obviously be referred for consultation to the appropriate surgeon, oncologist, and, possibly, radiotherapist. It is possible that she will require mastectomy and may then need a reconstruction. In my experience, this sequence is devastating. One patient, 48 years of age, went through this ordeal and said after she had been informed of the pathologist findings, "I loved my breasts just after operation. Now, this news is like you're taking away my child just after it is born." Not surprisingly, that patient required psychotherapy before she would undergo a modified radical mastectomy (nodes were uninvolved). She later had a reconstruction but never truly accepted her result. She wrote me a letter to thank me for what I had done, but said that she could never go into my office again because it reminded her of her "personal disaster."

As mentioned in Chapter 8, if a malignancy is recognized at the time of operation, the procedure must be terminated without any attempt made to reduce the opposite breast or to perform a mastectomy about which the patient has not been informed. The decision of how to treat breast cancer is not in the province of the plastic surgeon in most institutions.

MONDOR'S DISEASE

Mondor's disease is benign, self-limiting, superficial thrombophlebitis of a vein or veins of the anterolateral wall that can occur spontaneously or 3 to 7 weeks after trauma, such as reduction mammaplasty [13]. A visible, palpable, vertical cord is present, generally, but not always, in the submammary area and is made prominent when the patient

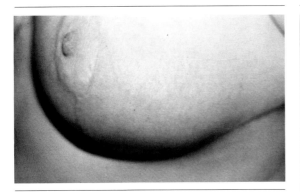

Fig. 34-10. *Mondor's disease in a 23-year-old woman. Three weeks after reduction mammaplasty, a vein going obliquely from the areola (2 o'clock) to the submammary fold was hard. No treatment was performed. The patient was reassured and after 5 months there were no signs of this condition.*

raises her arms, putting the skin under tension (Fig. 34-10). Since Mondor's disease disappears by recannulation and remodeling of collagen, no treatment is indicated [9]. Only rarely, however, because of pain or cosmesis, is it necessary to divide or remove the thrombosed vein [9].

SYSTEMIC PROBLEMS
This is not the place to detail the many possible problems, medical and surgical, that the patient might develop postoperatively (Fig. 34-11). It is, however, important to be on the alert for atelectasis and pneumonia, urinary infection, cardiac arrhythmia and ischemia, deep phlebitis, and pulmonary embolism. The application of basic knowledge of surgery and medicine is always necessary for treating patients.

Later Complications and Unfavorable Results
I agree entirely with McKissock, who stated, "For the most part, late complications represent those that result when the passage of time has failed to work its magic. Usually, they are the late manifestations of improper preoperative planning [12]." Usually, he says, but not always.

BAD SCARRING
Although scars are inevitable, some are worse than others; those especially prone to becoming hypertrophic are the ends of the inframammary incision, particularly lateral (Fig. 34-12), and the circumareolar incision [1]. The last is more likely to occur if there has been partial loss of the areola in a

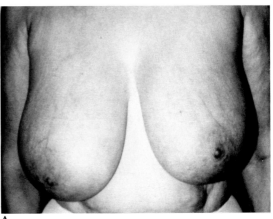

A

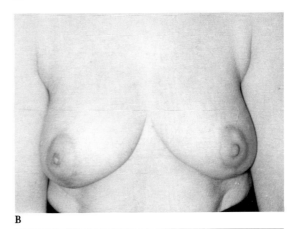

B

Fig. 34-11. *A. Preoperative view of a 68-year-old woman. B. Postoperative view at 1 year. The patient was pleased with the result. However, 8 days after operation, she had severe diarrhea and abdominal cramps but attributed this to "food poisoning." She was nevertheless referred to a gastroenterologist, who found partially obstructing cancer of the descending colon in an otherwise asymptomatic patient without change in bowel habits and without anemia. She had a left colectomy and has remained free of disease 10 years later.*

young patient, more prone to develop hypertrophic, thick, red scars.

The secondary healing that commonly occurs at the junction of the inverted T does not usually produce a thick scar, but if it should occur, it is in a hidden location.

Steroid injection with triamcinolone, 25 mg/ml once, twice, or even three times over intervals of 4 to 6 weeks, is usually helpful. The patient must be warned that the scar may turn purple, but it is hoped it will flatten. The hypertrophic scar that

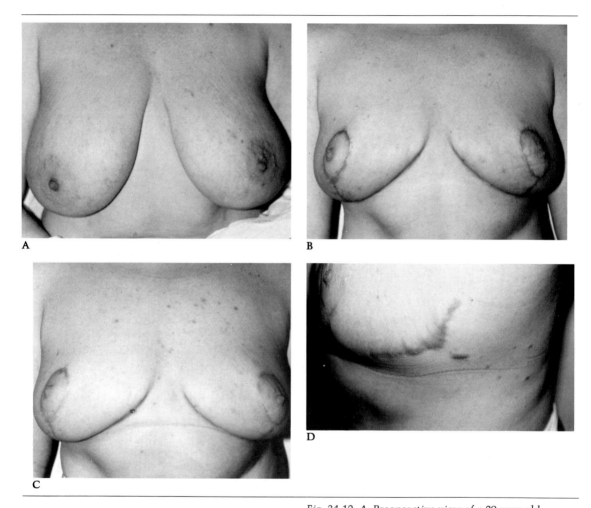

Fig. 34-12. A. Preoperative view of a 29-year-old woman. B. Postoperative view at 3 months. C,D. Postoperative view at 12 months. Wounds have healed well except for lateral scar.

"itches" is a good candidate for steroids, which usually provide quick relief.

Surgical revision of scars is disappointing in young patients who have healed primarily without infection. Patients should be informed about the possible futility of scar revision. McKissock [11] reported that 65 percent of his patients developed some degree of hypertrophy and that surgical revision was usually unsuccessful.

Revision should not be attempted until 9 to 12 months have elapsed. If extensive areas are to be revised, it is wiser, in my experience, to attempt a small portion of the scar under local anesthesia rather than submitting the patient to an extensive procedure whose outcome is dubious.

Strömbeck [23], in a 10-year retrospective study,

found that 30 percent of his patients consider their scars poor; 17 percent, ugly; and only 23 percent, excellent. Despite those sentiments, the majority of his patients would still have the procedure again.

ASYMMETRY AND UNDESIRABLE SHAPE OR SIZE

Unfavorable results in terms of contour and shape can be judged only after a sufficient time has passed—at least 18 months and even longer (Fig. 34-13). Occasionally, it may be necessary to re-

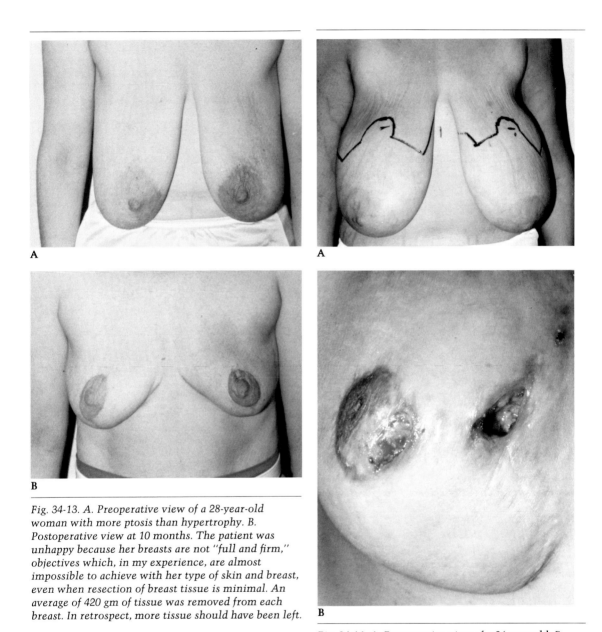

Fig. 34-13. A. Preoperative view of a 28-year-old
woman with more ptosis than hypertrophy. B.
Postoperative view at 10 months. The patient was
unhappy because her breasts are not "full and firm,"
objectives which, in my experience, are almost
impossible to achieve with her type of skin and breast,
even when resection of breast tissue is minimal. An
average of 420 gm of tissue was removed from each
breast. In retrospect, more tissue should have been left.

Fig. 34-14. A. Preoperative view of a 26-year-old. B.
Postoperative view showing fat necrosis after removal
of 1,800 gm of tissue using the original Strömbeck
procedure. Debridement and frequent daily changes of
saline dressings packed into the wound were required.
Healing took longer than patient wanted and surgeon
believes that the fat necrosis is even modest.

move more tissue. This can usually be done under
local anesthesia, very often with liposuction, since
what remains is more likely to be fat rather than
breast tissue. It may, of course, be both; then,
sharp dissection may be necessary.

It is my practice not to charge a patient for these
secondary procedures; they have to pay the hospital costs.

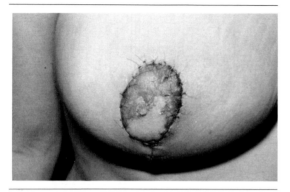

Fig. 34-15. A 22-year-old patient 10 days postoperatively. Impending necrosis proved to be superficial.

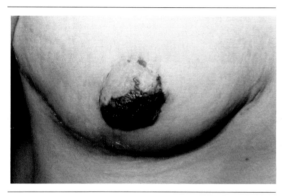

Fig. 34-16. A 25-year-old patient 14 days postoperatively. Full-thickness necrosis of the nipple and lower half of areola is seen. The patient never returned for reconstruction.

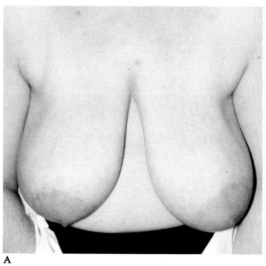

A

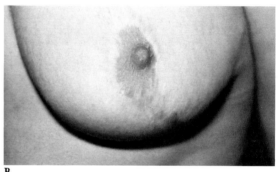

B

Fig. 34-17. A. Preoperative view of a 16-year-old girl. Note the very large areolae. B. Postoperative view at 2 years showing distortion of the areola with some loss superiorly and residual areola along the vertical scar.

FAT NECROSIS

If fat has been left attached but lying beyond the pedicle, it may later necrose because of its insufficient blood supply (Fig. 34-14). Drainage or a sterile abscess or even a hard mass may result. A lump that persists a few months despite the normal pathology report of the tissue previously removed should be biopsied to be certain of the diagnosis. There is the possibility of a malignancy in any breast at any time.

Strömbeck [22] reported a 16 percent incidence rate of fat necrosis in obese patients having a resection greater than 1000 gm. In my experience, with the inferior pedicle technique, necrotic fat drainage is rare unless nipple-areola necrosis has occurred; then, some of the pedicle has also died and must be debrided, with daily wound dressings and packing. If one is aggressive about getting rid of dead tissue, the patient's recovery time is shortened considerably.

NIPPLE-AREOLA NECROSIS AND THE UNHEALED WOUND

Although nipple-areola necrosis usually happens within the first 10 days after operation (Figs. 34-15 and 34-16), its effects may last many months if necrosis has been extensive in terms of the pedicle, as just mentioned. In Chapter 8, I discussed the necessity of enlisting the patient in caring for her own wound. This decreases her dependency and helps her to improve physically and emotionally. Occasionally, visiting nurses are helpful in this regard. The surgeon, however, is still responsible for the patient and must see her frequently, not simply to offer support, which is extremely important, but also to debride the wound. I usually have the patient use wet-to-dry dressings of saline or even tapwater, 3 to 4 times a day. I believe strongly in having the patient shower or tub bathe frequently using soap and water to clean the wound.

If the nipple or areola or both have undergone significant loss, reconstruction and replacement are necessary. The same kinds of techniques used in nipple-areola reconstruction after breast reconstruction are applicable here. At this writing, I use a modification of Little's quadropod method for rebuilding the nipple and a full-thickness skin graft from the upper inner thigh to reconstruct the areola. Tattooing is a helpful adjunct to get a better match.

INVERSION OF THE NIPPLES
Inversion of the nipples cannot always be avoided at operation. It can never be avoided if the patient has inverted nipples prior to operation—a fact that must be explained to her. Some techniques, such as that of Strömbeck, are associated with this problem more than other methods of reduction mammaplasty.

McKissock [12] states that with his vertical bipedicle flap technique, areolar retraction usually results from an excessively broad-based superior flap. Correction is possible by narrowing the attachment with incisions around the areola made to 11 o'clock and to 1 o'clock.

Every surgeon has his or her technique or techniques for correcting nipple inversion. I have found the method of Teimourian and Adham [24] to be usually reliable; it involves essentially the use of triangular flaps of dermis, one on each side of the nipple, slid under the nipple and joined together. This method provides needed bulk to aid and ensure nipple projection.

RESIDUAL AREOLA
Patients with very large areolae should be told preoperatively that it may be impossible to remove as much of the areola as is aesthetically desirable, since it would compromise closure and create unsafe tension (Fig. 34-17). As a secondary procedure, taking out the remaining areola is not usu-

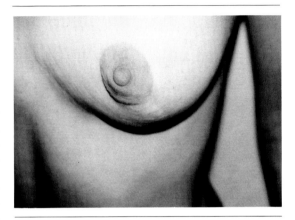

Fig. 34-18. Pouting, redundant areola in an 18-year-old woman at 8 months following operation. Sensation was normal and the patient did not wish to risk possible interference with sensation by revision.

ally difficult, since it lies adjacent in most instances to the vertical incision areola to inframammary fold.

POUTING NIPPLE-AREOLA
Occasionally the nipple-areola complex will look redundant and pouting (Fig. 34-18). An intimation of this sequela may have been noted at operation, where it can usually but not always be eliminated by trimming more fat and glandular tissue from the nipple-areola undersurface. However, it is better to accept the problem and not whittle away to the point of jeopardizing vascularity.

Postoperatively, after six to eight months, this relatively minor but exasperating problem can be resolved by trimming excess areola and/or increasing the diameter of the keyhole if it is less than that on the other side. Tacking the undersurface down to the deeper tissue with nonabsorbable sutures of nylon is also helpful. In one patient, however, all these maneuvers failed to work after two attempts. The cause might have been excess tissue tension at the initial closure and subsequent scarring at the junction of the vertical incision. Since neither the patient nor I tried again, I do not know whether this supposition is correct.

CONVERGENT AREOLAE
Areolae that are too medial and point inward toward each other present a difficult problem. However, a useful technique for correction has been described by Salema et al [19]. They make use

of an inferior dermal-fat curve flap that accomplishes the purpose and also preserves the blood supply to the nipple-areola.

Occasionally, a semicircular excision of skin may be all that is necessary if the nipple-areola is not too far toward the midline.

NIPPLE TOO HIGH

Nipple placement that is too high is one of the most challenging and exasperating problems (see Fig. 34-3) [21]. Resecting an inferior segment of tissue above the inframammary sulcus may lower the nipple-areola somewhat, but if its position is very high, it is not possible to lower it without leaving a scar above it. This is a vertical scar that results from closing the window that previously held the nipple and areola, now located more inferiorly.

One idea that I have had but never attempted is to place a slightly curve-shaped expander above the areola, and, after a suitable interval of filling it, removing it, then draping the excess skin around the nipple in its new, lower position.

NIPPLE TOO LOW

The unfavorable result of a nipple that is too low is less disturbing to the patient because her nipple(s) stays in the brassiere. Yet, it is not an outcome that pleases either the patient or the surgeon (Fig. 34-18). Unless the nipple is excessively low, a simple crescent excision of skin superiorly is sufficient to raise the nipple-areola. If more length is required, a Z-plasty can be effective. The angle and length of the limbs have to be calculated to match the other side if it is not necessary to operate on both breasts.

I have never needed to resort to a skin graft or a flap from below the inframammary fold. I would try to avoid those procedures.

INABILITY TO LACTATE

Despite the large numbers of women having had reduction mammaplasty, only a few studies of lactation have been reported [22]. These studies indicate a 50 to 70 percent chance of nursing in patients who have had breast reduction by transposition techniques.

GALACTORRHEA

Instances of galactorrhea immediately after reduction mammaplasty have been reported by Sandler et al [20] and by Bruck [3]. The reason for its occurrence is postulated by Bruck to be a combination of several factors: (1) prolactin, which is a stress hormone, and its secretion increased after operation; (2) a rebound phenomenon following discontinued birth control pills, if the patient is on them, could result in decreased progesterone, which might increase prolactin-releasing factors; (3) stimulation of prolactin production by means of a sucking reflex is well known and may be mimicked by transposing the mammilla on its pedicle; (4) sufficient elevation of steroid concentration as a result of surgical stress may stimulate prolactin receptors; and (5) there is a hypersensitivity to prolactin receptors. Obviously, this sequence is still conjecture. However, galactorrhea can be managed successfully by giving the patient bromocriptine, a prolactin inhibitor, which induces cessation of galactorrhea.

RECURRENT HYPERTROPHY

The recurrence of hypertrophy after reduction mammaplasty is extremely rare except in patients who are very young, aged 12 to 14 years (Fig. 34-19), whose breasts are massive and whose operation had to be performed because of very large, rapid growth whose consequences psychologically and socially were compelling.

LATE CHANGES OF SHAPE AND VOLUME

Vilain and Mitz [29] reported that patients followed for more than 20 years after reduction mammaplasty by the Biesenberger method showed little change in the appearance of their breasts despite the patients having weight fluctuations and having undergone pregnancies as well as the effects of aging. Changes in the breast, moreover, in the series of Vilain and Mitz were more likely to occur within 2 years of the procedure. Hoffman [10], however, found unexpected changes after 5 years or longer, including descent of the breast, ptosis, and asymmetry aggravated by failure at operation to resect enough breast tissue and by placing the nipple too high.

In my experience, it is a rare patient who returns years after reduction to have a revision. This does not necessarily mean that the appearance of the breast would not be helped by an additional operation. What it does suggest is that patients adapt well to changes in the breast that are slow to develop unless they are severe.

IMPAIRED SENSATION

In their study of the effects of plastic surgery on breast sensation, Courtiss and Goldwyn [6] found

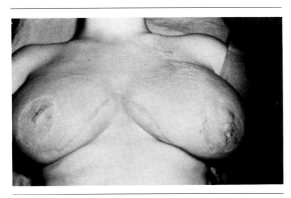

Fig. 34-19. Postoperative view after two reduction mammaplasties requiring eventual subcutaneous mastectomy with implants. (Courtesy of Joseph E. Murray, M.D.)

that after reduction mammaplasty by dermal pedicle transposition, almost all breasts had decreased sensibility to pain (measured by a dental pulp voltimeter), crude touch, and light pressure for about 6 months. At 1 year, the skin of the breast in most patients had regained its sensitivity, but the nipple had decreased sensation in 35 percent of patients, even at 2 years. These changes related more to amount of tissue removed rather than type of technique used. Even though the nipple objectively had some degree of numbness, women subjectively reported a higher degree of sensibility in their breasts, a finding that suggested that their better body image permitted them to enjoy sex more.

Nipple erectility was almost always normal. Erectility depends on sympathetic fibers to the areolar muscle [4] and precedes return of all sensory modalities; erectility may persist and usually does even in a nipple-areola that is numb. As surgeons, we note nipple-areola contractility when we stimulate it during operation when the patient is unconscious, as we prep her or mark out the new areolar diameter.

In a review of 362 breast reductions, McKissock [12] reported similar findings to those of Courtiss and Goldwyn: Immediately after reduction, about 90 percent of patients had some loss of sensation; by 6 months, 80 percent had regained some sensation, but at 2 years, 70 percent had reduced sensation; 22 percent had normal sensation, but 8 percent had no sensation. Although two thirds of McKissock's patients did not consider these sensory changes significant, patients with complete

numbness are not usually pleased with that aspect of the reduction mammaplasty. As noted in Chapter 8, sensation is likely to remain what it was preoperatively in a higher percentage of patients than when other reduction methods are used, but altered sensation and frank numbness of the nipple do occur unless great care is exerted to avoid the branches of the intercostal nerves [8], especially those of the fourth nerve, so clearly dissected by Astley Cooper [5] a century and a half ago. Terzis et al [25], by a quantitative neurophysiologic appraisal of normal breast sensibility, were able to subdivide the breast into distinct cutaneous areas with differing mechanoreceptive characteristics. They found, as did Courtiss and Goldwyn preoperatively in their patients, that although most women report the nipple to be the most sensitive part of their breasts, objectively, it is much less sensitive, a finding that led Courtiss and Goldwyn to postulate that these neurophysiologic features of the breast permit suckling by the baby without pain to the mother. However, all receptors, except nociroceptors, are high in the nipple region and may explain why the majority of women perceive the nipple to be the most sensitive part of the breast. Terzis et al [25] suggest that since the nipple "supplies visual evidence of temperature and sexual arousal . . . ," this "also contributes to a woman's perception that the nipple is the most sensitive area."

For the woman in whom reduction mammaplasty has caused nipple numbness, nothing now known can be done to improve sensation.

In my experience seeing women who had their reductions done elsewhere and complained of the result, more often than not, it is not the appearance of the breast or even the numbness of the nipples that bothers them, but, so they allege, the fact that the surgeon had not warned them of the possibility of altered sensation. This postoperative problem should be part of the informed consent, and I list it on the form that the patient signs. I also dictate in the chart that I have discussed it with her.

CYSTS

This problem, which should be avoidable, is more common than is recognized or admitted. If the procedure had involved a dermal pedicle, the surgeon should have inspected it carefully, with magnification lenses if necessary, to be sure that all epidermis had been removed, whether by knife or _c_, from the areas to be buried. Many of _remnants_ will disappear, but some can pro-_ce_ exasperating cysts and recurrent infection, necessitating a full-thickness excision of the area. Primary closure without additional tissue in the form of a flap or graft is usually but not always possible.

REGROWTH

Fortunately, recurrence of breast hypertrophy is unusual. It is more likely to happen in patients who are very young, between ages 12 and 15, who have experienced rapid development of their breasts (see Fig. 34-19). In this age, it is always important to discuss with the patient and her parents the possibility of recurrence of the macromastia. Sometimes administration of hormones, such as progesterone, is helpful in this difficult situation, but the effects of these medications may be hazardous to the patient in the future. Subcutaneous mastectomy with insertion of implants may be the only recourse for persistent, invidious regrowth.

PATIENT DISSATISFACTION

Although most patients are satisfied with their result, not all are. Some patients are unhappy when they should not be, at least from the surgeon's standpoint; however, some are justifiably displeased because of an obvious problem, such as bad scarring, significant nipple-areola deformity or asymmetry, or loss of sensation. Strömbeck found that satisfaction was related to age: the older the patient, the happier she was with the result. My experience has been that the older patients accept the problems of wound healing better than do younger patients, but not necessarily the rapid change in their breast size and body image.

Although the surgeon justifiably dreads nipple-areola necrosis, the few patients in whom this has happened have never returned to have a nipple-areola rebuilt and, in follow-up communication, have decided not to have it done by anyone else either.

When a complication or an unfavorable result produces noticeable asymmetry of breast size, women have problems in adaptation because of buying clothes or interpersonal relations. In this regard, what an "important other" says or how he or she reacts becomes the determining factor in persistent dissatisfaction.

If a patient has persistent pain, this usually indicates deep dissatisfaction with the surgical outcome and may be based in depression (see Fig. 34-1). With regard to sensation, the usual complaint is not pain but numbness. When a patient says that she cannot have sexual relations or go to work because of breast pain, she must be referred to a psychotherapist for evaluation.

If a patient has achieved a result that most patients and surgeons would consider good or even very good and she is still dissatisfied, one should arrange a consultation with another plastic surgeon. A patient who is unhappy with a surgical result is generally angry with the surgeon and is likely to seek legal action (see Chap. 7).

Conclusion

Reduction mammaplasty is usually but not always accompanied by a high degree of patient and surgeon satisfaction. The fact that a complication or unfavorable result can occur must be stressed to the patient preoperatively. The surgeon must take every means to emphasize that he or she cannot guarantee a result. In an effort to allay a patient's anxiety, it is easy to minimize the realities of the surgical act, many of whose consequences are beyond human control and repair.

References

1. Arion, H-G. _La Reduction Mammaire._ Paris: Maloine, 1974. Pp. 61–68.
2. Batchelor, G.G., Davison, P., and Sully, L. The salvage of congested skin flap by the application of leeches. _Br. J. Plast. Surg._ 37:358, 1984.
3. Bruck, J.C. Galactorrhea: A rare complication following reduction mammaplasty. _Ann. Plast. Surg._ 19:384, 1987.
4. Cathcart, E.P., Gairns, F.W., and Garven, H.S.D. The innervation of the human quiescent nipple, with notes on pigmentation, erection, and hyperneury. _Trans. R. Soc. Edinb._ 61:689, 1948.
5. Cooper, A. _The Anatomy of the Breast._ London: Longman's, 1840.
6. Courtiss, E.H., and Goldwyn, R.M. Breast sensation before and after plastic surgery. _Plast. Reconstr. Surg._ 58:1, 1976.
7. Cruse, P.J.E., and Foord, R. A five-year prospective study of 23,649 wounds. _Arch. Surg._ 107:206, 1973.
8. Craig, R.D.P., and Sykes, P.A. Nipple sensitivity following reduction mammaplasty. _Br. J. Plast. Surg._ 23:165, 1970.
9. Green, R.A., and Dowden, R.V. Mondor's disease in plastic surgery patients. _Ann. Plast. Surg._ 20:231, 1988.
10. Hoffman, S. Recurrent deformities following reduction mammaplasty and correction of breast asymmetry. _Plast. Reconstr. Surg._ 78:55, 1986.

11. McKissock, P.K. Complications and Undesirable Results with Reduction Mammaplasty. In R.M. Goldwyn (ed.), *The Unfavorable Result in Plastic Surgery: Avoidance and Treatment* (2nd ed.). Boston: Little, Brown, 1984. Pp. 739–759.

12. McKissock, P.K. Reduction Mammaplasty. In E.H. Courtiss (ed.), *Aesthetic Surgery. Trouble: How to Avoid it and How to Treat it.* St. Louis: Mosby, 1978. Pp. 189–203.

13. Mondor, M.H. Tronculite sous-cutanée subaigue de la paroi thoracique antero-laterale. *Mem. Acad. Chir.* 65:127, 1939.

14. Perpere, C., Forli, V., Inbert-Emperaire, M., et al. Coagulopathie et plastie mammaire. *Ann. Chir. Plast. Esthet.* 27:175, 1982.

15. Rand, R.P., and Bostwick, J. III. Pyoderma gangrenosum. *Perspect. Surg.* 2:176, 1988.

16. Ransjo, U., Asplund, O.A., Gylbert, L., and Jurell, G. Bacteria in the female breast. *Scand. J. Plast. Reconstr. Surg.* 19:87, 1985.

17. Rees, T.D., and Coburn, R. Breast reduction: Is it an aid to cancer detection? *Br. J. Plast. Surg.* 25:144, 1972.

18. Regnault, P., and Daniel, R.K. *Aesthetic Plastic Surgery.* Boston: Little, Brown, 1984. Pp. 530–536.

19. Salema, R., Aboudib, J.H., and DeCastro, C.C. Convergent nipple-areolar complexes corrected by inferior curve pedicle technique. *Ann. Plast. Surg.* 19:555, 1987.

20. Sandler, M.D., Forman, M.B., Lopis, R., and Kalk, W.I. Galactorrhea, amenorrhea and hyperprolactinemia after an operation on the breast: A case report. *S. Afr. Med. J.* 57:95, 1980.

21. Smith, J.W., and Gillen, F.J. Repairing errors of nipple-areola placement following reduction mammaplasty. *Aesth. Plast. Surg.* 4:179, 1980.

22. Strömbeck, J.L. Reduction Mammaplasty by Strömbeck Technique. In R.M. Goldwyn (ed.), *Plastic and Reconstructive Surgery of the Breast.* Boston: Little, Brown, 1976. P. 209.

23. Strömbeck, J.L. Late Results After Reduction Mammaplasty. In R.M. Goldwyn (ed.), *Long-Term Results in Plastic Surgery.* Boston: Little, Brown, 1980. Pp. 722–732.

24. Teimourian, B., and Adham, M.M. Simple technique for correction of inverted nipple. *Plast. Reconstr. Surg.* 65:504, 1980.

25. Terzis, J.K., Vincent, M.P., Wilkins, L.M., et al. Breast sensibility: A neurophysiological appraisal in the normal breast. *Ann. Plast. Surg.* 19:318, 1987.

26. Thornton, J.W., Argenta, L.C., McClatchy, K.D., and Marks, M.W. Studies on the endogenous flora of the human breast. *Ann. Plast. Surg.* 20:39, 1988.

27. Vandenbussche, F., Vandevord, J., Robbe, N., and DeCoopman, B. Plasties mammaires de reduction aleas et malfacons des techniques a cicatrice en T renverse. *Ann. Chir. Plast. Esthet.* 24:319, 1979.

28. Vilain, R., and Mitz, V. The Biesenberger Technique for Mammary Ptosis and Hypertrophy. In R.M. Goldwyn (ed.), *Long-Term Results in Plastic and Reconstructive Surgery.* Boston, Little, Brown, 1980. Pp. 708–734.

29. Whitlock, M.R., O'Hare, P.N., Sanders, R., and Morrow, M.C. The medicinal leech and its use in plastic surgery: A possible cause for infection. *Br. J. Plast. Surg.* 36:240, 1983.

30. Wray, R.C., and Luce, E.A. Treatment of impending nipple necrosis following reduction mammaplasty. *Plast. Reconstr. Surg.* 68:242, 1981.

35

Frederick M. Grazer

Suction-Assisted Lipectomy as an Adjunct to Reduction Mammaplasty and Removal of Axillary Breasts

With the advent of suction-assisted lipectomy (SAL), a variety of refinements have been made possible to improve the contour of the breast in relation to size reduction [1,2].

Breast Reduction

Most patients with breast hypertrophy have axillary fullness. Suction at the time of reduction can be accomplished through the incision site. Suctioning is also helpful to eliminate the dog-ears and to reduce the length of the transverse incision site.

AXILLARY FULLNESS

Reduction of axillary breast fullness can frequently be accomplished with suction alone. The approach is made through the axilla; however, the approach can be made through the breast if breast surgery is being performed for reduction, reconstruction, or augmentation (Figs. 35-1 and 35-2).

REDUCING THE PEDICLE

Another advantage of utilizing suctioning is that with a small cannula, one can reduce the size of the pedicle without affecting the circulation. Figures 35-3 and 35-4 demonstrate breast reduction with reduction of the axilla by suction.

ASYMMETRY DURING AND AFTER BREAST REDUCTION

Occasionally, after breast reduction is completed, the surgeon notes that there is a discrepancy in the sizes of the breasts. Suction-assisted lipectomy can be utilized to restore symmetry by suctioning for contour and without opening up the suture line (Fig. 35-5; preoperatively note the asymmetry, and postoperatively note that the symmetry is restored after the suctioning of approximately 75 to 100 ml of fatty tissue).

If the asymmetry is not noted at the time of surgery, suction contouring can be performed as a secondary procedure, usually under local anesthesia.

BREAST AUGMENTATION WITH CONTOUR REDUCTION OF THE AXILLARY BREAST

Breast augmentation may be done either with the traditional approaches through the nipple-areola complex or axilla or under the breast, or through the abdomen during an abdominoplasty. If contouring is required, suctioning of the axilla may be done directly through any of the incision sites (Fig. 35-6).

BREAST REDUCTION AS A RESULT OF SUBCUTANEOUS MASTECTOMY

Contouring can also be used in the patient who has had subcutaneous mastectomies where there are some irregularities. In such cases, secondary contouring can be accomplished without entering the capsule where the breast prosthesis is in place (Fig. 35-7).

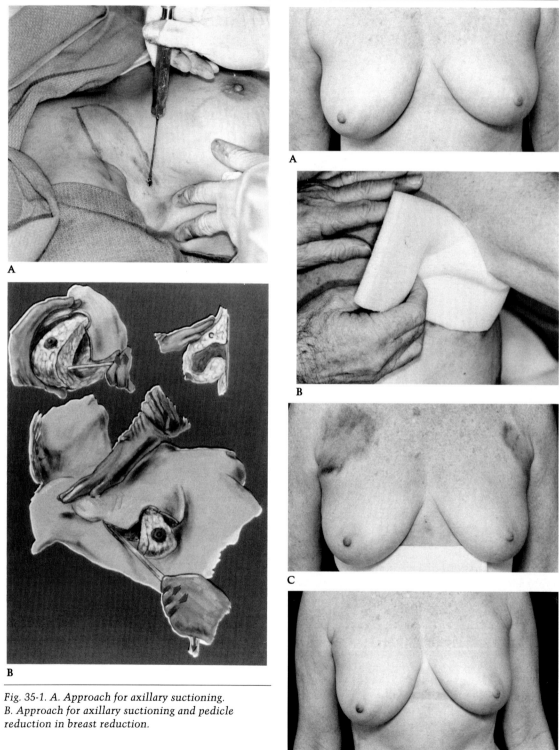

Fig. 35-1. A. Approach for axillary suctioning.
B. Approach for axillary suctioning and pedicle
reduction in breast reduction.

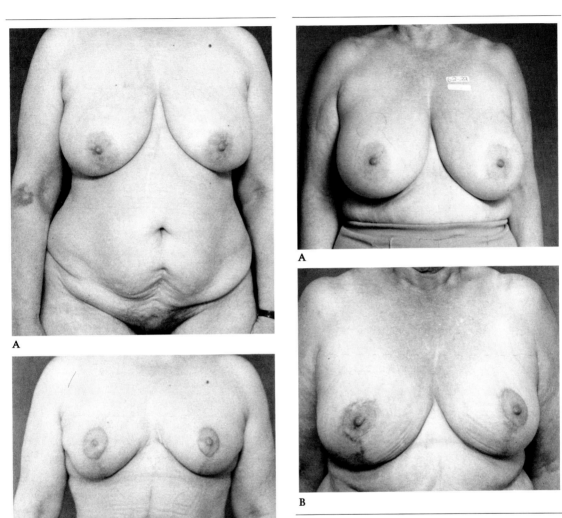

A

B

A

B

Fig. 35-4. A. Preoperative photograph of a 71-year-old
patient. B. One year postoperatively after breast
reduction and suctioning of the axilla.

Fig. 35-3. A. Preoperative photograph of a 61-year-old
patient who underwent abdominoplasty and breast
reduction with suctioning of the axilla.
B. Postoperative result.

Fig. 35-2. A. Preoperative photograph of a 47-year-old
patient with axillary fullness. B. Dressing with Reston
sponge. C. Postoperative bruising. D. Final result.

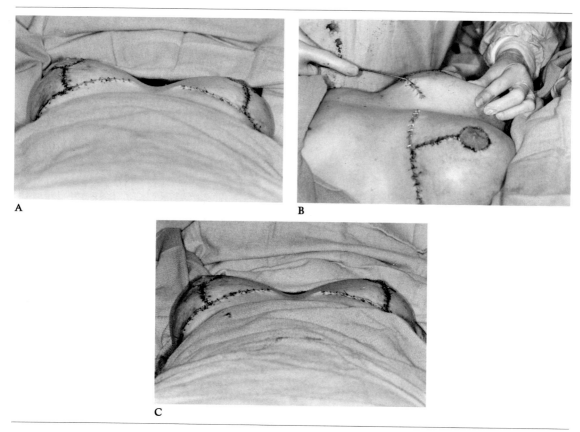

Fig. 35-5. A. This patient underwent breast reduction with the right breast being larger than the left. B. Operative procedure. C. Patient after 100 ml of fatty tissue was aspirated.

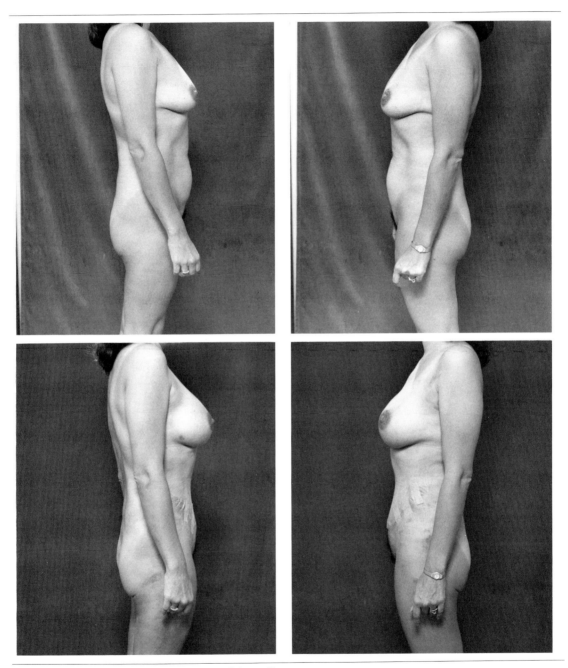

35-6. Breast augmentation with suctioning of the axilla
through the abdominoplasty incisions.

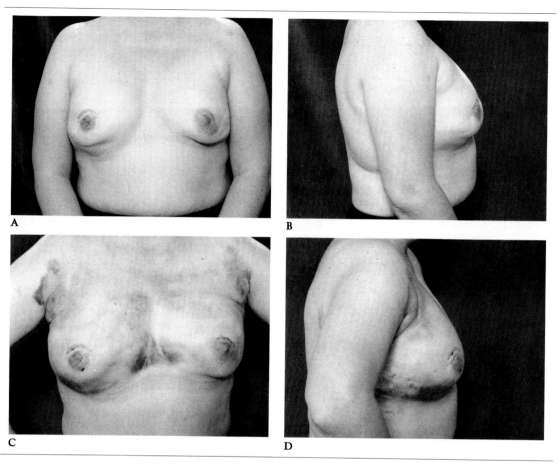

A

B

C

D

Fig. 35-7. A, B. Breast reduction as a result of subcutaneous mastectomy. Ten years previously, this patient underwent subcutaneous mastectomy resulting in whole breast asymmetry and axillary fullness. C, D. Photographs following suctioning for contour.

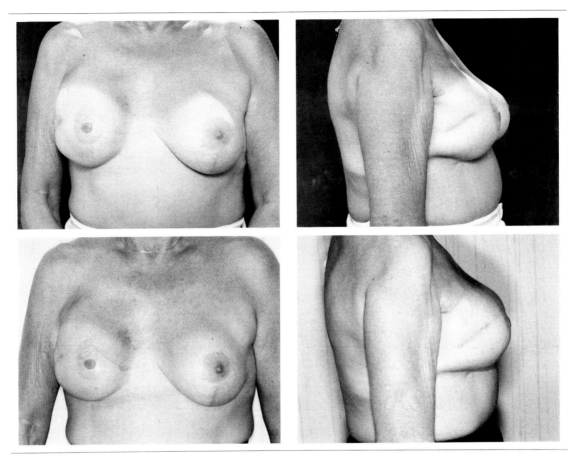

Fig. 35-8. Breast reconstruction and contouring of the axillary area with suctioning.

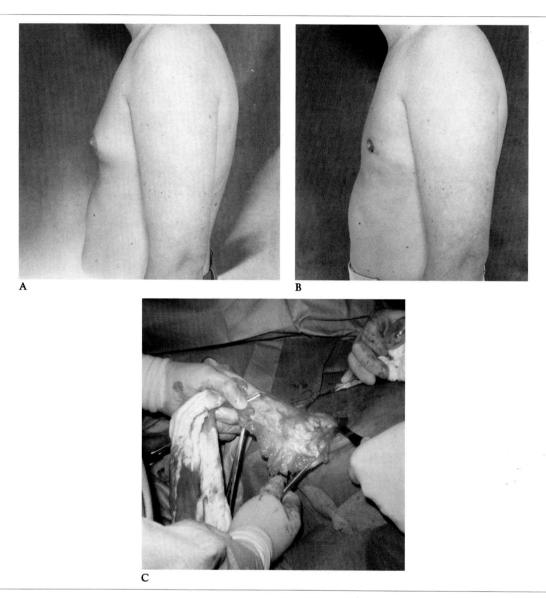

Fig. 35-9. A. Male gynecomastia with glandular component. B. Postoperative result following combined suctioning and reduction. C. Intraoperative photograph of glandular tissue.

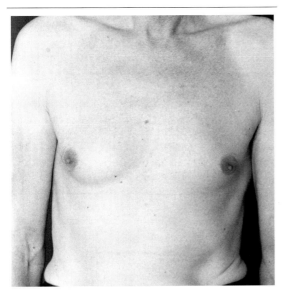

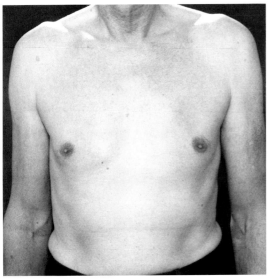

Fig. 35-10. Pre- and postoperative photographs of straight suction reduction.

CONTOUR REDUCTION OF THE RECONSTRUCTED BREAST

Another area of benefit is in the reconstructed breast where flaps, such as the latissimus dorsi or transverse rectus abdominis myocutaneous (TRAM) flap, have been used and can be contoured by SAL (Fig. 35-8).

GYNECOMASTIA AND PSEUDOGYNECOMASTIA

In the young man who has any component of glandular tissue, suctioning should be done, followed by glandular resection (Fig. 35-9).

Since most men have relatively little breast tissue in the middle and later years of life, suctioning can frequently be used to reduce pseudogynecomastia (Fig. 35-10).

In summary, all phases of breast reduction and, in fact, in breast surgery in general, whether cosmetic or reconstructive, can be influenced by SAL with the use of the appropriately sized suction cannula. I prefer to use cannulas that are 3.7 mm in diameter or smaller.

References

1. Grazer, F.M. Body Contouring. In J.G. McCarthy (ed.), *Plastic Surgery*. Philadelphia: Saunders, 1989 (in press).
2. Grazer, F.M. Suction Assisted Lipectomy — Its Indications, Contraindications, and Complications. In M.B. Habal (ed.), *Advances in Plastic and Reconstructive Surgery* (Vol. 1). Chicago: Year Book, 1984.

COMMENTS ON CHAPTER 35 *Robert M. Goldwyn*

With commendable brevity, Grazer has graphically demonstrated the various uses of liposuction as an adjunct to reduction mammaplasty. As most plastic surgeons know, Grazer has been a leader in the concepts and techniques of body contouring. He was well prepared to adopt and adapt liposuction to improve his results in many different areas of the body. The liposuction apparatus is integral to his operating room; it is ready whenever needed.

Many of us, however, think of the possibility of liposuction too seldom and too late. If the machine and cannulas are not already set up, many surgeons, including myself, may be too impatient to wait to use it.

Grazer has mentioned the most frequent ways liposuction can aid the surgeon in getting a better result: (1) reducing the length of the horizontal scar by eliminating fat at either end to avoid excising of dog-ears; (2) getting rid of axillary breasts, easily done when fat predominates over firm, glandular tissue, which might require excision by knife; and (3) revising initial results — secondarily doing away with dog-ears or improving symmetry and contour.

Again, the point to emphasize is to think of liposuction and have the equipment ready.

36

Robert M. Goldwyn

Concluding Thoughts

" . . . Breasts are only in the way, no matter what the situation. My solution will be to make women look like angels. From now on, breasts will be worn in the back and will be collapsible. With the aide of a helium tank, they will rise when we wish them to do so."
—*Salvador Dali, quoted in his obituary in the* International Herald Tribune, *Tuesday, January 24, 1989*

What do I, as editor and as one of the authors of this book, want an assiduous reader to gain from it?

The first is the realization that the surgeon who serves the patient best is the one who does not focus on the enlarged breasts to the exclusion of the patient as a totality: her personality, motivations, expectations, and medical and social history as well as the precise characteristics of her breasts in terms of shape, size, and possible disease. Careful examination, clinical and, if necessary, radiologic, is necessary to plan the operation intelligently and optimally.

In addition to providing proper treatment, the surgeon should try to establish a positive relationship with the patient. Ideally, their interaction should be gratifying to each of them. Although that achievement should be in itself rewarding emotionally to the surgeon, there are also practical benefits. If something goes wrong, and if one operates frequently, it occasionally will, having a strong bond with the patient helps her and the surgeon weather the tempest.

What I also hope the reader has by now concluded is that different surgeons are likely to use different methods for the same patient. There is no one way to perform reduction mammaplasty. However, what is also true is that a satisfactory procedure, if poorly done, will not give a satisfactory result.

Although this book includes many methods of reduction mammaplasty — indeed, most of the better known — other techniques do exist. Whatever the procedure the surgeon chooses, the decision should be based on the patient's requirements as well as the surgeon's preferences and, practically speaking, to a lesser extent, the patient's preferences. Too often, the surgeon automatically executes his or her favorite method without thinking why and at each step without asking himself or herself, "What am I doing now?" or "What should I be doing next and why?"

I do not expect the reader to become proficient in all or even most of the operations described in this book. I hope, however, that he or she would have mastered more than one technique for responding flexibly and optimally to the needs of the patient. Furthermore, a surgeon whose repertoire has some variety is more likely to be a thoughtful surgeon, to the benefit of the patient. That individual will probably also perform his or her preferred operation better. This does not mean that we should become surgical butterflies, flitting from one technique to another without spending sufficient time understanding it thoroughly and learning to perform it well.

Throughout our surgical careers, each of us must evaluate our results objectively in order to improve our efforts for the good of the patient. The conflict, all too familiar, is when to exchange the old for the new, the security that comes from the familiar with the insecurity that accompanies the unfamiliar. I hope that in this quest that we surgeons should be making, this book helps to give the reader a good idea of not only how to do a procedure but also information concerning its rationale, its indications — for what type of breast is it well- or ill-suited — its advantages, its disadvantages, and any complications or unfavorable results pertinent to that particular method. With regard to a technique's possible deficits, the comments that follow the chapters hopefully will have furnished a perspective.

Finally, I hope that this book will stimulate others to think more about reduction mammaplasty, so that we may evolve better techniques for answering our patients' needs.

Index